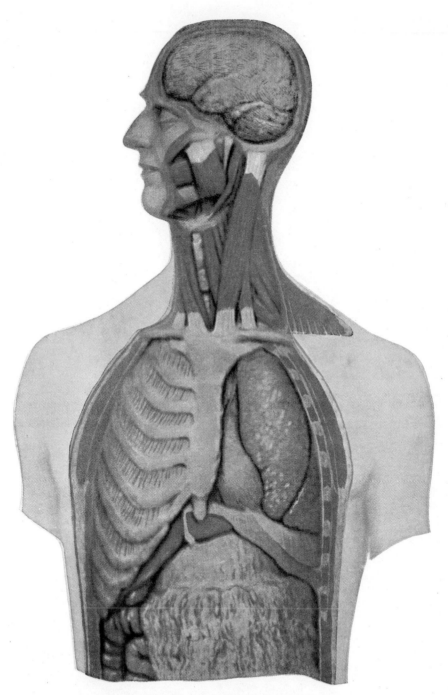

I. Cranial and thoracic cavities.

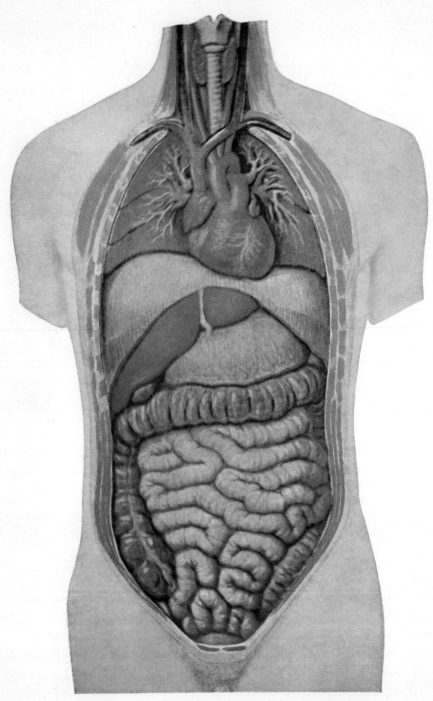

II. Thoracic and abdominal cavities, external layer.

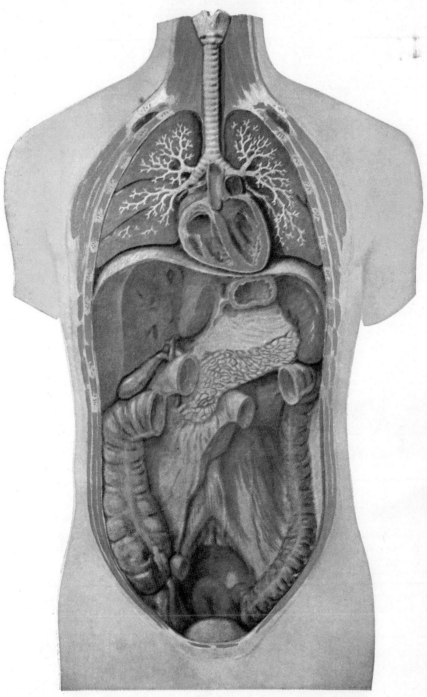

III. Thoracic and abdominal cavities, median layer.

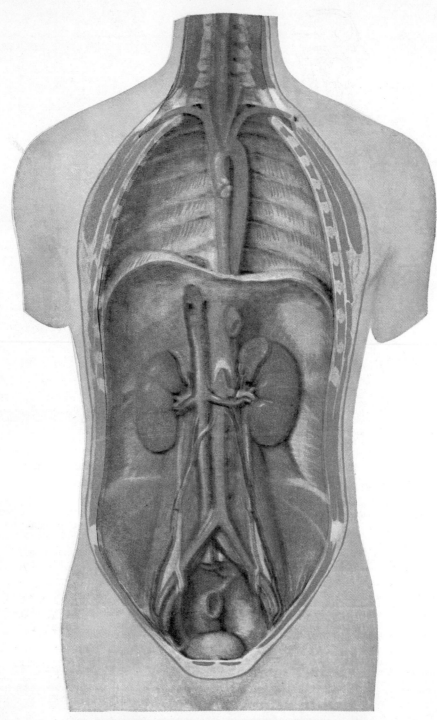

IV. Thoracic and abdominal cavities, posterior wall.

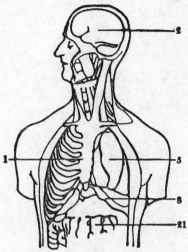

I. Head and chest. (*Explanation to color plate 1*)

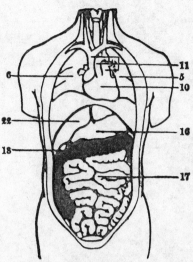

II. Thoracic and abdominal cavities. External layer. (*Explanation to color plate 2*)

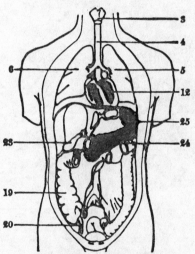

III. Thoracic and abdominal cavities. Median layer. (*Explanation to color plate 3*)

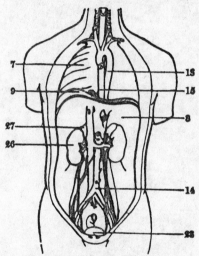

IV. Thoracic and abdominal cavities. Posterior wall. (*Explanation to color plate 4*)

1. Sternum. 2. Brain. 3. Larynx. 4. Trachea. 5. Left lung. 6. Right lung. 7. Right thorax. 8. Diaphragm. 9. Right dome of the diaphragm. 10. Heart. 11. Large cardiac vessels. 12. Cavities of the heart (shaded). 13. Large thoracic artery. 14. Large abdominal artery. 15. Esophagus. 16. Stomach. 17. Small intestine. 18. Large intestine (shaded). 19. Cecum. 20. Vermiform appendix of the cecum. 21. Omentum. 22. Liver. 23. Gall bladder. 24. Pancreas (shaded). 25. Spleen (shaded). 26. Right kidney. 27. Adrenal. 28. Urinary bladder.

These diagrams and the following four color plates are reproduced from *Man: Development, Nature and Function of Human Organism* (*Der Mensch: Von Werden, Wessen und Wirken der menschlichen Organismus*). Martin Vogel, Editor. Published by the German Hygiene Museum, Leipzig, 1930. Used by permission of Johann Ambrosius Barth.

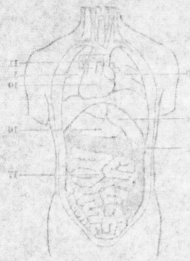

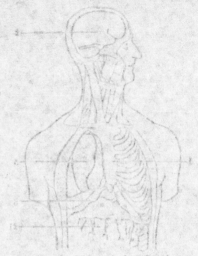

II. Thoracic and abdominal cavities.
External layers (Explanation to color
plate 2).

I. Head and chest. (Explanation to
color plate 1.)

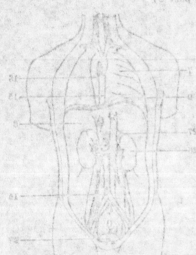

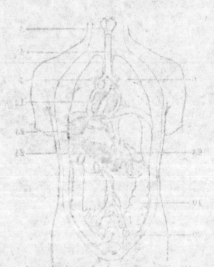

IV. Thoracic and abdominal cavities. Posterior wall. (Explanation to
color plate 4)

III. Thoracic and abdominal cavities. Medism layer. (Explanation to
color plate 3.)

1. Septum. 2. Brain. 3. Larynx. 4. Trachea. 5. Left lung. 6. Right lung. 7. Right
thorax. 8. Diaphragm. 9. Right dome of the diaphragm. 10. Heart. 11. Large cardiac vessels. 12. Cavities of the heart (shaded). 13. Large thoracic artery. 14. Large abdominal
artery. 15. Esophagus. 16. Stomach. 17. Small intestine. 18. Large intestine (shaded). 19.
Organs. 20. Vermiform appendix of the caecum. 21. Omentum. 22. Liver. 23. Gall bladder. 24. Pancreas (shaded). 25. Spleen (shaded). 26. Right kidney. 27. Adrenal. 28.
Urinary bladder.

These diagrams and the following four color plates are reproduced from *Man: Development, Nature and Function of Human Organs* (*Der Mensch. Von Werden, Wesen
und Wirken des menschlichen Organismus*), Martin Vogel. Published by the German Hygiene Museum, Leipzig, 1940. Used by permission of Johann Ambrosius Barth.

MODERN HOME MEDICAL ADVISER

BOOKS BY MORRIS FISHBEIN, M.D.

AUTHOR:

Handbook of Therapy (1925) with Dr. Oliver T. Osborne
The Medical Follies (1925)
Mirrors of Medicine (1925)
The New Medical Follies (1927)
The Human Body and Its Care (1929)
An Hour of Health (1929)
Doctors and Specialists (1930)
Shattering Health Superstitions (1930)
Fads and Quackery in Healing (1932)
Frontiers of Medicine (1933)
Syphilis (1937)
Your Diet and Your Health (1937)
Do You Want to Become a Doctor? (1939)
The National Nutrition (1942)
First Aid Training (1943), with Leslie W. Irwin
Health and First Aid (1944), with Leslie W. Irwin
Popular Medical Encyclopedia (1946)
History of the American Medical Association (1947)
The Technic and Art of Medical Writing (1948)
The Handy Home Medical Adviser (1952)

EDITOR:

Your Weight and How to Control It (1927)
Why Men Fail (1928), with William A. White
Doctors at War (1945)
Medical Uses of Soap (1946)
Successful Marriage (1948)
Your Weight and How to Control It (1949)
Modern Home Medical Adviser (1956)

MODERN HOME

MEDICAL ADVISER

YOUR HEALTH AND HOW TO PRESERVE IT

Edited by

MORRIS FISHBEIN, M.D.

COMPLETELY REVISED AND RE-EDITED

With over 150 Line and Halftone Illustrations

Garden City Books, Garden City, New York

Preface

THE SPEED of medical progress is one of the marvels of our scientific century. A simple comparison of what was known five or ten years ago with the knowledge of today creates amazement. Teaching of health in most of our schools has not begun to catch up with the minimum essentials that should be as familiar to every person as the multiplication table.

This book is offered to answer significant questions concerning all the common and even some of the extraordinary illnesses that may develop in any family. Included are the infectious diseases caused by viruses and bacteria and parasites, deficiency diseases, diseases of metabolism and digestion, disorders of the glands, allergy, industrial diseases and conditions affecting the skin, eyes, ears, nose and throat.

Prevention is better than cure! Here also are adequate considerations of first aid, prenatal care, and care and feeding of the child, sex hygiene, suitable diet, care of the feet, posture, mental hygiene and old age.

The book provides first the considerations in making choice of a family doctor and the materials that ought to be regularly available in the family medicine chest.

A knowledge of the structure of the body and the way it works—anatomy and physiology—is necessary for understanding. This is provided through charts, diagrams and descriptions.

The years of use of the MODERN HOME MEDICAL ADVISER have indicated possibilities for improving it as a tool for teaching and furnishing information. Many of the articles and most of the pictures are entirely new; all of them are thoroughly revised.

Many new and brilliant young authors have kindly associated themselves with me in this work. I express appreciation to them.

MORRIS FISHBEIN, M.D.

Collaborators

HOWARD T. BEHRMAN, M.D.

Chief of Clinic in Dermatology and Syphilology, Mount Sinai Hospital, New York. Assistant Attending Dermatologist, University Hospital, New York University and Bellevue Medical Center, New York.

HUGH R. BUTT, M.D.

Associate Professor of Medicine, Mayo Foundation, University of Minnesota Graduate School, Rochester, Minn.

CHARLES S. CAMERON, M.D.

Medical and Scientific Director, American Cancer Society, Inc., New York City.

LEO H. CRIEP, M.D.

Associate Professor in Medicine, Lecturer in Immunology and Chief of the Allergy Clinic, University of Pittsburgh School of Medicine.

EDWARD E. DART, M.D.

Consultant in Occupational Medicine and former associate of Dr. Carey P. McCord, San Lorenzo, California.

MORRIS FISHBEIN, M.D.

Former Editor, *Journal American Medical Association*, Chicago; Editor, *Excerpta Medica; Post-graduate Medicine.*

NEWELL C. GILBERT, M.D.

Late Chairman, Department of Medicine, Northwestern University Medical School, Chicago.

J. P. GREENHILL, M.D.

Professor of Gynecology, Cook County Graduate School of Medicine.

HARRY L. JAFFE, M.D.

Associate of Dr. Arthur M. Master, New York City.

PHILIP C. JEANS, M.D.

Late Head Pediatric Division, University Hospitals and Prof. of Pediatrics and Head Dept., State University of Iowa College of Medicine, Iowa City, Ia.

ELLIOTT P. JOSLIN, M.D.
Professor Emeritus of Clinical Medicine, Harvard University, Medical School, Boston, Mass.

PHILIP LEWIN, M.D.
Professor of Bone and Joint Surgery, Northwestern University Medical School, Chicago.

ARTHUR M. MASTER, M.D.
Consultant in Cardiology, U.S. Navy. Cardiologist, Mount Sinai Hospital, New York.

CAREY P. McCORD, M.D.
Consultant, Institute of Industrial Health, University of Michigan, Ann Arbor.

HOWARD M. ODEL, M.D.
Assistant Professor of Medicine, Mayo Foundation. Consultant in Medicine, Mayo Clinic, Rochester, Minnesota.

HOWARD F. POLLEY, M.D.
Associate Professor, Graduate School of Medicine, University of Minnesota; Consultant in Medicine, St. Mary's Hospital, Rochester, Minnesota.

SIDNEY A. PORTIS, M.D.
Late Clinical Associate Professor of Medicine, University of Illinois College of Medicine, Chicago.

GEORGE K. PRATT, M.D.
Associate in Neuropsychiatry, Bridgeport Hospital, Bridgeport, Conn.

THURMAN B. RICE, M.D.
Late Professor of Bacteriology and Public Health, Indiana Univ. School of Medicine, Indianapolis, Ind.

ELMER L. SEVRINGHAUS, M.D.
Nutley, New Jersey.

KARL SINGER, M.D.
Director, Department of Hematologic Research, Medical Research Institute, Michael Reese Hospital, Chicago.

CARL D. STROUSE, M.D.
Junior Attending Staff, Department of Medicine, Los Angeles County Hospital. Instructor in Medicine, University of Southern California Medical School, Los Angeles.

SOLOMON STROUSE, M.D.
Clinical Professor of Medicine, Univ. Southern California School of Medicine, Los Angeles.

RUSSELL M. WILDER, M.D.
Head of Section in Division of Medicine, Mayo Clinic; Professor of Medicine and Nutrition, Mayo Foundation for Medical Education and Research, Graduate School, University of Minnesota, Rochester, Minn.

HAROLD G. WOLFF, M.D.
Professor of Medicine (Neurology), Cornell University Medical College, New York City.

Contents

Illustrations

PLATES

CHAPTER I

The Choice of a Physician

MORRIS FISHBEIN, M.D.

THE FAMILY DOCTOR

OF ALL THE PROBLEMS that may concern the average family, there is probably not one in which the decision is of more ultimate importance for the health and happiness of the family than the choice of the family physician. The family doctor of an earlier day was mostly learned in the school of experience. In many instances he had studied with a preceptor and perhaps had a course of lectures in some medical school lasting six months and devoted but slightly to the practical side of medicine. Such knowledge he obtained by studying cases with his preceptor. He did, however, develop an intimate personal relationship with those whom he served, which is recognized today as the basic feature of the best type of medical practice.

In the old days the family loved, indeed almost worshiped, the family doctor. He was their guide in health as well as in sickness. He alone, of all the community, knew the family secrets, and he could be depended on to keep the faith. True, his remedies were occasionally harsh and his diagnosis largely guesswork, but his record of cures is surprising. He was especially known for his ability to practise the art of scientific observation, using to the utmost his five senses. The physician of today has available innumerable scientific devices for aiding, prolonging, and extending these senses, but unless brains are carefully mixed with the application of the devices the end result may be confusion rather than scientific diagnosis, and the cost far beyond the necessary cost for first-class medical practice.

GRADUATION FROM A MEDICAL COLLEGE

In choosing a physician be sure you know the answers to the following questions: First, is he a graduate of a recognized medical school that requires at least four years of thorough training? There was a time when there were more medical schools in the United States than in all the rest of the world. We had almost 200 medical schools in this country around 1900. Today there are more than 80 medical colleges in the United States. Now all of these are rated as Class A by the Council on Medical Education and Hospitals of the American Medical Association. A Class A college is one with a certain definite number of full-time teachers and with a well-established graded curriculum. At least two years of college education are required previous to studying medicine, four years of medical education of approximately nine months each, and around one year or two years of internship after graduation before the prospective physician can get his diploma.

LICENSE BY THE STATE

Is the doctor licensed to practice medicine in the state in which he has his office? The majority of the states conduct regular examinations for a license to practise, these examinations being given by a group of physicians known as the State Medical Board of Registration and Licensure. In some states the doctor is required to renew his license every year. Before he can get a license he must usually show evidence of his graduation and also undergo a written and practical examination in the basic medical subjects. He must also present certificates of good moral character from at least two physicians who know him.

THE DOCTOR'S INTERNSHIP

Has the doctor had actual training as an intern in a hospital? Or has he been associated with a practising physician long enough to obtain practical education in medicine? Has he at the time of consultation a direct connection with a good hospital? There are in the United States almost 7,000 hospitals acceptable to the joint rating board of the American Hospital Association, the American Medical Association, the American College of Physicians and the American College of Surgeons. Of the 220,000 physicians in the United States more than 130,000 are directly affiliated with these hospitals as members of the staff. The appointment of a physician to the staff of a good hospital indicates that he has been passed upon according to his qualifications by the medical staff of the hospital and frequently also by the board of directors of the institution.

MEMBERSHIP IN THE COUNTY MEDICAL SOCIETY

Is the doctor a member of his county medical society, of his state medical society, of the American Medical Association, or of any other recognized, organized body of physicians? The American Medical Association is organized like the United States government. It has county societies which pass carefully on physicians who wish to join. Before a man can belong to his state medical society he must belong to his county medical society. Before he can belong to the American Medical Association he must belong to both county and state medical societies. Before he can belong to any of the recognized special societies, such as those in surgery, diseases of the eye, ear, nose and throat, skin, and other specialties, he must belong to the American Medical Association or to his state and county medical societies.

While membership in a medical society is not an absolute guarantee of honesty or of good faith, the physician who belongs to such a society is subject to the criticism of his colleagues and subject also to being called before special committees to explain actions that are not considered ethical or satisfactory. A patient is much better off with a doctor who belongs to a recognized medical society than in the hands of one who is utterly independent of such organizational control. There are, of course, numerous medical organizations which are not recognized or established or scientific. There is even an organization composed of innumerable quacks who practise all sorts of strange medical cults and promote many unestablished notions.

CHARACTERISTICS OF AN ETHICAL DOCTOR

An ethical physician may be differentiated from a quack by certain well-established characteristics. An ethical physician does not advertise his methods or cures in a newspaper. He does not give out circulars concerning his work or his fees. He does not indiscriminately distribute his picture. He does not put large signboards on his windows or outside his office, advertising his extraordinary merits, or otherwise promoting his wares. A competent ethical physician seldom finds it necessary to travel from town to town to secure patients. He usually has an established place of residence and of work to which patients come when they require his services or to which they send, requesting his attendance when they themselves are unable to travel. The traveling doctor who moves from town to town is not to be consulted or to be considered a safe family physician.

There has been for years a tradition in medicine that new discoveries are freely published to the profession in the various medical periodicals and are not held as secrets by certain men which only they can apply. The public may therefore well beware of any doctor or group of doctors who advertise or publish broadcast the fact that they have discovered a new cure or method of treatment that other doctors do not know about, or who claim they can cure such serious conditions as cancer, tuberculosis, the venereal diseases, or rheumatic disease in a short time by some secret manipulation or by some unestablished method.

THE SCIENTIFIC ADVANCEMENT OF MEDICINE

The advancement of medicine has been associated with the introduction of innumerable complicated devices used not only in the diagnosis of disease but also in treatment. The sense of vision is aided by the microscope which enlarges invisible objects so that they may be seen. There are other instruments such as the cystoscope, the otoscope, the laryngoscope, and the ophthalmoscope which enable the physician competent in their use to look directly into various body cavities. By means of the X-ray, opaque tissues are brought into the field of vision, and by the use of various dye substances combined with the

X-ray most of the organs and tissues of the body can now be seen during life.

The development of physics, of chemistry, of bacteriology, and of many sciences on which medicine rests has made it possible for physicians to determine to the thousandth of a gram the content of the blood and of various secretions and excretions of the body, determining thus the presence of sugar, of protein, of various salts, and of other substances related to the functions of the body in health and in disease. In surgery new devices have been developed for cutting tissues without hemorrhage, for keeping the patient quiet or anesthetized during operation, and for keeping conditions so clean that there is no danger of infection.

New methods have been discovered which aid the specialist in diseases of the nose and throat in looking into the sinuses, in determining their contours, in examining the ear externally and internally, and in peering into the very depths not only of the larynx but even of the lungs.

DEVELOPMENT OF SPECIALISTS

The employment of the special devices used in medical practice requires hours of study and practice for the development of proper technic. As a result of the tremendous expansion of medical knowledge specialization entered the field, so that today not only is medicine practised by general practitioners who, it has been determined, can easily take care of 85 per cent of the conditions for which patients consult physicians, but it is practised in some eighteen to twenty specialties of various types, such as those which concern themselves wholly with internal medicine and diagnosis; surgery, which is divided into orthopedic surgery, genito-urinary surgery, brain surgery, abdominal surgery, and similar branches. There are also specialists in diseases of the skin, in diseases of women, in diseases of children, in obstetrics, in nervous and mental diseases, in diseases of the stomach and intestines, in industrial medicine, in preventive medicine, in anesthesia, and in several other more confined branches.

There is not as yet any legal method for determining who shall be considered competent to practise a specialty in medicine and who shall not. It therefore becomes possible for any physician who wishes to do so to set himself up as a specialist in any medical field. The rewards of specialization are usually beyond those of general practice in the form of shorter hours of work, more time for research, higher pay for work accomplished and, no doubt, much more interest in the work. Various means have been developed by the medical profession itself for limiting, if possible, entrance of unworthy men into various specialties. Some of the specialistic societies will not admit any man until he has had at least five years of experience in a specialty and until he has done sufficient research work and published enough scientific papers to prove his competence.

Moreover, the medical profession has itself established examining and certifying boards which now undertake, after a young man has been at least five years in practice, to give him both a written and a practical examination and, provided he is qualified, to issue to him a certificate of competence.

CONSULT THE FAMILY DOCTOR FIRST

In the vast majority of cases people who wish to consult a specialist will do well to go first to their family doctor or general practitioner so that he may, after a study of the case, select for the patient such specialists as may be necessary for consultation as to diagnosis or for specialistic treatment. In this way the patient may save himself a great deal of time and money. Numerous instances are recorded in which a patient with a pain in some portion of the body went directly to a specialist, only to find out that the pain which concerned him was not due to an organ within the field of that specialist but perhaps to some entirely different cause.

For instance, such a condition as ordinary dizziness may be due to causes arising in the digestive tract, in the heart and circulation, in the internal ear, or in the brain. Only a careful study of the history of the case, the nature of the symptoms, and similar factors, will enable a physician to see which one of these organs or systems may be concerned. Similarly, bleeding from the throat may be due to conditions in the throat, in which case a general practitioner or a specialist in diseases of the throat might be consulted. On the other hand, it might be due to tuberculosis of the lungs, to a tumor of the esophagus or to hemorrhage taking place in the stomach, in which case a specialist concerned with those organs might be needed. Hence, for the vast majority of complaints the patient should first of all consult a family physician, preferably one to whom he has gone for some time. He may confidently be guided by his advice.

PICKING A FAMILY DOCTOR

When coming into a community you may select your physician in various ways. If you will call the secretary of the county medical society the secretary will probably be willing to give you a list of general practitioners in his vicinity. You may then determine by meeting these men and by inquiry into their qualifications whether or not you care to commit the illnesses of yourself and of your family to their care. If you are a member of any well-established fraternal organization or church, association of commerce, business organization, or similar group, you may on inquiry among your associates in these groups find out who are the competent physicians in the community, and then, by making your own inquiries as to competence along the lines of the questions that have been suggested earlier in this chapter, determine which of those that have been recommended is suitable to your needs.

Once a physician has been selected and has been found competent to give not only the type of scientific advice needed for ordinary cases, but also to give the personal intimate attention that is the distinguishing characteristic of the best type of family doctor, you will do well to cling to that family physician and to recognize in him a friend and a counselor. Remember also that the servant is worthy of his hire. Far too often physicians' bills are the last to be paid because the very nature of the profession has in the past made the physician willing to wait until the bills for food, for clothing, for shelter, for fuel, and the other necessities of life have been taken care of. The physician must himself provide these things for his family. A physician who receives from his patient conscientious and responsible treatment is likely to return to that patient even more conscientious and responsible attention than he himself has received.

CHAPTER II

The Family Medicine Chest
MORRIS FISHBEIN, M.D.

Most Americans, being independent and individualistic, feel themselves competent to fix defects in the plumbing and almost equally competent to take care of their own disturbances of health, as well as to prescribe for more complicated disturbances which really ought to have prompt medical attention.

A household remedy should be one with a certain definite action; usually it should contain but one active ingredient. If the thing is worth keeping in the medicine chest it should be something which is used fairly frequently. Dangerous poisons have no place in the family medicine chest. A dangerous poison is one which is likely to produce serious symptoms or death if taken in even moderate amounts. Prescriptions ordered by the family doctor for a certain illness should never be kept for the future. If any of the material remains in the bottle it should be poured promptly into a safe place of disposal. Since useful bottles are rare around most homes, the bottle may be thoroughly washed with hot water, dried, and stored away. Few people realize that most drugs deteriorate with age and that a prescription for a certain illness is not likely to be useful for the future.

The wise person will go over the family medicine chest at least once every three months and at that time discard all materials not constantly in use. It might also be well to have the family doctor look at the materials once in a while to offer his advice as to the materials worth keeping.

TAKING MEDICINE

Medicines rightly used can be of immense aid and comfort to the afflicted; wrongly used, they may cause serious damage to the human body. When a doctor prescribes medicines for a patient, they are for that particular patient and not for anybody else in the family. Hence, old prescriptions should not be saved but should be disposed of as soon as possible after they are no longer necessary for the patient for whom they were prescribed.

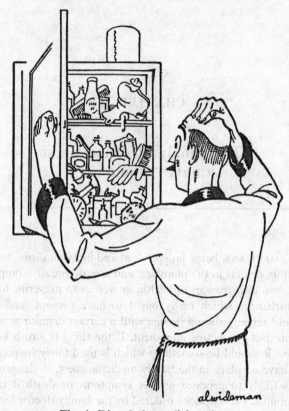

Fig. 1. Disorderly medicine chest.

The doctor usually writes on his prescription, and the druggist recopies on the label, the directions for taking the medicine. It is, therefore, well when giving medicine to a sick person to be sure you know exactly what is on the label of the bottle. If necessary, take the bottle into another room to read the label so as not to be disturbed by conversation with the patient or with anyone else.

Then, when you measure out the medicine, think of what you are doing and pay no attention to anything else. Medicines are usually prescribed in dosages of drops, teaspoons, fractions of teaspoons, and spoons of larger sizes. Because spoons are nowadays in many fanciful shapes and sizes, each family should have a medicine glass with measures of various spoons recorded. When a doctor says any number of drops, the drops should be measured with a medicine dropper and not by guesswork.

If liquid medicine is being prescribed, the bottle should be thoroughly shaken each time before the medicine is measured. When medicine is poured out of the bottle, the cork should be deposited with its top down on the table and immediately put back in the bottle after the medicine has been poured.

Most medicine should be mixed with a little water when taken, but sometimes the medicine may be put in the mouth and washed down with a swallow of water. Pills and capsules should either be handed to the patient from the original package so that he may help himself, putting the pill or capsule on the back of the tongue and washing it down with a drink of water, or else brought to the patient on a spoon so that he may take the pill or capsule from the spoon. In other words, the person who is waiting on the patient should not carry the capsules or pills in the palm of the hand, where they may be softened or disintegrated by moisture or contaminated from the hands.

There are several ways in which medicines of unpleasant taste may be made more palatable. If very cold water is taken, it will serve to cover the taste. It is not advisable to give medicine to children in foods, particularly in milk, as this may create a distaste for the food or milk which lasts for a long time thereafter.

There are very few remedies which should be kept regularly in the family medicine chest. American people suffer today with overdosage of cathartics and laxatives, and with overdosage of medicine to relieve pain and produce sleep. Physicians are beginning to notice some serious results particularly from overdosing with drugs of the last mentioned type. No one should take such remedies regularly without the physician's directions.

Let us consider now the items that are most commonly found in any first-class family medicine chest. Most families want something to use for moving the bowels in the occasional case of temporary obstruction or slowness of action. Under certain circumstances any laxative or cathartic may be exceedingly dangerous. The most conspicuous example is appendicitis. This is at first just an infected spot on a little organ which comes off the large bowel and which apparently has no serious function in the human body. If this infection develops the way a boil develops from a pimple, it is in danger of bursting and spreading throughout the body. When infection is spread in the abdomen the result is peritonitis. Therefore, a laxative or cathartic should never be taken when the abdomen is exceedingly painful.

The most common laxatives found in a family medicine chest include liquid petrolatum, or mineral oil, which is a mechanical lubricant that may interfere with absorption of Vitamin A. Other preparations commonly used include castor oil, seidlitz powders, milk of magnesia, Epsom salts, sodium phosphate, phenolphthalein, aromatic cascara, and bulk formers like cellulose and psyllium seed preparations. For the people who use the medicine chest a large sign should be placed indicating that none of these preparations is ever to be used for abdominal pain of unknown cause.

The next most commonly found preparations in a family medicine chest, aside from the cosmetics, are pain relievers. Most of these are used for headaches, although sometimes they are used for what are called neuritis, neuralgia, toothache, and other pains of unknown origin, as well as to produce sleep. Most headache powders bought under patent trade marks contain phenacetin

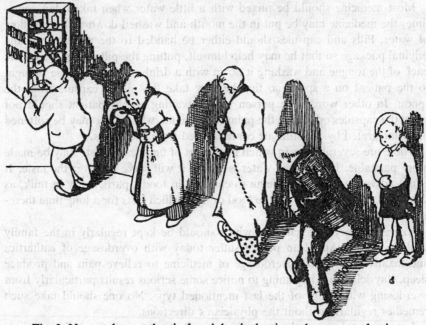

Fig. 2. Never take a cathartic for abdominal pain, unless cause of pain
is known. It may be appendicitis.

or acetanilid, sometimes in considerable dosage. Don't experiment with acetanilid because it may, in large dosage, have serious effects on the body. Too
large or too frequently repeated doses will poison anyone who uses them.
Moreover, people tend to form the habit of taking such preparations, and such
habits are dangerous, since they temporize with what may eventually become a
serious condition. Least harmful of the pain relievers is aspirin.

Other drugs much used to produce sleep nowadays are derivatives of barbituric acid of which some of the best examples are phenobarbital, nembutal,
and ipral. In some states druggists are not permitted to sell such preparations
to anyone without a physician's prescription. This should be sufficient indication of their danger as used by many people without medical knowledge. The
family medicine chest is better off without preparations of this character. The
possibilities for harm are sufficiently great to suggest that these preparations
be not used except on medical advice. Thousands of deaths have resulted from
accidental overdosage.

The most commonly used general pain reliever throughout the country
today is acetylsalicylic acid, commonly called aspirin. It is relatively harmless
except for a few people who are especially sensitive to it. Such people cannot
take even small doses. One aspirin is as good as another, provided it is up to
the standard of the United States Pharmacopeia. Special claims are made for
aspirins that dissolve more quickly in the stomach. Old tablets become dry and
harden and may not be absorbed.

Among the strongest of medicinal preparations are the narcotics and anesthetics. Narcotics should never be used by anyone without a physician's prescription and, indeed, no drug that has to be administered with a hypodermic syringe should find a place in the average family medicine chest. Some people with diabetes have been taught by their doctors to inject themselves with insulin. Even these people should keep their syringe outfit separate from the materials in the family medicine chest.

All sorts of antiseptics are available for use on the skin, in first aid and also for gargling and for washing various portions of the body. The Council on Drugs of the American Medical Association is not opposed to advertising recognized antiseptics for first aid to the public, and tincture of iodine and mercurochrome are included among the preparations that may be so advertised. Others commonly used are merthiolates, metaphen, and zephiran.

There is no scientific evidence that any of the widely advertised antiseptic solutions used as gargles, sprays, or in any other manner will prevent the onset of a common cold. One of the best old-fashioned antiseptic solutions for common use around the home is boric acid solution. Most people prefer to have packages of crystals of boric acid, and to make up the solution fresh just before use. Poisoning of children with boric acid taken internally is possible.

The family medicine chest may also contain aromatic spirits of ammonia which is sometimes given when a prompt stimulant is needed following fainting. Half a teaspoonful in water, in a sudden fainting spell, is a fairly safe thing to give in most cases of emergency. The widely publicized milk of magnesia and sodium bicarbonate, or baking soda, are two preparations which can safely be kept in the family medicine chest and which are frequently advised by physicians for alkaline purposes. Some families keep paregoric as a useful preparation in case of cramps that disturb women at periodic intervals. Really these constitute practically all of the drugs that need to be in any family medicine chest because they are the few materials that can be used safely by most people.

SURGICAL SUPPLIES

In these days when everybody takes the chance of needing emergency first-aid treatment because of the common use of the automobile and wide indulgence in sports and gardening, it is well to have a certain minimum quantity of useful supplies around the home.

Among the materials needed for first aid are packages of adhesive tape of various widths, sterile cotton, sterile gauze bandages, sterile gauze pads, scissors which should be kept in the medicine chest and not used for the family sewing or for other emergencies around the home, and the ready-made combinations of a piece of adhesive tape with a tiny piece of sterilized bandage that can be used to cover small wounds or wounds after they have been treated with iodine or mercurochrome.

Most people should know that the proper way to stop bleeding of small wounds on the surface of the body is simply to press upon them with a sterile piece of gauze. In case of very serious wounds affecting arteries, and thereby difficult to control, it may be necessary to put a tourniquet around the limb. The tourniquet should be fastened just tight enough to stop the bleeding. An ordinary piece of rubber tubing or a narrow towel tied and twisted with a stick will serve most purposes satisfactorily. It should be temporarily released every ten or fifteen minutes.

In addition to the materials used for first aid, most families will have bed pans for use in cases of illness, glass drinking tubes, syringes for giving enemas, atomizers, and sometimes special devices for creating steam to be medicated with small amounts of tincture of benzoin for relief in various forms of hoarseness or other conditions affecting the larynx and the lungs.

The final materials to be included are the cosmetics. Most modern women prefer to keep their cosmetics in their own boudoirs or sleeping apartments. The man of the house is likely to put his into the family medicine chest. They should include, in most instances, a razor which should be kept in its box and not permitted to lie around loose; also some shaving soap or cream, some face lotion, which may be either witch hazel or any special lotion that he prefers.

Do not use a styptic in the form of a stick of alum to stop slight bleeding points after shaving. Much better are any of the stringent surgical powders, of which a small amount may be taken from the box at each occasion and applied directly to the bleeding point.

Finally, any good talcum powder may be used with satisfaction after shaving and after bathing, according to the individual preferences of the users.

Every modern household should have a good clinical thermometer, a hot-water bottle, and an ice bag. When these are available in an emergency the comfort they give is tremendous.

WARNINGS

Do not save poisonous preparations of any kind, including particularly bichloride of mercury, pills containing strychnine, or solutions containing wood alcohol. Do not keep samples of patent medicines of unknown composition recommended beyond their actual virtues. Never permit any preparation of opium or morphine to be loose in the family medicine chest. Never save any prepared prescription after the specific use for which it was ordered by the physician has disappeared.

EQUIPMENT OF THE FAMILY MEDICINE CHEST

A *fountain syringe:* This should be of rubber or of metal. Capacity about two quarts. It will have a long rubber tube and several nozzles of assorted sizes.

A *bed pan:* In many illnesses it is not safe for the patient to get up even to attend to the usual body needs.

A rubber sheet: This is to be placed under the sheet to prevent soiling of the mattress. A piece of oilcloth will service the purpose satisfactorily for a short time.

Bandages: These are cheaply purchased. They should be in various sizes from one-inch width to three-inch width.

Adhesive tape: This can also be purchased in spools of various widths and lengths.

Scissors: These should always be kept available in the medicine chest.

Thermometer: A good clinical thermometer should be available, and preferably two, one for taking temperature by mouth and another for temperature by rectum.

Ice bag: The ice bag applied to the sore throat is frequently recommended by doctors.

Atomizer: For spraying nose and throat. A graduated medicine glass for measuring dosages.

THE DRUGS AND MEDICAL SUPPLIES

CATHARTICS AND LAXATIVES:

Epsom salts: An old-fashioned remedy with lots of power. Best taken in the morning on arising. About a tablespoonful in a half-glass of warm water.

Citrate of magnesia: A milder saline laxative. Order a bottle from the druggist. Take a half bottle on arising and the rest later if needed. Anywhere from six to twelve ounces of the solution of magnesium citrate is a dose.

Castor oil: An effective and prompt cathartic but likely to be followed by constipation and therefore not indicated in chronic constipation. A dose is four teaspoonfuls. This can now be had in tasteless and flavored forms.

Mineral oil: A lubricant much used in chronic cases of constipation. Dose: One or two tablespoonfuls. Mineral oil should not be used habitually since it absorbs vitamin A.

Other cathartics: Other cathartics and laxatives much used include sodium acid phosphate, phenolphthalein, which is the active substance of such advertised laxatives as Feenamint, Ex-lax, and similar products, also the Hinkle pill, the compound cathartic pill, and other mixtures. Bulk laxatives are psyllium seed, agar, cellothyl. It is not well to develop a cathartic habit. It is not safe to take cathartics in the presence of undiagnosed pains in the abdomen.

GENERAL DRUGS AND SUPPLIES

Glycerine: Useful for many purposes. A few drops warmed and dropped into the ear are frequently advised for earache.

Vaseline petroleum jelly, Cold cream, Zinc oxide ointment: These are useful for abrasions of the skin, chafing, sunburn, etc.

Tincture of iodine: An ideal antiseptic for application to cuts or small wounds of the skin. It is usually painted on, using a toothpick wrapped with cotton.

Boric acid: A concentrated solution is a good home antiseptic solution.

Hydrogen peroxide solution: Diluted about one half with water makes a good cleansing wash for wounds. Diluted one to three with water, can be used as a gargle.

Sodium bicarbonate: Baking soda. Useful as a gargle. Much used for so-called "sour stomach." Good in the bath for itching of the skin.

Aspirin: The great American pain reliever. Much used for headaches. Much safer than pyramidon, barbituric acid derivatives, acetanilid, phenacetin, and all the other coal-tar derivatives. Dosage: one or two five-grain tablets, repeated in about three hours.

Aromatic spirits of ammonia: Used to bring about recovery after fainting spells.

Surgical powder: A styptic powder, best used on small cuts after shaving.

Petrolatum eucalyptus menthol compound: A nice mixture for use in the nose as a spray.

Paper towels, Paper handkerchiefs: Most useful in sickness. Can be destroyed after use.

The medicine chest should always be kept out of reach of the children. Prescriptions in current use may be kept in the chest, but should be destroyed after the patient is well. Every bottle and package should be clearly labeled. Do not stock up with a lot of cathartics and laxatives, cough and cold remedies. Keep only those regularly used and called for by members of the family.

CHAPTER III

First Aid

MORRIS FISHBEIN, M.D.

WHEN ILLNESS or accidents occur in any home someone should know what can be done immediately. The certainty of knowledge will avoid the confusion, alarm, and distress that inevitably occur when no one knows just what to do in an emergency.

The emergencies that may occur range alphabetically from accidents to zebra-kick. No one can be fully prepared for all of these any more than any family is fully prepared for twins or triplets. Certain supplies may be kept in every home pending the occurrence of various accidents. The knowledge of the availability of these supplies and what to do with them by the mother, father, or the nurse will be found exceedingly helpful when the emergency arises.

ACCIDENTS

In the United States almost one hundred thousand people lose their lives in accidents each year, and it is said that ten million people every year have accidents sufficiently severe to take them from their work. Of the accidents which occur in the home, falls constitute 40 per cent of the total; after falls come accidents from burns, scalds, and explosions; then asphyxiation or strangulation and, finally, cuts and scratches. Most of these accidents are preventable with care, but it is in the nature of the human being not to be as careful as he might.

FALLS

When a person is injured in a fall the first step should be a consideration of the extent of the injury. It is necessary to determine whether or not bones have been broken, if there is bruising or hemorrhage and, finally, the extent to which the skin has been damaged. A broken bone usually reveals itself by inability to function. However, the only safe procedure is to call a physician who will take an X-ray picture and ascertain the actual extent of the damage.

Pending the arrival of a doctor it is well to place the injured part completely at rest and, if necessary, to hold it quiet with some suitable splint. A good splint is frequently made by wrapping a large-size magazine, or a newspaper folded many times, with handkerchiefs around the arm or leg to hold the tissues in place. However, unless the person who is applying the first-aid measure knows exactly what he or she is doing, it is better merely to put the injured person at rest and to keep him quiet.

Bleeding or Hemorrhage

In the case of bleeding certain measures may be undertaken at once. Ordinary wounds can be controlled by pressure with a clean piece of sterile gauze. In case of severe hemorrhages it is possible to wrap a cloth tightly around the arm or leg above the place of the bleeding. However, tourniquets are so little needed in ordinary accidents about the home that it is hardly worth while to keep a constant supply on hand. A tourniquet is easily improvised by merely tying a loop in a small towel or handkerchief and twisting with a rod of any kind.

If there is hemorrhage from a tooth socket following the extraction of a tooth it can usually be controlled by plugging the socket with sterile cotton or by the application of hot water. Under such circumstances care must be taken to avoid burning or scalding.

NOSEBLEED

Bleeding from the nose is fairly frequent, due either to a purposeful "sock" or to an accident such as running into a door. The simplest measure to stop bleeding from the nose is to place the bleeder in a recumbent position, preferably with the face down. The application of ice water or of hot water to the nose or temporarily packing with sterile clean gauze will help. It will not help particularly, except to distract attention, to pass a key down the back, to inhale smoke, to apply ice to the back of the neck, or to collect cobwebs and stuff them into the nose. If bleeding from the nose is frequent or continuous, a physician should make a careful examination of the blood to determine whether or not clotting, or coagulation, of the blood is delayed because of some deficiency. There is no way to strengthen blood vessels to prevent hemorrhage. If there is frequent hemorrhage from the nose a competent specialist in diseases of the nose will be able to look directly into it and to find out whether a dilated blood vessel or an ulcer of any kind is responsible. He can control such a condition by cauterizing the bleeding point or otherwise modifying the conditions responsible.

CONTROL OF BLEEDING

In addition to bleeding from the nose, there may be oozing from wounds elsewhere in the body. If this is continuous it can usually be controlled by

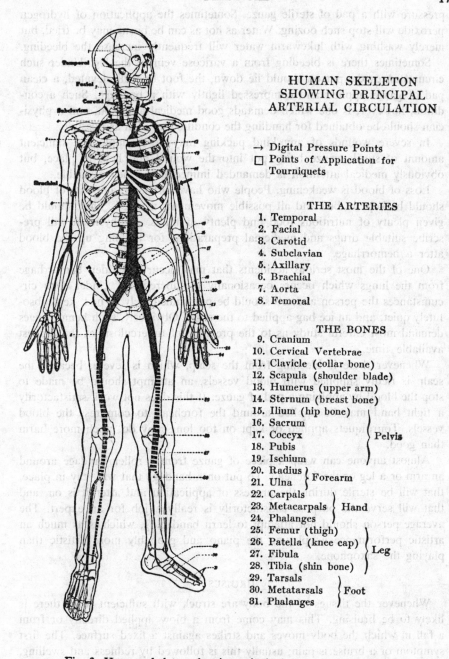

HUMAN SKELETON SHOWING PRINCIPAL ARTERIAL CIRCULATION

→ Digital Pressure Points
☐ Points of Application for Tourniquets

THE ARTERIES

1. Temporal
2. Facial
3. Carotid
4. Subclavian
5. Axillary
6. Brachial
7. Aorta
8. Femoral

THE BONES

9. Cranium
10. Cervical Vertebrae
11. Clavicle (collar bone)
12. Scapula (shoulder blade)
13. Humerus (upper arm)
14. Sternum (breast bone)
15. Ilium (hip bone)
16. Sacrum
17. Coccyx ⎱
18. Pubis ⎰ Pelvis
19. Ischium
20. Radius ⎱
21. Ulna ⎰ Forearm
22. Carpals
23. Metacarpals ⎱ Hand
24. Phalanges ⎰
25. Femur (thigh)
26. Patella (knee cap) ⎱
27. Fibula ⎰ Leg
28. Tibia (shin bone)
29. Tarsals
30. Metatarsals ⎱ Foot
31. Phalanges ⎰

Fig. 3. Human skeleton showing principal arterial circulation.
(Copyright, 1942, Clay-Adams Co., Inc.)

pressure with a pad of sterile gauze. Sometimes the application of hydrogen peroxide will stop such oozing. Water as hot as can be borne may be tried, but merely washing with lukewarm water will frequently increase the bleeding.

Sometimes there is bleeding from a varicose vein of the leg. Under such circumstances the person should lie down, the foot be well elevated, a clean pad of gauze applied and compressed lightly with a bandage. Such a condition, however, is one which demands good medical attention, and a physician should be obtained for handling the condition as soon as possible.

In severe wounds of any kind packing may be attempted, a sufficient amount of sterile gauze being put into the wound and held in place, but obviously medical attention is demanded immediately when available.

Loss of blood is weakening. People who have lost large amounts of blood should be kept in bed and all possible movements avoided. They should be given plenty of nutritious food and plenty of fluids. A physician will prescribe suitable drugs and medicinal preparations for building up the blood after a hemorrhage.

One of the most serious accidents that may occur is sudden hemorrhage from the lungs which occurs occasionally in tuberculosis. Under such circumstances the person affected should be put immediately to bed, kept absolutely quiet, and an ice bag applied to the chest. Obviously, such hemorrhages demand most careful study as to the presence of tuberculosis at the earliest available time.

Whenever there is bleeding from the scalp, which is severe, because the scalp is richly supplied with blood vessels, an attempt should be made to stop the blood by applying a pad of gauze. If this does not work satisfactorily a tight band may be applied around the forehead to compress the blood vessels. Tourniquets applied or kept on too long may do much more harm than good.

Almost anyone can wrap a piece of gauze from a roller bandage around an arm or a leg or the forehead. To put on a bandage that will stay in place, that will be sterile during the process of application and after it is on, and that will serve the purpose satisfactorily is really a job for an expert. The average person should not attempt to learn bandaging, which is as much an artistic performance as playing the piano and probably more artistic than playing the saxophone.

BRUISES

Whenever the tissues of the body are struck with sufficient force there is likely to be bruising. This may come from a blow applied directly or from a fall in which the body moves and strikes against a fixed surface. The first symptom of a bruise is pain; usually this is followed by redness and swelling. Later, due to the blood that has poured out from the blood vessels into the skin, the tissues become black and blue. As the blood is gradually absorbed this changes from brown to yellow and gradually disappears. For most bruises little immediate treatment is necessary. The application of pads wrung out of ice water will lessen pain.

A black eye is a form of bruise especially unsightly and likely to arouse ridicule. The application of iced compresses to the eye will stop the pain and perhaps, to some extent, prevent discoloration. After the blackness appears, the application of heat in the form of hot compresses kept on for half an hour three times a day will hasten the disappearance of the swelling and discoloration. Among things that are not to be done to a black eye are the application of a slice of raw beefsteak, pressure with the handle of a knife, and the application of any kind of strong medicinal lotion or solution.

The danger of injury to the eyeball is far more serious than either the mental or physical pain associated with the ordinary black eye. It is well to have the eye looked at promptly to make certain that the eyeball has not been injured in any way.

FOREIGN BODIES

Among the emergencies demanding first aid is the presence of foreign bodies in the eye, ear, nose, throat, or esophagus. Regardless of how careful mothers may be, children occasionally push foreign substances into various body cavities. When a child chokes there is no time to call a doctor. The mother must act promptly. The mother should remember that the attempt to remove any object in the throat by rough methods may do more harm than good. If the baby is small it should be put face downward, or head downward, and given an opportunity to cough the object out. A very large object can, of course, be pulled out with the finger. A physician removes objects from the throat by the use of special devices developed for this purpose. He has "scopes" of every type with which he may look into the various cavities. He has also special lighted tubes with forceps and hooks for the withdrawal of foreign substances.

When foreign substances get into the nose, more harm is usually done by attempts to dislodge them with improper instruments than by letting them alone until competent advice can be had. If blowing the nose will not remove a foreign substance, sneezing may accomplish it. The physician may wash out foreign substances or by the use of proper forceps seize and remove them.

Another type of emergency is the foreign substance in the ear, particularly an insect. An insect in the ear may be removed by turning the head to one side and filling the ear with warm sweet oil poured into it by means of a spoon. The insect is unable to live in the oil, and it promptly dies, and then can be floated out with warm water. In syringing the ear with warm water it is best to spray the water against the side at the entrance of the ear rather than directly against the eardrum.

If a child swallows any sharp-pointed object, such as a piece of glass, a bone, or a pin, relief is sometimes had by eating mashed potatoes and bread thoroughly chewed, which aid the passage of the substance down the gullet into the stomach. It is well then to obtain medical advice immediately. By the use of the X-ray the substance may be located and a decision made as to the best method for its removal. Experience shows that in many instances foreign substances that are swallowed will pass from the body by way of the bowel without undue harm.

Foreign substances in the eyes are particularly annoying. With experience, it is possible to locate such foreign substances on the lower or upper lid and to remove cinders or tiny specks with the point of a clean pocket handker-chief. With a little experience it becomes possible for anyone to turn back the upper lid. The simplest method is, first to wash the hands thoroughly; then, with a small match stick or some similar rod laid across the lid, the patient looks down, the attendant grasps the eyelashes, and turns the lid upside down by pulling the eyelashes over the match stick or rod.

Do not attempt to remove a foreign substance from the surface of the eyeball without special training in such first aid measures. It is safer, pending the arrival of expert attention, to merely place a small pad of wet gauze over the eye and to restrain the motion of the eye until attention is available. If any foreign substance has been removed from the eye it may be washed out with a saturated solution of boric acid, made by adding a flat teaspoonful of boric acid powder to a glassful of warm water and stirring until dissolved.

The simplest way to put drops in the eye is with the use of an eye dropper. A small quantity of the drops is drawn into the dropper, the patient sits on a chair facing a good light, the person who is putting the drops in stands in front, pulls down the lower lid, and, while the patient looks away, places one or two drops of the fluid on the outer edge of the lower lid. This will run across the eye and wash the surface. The patient looks away in order to avoid seeing the dropper and jumping when it approaches the eye.

All sorts of suggestions are made for the removal of cinders or other specks from the eye, including rubbing the other eye, blowing the nose, and indulging in similar manipulations. The chief advantage of these manipulations is to avoid harm to the eye from too much inexpert attention.

FIREWORKS AND TOY FIREARMS

Among frequent emergencies demanding prompt attention are explosions of fireworks. Hundreds of people used to be killed or injured in celebrating the independence of the United States. Following great campaigns of edu-cation this type of celebration has been largely displaced by pageants, plays, and exhibits of fireworks under the control of expert showmen.

Air rifles, BB guns, shotguns, and other small-caliber rifles, blank cartridges and cap pistols, sling shots and rubber band flippers, arrows and stones, are responsible for one third of the accidents resulting in loss of eyesight to children. Firecrackers, torpedoes, bombs, and various types of fireworks are responsible for one fourth of the cases of blindness.

Lockjaw or tetanus is discussed elsewhere in this book. The germs of lockjaw develop in soil and in manure and on dirty clothing. Any time an injury occurs in which dirt is forced into a wound and sealed in there is danger of lockjaw. There is the kind of accident that occurs in explosions of cannon crackers, blank cartridges, and toy cannon. The size of the wound is not significant. The tiniest puncture may admit germs into the body.

Whenever an injury from fireworks occurs, get a doctor as soon as possible. He will open the wound, clean it, and treat it with suitable antiseptics, and in questionable cases inject the antitoxin against lockjaw to prevent that disease. Never wait until lockjaw develops. After the disease has developed it is one of the most serious affecting a human being. So serious is the possibility of lockjaw that in many cases health departments provide antitoxin without charge to make certain that cases of lockjaw do not develop.

WOUNDS

Whenever the skin is opened, torn, or punctured the injury is called a wound. Wounds may thus vary from the tiniest puncture, such as that of a needle, to severe injuries tearing open several inches of skin and penetrating into body cavities. The greatest danger from wounds, after the immediate danger of hemorrhage, lies in infection. Therefore, the first step of importance in first aid is to prevent infection. Infection may be prevented by disinfection.

In taking care of a wound be certain that your own hands are as clean as possible. Surgeons wash the hands thoroughly with soap and water and then wash them in antiseptics, and thereafter wear rubber gloves which have been sterilized by steam under pressure. In taking care of any small wound around the home, be certain that the hands of the person who is taking care of the wound are as clean as possible. Hence they should be washed thoroughly with soap and water and perhaps also in alcohol. All materials applied to the wound should be sterilized. Such materials are now available in any drug store in packages. If a sterile package of material is not available, it may be made by boiling thoroughly materials available in the home. A freshly laundered handkerchief or towel is likely to be relatively free from germs because laundering, heating, and ironing kill organisms on the surface.

Hundreds of antiseptic substances are now available and are widely advertised. Among the best of the antiseptics is alcohol. Tincture of iodine is widely used as a first aid dressing, as are also mercurochrome, saturated solution of boric acid, hydrogen peroxide, metaphen, merthiolates, zephiran, and hexylresorcinol solution. When a wound has been contaminated with dirt this should be washed out with a suitable solution. Do not apply hydrogen peroxide to a fresh wound because it may cause pain and unnecessary crusting with destruction of tissue.

After the wound has been disinfected by the application of a suitable antiseptic it should be covered with clean sterile gauze and suitably bound. No one should attempt to sew a wound unless he has had medical training. Whenever pus or infection occurs in a wound it should have prompt medical attention. If a person is far removed from medical attention he should realize that it is of the greatest importance to release the pus by opening the wound and then to apply the antiseptic. Wet dressings of concentrated boric acid solution applied for several days are helpful.

Certain types of wounds represent unusual emergencies, among them splinters entering the skin. Small splinters are best removed by using a needle which has been passed through a flame in order to sterilize it; large splinters by the use of a knife blade sterilized in a similar manner, and perhaps also with the aid of a forceps.

When a fishhook gets into the skin don't try to pull it out. In order to avoid tearing the tissues push the point onward and forward and let the end of the fishhook follow the point. The barbed end may then be cut off with a wire cutter, and when this is removed the fishhook may be removed by reversing the process.

BURNS

Burns of the skin may be produced by many different methods including the heat from a flame or hot iron, the heat from scalding water or steam, and the heat from electricity. Burns which involve more than one half of the surface of the body are usually fatal. When a person has been suddenly or severely burned he may suffer from shock. This demands immediate attention in order to stimulate him and to save life. He should, of course, be put at rest and the burn suitably covered to prevent continued irritation. Almost everyone now knows that when a person's clothing is actually burning it is well to smother the flames by the use of a blanket, a rug, or any other heavy material that is handy.

In the presence of slight burns or scalds it is preferable to cover the burned portion immediately with cold water, which will check the effect of the heat and stop the pain. Some recommend application of ordinary vinegar. If the foot or hand has been burned by spilling hot water, soup, or coffee over it, put the part burned immediately under water and keep it submerged until the first effects of the injury have passed. Thereafter it may be covered with Vaseline petroleum jelly. Loose cotton should not be put on a burn, nor should wide pieces of gauze be applied. It is practically impossible to remove such materials without great injury to the tissues. The gauze may be applied in narrow strips.

Modern methods of treating burns include application of liquid petrolatum, or the application of melted petrolatum, which hardens and covers the burn.

Burns from acids are among the most serious, particularly nitric and sulphuric acids. The first treatment following a burn by acid is to wash off the acid as quickly as possible with a solution of bicarbonate of soda and to leave the wound in the soda solution for some time. People who work in acids regularly should wear gloves whenever possible. Electric burns are usually deep and severe. They should be treated as are other burns.

RESUSCITATION

Among the most serious of emergencies which may occur, demanding first aid, is resuscitation after asphyxiation, which may result from drowning, from electric shock, and from exhaust-gas poison. Occasionally also there may be asphyxiation from other sources, such as gas escaping from electric refrigerators.

It has been estimated that 25 per cent of men and boys past twelve years of age do not know how to swim, and there are few women who would be capable of swimming long enough or far enough to save themselves in an emergency. When a person has been under water long enough to become unconscious—about four or five minutes—first aid measures are of greatest importance to save life. There are numerous devices for artificial resuscitation, but it is usually not well to wait until these come. Until 1952 the most commonly practiced method was the Schaefer technique. Then the American Red Cross, the American Medical Association and other agencies after extended research adapted a method called the Holger. Now recommended is mouth-to-mouth resuscitation. This new technique has the distinct advantage of allowing the rescuer to provide enough pressure immediately to inflate the lungs of the victim. Here are the steps recommended by Dr. Peter Safar and his associates at the Department of Anesthesiology, Baltimore City Hospitals.

Method 1 is recommended for adults and large children.
1. When the victim is found, place him on his back and kneel close to his left ear. If foreign material is visible at the mouth, turn the victim's head to the side and quickly clean the mouth and throat with your fingers or a piece of cloth. *Fig. 1.* This should take only a few seconds. If the mouth appears clean, tilt the head back so that the chin is pointing upward. *Fig. 2.* Repeat cleaning procedure during mouth-to-mouth breathing whenever necessary.

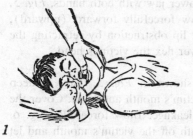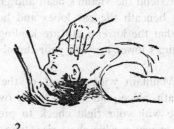

1   2

Fig.1, left. When the victim is found, place him on his back and kneel close to his left ear. If foreign material is visible at the mouth, turn the victim's head to the side and quickly clean the mouth and throat with your fingers or a piece of cloth. *Fig. 2, right.* Tilt head so that chin points upward.

2. Extend victim's head, insert your left thumb (which may be wrapped for protection) between his teeth, grasp the lower jaw at midline, and hold it forcefully forward (upward), so that the lower teeth are leading. *Fig. 3.*

3. Close the victim's nose with your right hand. Take a deep breath, place your mouth firmly over his mouth, and blow forcefully. *Fig. 4.* Watch the victim's chest, and when it rises, take your mouth off his mouth and let him exhale passively. Repeat the blowing effort at the rate of about 12 to 20 breaths per minute.

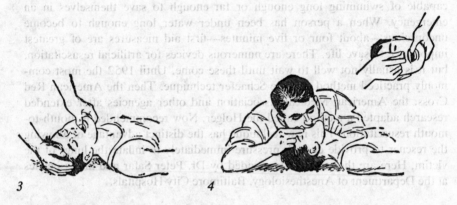

3   4

Fig. 3, left. Extend victim's head, insert your left thumb (which may be wrapped for protection) between his teeth, grasp the lower jaw at midline, and hold it forcefully forward (upward), so that lower teeth are leading. *Fig. 4, right.* Close the victim's nose with your right hand. Take a deep breath, place your mouth firmly over victim's mouth, and blow forcefully in adults (about 20 breaths per minute) and gently in children (about 12 breaths per minute).

Method 2 is recommended for adults whose mouths cannot be opened and for small children.

1. Extend the victim's head and grasp the lower jaw with both hands, *Fig. 5,* just beneath the ear lobes and hold the jaw forcefully forward (upward), so that the lower teeth are leading. Prevent lip obstruction by retracting the victim's lower lip with your thumbs, but never flex the victim's head.

2. Maintain your support of the jaw as shown in *Fig. 5.* Take a deep breath, place your mouth firmly over the victim's mouth and blow. Cover the nose with your right cheek to prevent air leakage. Blow forcefully. *Fig. 6.* When you see his chest rise, take your mouth off the victim's mouth and let him exhale passively. Repeat the blowing about 12 to 20 times per minute. Blow forcefully in adults, gently in children. Use only puffs from the cheeks in newborn babies. When you see the victim's chest rise, take your mouth off his mouth and let him exhale passively.

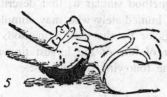
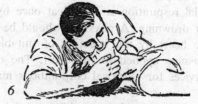

5   6

Fig. 5, left. Extend victim's head and grasp the lower jaw with
both hands just beneath the ear lobes and hold the jaw forcefully
forward (upward), so that lower teeth are leading. Prevent lip
obstruction by retracting victim's lower lip with your thumbs.
Never flex victim's head. *Fig. 6, right.* Take a deep breath, place
your mouth firmly over the victim's mouth and blow. Cover the
nose with your right cheek to prevent air leakage. Blow forcefully in adults, gently in children. Use only puffs from the cheeks
in newborn babies.

In infants and very small children, the technique of mouth-to-mouth *and
nose* resuscitation may be used. Follow instructions as shown in *Figs. 1, 2,* and
5. Place your mouth over child's mouth *and* nose making sure no air can escape.
Breathe into the child, using shallow puffs of air at about 12 breaths per minute. *Fig. 7.*

As an aid to rescuers, a new device for artificial resuscitation has become
available generally. Called the *Resusitube* (T.M. Johnson & Johnson), this
plastic device provides a breathing tube for the victim and a mouthpiece for
the rescuer, eliminating direct oral contact. *Fig. 8.*

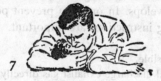
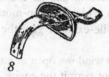

7   8

ELECTRIC SHOCK

Following electric shock it is first necessary to remove the electrocuted man
from the electric conductor. Employees of electrical corporations do not
stop to shut off the current. They take off a coat or wrap and throw it
around the patient's body so as to pull him away from the contact. They
are told never to put their hands near the pockets of an electrified man nor
near his shoes, because the presence of metal materials or nails in the shoes
will cause severe shock to the rescuer.

When a person has been shocked by electricity, death may occur instantaneously from paralysis of the centers of circulation of the heart because of
overexcitation of the heart muscle, perhaps due to suffocation from the
forcible contraction of the muscles of breathing. Sometimes death occurs from
burning, and sometimes the person who has been shocked by electricity
falls and dies from the fall.

The person is first removed from contact with the electrical current. Artificial respiration is started at once by the method similar to that described for drowning. A physician should be called immediately who may stimulate the heart by the injection of suitable drugs or by the use of methods of massage applied to the heart. The director of one of the largest first aid services for electrical corporations makes the following suggestions:

1. Release victim, avoiding sustaining a shock one's self. Any dry nonconductor may be used to move victim or the live conductor.
2. If both the victim's hands are grasping the live conductor, free them one at a time.
3. If necessary, shut off the current. Nearest switch should be opened.
4. If it is necessary to cut a live wire, use a wooden-handled axe, turning away the face to avoid the flash.
5. Put finger in victim's mouth to remove teeth, gum, or tobacco.
6. Place patient on back for giving mouth-to-mouth resuscitation.
7. Carry out artificial respiration.
8. When the patient revives, keep him lying down. Keep him warm.
9. Watch the respiration carefully, in case it fails again.

GAS POISONING

Most of the deaths from the inhalation of carbon-monoxide gas occur from running automobiles in closed garages. However, there may be suffocation from illuminating gas in the home or from working with various types of machines in which carbon-monoxide develops. In order to prevent poisoning by automobile-exhaust gas, the following instructions are important.

1. Keep windows open as much as possible.
2. Do not permit the engine to run and discharge exhaust gas directly into the air of the workroom. Every workroom should have a flexible tube which can be attached to the exhaust pipe and through which the exhaust gas may then be carried out of doors.
3. Remember that carbon-monoxide gas has no smell. You cannot, therefore, know if carbon-monoxide gas is in the air by the smell of the room or by the cloudiness of the air. These are produced by burning oil and gasoline.
4. If you suffer with headaches report this fact at once so that the conditions of the air may be investigated and proper ventilation established.
5. If you do not feel well, see a doctor at once. You may be particularly sensitive to carbon-monoxide gas, more so than the others. In that case you had better change your occupation. It is not safe for you to be exposed to even very small amounts of the gas.

The Bulletin of the New York State Department of Labor recommends these first aid measures:

If you get a headache, or feel faint, nervous, or irritable, go out into the fresh air at once and stay there until you feel better. When you go out go out slowly and when you get out sit down quietly. Do not go for a walk. You may not have enough oxygen in your blood to permit you to take any additional exercise or exert yourself in any way. Any added exertion at such a time is dangerous and may be sufficient to cause you to become unconscious. Wrap up warmly, therefore, and sit down out of doors until you feel better.

Do not hurry around unnecessarily at your work. The more exercise you take, the more carbon monoxide will get into your blood.

If one of your comrades faints, get him out into the fresh air at once. Put blankets under and over him and surround him with hot-water bottles or hot bricks. Keep him warm at all costs, or he may develop pneumonia. Persons who become asphyxiated with carbon-monoxide gas are peculiarly susceptible to pneumonia. Call up the gas company and an ambulance at once. You must always call both of these, because ambulances are not equipped with resuscitation apparatus. In the meantime the patient should be given artificial respiration. Everyone working in industries where there is a possibility of exposure to carbon-monoxide gas should be familiar with this method of resuscitation. It is very easily carried out. Anyone can learn how to do it. He may thus by his knowledge be able to save someone's life.

Recently the use of injections of methylene blue has been offered as a scientific means for treating patients with carbon-monoxide poisoning. In the presence of such poisoning a physician should be called immediately. He will then determine whether or not any remedies are to be injected. Of the greatest importance is the immediate application of the methods of artificial respiration already described.

FAINTING AND UNCONSCIOUSNESS

Few persons have the slightest idea of what is to be done when another person suddenly becomes unconscious. There are numerous causes for this condition: a blow on the head; pressure on the brain from a large blood clot; a lack of blood supply to the brain; the effects of such drugs as opium, ether, chloroform, or alcohol; or carbon-monoxide gas; but practically all of these are related in some manner to the brain, since the brain is the seat of consciousness.

A physician who is called to see a person who has suddenly become unconscious makes his decision as to the cause of unconsciousness from a number of factors. He feels the pulse to determine whether, by its rate and strength, the difficulty is affecting the circulation of the blood. If the pulse rate is between 76 and 90 and strong, he realizes that there is no immediate danger of death from failure of respiration. He studies the color of the face. If there is great pallor or blueness or a purple color he realizes that there are difficulties with the blood. He observes also if the skin is hot or cold and determines the presence or absence of perspiration. The eyes are noted to observe if the pupils are equal or unequal, if they are dilated or contracted.

Unequal size of the pupils is a common symptom of injury to the brain, such as a brain hemorrhage. It may also be desirable to feel the skull to determine whether or not there is a fracture or crushing injury beneath the surface of the scalp.

In the presence of excessive heat, sunstroke may be the cause of unconsciousness. The odor of the breath may indicate the presence of acidosis or the fact that the person has taken a large dose of alcohol or of ether.

Associated with the onset of fainting there may be dizziness or lightheadedness. The average human being walks erect and pays no attention to his sense of balance because that is controlled by a number of reflex sensations coming to the brain from various places. The semicircular canals of the internal ear give the human being a sense of his position in space. There is also a feeling associated with the muscles which aids the determination of presence in space. If the body tends to accumulate acid, dizziness is a prominent symptom. Anything that interferes with the coördination between the sense of vision, the muscle sense, and the sensations coming from the semicircular canals will produce dizziness.

If the sense of dizziness merely comes and goes and yields quickly to proper hygiene such as suitable attention to the diet, the digestion, the action of the kidneys, and correction of disorders of vision, one need not be disturbed. However, if dizziness is repeated again and again it may be due to insufficient blood supply to the brain, insufficient action of the heart, a tumor growing in connection with the semicircular canals, or some hidden disturbance elsewhere. A feeling of dizziness and fainting, if repeated, demands careful scientific study. Of course, some people faint more easily than do others. Some faint from the slightest emotional shock. Some people faint at the sight of blood, others faint quickly from exhaustion, weakness, lack of air, or similar conditions.

A person who is about to faint realizes it from a feeling of weakness, a blurring of vision, a failure of circulation so that the face becomes pale, and the presence of cold perspiration. The moment a person faints he should be placed flat on the back and his head lowered. The color of the face is an indicator to some extent of the blood supply to the brain. If the face is pale the head should be lowered until the color of the face improves. If, on the other hand, the face is extremely red, it may be desirable to keep the head raised.

A person who has fainted should have plenty of fresh, cool air, cold water applied to the face or chest as a stimulant to recuperative action. Sometimes the inhalation of smelling salts serves to stimulate the breathing of the patient and in that way to aid his recovery. The usual first aid remedy, found in most family medicine chests, for attacks of fainting is half a teaspoonful of aromatic spirits of ammonia given in water. A person who has fainted should be kept quiet and recumbent until fully recovered. If permitted to get up and walk too soon, serious results may follow.

Heat Stroke

Heat stroke occurs not only in tropical countries and in extremely hot weather in the temperate zone, but also at any time in factories, engine rooms, laundries, and kitchens, where people work in extreme heat associated with considerable moisture. For prevention, tablets of common salt may be taken every few hours in extremely hot weather.

The symptoms of heat stroke may come on suddenly but most frequently come on gradually. The person who is about to become affected feels weak and tired, gets dizzy and drowsy. The digestion may be disturbed, and there may even be pain in the abdomen. The temperature rises, the fever increases, the pulse becomes rapid, the skin dry, burning, and flushed; the pupils of the eyes are usually contracted, and the breathing fast and noisy. Just before death the pupils may dilate. It is important to be certain of a diagnosis of heat stroke and to make positive that the unconsciousness is not due to drugs, hemorrhage, epilepsy, or diabetes.

The ability to keep cool depends on common sense. One should wear light clothing, loose and porous. Cool baths at frequent intervals aid in making one feel much better. Adequate amounts of sleep keep the body prepared for unusual stress and strain. One should take plenty of water, because evaporation of water from the surface of the body aids the control of temperature. Traveling in hot weather is extremely difficult. It is better, under conditions of extreme heat, to sit in an open coach with a free circulation of air than in the smaller compartments and drawing rooms.

In case of heat exhaustion, the first thing to do is to get the person into a cool place and absolutely at rest, flat on the back. Sponging with cool water helps to control the temperature. It may be necessary to stimulate the circulation with stimulating drugs or coffee to help the patient over the acute condition. Tropical authorities recommend that the person be placed as soon as possible on a bed covered with a large rubber sheet, and then that ice and cold water be rubbed over the body. At the same time that the ice is rubbed, the friction or massage encourages the circulation.

The temperature should be taken regularly and when it falls to 101 degrees, as taken by the bowel instead of by the mouth, one stops the application of cold, covers the patient with blankets, and makes certain that collapse does not follow. If breathing stops it may be necessary to apply artificial respiration. After recovery from heat stroke, small quantities of nutritious food may be given repeatedly in order to aid recovery.

Bite Wounds

The bites of insects, snakes, cats, dogs, and other small animals frequently demand some attention in first aid. The sting of a bee, yellow jacket, or other wasp, should be pulled out, if still in the flesh, and a drop or two of diluted ammonia water applied to the wound. The application of cold compresses will help to stop pain. The sting of a centipede, spider, or scorpion may be more severe than that of a wasp or bee. Bleeding should be encouraged to wash out any material deposited by the bite; then tincture of iodine may be applied and a cold compress used to stop pain. Antihistaminic ointments have a slightly antiseptic effect, relieve itching and act against the sensitization to insect poisons.

Most spider bites in the United States are due to the shoe-button spider or the black widow. It is called shoe button because it looks like a black button; and black widow because the female frequently eats the male. The sting of a scorpion is not frequent. A physician usually treats such stings by injecting some anesthetic solution around the bite, including some adrenalin solution to constrict the blood vessels and prevent absorption of the poison.

Flea bites, if painful, may be treated with weak solutions of menthol or camphor.

Dog bites, or the bites of any small animal, must always be investigated to determine the possibility of hydrophobia in the animal that bites. The treatment of the bite itself is ordinarily the same as that for any infected wound. If it seems certain, however, that the animal has rabies, or hydrophobia, the wound should be thoroughly cauterized by a physician.

The scabies, or itch mite, travels rapidly from one person to another. The handling of infestation with the itch mite is really a problem for a physician. It demands thorough cleansing, the application of suitable drugs, and care of the clothing as well.

The bite of the bedbug seldom becomes infected but is an annoyance. The itching is, of course, easily treated by solutions of weak ammonia or very weak menthol.

In the case of every type of insect, prevention is far better than cure. It is necessary to know, first of all, the presence of the insects; second, their breeding habits; and third, special methods for destroying them. If they are once completely destroyed by fumigation or disinfestation methods they are not likely to return soon again, particularly if sufficient watchfulness is exercised to attack them while they are few in number.

HICCUPS

Hiccups to most people is just a temporary disagreeable symptom, but to the scientist who knows of all of the possible relationships of the hiccup as a symptom of various diseases, it constitutes a phenomenon of considerable significance. Between the chest and the abdomen lies a great muscular structure called the diaphragm. Above the diaphragm are the heart and lungs; below it, the stomach, intestines, liver, pancreas, spleen and other organs.

When one breathes, the diaphragm contracts, enlarging the chest cavity and helping the lungs to expand. In order for any muscle tissue to contract, a stimulus comes to it through a nerve. The nerve that controls the contractions of the diaphragm passes from the upper part of the spinal cord in the region of the neck. If this nerve is irritated at any spot it becomes stimulated, and the stimulation causes a sudden spasmodic contraction of the diaphragm that is called a hiccup.

In many cases hiccup is due to some infection involving the portion of the brain associated with the stimulation of contraction of the diaphragm. In such cases, the condition affects chiefly men more than forty-five years of age and it tends to follow operation on the colon, the prostate gland, the gall bladder, or the stomach. If there is an infection of the brain at the basis of an attack of hiccups, early diagnosis may mean the saving of life. Such diagnosis demands the services of a specialist in neurology.

Then there are cases which can be classed as chemical hiccup. In these cases hiccup occurs following the eating of highly irritating foods or liquids. Generally such hiccups last only a short time. It is also recognized that tumors of the brain, pressing on the areas associated with stimulation of the diaphragm, may produce hiccup. It is also possible by a sudden dilatation of the stomach to produce an irritation which will result in this symptom. Finally, there are cases of hiccup that have a nervous basis, exactly as hysteria may duplicate almost any disease known to medical science. Then there are cases of hiccup in which the origin cannot be easily determined even with the most careful study.

Everybody has his own cure for ordinary hiccups. In most instances it involves something that will fix the attention on anything except the hiccup. The physician who treats such cases may carry out certain procedures in persistent hiccups which frequently bring relief. One of these is to wash out the stomach; another to prescribe certain narcotics and sedatives that will give temporary relief; a third is to treat the specific infection from which the patient seems to be suffering. Another method involves the giving of enemas and doses of oil to clean out the entire intestinal tract. Breathing into a paper bag is also a helpful method.

In the case of a baby, it may be held on the shoulder and patted on the back, which will cause it to expel the air which may be distending its stomach or esophagus and thus leading to hiccups. In some cases the stimulation of the nerve results from poisons associated with infections such as infantile paralysis or epidemic encephalitis. The latter condition has been called American sleeping sickness. In these cases the hiccups may be severe and go on for long periods of time; indeed, actually to the point of exhaustion. The treatment of such conditions is a long and serious matter and it is only by the treatment of the fundamental condition that the hiccups are to be controlled.

When every method of treating hiccups has failed and the symptom persists there may, of course, be danger to life. In such cases the surgeon may expose the phrenic nerve and either cut it or place pressure upon it. This will invariably cause the hiccup to stop by interfering with the passing of the stimulus from the irritated center along the nerve to the diaphragm.

Migraine or Sick Headache

Migraine or sick headache is often called recurrent headache. It is called sick headache because it is sometimes accompanied with nausea or vomiting. Sometimes it is found to be dependent on uncorrected errors of vision or sinus disease or on various poisonings of the body. In other words, it seems to be associated with sensitivity to food of one kind or another, or even to serious diseases of the stomach and other organs of the body. On occasion, severe headache is associated with disturbance of the brain, such as tumor or hardening of the arteries. In some instances, the headaches may be wholly on a mental basis.

Every case of persistent headache should be carefully studied so that the physician may evaluate all of the different factors that may be concerned. The headache or the pain is the symptom of a disorder of the human body rather than a disease in itself.

Sometimes the headache is associated with the type of nausea that has been mentioned; sometimes with disturbances of vision in the form of blindness, dullness of vision, blinding flashes of light, or dizziness. In certain cases there are, associated with the pains in the head, emotional disturbances such as a feeling of depression or melancholia. In other cases the headaches are associated with restlessness and irritability, and in still another group with confusion, absent-mindedness, or a sense of unreality. In some cases there are pains in the abdomen which are of the same type as the pain in the head.

Women have their symptoms chiefly at the time of menstruation. In many cases the headaches occur frequently, but in the majority about once in two weeks. The type of headache called migraine occurs most often between the ages of eighteen and thirty-five, but may appear at any age. There was a time when it was thought primarily to be a disease affecting women, and some writers have said that it occurs four times as often in women as in men. More recently careful studies seem to show that headaches of this type occur just about as often in men as in women. The reason why it has seemed to be more frequent in women is that they are more likely to consult a physician about the condition than are men, and that the attacks in them may seem to be more severe.

Sometimes the headaches come on without any warning, but in most cases they are preceded by a feeling of depression, by an unwillingness to work or to go about the daily affairs of life. Since there seem to be many possible causes for headaches of this type, the attack on them must be made from various points of view. It is believed that they may on occasion be associated, as has been said, with eye strain or disease of the sinuses. Obviously in such cases careful examination must be made by a competent specialist in diseases of the eye to make certain that the vision is properly corrected with suitable glasses. It should be made certain that the eyes are not abused by working under conditions of improper illumination. The nose must be examined most carefully and, if necessary, X-ray pictures made of the sinuses to make certain that they do not contain polyps or infection.

The physician will use the ophthalmoscope to look in the back of the eye in order to make certain that there is no pressure within the skull due to any disorder. Sometimes it is necessary to X-ray the skull for possible observation of an abnormality in the brain.

It is believed that migraine is associated with such disorders of hypersensitivity as hay fever, eczema, asthma, and similar conditions. It is possible in such cases to test the reaction of the patient to various foods and proteins by skin sensitivity tests or perhaps to try elimination diets, in which food substances are eliminated from the diet when their consumption seems to be followed by an attack. Apparently not all cases are due to such sensitivity, but a considerable number may be.

In some instances the attacks seem to come on when the digestion of the person concerned is not working properly. In these instances, it is well to have a thorough study of the gastro-intestinal tract to make certain that there is neither constipation nor a residue of putrefactive matter in the bowel.

In other cases the glands of internal secretion may be involved, and it is necessary to make a thorough study of the body with a view to determining that all of the glands are neither overfunctioning nor underfunctioning. This is merely an indication of the necessity for studying every case of recurrent sick headache with all of the means known to modern medical science.

Almost every method of treatment known to medical science has been applied at one time or another in the treatment of recurrent headaches. In many instances some definite change should be made in the life habits of such a patient based on a complete survey of his work, his play, his food, his mental attitude, and his philosophy of life. An inequality of emphasis in the patient's interests and activities should be corrected. He should live a moderate existence, and all excesses should be prevented. This applies particularly to excess in work involving the eyes and to overeating.

A patient who is constantly indoors and gets insufficient exercise should change his habits in the right direction. Rest and change are particularly valuable for people who are constantly under physical, mental, or emotional pressure. Persons who suffer from recurrent sick headaches should not try to work all the time. They will do well to take at least one afternoon and one day a week for rest or recreation, and perhaps both winter and summer vacations.

In controlling the immediate attack, the room in which the patient rests should be darkened and everything be kept quiet. Most such patients are so intensely uncomfortable that they do not want to be touched or interfered with. In some instances, an ice bag to the head or a hot-water bottle to the feet may give relief.

The physician who is actively in charge of the treatment of such a patient can do much by controlling the diet, eliminating the substances to which the patient seems to respond with headache. The use of various glandular preparations to overcome deficiencies in glands or, in some instances, to oppose over-activity of certain glands is again experimental but is worthy of trial.

When drugs are given to control the pain, the constant attention of a physician who is thoroughly familiar with the patient, his habits, his emotional reactions, and particularly his headaches is desirable. It is easy to fall into the habit of taking strong drugs constantly, and the physician who understands the patient and his reactions will know how to avoid the danger of such habits. The drug called ergotamine in various forms, for instance, combined with caffeine as in "cafergone" has been found helpful. The drug is powerful and should be used only when prescribed and in the manner prescribed by the doctor.

METALLIC AND FOOD POISONING

The human being is subject to various kinds of possible poisoning from foods and drugs, from mushrooms, and all sorts of similar toxic substances. There are poisons constantly used in industry which may get into the body and thereby produce severe illness.

In any case of poisoning certain procedures are immediately desirable. First, try to ascertain the nature of the poison taken. An empty bottle in the vicinity, the presence of some of the substance in a cup or utensil, or the presence of the poison on the tablecloth or floor or clothing may be a valuable sign. By smelling the breath and examining the mouth of the patient, the physician may determine the presence of stains or burns characteristic of the action of certain poisons. If the patient has taken the poison accidentally he will probably be willing to tell the physician, if he is conscious.

If poisoning is suspected, a physician should be called immediately. Before the doctor comes, it is well to give white of eggs, milk, or strong tea, which are antagonistic to many poisons. In order to get the poison out of the system as rapidly as possible one should provoke vomiting, either by tickling the back of the throat, by giving a cup of warm water mixed with salt, or by washing out the stomach with a stomach tube, if one understands how this is done. If one puts a heaping teaspoonful of salt in a cupful of lukewarm water, stirs until dissolved, and has the patient drink the mixture, repeating the dose every ten minutes until three or four cupfuls have been taken, vomiting takes place promptly, serving to wash out the stomach.

Thereafter the person must be treated as in any case of fainting, dizziness, or shock, the symptoms being treated according to the nature of the case. If the patient is greatly weakened or prostrated he must be kept warm, recumbent, and his general strength sustained.

For many of the common poisons there are special antidotes. However, these are seldom present in the average home, and even when present, few people have time to consult tables of antidotes or know where the antidote is to be found. For poisoning with carbolic acid it is customary to wash out the mouth with whisky or alcohol diluted with water, to have the patient swallow three or four tablespoonfuls of diluted whisky or alcohol diluted with water, and to give a heaping tablespoonful of Epsom salts dissolved in water.

Bichloride of mercury is one of the most dangerous of poisons. The physician should be called at the earliest possible moment in order that he may supply antidotes and do everything possible to sustain the patient's circulation and elimination.

In case of poisoning by various narcotic drugs it is customary to provoke vomiting and then to give strong black coffee, at the same time doing everything possible to keep the patient awake. Sometimes it is necessary to walk him about forcefully. As long as he is awake he will continue to breathe, but if he is permitted to sleep, breathing may stop.

There follows a table of poisonings and methods of treatment summarized by the health department of San Francisco:

SYMPTOMS AND TREATMENT OF ACUTE POISONING

SYMPTOMS	ANTIDOTES AND TREATMENT
Acetanilid, Antipyrin, Acetphenetidin (Phenacetin)	
Vomiting (sometimes). Face cyanosed. Skin: cold; profuse sweat; sometimes rash simulating measles, scarlatina, or pemphigus. Collapse; feeble and irregular pulse; slow respiration.	Lavage or emetic. External heat; recumbent position. Caffeine, digitalis. Carbon dioxide-oxygen inhalation, if needed.
Aconite	
Tingling and numbness of tongue and mouth and sense of formication of the body. Nausea and vomiting; diarrhea with epigastric pain. Dyspnea. Pulse irregular and weak. Skin cold and clammy; features bloodless. Giddiness, staggering walk; feeling of heaviness. The mind remains clear.	Avoid emetics. Gastric lavage—stomach to be washed with 0.1 per cent (1:1000) potassium permanganate, 250 cc. Reflex stimulants: ether, alcohol (whisky), aromatic spirits of ammonia. Caffeine or atropine. Carbon dioxide-oxygen inhalation, if necessary. External heat; recumbent position with head lower than feet.
Alcohol (Ethyl Alcohol)	
Ataxia, cramps, coma, decreased respiration. Abolition of the superficial and deep reflexes.	Gastric lavage. Coffee enema. Carbon dioxide-oxygen inhalation. External heat. Aromatic spirits of ammonia, caffeine or atropine.
Alkalies, Fixed and Caustic (Sodium and Potassium Hydroxide—Lye), Sodium Carbonate (Washing Soda)	
Burning pain from mouth to stomach; difficulty in swallowing; sloughed tissues in mouth; vomiting and purging of mucus and blood. Collapse; skin cold and clammy; pulse feeble; anxious countenance; rapid exhaustion; dyspnea. Convulsions. Unconsciousness or coma.	Do not use stomach tube! Give from 100 to 500 cc. of 0.5 per cent hydrochloric acid. Eight ounces of olive oil by mouth. Demulcents such as gelatin, acacia, or flour in water. Caffeine or digitan hypodermically, if necessary. External heat.

Symptoms	Antidotes and Treatment

Ammonia

Gastro-intestinal symptoms, as in corrosive poisoning. Purging usual, with pain and straining. Body cold, with cold sweat. Countenance anxious. Pulse rapid and weak.

Eight ounces of olive oil by mouth. Large quantities of water. Neutralization with from 100 to 500 cc. of 0.5 per cent hydrochloric acid. *Do not use stomach tube.*

Anesthetics, Volatile (*Chloroform, Ether, Nitrous Oxide*)

Rapid heart rate, abolition of reflexes, stoppage of heart or respiration.

Withdrawal of anesthetic. If circulatory collapse persists, ouabain intravenously; epinephrine intravenously or intracardially. If respiration stops, artificial respiration; carbon dioxide-oxygen inhalation; caffeine given intravenously or intramuscularly; atropine hypodermically.

Arsenic

Symptoms usually appear in from a quarter of an hour to one hour. Vomiting profuse, painful diarrhea; thirst; sense of constriction in throat, rendering swallowing difficult; cyanosis; coma.

Abundant gastric lavage with warm water. External heat. Opiate for diarrhea and colic. Infusion of solution of sodium chloride containing sodium bicarbonate (5 per cent), if necessary. Milk diet. Treat patient as potential nephritic patient.

Atropine, Belladonna

Dryness of mouth. Difficulty in swallowing and articulation; thirst. Skin flushed. Temperature raised. Pulse quick. Pupils widely dilated. Purging. Delirium.

Purified animal charcoal as antidote (2 tablespoonfuls in 250 cc. of water). Evacuation of stomach. Caffeine. Potassium permanganate in 1:1,000 solution, 250 cc.; lavage with the same preparation. Catheterization if necessary. If excitation persists, barbital or paraldehyde. Physostigmine.

Barbituric Acid Derivatives (*Phenobarbital, Barbital, etc.*)

Coma, circulatory collapse, pulmonary edema, cold skin, cyanosis. Sometimes delirium, twitching and increased reflexes.

Cover patient warmly; apply hot-water bottles. Gastric lavage. Caffeine. Ephedrine. Carbon dioxide-oxygen inhalation.

Bichloride of Mercury

Metallic taste, choking sensation. Pain in stomach, vomiting and purging of stringy mucus and blood. Tongue may be white and shriveled. Skin cold and clammy. Pulse feeble and rapid.

Treatment in Emergency Room: Antidote (by mouth): 10 cc. of 10 per cent sodium hypophosphite in water and then add 5 cc. hydrogen peroxide for each gram (15 grains) of bichloride of mercury. One glass of water. Lavage with antidote (one dose per hundred cubic centimeters of water). Two egg whites, or liberal dry egg albumin in water, and one glass of milk, followed by lavage with water.
Treatment in the Ward: Gastric lavage twice a day with 6 quarts of sodium bicarbonate solution. Sodium acetate by

mouth (amount to keep urine alkaline). Use low pressure colonic irrigation twice a day with 6 quarts of solution. (2 drachms sodium acetate to 1 pint of water.) Send urine, vomitus and colonic washings to the laboratory daily for examination for mercury (500 cc. of each). Daily specimens of urine to internes' laboratory. Daily chemical examination of the blood. Administration of stimulants and sedatives as indicated. Treatment continued until symptoms have abated and mercury has disappeared from urine and colonic and gastric washings.

Boron (Boric Acid, Borax Solutions)

Epigastric pain, abdominal cramps, vomiting, diarrhea, weak pulse, cold clammy skin, sometimes cyanosis and collapse. (Boric acid, 3 to 6 gm., has been fatal to infants, and 15 grams has been fatal to adults. Thirty gm. of borax, likewise, has been fatal to adults.)

Keep patient warm, in recumbent position. If taken by mouth, gastric lavage; or, if given by rectum in enema, rectal lavage, warm water. Caffeine may be given, and the kidneys should be protected by the administration of alkali (1.0 to 5.0 gm. sodium bicarbonate and alkaline drinks or fruit juices) and by the administration of sodium thiosulphate.

Camphor (Camphor Oil; Spirit of Camphor)

Characteristic odor of breath; burning pain in stomach; colic; giddiness; pulse rapid and weak. Impulsive movements; delirium. Face flushed. Sometimes convulsions. Collapse. Coma.

Apomorphine, hypodermically. Gastric lavage repeatedly with warm water. Inhalation anesthesia to check convulsions; then barbital by mouth or intramuscularly to check excitation. Caffeine or digitan hypodermically, if necessary. External heat. Artificial respiration, if required. Convalescence may be prolonged.

Cantharides

Burning pain in throat and stomach; difficulty in swallowing. Vomiting and diarrhea; mucus and blood may contain shining particles of the powder. Salivation and swelling of the salivary glands. Burning in urethra; frequent micturition. Urine contains albumin, casts, and blood. Pulse weak and slow; collapse.

Gastric lavage; mucilaginous drinks; opiate for pain. No oil by mouth. Treat as for potential nephritis (alkalies and milk diet).

Chloral Hydrate

Vomiting, collapse, delirium, fall of temperature, cyanosis, dyspnea or slow respirations. Coma.

Gastric lavage with potassium permanganate 1:1,000, 250 cc. External heat. Caffeine, then digitalis. Carbon dioxide-oxygen inhalation, or artificial respiration, as needed.

Cinchophen (Atophan)

Poisoning generally subacute or chronic, but toxic symptoms may become rapidly

Gastric lavage. Magnesium sulphate. Withdrawal of administration of drug.

SYMPTOMS   ANTIDOTES AND TREATMENT

Cinchophen (Atophan) (continued)

severe during or in absence of administration of drug.

Symptoms of cinchonism; nausea and vomiting; persistent abdominal pain; diarrhea. Jaundice; liver pain or tenderness; stupor. Urine colored red to brown. Collapse. Coma.

Camphor oil, caffeine or digitan, if necessary. Continue with treatment for hepatitis; injections of dextrose and insulin; carbohydrate diet; bicarbonate by mouth for acidosis.

Cocaine and Procaine Hydrochloride

Anxiety, fainting, pallor, dyspnea, brief convulsions and apnea. With smaller doses, confusion, laughter, vertigo, motor excitement, tachycardia, irregular respiration, pallor, dilated pupils and exophthalmos, paresthesia, delirium and dyspnea. If death does not occur in a few minutes, recovery always follows.

Gastric lavage with 1 liter of 0.1 per cent (1:1,000) potassium permanganate (if taken by mouth). One-half per cent potassium permanganate solution if stomach is empty; otherwise, tannic acid (5 gm.). Soluble barbital intravenously.

Cyanides (Sodium or Potassium; Hydrocyanic Acid)

Characteristic odor of poison. Dyspnea; rapid pulse; unconsciousness; tremors; violent convulsions; dilated pupils; absence of cyanosis. If patient survives an hour, recovery may occur.

If poison has been swallowed, give sodium thiosulphate, 10 per cent in water, 500 cc., using stomach tube if necessary. Inject intravenously 50 cc. methylene blue (1 per cent in 1.8 per cent sodium sulphate solution), repeat in 15 minutes, if necessary. Or, try sodium nitrite, 10 to 20 mgm. per kg. body weight (12 to 24 cc. 5 per cent sodium nitrite solution) intravenously. Epinephrine into heart.

Digitalis

Vomiting; diarrhea. Slow pulse; cardiac irregularity. Lassitude; muscular and sensory derangements.

Gastric lavage with potassium permanganate 0.1 per cent (1:1,000) or tannic acid, 1 per cent. Horizontal position. External heat. Atropine hypodermically. Quinidine for cardiac irregularity.

Ergot

Pale skin, small and rapid pulse, constricted arteries. Hallucinations. Cyanosis of the finger tips and toes. Sensory disturbances. Ascending gangrene of the extremities.

Gastric lavage in acute poisoning; withdrawal of administration of ergot. Nitrites. Warm room. Periodic inhalation of carbon dioxide and oxygen.

Fluoride (Roach and Insect Powders)

Nausea and vomiting; burning, cramplike abdominal pains; diarrhea. Sometimes tremors or convulsions. Grayish blue cyanosis. Urine and blood show presence of fluoride.

Copious gastric lavage with limewater or weak calcium chloride solution. Calcium gluconate intramuscularly, or calcium chloride, 10 cc. of 10 per cent in water, intravenously. Digitan hypodermically; artificial respiration, if necessary. External heat.

SYMPTOMS | ANTIDOTES AND TREATMENT

Formaldehyde

Odor. Sore mouth. Dysphagia. Severe abdominal pain. Unconsciousness and collapse. Later diarrhea and tenesmus.

Swallow a tumblerful of 0.2 per cent ammonia. Lavage with dilute ammonia followed by raw egg, or egg albumin in water.

Gas (Garage Gas, or from Defective Flue Fumes, Carbon Monoxide)

Giddiness and singing in the ears. Lividity of face and body. Loss of muscular power. Unconsciousness and collapse.

Carbon dioxide-oxygen inhalation, or artificial respiration, if needed. Bleeding followed by transfusion if indicated. External heat. Oxygen tent if available. Digitalis.

Hydrochloric Acid

Gastro-intestinal symptoms, coffee-ground vomitus. Purging usual, with pain and straining. Body cold, with cold sweat. Countenance anxious. Pulse rapid and weak.

Magnesia magma 100 to 400 cc. White of egg or olive oil as a demulcent; external heat; camphor oil, caffeine or digitan hypodermically, if necessary.

Iodine

Pain and heat in throat and stomach. Vomiting and purging, vomitus being yellow or blue if starchy matter is present in the stomach. Stools may contain blood. Intense thirst. Giddiness, faintness and convulsions.

Sodium thiosulphate by mouth (1 to 10 gm. in water) as an antidote. Then lavage with 1 per cent sodium thiosulphate. Later, thin starch paste or flour soup. External heat; camphor oil, caffeine or digitan hypodermically, if necessary.

Lead

Metallic taste, dry throat, intense thirst. Abdominal colic. Constipation, dark feces. Vomiting may occur. Giddiness, stupor, convulsions, coma.

Magnesium sulphate in solution as antidote. Lavage with 1 per cent sodium sulphate, mucilaginous (acacia) or egg albumin drinks. External heat. Cathartic after lavage. Calcium gluconate intramuscularly. Opiate for colic.

Morphine, Opium

Coma, gradual in onset. Symmetrical pinpoint pupils that dilate terminally. Respirations slow and shallow. Body cold. Cyanosis; convulsions.

Potassium permanganate 0.1 per cent (1:1,000), 250 cc. by mouth. Gastric lavage with some solution of potassium permanganate. Black coffee. Try to keep the patient awake by suggestion. Carbon dioxide-oxygen inhalation. Artificial respiration, if necessary. External heat. Caffeine or atropine hypodermically, if respiration fails to improve.

Mushrooms

Colic, vomiting, purging. Mental excitement followed by coma. Extremities cold. Pulse slow. Respiration stertorous. Pulmonary edema. Pupils dilated.

Gastric lavage. External heat. Atropine.

Symptoms	Antidotes and Treatment

Nicotine and Tobacco

Severe depression, prostration and muscular weakness; severe nausea and vomiting. Marked dyspnea. Weak rapid pulse. Pupils first contracted then dilated. Muscular tremors, followed rapidly by convulsions. Coma.	If free vomiting has not occurred, wash out stomach repeatedly with potassium permanganate, 0.1 per cent (1:1,000), and warm water. Strong coffee. Caffeine or digitan hypodermically, if necessary. External heat. Artificial respiration, if necessary.

Nitric Acid

Pain in throat and stomach. Vomiting of whitish, flaky matter that blackens on exposure to light.	Magnesia magma, from 100 to 400 cc. White of egg, or egg albumin in water, or olive oil (250 cc.) as a demulcent. External heat. Camphor oil, caffeine or digitan hypodermically, if necessary.

Nitrites and Nitroglycerine

Collapse, unconsciousness, cyanosis or pallor, low blood pressure, slow pulse, irregular respiration. Sometimes vomiting and convulsions. Persistent cyanosis. Methemoglobinuria.	Recumbent position. Gastric lavage if poison has been swallowed. Guaiacol 0.5 gm. and Berlin blue 0.5 gm. together, gastrically or orally, 3 to 6 times daily. If necessary, epinephrine intravenously; digitan hypodermically; oxygen inhalation. External heat.

Oils, Volatile and Ecbolic (Tansy, Pennyroyal, Santal, Absinthe, Turpentine)

Characteristic odor of breath; burning, nausea, vomiting; eructations; colic; diarrhea. Skin rash; jaundice. Convulsions; dilated pupils; rapid stertorous respiration; pulse slow and feeble. Unconsciousness. Coma. Sometimes, uterine hemorrhage, abortion, hematuria.	If vomiting has not occurred, repeatedly wash out stomach with warm water. Demulcents: acacia, starch, or flour in water. Magnesium sulphate unless diarrhea is present. Opiate for colic. Camphor oil, caffeine or digitan, if necessary. External heat. Barbital for excitation. Later, treatments for nephritis and hepatitis; abortion.

Oxalic Acid

Gastro-intestinal symptoms as in corrosive poisoning. Purging, in most cases, with pain and straining. Body cold, with cold sweat. Countenance anxious. Pulse rapid and weak.	Calcium lactate (10 to 20 gm. in 250 cc. of water). Potassium permanganate, 0.1 per cent (1:1,000), 250 cc. by mouth. Gastric lavage with same permanganate solution. Demulcents. Heat applied to abdomen. Camphor oil, caffeine or digitan hypodermically, if necessary.

Paris Green

Symptoms usually appear in from a quarter of an hour to one hour. Burning heat and constriction or choking in throat, rendering swallowing difficult. Nausea and incessant vomiting and purging. The vomiting matter may be green from bile, or, in the case of arsenic, black from the ad-	Abundant gastric lavage with warm water. Infusion of solution of sodium chloride if necessary. Tincture of opium for diarrhea and colic. Caffeine, strychnine or atropine, as needed, for circulatory and respiratory stimulation. Milk diet. Treat as for potential nephritis.

SYMPTOMS

ANTIDOTES AND TREATMENT

mixture of soda, or blue from indigo. Pain in the stomach and abdomen. Cramps in the calves of the legs. Urine may be suppressed. There may be delirium or paralysis. Collapse; skin cold and clammy, sometimes showing eczematous rash. Pulse small, quick and irregular, or imperceptible.

Phenols (Carbolic Acid, Lysol, Cresols, "Sheep-Dip")

Characteristic odor present. Burning sensation in mouth and throat; burns on lips and in mouth; nausea and vomiting. Abdominal pain. Faintness; collapse; pulse slow and weak; face livid; cold sweat; respiration depressed; unconsciousness. Coma. Urine scanty with smoky color.

Gastric lavage with 10 per cent ethyl alcohol in water, 1 quart; continuous lavage with warm water. Infusion of physiological salt solution; epinephrine intravenously or intracardially. Caffeine or digitan hypodermically. External heat. Artificial respiration if necessary. Later treatment same as for aftereffects of corrosives.

Phosphorus

Symptoms usually appear in three stages: (1) A few hours after administration, there develops a garlic taste, gastrointestinal irritation, burning pain, thirst, swelling of the abdomen and vomiting of blood (green or black). The vomit has a garlic odor and in the dark may be phosphorescent. The patient may die, or there may be: (2) An intermission of symptoms for three days or more, with a feeling of malaise followed by: (3) The final stage, characterized by intense jaundice, enlarged liver and distended abdomen; great prostration, cold sweat, an anxious look, feeble pulse, muscular twitching, coma.

Two hundred cubic centimeters of 0.2 per cent solution of copper sulphate by mouth. Lavage with from 5 to 10 liters of the same solution followed by lavage with 1 liter of 0.1 per cent potassium permanganate; followed by the administration of 100 cc. of liquid petrolatum. No fats or oils should be given, as they aid absorption. External heat. Treatment continued for liver injury—high carbohydrate diet; dextrose and insulin.

Quinine and Quinidine

Ringing in ears, disturbed vision, photophobia. (Later deafness and blindness.) Nausea; vomiting. Faintness. Difficulty of speech, somnolence; unconsciousness, alternating with delirium and coma. Pulse slow and feeble. Sometimes convulsions.

Tannic acid by mouth. Gastric lavage with potassium permanganate 0.1 per cent (1:1,000). Epinephrine intravenously or intracardially, if necessary. Caffeine or digitan hypodermically. If excitation persists, barbital by mouth.

Strychnine, Nux Vomica

Feeling of suffocation and lividity of the face. Tetanic convulsions, with short intermission, causing sweating and exhaustion, opisthotonus, risus sardonicus, staring eyes, fixed chest, and hard abdominal muscles. Hearing and sight are acute, and consciousness is retained. The muscles of the jaw are not affected until late.

Early: Give by mouth or with stomach tube purified animal charcoal, from 1 to 2 tablespoonfuls in a glass of water. Gastric lavage with potassium permanganate, 0.1 per cent solution (1:1,000). Later (with muscular hypertonicity): Arrest hyperexcitability or convulsions with inhalation anesthesia (ether or chloroform) and then

Strychnine, Nux Vomica (continued)

inject intramuscularly soluble barbital, 1 gm. (20 cc. of 5 per cent), later by mouth; or pentobarbital, 1/10 gr. (6 mgms.) per pound body weight as the first dose and one half this amount for succeeding doses. Do not use any methods that excite spasm, such as attempting intravenous injection. The patient should be isolated and kept absolutely quiet. Ether inhalation should be given if convulsions continue. Artificial respiration, if respiration fails.

Thallium (Depilatories; Rodent Poisons—"Thalgrain")

Abdominal colic, nausea, vomiting, and diarrhea; constipation; stomatitis; alopecia; peripheral neuritis; central nervous involvement (ptosis, strabismus, convulsions, choreiform movements, optic atrophy). Evidences of liver damage, nephritis; sometimes pulmonary edema. Thallium in urine.

Early: If emesis has not occurred, copious gastric lavage with 1 per cent sodium or potassium iodide (in water); catharsis (avoid sulphates). If shock is present, 25 gm. (50 cc. of 50 per cent) dextrose intravenously; external heat; reflex stimulants, epinephrine, caffeine, or digitan hypodermically; artificial respiration if necessary. *Later:* Rest in bed; control mobilization of thallium in body by daily intravenous injections of sodium iodide, about 15 to 40 cc. of 2.3 per cent, in water (freshly prepared) (about 0.3 to 1 gm. NaI) until urine test shows absence of thallium; dose of iodide may gradually be doubled. Daily chemical examination of urine: collect and evaporate to dryness 24-hour urines for thallium test—absence of, or only slight, green color on flaming residue. When symptoms of thallitoxicosis subside, proceed cautiously to increase elimination of thallium by intravenous injection of sodium thiosulphate, 0.3 to 1 gm. (6 to 20 cc. of 5 per cent in water; freshly prepared) for adult, alternating with sodium iodide solution intravenously, if necessary. Pilocarpine (promotes secretion), calcium lactate, if necessary; dilute with hydrochloric acid for achlorhydria; bland ointments for dermatitis; barbital or codeine for restlessness and pain; treatments for liver injury and nephritis, if necessary.

CHAPTER IV

Hygiene of Women
MORRIS FISHBEIN, M.D.

THE BOY AND GIRL, until the age of twelve, may be reared in much the same manner. Their health problems are approximately the same. Thereafter, however, the problems of the girl are distinctive. At this period in her life her organs begin to differentiate to prepare her for her functions as a mother. It is taken for granted that the mother will have prepared the daughter suitably for recognition of the changes that are to come. In the majority of girls these changes take place so gradually that they are not noticed.

The startling change which appears is the development of the menstrual flow. In far too many instances, notwithstanding the advance in health education that has been made in the last quarter century, girls still come to this phenomenon without any knowledge, and some of them sustain mental shocks which mark their lives thereafter. Until menstruation appears, the girl is not likely to bear children; with the coming of menstruation, the organs develop and the possibility exists.

Before that time, the body configuration of most girls has been much like that of the boy. After puberty, which is the time when the menstrual flow appears, the breasts, the pelvis and neck enlarge, hair develops in the armpits and over the sexual area, and the voice changes.

The onset of the menstrual flow is not always an abrupt and complete development. The first flow may be very brief; it may disappear and not appear again for weeks or months; it may, at first, be irregular and then later regular. Just as soon as the flow appears regularly at a definite interval for several months, the menstruation may be said to be established.

Associated with this physical change are also mental changes. Many of these changes are associated with interests in the male sex, in more mature occupations, in a different type of reading, and in many new interests. For this reason, parents should have surveillance over their daughters and use proper understanding of the nature of the change that is occurring.

Our views have greatly changed in the last quarter century. Girls used to be sick in every sense of the word during the menstrual period. Nowadays they are likely to go through without the slightest alteration in their habits. There are, of course, instances in which the function is accompanied with severe pain or with physical disturbance. When these occur, they should have the attention of a physician.

The adolescent girl is undergoing rapid development. For this reason her posture must be carefully watched. If she grows too rapidly and is somewhat tall, there may be an inclination to slump the shoulders forward, the abdomen out and the chest in. Such posture is bound to lead to a poor figure later in life. Exercises, described in the article on posture in this book, will help to develop a proper position when standing and when sitting. The chin and abdomen should be kept in and the chest forward. Many young girls worry about the development of the breasts and, not understanding the changes that occur, attempt to hide them. Poor posture may result from holding the shoulders in such a manner as to draw in the chest.

The girl, at this period of life, needs plenty of sleep; ten or eleven hours in twenty-four is not too much. Extra relaxation in the form of a nap in the middle of the day, such as is given to smaller children, may be exceedingly useful in maintaining her body tone. There need be no special attention to the diet other than the certainty that it contains the necessary proteins, carbohydrates and fats, mineral salts and vitamins that are necessary in any well-balanced diet.

Many girls passing from adolescence into adult age feel that it is necessary for them to adopt sophisticated habits. Whereas they have formerly avoided tea and coffee in favor of milk, they want to partake of these and even of alcoholic beverages as giving them somewhat more of an adult status in the family. Smoking cigarettes is not necessary, and again may be considered as a habit to be controlled until it can be indulged in at a later date with intelligence and restraint.

Some girls at this age put on so much weight that they are seriously disturbed. The weight may increase so rapidly that the skin of the abdomen stretches and red marks appear along the curves of the hips. These should not cause worry because they will fade when the weight of the body is more definitely adjusted. For the control of the tendency to overweight, a suitable diet with a lowered amount of carbohydrates is desirable. Nowadays most people have learned enough about calories and carbohydrates in relationship to overweight to exercise a certain amount of control over this danger.

Special attention should also be given at this period to the condition of the thyroid gland. In some children there is a tendency to overactivity of the gland, which is marked also by rapid heart, nervousness, perspiration, and similar symptoms. If any sign appears of overactivity of the thyroid gland, the basal metabolism should be determined by a competent doctor and the condition of the thyroid gland controlled in relationship to the results. If there is overweight or underweight, the basal metabolism test should also be made to determine whether or not the activity of the thyroid gland is related in any way to this unusual development.

In the Great Lakes area and in the Northwest, the water and the soil lack iodine, hence there is a tendency among young children to develop simple enlargement of the thyroid gland that is known as simple goiter. There is a special chapter on this condition elsewhere in this book. Any tendency of the thyroid gland toward enlargement should, of course, be studied by the family doctor. In most cases, however, intelligent parents nowadays give small doses of iodine regularly each week to supply the iodine deficiency and thus effectively prevent the appearance of simple goiter.

DISORDERS OF MENSTRUATION

As I have already said, menstruation may be occasionally irregular during the first year without causing any anxiety. Certainly, by the end of the first year it should be regular, in the majority of women, occurring every twenty-eight days. Menstruation occurring regularly anywhere from twenty-one days to five-week intervals may be considered within normal limits.

Sometimes, in connection with the first appearance of menstruation, the usual signs of adolescence appear, including pimples and blackheads on the face, back, and chest, soreness and swelling of the breasts, and headache. These may appear as the result of the changes in the glands that occur at this time.

Ordinarily menstruation should cause no more pain than any of the other functions of the body. When the pain occurs, it is usually associated with a disturbance of the circulation or of the glands. Sometimes failure of the bowels to act properly is a complication, which may be easily corrected by establishment of regular habits, sufficient rest, drinking of plenty of water, and the other measures suggested in the section on digestion.

Doctors now recognize a period of a few days before menstruation when symptoms of distress, irritability, anxiety, flushing, nausea and such, make what is called premenstrual tension. Control may involve study of the glandular condition and prescription of suitable drugs, vitamins and glandular substances.

EXERCISES

Various exercises have been described for use by growing girls at this time. Some of these simple exercises involve not only the usual bending and standing, which are good for posture, but also kneeling in the knee-chest position, walking on the hands and feet as the monkey or cat walks, and other postures which help to develop the ligaments which hold the organs of the pelvis in position. Since menstruation is a normal function of women and involves several different organs, its control must involve study of the organs concerned.

Emotional shocks and nerve shocks may tend to be associated with pain at this time. A change in the altitude, extraordinary changes in the diet, over- and under-exercise, and many similar factors may yield difficult symptoms. For this reason, the routine of the girl's life during the menstrual period should be disturbed as little as possible.

She may take her baths daily as always, preferably a warm bath; but if she is in the habit of taking cold baths, she may take these also. There is no good reason why most women should not take a bath during the menstrual period. If the flow of blood is profuse, strenuous swimming may make it excessive; also a very hot tub bath may increase the amount of blood lost. A very cold bath taken just before or at the beginning of menstruation may occasionally stop the bleeding. The danger of infection from the water is very slight.

Indulgence in competitive games during the menstrual period should, of course, be carefully controlled. Such games involve emotional stress and high tension. They place a considerable burden upon the heart. They bring about shocks and jolts to the internal organs for which these organs are not competent. It is particularly important that every girl indulging in athletic sports have a physical examination in relationship to her feminine constitution.

PAINFUL MENSTRUATION

A tremendous number of remedies have been suggested for painful menstruation. Sufficient rest and sleep, proper hygiene and treatment for anemia, if that is present, are especially important. Some patients get immediate help from rest in bed and the use of an enema for emptying the bowels. Others are relieved by placing a hot-water bag over the painful area. Aspirin and similar drugs which relieve pain are used by many girls and are not harmful, if taken in small doses and preferably under the direction of a physician.

Sometimes it is necessary for the doctor to make certain modifications of the glandular mechanism of the patient. The administration of suitable glandular substances which are known to have control over the menstrual functions sometimes yields successful results in eliminating pain.

In the process of menstruation several organs are involved: the pituitary gland, adrenals, ovaries, and the uterus. Regular bleeding from the uterus, called menstruation, is nearly always dependent on proper functioning of the ovaries. These, in turn, are controlled by a portion of the pituitary gland in the brain. The pituitary gland has been called the motor of the ovaries. When there are unusual symptoms during the menstrual period, such as flushing, numbness of the finger tips, fainting spells, and crying, the glands and their secretions are ordinarily responsible, related in turn to various mental influences.

Because of the tendency to bleed at this period, some women bruise more easily during the menstrual time; others suffer with nosebleeds. These symptoms usually disappear when the menstruation ends.

When menstruation is exceedingly scanty, the state of the blood should be studied as to whether or not there is anemia. There should also be an investigation of the basal metabolism and the general nutrition.

During menstruation the vast majority of women wear a simple cotton pad, such as is now commercially available in many different forms. Vaginal tampons are also used satisfactorily and safely. Where there are unusual odors of any kind, a careful investigation should be made by a competent doctor to determine the presence or absence of infection. In most cases, annoying odors are a sign of infection, and they cannot be corrected by application of deodorants or powders of any kind.

The tampons do not seem to be quite dependable for women who have a profuse flow. This applies also to various types of rubber cups that have been devised for controlling the menstrual flow. For persons in the theatrical profession, for acrobats, and women who indulge in sports of various kinds, such devices may be especially desirable.

The medical profession has not settled definitely the question of the advisability of using douches before and after the menstrual period or at any other time. About an equal number of specialists in diseases of women are arrayed on each side of this question. Women who are not infected in any manner and who do not have excessive discharges of mucus and other material from the genital tract need not employ douches regularly. Ordinary bathing will suffice for the purpose. However, in cases in which there are excessive discharges, or in which, as has been mentioned, an odor is present, a physician should be consulted in order to determine the presence and nature of the infection. The infection should be treated by the means that the physician will recommend. This recommendation will in most instances involve the use of suitable cleansing and antiseptic agents used in the form of douches and in similar ways.

ABSENCE OF MENSTRUATION

Most people know that menstruation disappears when a woman becomes pregnant and is to have a child. It disappears also at a period known as the climacteric, which is also an important epoch in the life of women. This period is also called the menopause, as an indication of the fact that the menstruation disappears at this time.

There are, of course, other factors which occasionally produce a change in menstruation and in some instances even a temporary absence. A change of geographical location, which involves chiefly a change of climate and perhaps of altitude, not infrequently produces alterations in menstruation. Usually the flow may stop, but in some cases the amount of blood lost is excessive. Because the process of menstruation is controlled by glandular action, disorders of menstruation, including stopping for no apparent reason, are generally assumed to be due to some glandular difficulty.

Women who do not menstruate are not in any way inferior to those who do. They rarely show any abnormal symptoms, and their sex life is about the same. The whole difficulty lies in the minds of such women. They feel they are subnormal; they may become exceedingly disturbed mentally worrying over the condition. Frequently a physician can bring about menstruation in such patients by the experimental use of various glandular preparations.

The discontinuance of menstruation at the menopause is, of course, a different matter. The average duration of menstruation in women is from 30 to 32 years. The average age for the beginning of the climacteric or menopause in the temperate zone is about 47 years. However, there is an enormous variation in the ages at which the symptoms of climacteric may arise. Cases are known in which the change of life occurred as early as 27 years of age and as late as 59 years. Usually in the United States the discontinuance of menstruation occurs between 45 and 50 years of age in 50 per cent of women; between 40 and 45 in 25 per cent; between 35 and 40 in 12½ per cent, and between 50 and 55 years in 12½ per cent.

In most instances there is a definite association between the onset of puberty, or the beginning of menstruation, and the time of the appearance of the menopause. In general, the earlier the menstrual function begins, the longer it will continue. Girls who have an early puberty will have a long, potential, reproductive career and a late menopause. A physician named Gallant published a chart of approximate ages as to when the menopause would appear, based on the age of the onset of puberty. The table, which is for healthy women, follows on the next page:

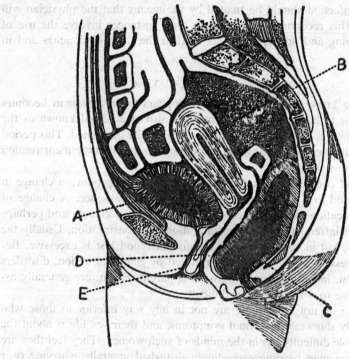

Fig. 7. Lateral view of female pelvic organs.
A. Bladder. B. Uterus or womb. C. Rectum.
D. Vagina. E. Urethra.

Year in Which *Menstruation Appears*	*Menopause* *Should Occur*
10............................	Between 50 and 52 years
11............................	Between 48 and 50 years
12............................	Between 46 and 48 years
13............................	Between 44 and 46 years
14............................	Between 42 and 44 years
15............................	Between 40 and 42 years
16............................	Between 38 and 40 years
17............................	Between 36 and 38 years
18............................	Between 34 and 36 years
19............................	Between 32 and 34 years
20............................	Between 30 and 32 years

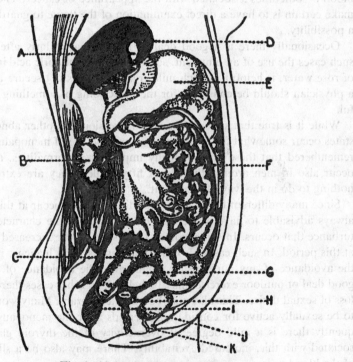

Fig. 8. Abdominal female organs.
A. Gall bladder. B. Kidney. C. Large intestine.
D. Liver. E. Stomach. F. Small intestine.
G. Uterus or womb. H. Vagina. I. Rectum.
J. Bladder. K. Urethra.

Exactly as parts of the body change at the onset of puberty, so also do similar changes occur at the menopause. Usually the spleen and lymphatic glands decrease in size. There is an increased tendency to constipation, because of changes in the wall of the intestine. Most women have some physical discomfort and some mild mental or nervous changes, but some women cease menstruating with slight inconvenience. As a rule, the woman may miss one or two or more periods, then will have menstrual periods that seem almost normal; then she will miss other periods, and finally the periodic flow will cease altogether. This variability is due to the fact that the glandular changes which are occurring take place gradually.

There may be, during this period, slight inflammation and swelling of the sexual parts. These are, however, of little significance. The most difficult symptom which may develop at this time is excessive bleeding. Whenever excessive bleeding occurs, however, either at the menopause or at any other time, a physician should be consulted immediately so that he may make a study of the condition and determine its cause. It is well established that the appearance of blood is sometimes associated with the appearance of cancer. The only way to make certain is to have a direct examination of the tissue to guard against such a possibility.

Occasionally there is a good deal of itching, particularly after bathing. In such cases the use of an ointment, such as 12 per cent boric acid in an ointment of rose water, is helpful. If such mild treatment does not secure a good result, a physician should be consulted for the prescribing of something more powerful.

While it is true that states of mental depression and other abnormal mental states occur somewhat frequently at or about the age of menopause, it must be remembered that these are not really important abnormalities, and that they occur also in men around the age of fifty. Unless they are extreme, there is nothing to do in the way of treatment.

Since many different forms of mental disorder may occur at this period, it is always advisable to have a scientific diagnosis as to the character of the disturbance that occurs. In some women there seems to be increased sexual desire at this period. In such cases also the treatment is good hygiene, including also the avoidance of any unnecessary stimulants. The avoidance of coffee, and a good deal of outdoor exercise, may be helpful. In other cases there is a gradual loss of sexual desire. This also may be quite temporary. Many women continue to be sexually active for considerable periods after the menopause. Not infrequently there is a mild degree of overactivity of the thyroid gland, and, associated with this, increased excitability. There may also be a slight elevation of the blood pressure.

All of these symptoms, however, are associated with the gradual change in the glandular mechanism and, unless severe, need not be considered seriously. New substitutes for missing glandular substances may be prescribed by the doctor to overcome symptoms.

The changes associated with this period demand slight modification of the general hygiene of the body. Usually older people will want less food. Because of the difficulties of digestion, foods rich in carbohydrates, including sugars, cake, candy, preserves, and jelly, should be taken with moderation, as also foods that are known to cause indigestion in many cases; for example, foods fried in a good deal of grease, hot breads, pastry, cheese, and similar substances.

Since there is a considerable amount of congestion in the abdomen, the care of the bowels should be a special problem. A daily, free evacuation of the bowels is essential to health. The use of mild laxatives may bring a good deal of relief. The kidneys must be especially watched for the onset of any degenerative changes.

It is necessary to keep the skin in good condition by bathing—sometimes alternate hot and cold baths. Massage is helpful in toning up the nervous system and the circulation. Exercise daily in the open air is helpful in steadying the nerves and stimulating the body generally.

From the point of view of the mind, it is particularly necessary at this time of life that some pleasant occupation be followed. Usually by this time children will have passed the age when they need constant supervision, and the mother must take relaxation from her home cares. Many women at this time of life become expert bridge players or golfers, although previously they may have taken but little interest in such diversions. Any mental occupation that will take the woman into a new interest is the best possible safeguard against the slight mental difficulty which develops in some women at this period.

The estrogenic hormones including the natural and the synthetic, stilbestrol, will aid in overcoming headache, hot flashes, and melancholia, which are so distressing at this time. These substances should never be taken except when prescribed by the doctor. Physicians also prescribe some androgen or male sex hormone particularly when there is depression or fear of loss of sex-life.

The Rhythm of Menstruation and the Safe Period for Prevention of Conception

A definite relationship exists between the time a woman menstruates and the time when an egg cell or ovum passes from the ovary into the uterus. If a woman menstruates regularly every twenty-eight days, it is usually impossible for her to conceive between the first and tenth day of her menstrual cycle, the first day being the one on which the menstrual flow begins. She can conceive on the eleventh day and up to and including the seventeenth day, but she will not be able to conceive from the seventeenth day on. Therefore, the days on which conception is most likely are the days from the fourteenth to the sixteenth day after the first day of menstruation. This is the period in which the mother cell or egg cell is produced by the ovary. In a woman who menstruates every twenty-eight days, the egg cell comes from the ovary on the fourteenth day.

The period of nine days, referred to as the period when conception is most likely, includes three days for the production and discharge of the egg cell, one day allowed for variability, and two to three days for the survival of the fertilizing power of the male cell. It has been definitely shown that the male cell will not survive much over three days, unless it meets the egg cell of the female and brings about conception. The extra three days added to these seven are in the interests of safety against any irregularities.

Records have now been kept of many thousands of cases in which women have observed this safe period, and failures, when absolute observance prevailed, are exceedingly few. Of course, the matter is complicated when the menstrual cycle in the woman is more or less than twenty-eight days. For the majority of women, therefore, it will be necessary to determine the exact dates and variations of the menstrual cycle. This is done by keeping an accurate record for several months of the exact dates on which menstruation begins, how many days it continues, and the number of days from the first day of menstruation to the first day of the next menstruation. All sorts of calendars and devices have now been developed for keeping records of this kind.

It is known that a good many women have occasional variations in their menstrual cycle. Thus one authority said, "The only regular thing about menstruation is its own irregularity." Just as soon as the cycle is definitely established, it becomes possible for the woman to calculate the periods when she is likely to conceive, or the fertile period, and the period when she is not likely to conceive, or the sterile period.

THE TEMPERATURE CONTROL METHOD

Many people think there is a chance for conception whenever the male sperm cell is deposited in the woman's genital tract. Actually, the sperm cannot fertilize an egg cell or ovum unless the ovum is there when the sperm reaches the Fallopian tube. Only one ovum, smaller than a pin point in size, is released by the ovary during the woman's periodic cycle. This takes place about 14 days before the beginning of the next cycle. If pregnancy is to occur, intercourse must take place within 24 hours of ovulation, since the life of the ovum is not more than 24 hours, and the sperm cells have fertilizing power for only 24 to 36 hours. Hence, if a woman can determine the exact time of ovulation, she can increase her chances of conception by having intercourse then.

The most practical method of achieving this is to keep a careful record of body temperature on arising each morning. Whereas a man's temperature follows a regular pattern day after day, the temperature of a woman is altered by the normal functioning of the ovaries. For several years thousands of women have kept daily temperature records, which physicians have studied and interpreted. We now know that the release of the ovum raises the level of a woman's temperature during the latter half of the menstrual cycle.

Your doctor can help you get charts especially designed for daily temperature records and show you how to use them.

Take your temperature immediately after waking up in the morning. Do not get up to go to the bathroom first, or drink water or smoke a cigarette. Just reach over, get the thermometer, put it under your tongue, lie back and remain quiet for five minutes. Then record the temperature on your chart. If it differs from those recorded before, and particularly if it is lower, shake the thermometer down, put it back under your tongue and hold it for another five minutes to verify the reading.

Temperature drops 24 to 36 hours before the onset of the menstrual flow, reaching a low point during the first day or two after the flow begins. This low level continues until the middle of the interval between two menstruations. This is the time when ovulation usually occurs in the woman who has a 27- to 31-day cycle. A sharp drop often takes place just before the rise that indicates the ovulation is occurring. During the next 24 to 36 hours, the temperature goes up abruptly. It stays at the higher level until one to two days before the beginning of the next flow. Start a new chart when the next period begins. You should have records of two consecutive cycles to establish your personal cycle. Then you can be reasonably sure when the next shift in temperature, and ovulation, will occur.

After childbirth or a miscarriage, about three months are required for the cycle to return to normal.

At least four out of five women find that the temperature record is an accurate guide to the time of ovulation if it is recorded and evaluated intelligently. Emotional upheavals, infections, dissipation, overeating and colds can cause an irregularity in temperature; barring such disturbances, the record pursues a remarkably constant course.

A couple wanting a child should have intercourse at the time the temperature falls, just before the rise that precedes ovulation. Intercourse should be continued daily during the rise of the temperature and when it has reached its peak after ovulation; however, too frequent intercourse causes a decrease in the number of sperm cells and lessens a man's fertility.

A carefully kept temperature record will also indicate the beginning of pregnancy. If the elevated temperature that develops after ovulation does not drop in its customary fashion, the woman is pregnant. Failure of the temperature to drop during the first week of the missed menstrual period is reliable evidence.

This natural method of child-planning is within the normal range of human functions, and it does not require procedures that might cause objections for religious or esthetic reasons. An intelligent young couple can plan to have their babies when they want them. When a baby is born, the mother can be given full opportunity to recover from the stress of that birth before undertaking another pregnancy. This will mean healthier mothers, healthier babies, happier families.*

* The section on "The Temperature Control Method" is a condensation of the article "The Natural Method of Child Planning," by Dr. Morris Fishbein, and is reprinted by permission of *Cosmopolitan Magazine* (May, 1951).

PREVENTION OF CONCEPTION

There are many different reasons to be considered when a woman wishes to avoid pregnancy. These reasons may be related to a possible illness of the prospective mother or father. The physician who is fully familiar with the physical condition of the prospective parent will be able to advise whether or not any of the available methods for the avoidance of pregnancy is to be tried. Frequently childbirth may be difficult so that the mother's health needs to be fully restored before another pregnancy. If she is nursing a baby that is still small and dependent on her, it may be harmful for both mother and child as well as for the prospective child to have another pregnancy too soon. Sometimes after a difficult childbirth the tissues of the mother will be injured and surgical repair may be necessary before she is to become pregnant again. When the health and even the life of the prospective mother may be threatened by another pregnancy, most specialists in the care of women do not consider it wise to depend on the so-called "safe period." In such instances they are likely to advise the use of some of the techniques which are much more certain to prevent the contact between the sperm cell of the male and the egg cell of the female that is necessary to begin a pregnancy.

The method to be used must be practically certain to succeed and it must be free from harmful psychic as well as physical effects. Many marriages are endangered by the use of methods for the control of births that do not meet with all of the objections that arise from both psychic and physical considerations.

Whenever any method of birth control is used that conflicts with the religious beliefs of either of the partners to a marriage, serious conflicts may arise in the minds of those concerned. Indeed, marital discord as a result of such conflicts is not unusual. Any method that interferes greatly with the normal conduct of sex contact may be distasteful to the married partners and may even be physically harmful. Almost every physician condemns techniques which involve separation of the partners before culmination. Moreover, several widely observed religions are definitely opposed to this practice. Finally, the method is not at all dependable because it is difficult to practice and the percentage of failures is very high. Physically it may leave the tissues congested and the nervous system in a state of unrest.

All the methods mentioned by Dr. Thurman Rice in his chapter on this subject must be used, if at all, with a full understanding of the physical and mental possibilities. Those methods which involve materials placed over the male organ of sex are not always successful because of the possible breakage or faulty character of the device. Even when such devices are ample in size and properly lubricated, they are difficult to use artistically, and their obvious character sometimes sets up resistances and deters the emotional response in the female partner. Frequently the male partner will complain that such material interferes with the feeling of release and gratification.

The use of various chemicals and washes and pastes should be attempted only with the advice of the family physician because many such materials are harmful and even more are quite without dependability. After the male egg cell has once entered the uterus no such material can reach it. The American Medical Association has accepted a number of products as suitable for safe use when prescribed by the doctor. The list includes "Contra-creme," "Laktikal Creme," "Lorophyn Jelly," "Koromex Cream," "Lanteen Jelly," "Lygel Cream," "Lygel Jelly," "Ortho-Creme," "Ortho-Gynol Vaginal Jelly," "Ramses Vaginal Jelly," "Marvasan Creme," "Veritas Kreme," "Cooper Creme," and also "Lorophyn Suppositories" and "Pernox Vaginal Capsules."

Many women have the superstition that pregnancy is not possible unless the female receives complete sex gratification during the sexual act. This is a superstition without the slightest scientific basis.

A new glandular material called Enovid can be taken in pill form as prescribed by the doctor. When taken from the fifth to the twenty-fifth day of the cycle, ovulation is prevented and the woman cannot become pregnant. When the pill is stopped, the cycle promptly returns.

Even women in some of the savage tribes of Africa and South America have attempted to prevent the entrance of the male sperm cell by obstructive devices made of wool, sponge, metal or rubber. Such devices are frequently prescribed by physicians when they are necessary for reasons of health. The device which is prescribed and carefully fitted by the doctor who also gives instructions as to its proper use is the technique now most frequently approved. This method it must be remembered is only dependable when the doctor has made an individual examination, selected the proper device and given the necessary information.

A successful marriage depends on the presence of children. Methods for the prevention of conception should be used only when they are definitely indicated, and most marriages are far more likely to be permanent and happy if children come soon to complete the marriage bond.

CHAPTER V

Sex Hygiene

THURMAN B. RICE, M.D.

Revised by M. F.

INTRODUCTION

THE INVESTIGATIONS *of recent years indicate how profoundly various aspects of sex hygiene affect our lives not only from the physical but also from the mental point of view. The chief contribution of the Freudian psychology has been the emphasis which it has placed on the extent to which the inhibitions of previous generations have operated to establish many neuroses and sexual disorders. Certainly, there is good evidence that some conditions which were formerly thought to be wholly physical in character have a mental basis, and that this mental basis is established by failure to develop proper relationship between the sexes.*

Much of the background of these disorders is established in childhood and in adolescence. It is therefore important to recognize the significance of proper education in the facts of sex early in life. In the section which follows, the whole problem of sex education beginning with the instruction of the child in these important matters and carrying his subject through to relationship during courtship, marriage, and wedded life is considered.

A proper appreciation of the relationship of sex to health and to daily life is essential for satisfactory living.

The continuation of our basic culture and the propagation of life itself is directly dependent on the functioning of the fundamental instincts which bring men and women together in an infinitely important relation known as the family or the home, and into which are born other human beings like unto themselves. Sex is everywhere about us. We see it in the clothes we wear, in the occupations we serve, and in the sports and games by which we seek relaxation. Short stories, novels, poetry, art, sculpture, music, and the drama constantly remind us of the fact that men and women are different but closely interrelated and that they behave as they do largely because of this difference. If we would know what it is that motivates men and women and boys and girls; if we would understand the psychology, the hopes, the fears, the desires, the lusts, the passions of our neighbors; if we would know what it is that makes one man a hero and another a beast, we will do well to look into this matter of sex. Sex is omnipresent; it is everywhere about us; it touches us from a dozen angles; it is actually the *sine qua non* of our existence, the priceless ingredient of our daily life.

Is it not strange, then, that there should be so much misunderstanding of this vital subject? Is it not rather amazing that intelligent men and women should be in so many instances utterly ignorant of the true significance of this, the basic fact of life?

THE IDEALS AND PURPOSES OF SEX EDUCATION

There are many reasons why every child and every adult should understand, as well as he may or can, the various complicated functions by which the race reproduces itself and by which the family comes into existence and is held together as a unit. How this information may be transmitted correctly and decently to the younger generation is a problem of the utmost consequence to the success of the family and the nation.

The layman needs comparatively little detailed information concerning the minutiæ of the process of reproduction. He needs rather a broad understanding of the general principles involved. He should regard the understanding of sex as being of the nature of an art rather than a science, the science being needed only that he may practise the better the fine art of living broadly, deeply, and well. Sex and life are inseparable; each is the origin and the end of the other. Happy is the man or woman, the boy or girl, in whom sex is a well integrated part—*and nothing more*—of the whole purpose and philosophy of life.

Sexuality has been confused with sensuality. A mere incident in the program —an incident that corresponds to the carrying of the pollen by the bee—has been regarded as the *whole* program. It has been supposed that sex is selfish and seeks only its own self-gratification when actually nothing is so unselfish as the love of a mate for a mate or a parent for a child. It has been said that sex has ruined many a man or woman, but it has been forgotten that it has brought out the best that was in countless millions of others. It has made men and women of foolish boys and giddy girls. Sex can inspire an ordinary swain to poetry; it can make heroes of us all when our children or loved ones are in danger. Sex endangers us only when it is misunderstood or misused.

Our young people are demanding a positive education. They will not take "don't" as a rule for conduct. If "mother knows best," they think that mother should be able to give a reason for thinking that she knows best. Negative education tends to produce a pedagogic vacuum which will speedily be filled with something, be it good, bad or indifferent. When the minds of children—and adults—are loaded high with positive facts and principles based on the assumption that sex is natural, good, beautiful, and entirely proper when in its proper place, there will be little to be feared from the untruths and half truths which may otherwise be so disastrous. Once the mind is filled with pertinent facts it is satisfied and goes about its legitimate business untempted by morbid or lascivious curiosity. We much prefer to have our children turning toward the beauties of virtue rather than fleeing from the ugly face of sin. It is most unfortunate that virtue has so often been made to appear dull and prosaic while dangerous and immoral practises have been made most enticing.

Particularly is it important that the child should never be frightened when this subject is discussed. The method of imparting sex education whereby the mother calls the child to her side and tells him or her that she went down to death's door in order that the child might be born is most vicious. Children cannot understand the fact that suffering and sacrifice may make a thing precious. The normal child may be told that the benefits of a dental operation are immeasurable, but, just the same, the fact that "it will hurt" when he goes to the dentist outweighs, to him, every conceivable gain. The mother who associates sex with pain and danger is often laying the foundation for an unsatisfactory or even destructive attitude toward life. Likewise, the parent who makes the subject ugly or disgusting or vulgar is injuring the child instead of helping him. Some suppose that it is necessary to do this in order to guard the virtue of the unmarried young person. Virtue is far better guarded by those who have a thorough understanding and appreciation of its worth.

Sex is a red-blooded thing; it throbs with high passion; it lives, and loves, and fights. It is a giant who constructs or destroys, makes or breaks, according as it is understood or not. Pink pamphlets for pale people will hardly serve the needs of the robust men and women who make the world go around. As well say "naughty, naughty" to a hurricane as to prescribe certain anemic books as a means of helping young people to control the powerful forces which surge within them. Most publications of this sort have been written by persons who have never known *la grande passion* or who, having seared themselves in its flame, are now devoutly wishing "to save the young people from what I have gone through." The services of such are not needed in the present purpose. This is a task for men and women who have felt the divine urge to create, have gladly accepted the challenge, and have not betrayed the trust.

We shall make no attempt to anticipate the questions which some bright-eyed child may ask, but are merely hoping that we may be of aid in preparing the parent so thoroughly in the basic principles of the subject that he or she may be able to feed and to satisfy the perfectly natural childish curiosity which brings a child to his parent with vital questions. Possibly the choice of words which we use may be of value, inasmuch as the lack of the proper word to use is often a serious difficulty. The method of approach may be of value to some who know well enough the subject matter but not the pedagogic methods for putting it across. The parent need not expect to learn or build up a philosophy of sex and life in a moment. Nor can he acquire one second hand by reading a book on the subject. He will need to study long and seriously before he will be skillful in the handling of so delicate a matter. Unless the parent has had a reasonably satisfactory understanding of, and attitude toward, the subject, he need hardly expect to become expert in teaching his children concerning it. This is particularly a subject to be taught by example as well as precept. The man who treats his wife as if she were an inferior creature will have difficulty in instructing his boys, and the nagging wife will fail utterly in leading her offspring to a beautiful conception of sex life.

REPRODUCTION IN THE PLANT AND ANIMAL KINGDOMS

Those who would understand the marvelous process by which plants and animals may produce other plants and animals of the same sort, and, in particular, would like to understand the matter of sex as it is manifested in the reproduction of the human race, can do no better than to study the phenomenon as it is manifested in simpler forms of life. The process as it is observed in man is so complicated as a result of various social, moral, and ethical relations that it is necessary first to study the subject in some easier form. As a matter of fact, every phase of the process may be scrutinized in this way without arousing the various prejudices and suspicions which have so clouded the issue. Many parents are anxious to initiate their children into the mysteries of the subject, but are deterred by the lack of suitable means of expression. They need elementary examples of sex life before attempting to instruct in the extremely complex relations of modern human society.

A fairly complete understanding of the phenomenon in lower forms of life will give the parent or teacher poise and resourcefulness which will be greatly needed in teaching the subject and in developing a satisfactory philosophy of life. Not infrequently the parent or teacher needs more than anything else concrete illustrations for the explanation of the various difficult points. Very frequently an accurate and dignified vocabulary is needed. It is impossible to suppose that the vulgar words of the alley can be used in good sex instruction. We insist that he or she who teaches must himself or herself have reached some degree of mental poise and decision on these matters. There is no better way to do this than to become acquainted with the elementary biology of sex as it is manifest everywhere about us.

Obviously each species must have some adequate way of reproducing itself, otherwise it would long since have perished from the earth. The continuation of the species is the most fundamental instinct of every plant and every animal species. Most plants begin to die as soon as the seeds are well along toward maturity, and all animals except man are ready to die as soon as the end of the reproductive cycle has been reached. It is sometimes supposed that the self-preservative instinct is strongest in man and beast, but everyone must have seen men and women risking life, reputation, health, social standing, wealth—everything—in order that they might express themselves sexually or take care of their offspring. In such case we must conclude that the instinct for reproduction is really basic.

Two general methods by which the species may be reproduced are observed in nature: the sexual and the asexual. Animals, except in the very lowest forms, use the sexual method. The same is true of most plants, but there are a considerable number of them which have dispensed with sex as a means of procreation. The bacteria, for example, merely divide in the middle, making two new individuals which are exactly alike and like the parent cell. In a sense the different individuals in a bacterial culture are really different fragments of the same original germ. Even high in the plant kingdom we see essentially the same thing. A twig from a willow tree becomes itself a willow tree. It is like the parent tree for the good reason that it is a detached part of the parent tree. A number of cultivated species of plants are propagated by tubers, roots, bulbs, cuttings, and grafts, which are all asexual means, though these plants have sexual organs as well. Seed *potatoes* represent a use of the asexual method, while potato *seeds* (occasionally found in small pods where the flowers have been) are of sexual origin. Several of the very low forms of animal life can reproduce themselves merely by dividing or being divided. We need not discuss this phase of the subject, however, for the good reason that we are wishing as quickly as possible to make the application to the human race.

Even though some forms of life may use the asexual method of reproduction, it is now believed that all of them have some sort of sex, rudimentary though it may be. Bacteria, until recently, have been considered as being exceptions to this general rule, but now a great many authorities believe that even they manifest an extremely primitive activity which is to be regarded as being essentially sexual. Inasmuch as Nature has used this particular plan in the life of every one of her products, the conclusion is inevitably forced upon us that there must be some most excellent reason for the phenomenon. Let us suppose that every individual of a given species were free to reproduce himself by asexual means for an unlimited number of generations. It is easy to see that a given strain might come rather soon to be quite different from the original species. In this way there would arise an enormous number of varieties, and a condition approaching chaos would result. This is, indeed, exemplified by the fact that those plants which are reproduced by bulbs, cuttings, and tubers commonly have a great number of varieties: roses, dahlias, gladioli, etc. Nature seems, however, to hold the majority of species more constant, and so each time the act of reproduction is repeated it is necessary that a given individual fuse his heredity with that of another individual of the same species. In this way each separate drop of living matter is merged with the great ocean of related living matter, and wide deviations from the type species are rendered much less likely to occur.

However that may be from a theoretical standpoint, it certainly is a practical fact that sex is fundamental to the continuation of all higher forms of life. It is the warp of life into which an infinite variety of patterns may be woven by manipulation of other factors which may be called the woof. Sexual reproduction is the masterpiece of Nature. Into this process she has poured her sweetest perfumes: the flower, for example, is the sex organ of the plant. About it she has drawn her most beautiful patterns. Into it she has dumped her paint pots, as witness the colors of the mating bird, the butterfly, and the flower. On the human level music and poetry are called upon to adorn it. Sex is motivated by the most precious of all passions, conjugal and parental love. Young girls are as enticing as it is possible to be; young men are handsome and valiant. The young of most species are charming—or, if not that, are at least interesting. Everyone loves the puppy, the colt, the kitten, and most of all, the baby. Who can be so blind as to fail to see in this thing the very essence of life itself? If life be good then this is the very best thing in life—or the worst when it has gone sour.

If we look into even the simpler and most familiar forms of sex, we may discern opportunities for the teaching of human problems to children. There is the flowering plant; for example, the bean. Every child is familiar with the seed of the bean, and if not accustomed to seeing the growing plant, it is quite a simple matter to plant a few beans and see them grow. (Beans bought for food purposes have often been heated so that the germ of life has been killed; therefore beans intended for planting should be used for this purpose.) A flower pot in the window will serve if there is no room for a garden. The child will be much interested in planting the seed and in seeing it grow. Finally the buds and then the flowers will appear. They are the most beautiful part of the plant. Insects will visit the flowers and will go from one to another sipping the nectar and transferring the pollen as it sticks to their legs. Even a crude dissection of the flower will reveal two sets of organs in the heart of the blossom. The one set, the stamens, carry at their tips a yellow powder (pollen) which is the male element; while the other, the pistil, is the female portion of the plant and has a sticky spot on the end to which pollen will adhere if it touches.

The insect, in visiting one flower after another, carries the pollen of one plant to the pistil of another. The pollen grains sprout and grow down the entire length of the pistil and carry the tiny cells which unite with the egg cells to form the seeds which are essentially new individuals. The growth of the seeds in the pod—the body of the mother plant—may be easily followed. Essentially the process is the same as is observed in the higher animals, except that the points that are hardest to get across to children are much more simply explained. Most important is the fact that the part of the process which corresponds to the mating of the sexes is the apparently trivial visit of the bee who carries the male element to the female organ of the next flower. In teaching children it is usually this point that puzzles and deters most parents. Possibly the use of the bean plant as an example may make it easier to explain this part of the process. Emphasis must, of course, be put upon the significance of *the whole program* and not upon this particular episode. The purpose of the process is the reproduction of the species—a very important matter indeed—rather than the making of an opportunity for the bees. The whole process is magnificent while the transfer of the pollen—except as it is part of the whole—is trivial.

Other plants may be used in somewhat the same way. For example, the flowers of the members of the melon family—muskmelons, pumpkins, cucumbers—are not all alike. Some of them have only the female organs, while others have only the male. In this respect they are more like the higher animals with which we are particularly concerned. In the case of strawberries and certain fruit trees there are some barren plants which are male. These plants never have fruit, but if they are all pulled out the other plants will be worthless as well.

The nesting habits of fish furnish an excellent example for teaching purposes. The females lay their unfertilized eggs over a clean spot on the bottom of the lake or stream. The male then comes to the nest and pours over the eggs a secretion known as "milt," which consists of millions of the sperm cells. When one of these sperm cells unites with an egg cell a new individual life begins. Obviously the method is exceedingly wasteful, but it is the best that fish can do. The young are compelled to get along as best they can after they are hatched, and, as a matter of fact, great numbers of them perish. In consequence, it is necessary that thousands or even millions of eggs be laid. By paddling slowly in a boat about the edge of a lake during the spawning season, the nests of sunfish may easily be found as clean round spots on the gravelly or sandy bottom, over which the parent usually hovers. The parent fish keeps the area clean and will chase away enemies who may come to destroy.

The mother frog does somewhat better. Her eggs are put out in a gelatinous material that protects them considerably. Then, too, they are black above and light below, making them harder to see. The dark color absorbs the heat of the sun and hastens the hatching process. The male fertilizes the eggs at about the time they leave the female's body. When the young tadpoles are finally hatched they are usually compelled to get along as best they may in a cruel world and many of them serve as juicy tidbits for birds, fish, and other animals.

The turtle illustrates a marked step in advance. The eggs are fertilized before they are laid and are held in the body of the female until a considerable quantity of food has been stored up in them and a firm shell is built about the food and the living portion of the egg. The eggs are then laid in and covered with the sand near the water's edge. There the heat of the sun stimulates growth. They will not be hatched until they are in a rather advanced state of development as compared with the young of the fish and the frog. Far fewer eggs are laid, for the good reason that the few that are laid are better equipped for survival. Even so, there is no further care on the part of the parents, and the young have strenuous times finding food and escaping the myriad dangers which beset their paths.

Birds do still better by their young. The parent birds mate and build a home—a most interesting home, indeed, as may be found by the simple expedient of sitting quietly and watching. The egg is retained in the mother's body until it is large and loaded with food for the young bird. It is then laid in the carefully prepared and concealed nest, where it is faithfully guarded for days by the mother, who hatches it with the heat of her own body. In the meantime, the father bird has protected the nest by driving away enemies, or has attracted attention and danger away from the nest and to himself by flashing his bright colors and brilliant song from a tree safely remote from the nest. When the young are hatched, the parents bring food, the mother keeps the nest clean and picks lice and other vermin off the young. She hovers over them when they are cold or when it is storming; she powders them with dust from the road, thereby discouraging insect pests; she never rests in her untiring efforts to feed and protect them; she teaches them to fly and to find food for themselves.

A most interesting subject for children to study is the nesting habits of the birds. City children need not often be at a disadvantage in this respect, for robins nest everywhere, and canaries can be had for a small sum. The larger cities may have fewer natural facilities, but such cities have zoölogical gardens and museums where there are unusual opportunities for such study. Parents who are awake to the possibilities can always find opportunity for such instruction in nature.

Higher in the scale the mammal takes even better and longer care of the young. The egg is developed as in the case of the other animals mentioned, but is never entrusted to the dangers of the outside environment—being far too precious—and so the young develop in the body of the mother. When the time comes that they must be delivered, Nature has provided for them a food which is taken from the mother's body and is the perfect food for the growing baby animal. The protective instincts of the mother are easily observed. Here is an example of parental love which is easily recognized even by a young child. Unfortunately, the function of the father is often much less inspiring, inasmuch as the male of the most easily studied mammals is generally apparently little interested in his offspring. There are, to be sure, instances in which the mammals have something somewhat like a human family, but most of these are in animals not easily observed by the child.

It is for this reason, in our opinion, a mistake to say too much about the male parent when referring to mammals. The example of the birds is better and more easily observed. By this we do not mean that the act of fertilization is any the less proper, but as we are teaching human children it is better to use examples which are more nearly like human customs. It is not that we would attempt to conceal the facts, but only that we would not call attention to them as they may be observed in the polygamous animals. There are authorities on sex education who advise that children be deliberately shown every phase of reproduction, as may be easily shown in dogs, for example. Personally, we are inclined to think that it must be rather hard to make the demonstration edifying. We believe that this is a phase of mammalian life that had best be left to accidental observation. If the child, after having been properly instructed in such matters as indicated above, asks questions about the more obvious facts of mammalian life, the whole matter should be discussed with him, and the social need for discretion in the mentioning of such matters should be explained. The subject is not of itself improper, but it has been treated in such a way that the child might easily get the wrong impression if he talks about it outside his own family.

Even a child must have observed that the human being is an animal, and as such has many of the ways of an animal. Even a child must learn early that the human being is *much more than a mere animal,* however, and should conduct himself or herself accordingly. Human children are precious. They must be given tender care over a long period of time. In this way the child can be made to see the reason for the family as we have it. In this way he comes to appreciate the rôle of the father and the mother, who have built about him a home that is stable, safe, and the very core of his existence. The functions of the father and the mother in that home seem widely different, but each is equally important and each has for its purpose the preservation of the child himself. The child sees his father working, bringing home food, paying for coal, furnishing a house in which to live, protecting him from injury, giving elemental care, playing and romping with him, planning with him, helping him, and advising him in ways that help tremendously. Every boy and girl should believe that his or her father is of the nature of a god, and so in this way the human father lifts himself above the level of the father of a puppy. The child sees—or should see—the father and mother exchanging embraces and words of affection. He realizes that sacrifices are being made, and so he comes to the way of thinking that anything that his father does must be quite all right—and as a matter of fact the father's position in the family will be much easier taught when everything that the father does *is* quite all right.

We are here giving much attention to the father for the reason that his rôle is commonly considered to be the hard part to explain. It is hard to explain, probably, for the reason that the male of most of the lower species have so little to do that is exemplary in terms of human conduct. Unfortunately, for one reason or another, a considerable number of human fathers also do little that is exemplary by the same standards, and so their purpose is rather hard to explain to the innocent child.

The function of the mother is much more obvious and needs no particular elaboration here. One point is important: The actual deliverance of the child from the body of the mother is usually a considerable ordeal and may easily become a family catastrophe. It is hard to make the child understand why such a process is necessary if he knows all of the sordid details. For that matter, it is hard to make adults understand why the bearing of children should be so difficult. We are happy to report that a great deal has been done by the medical and nursing professions to relieve that difficulty and danger.

Why must childbirth in the human be so much more difficult and dangerous than in the lower animals? The reason is to be found in several relations which are not very obscure. In the first place, there is the matter of the erect posture, which has done so much to change the configuration of the pelvis in many women, and particularly in those who may have suffered as children from the disease known as rickets. This disease allows the abnormally soft bones to be excessively distorted by the weight of the body, and, in consequence, the birth canal is made too narrow. Erect posture is, however, a fundamental advantage to the human race and is not to be lamented. Secondly, the nervous development of the human mother makes her much more susceptible to pain than are the lower animals. Human beings are not clods, and so they feel more keenly. Frankly, we would not have it otherwise. In the third place, the human child is so precious that Nature strives to hold it as long as possible in the place where it is safest. The newly born human infant is exceedingly helpless even then, and would be dangerously so if it were born any sooner. For this reason the mother must carry the child a relatively longer time. Finally, the development of the head which is made necessary by the large size of the brain enormously complicates the act of delivery. But that marvelous brain is the one really great characteristic of man, and we must not find fault with that which makes us great among the creatures of Nature. Thousands of those brains are now actively engaged in devising means of making childbirth easier and safer, and they are succeeding, too.

We are presenting these facts for the enlightenment and instruction of adults, but *for the sake of the child.* As mentioned previously nothing is gained by telling the child of Mother's travail and sacrifice. The child knows nothing, and can understand very little, of sacrifice and suffering. He does not know that things that are precious are also expensive. He is often shocked and frightened. Pain is always bad to the child and to be avoided. Entirely too much has been said about the *sacrifices* of motherhood, and far too little about the *privileges* and compensations. No parent worthy of the name begrudges a reasonable personal sacrifice which he or she has been compelled to make for the sake of a bright and healthy child. Then why talk about it? Particularly is it bad to throw the matter in the face of the child itself, as if he or she were somehow to blame.

We are in great need of an understanding of sex as a *normal* physiological function of the greatest consequence to the perpetuation of life on the earth.

When assigned to its proper place in the scheme of things, and when interpreted properly, the understanding of this subject adds enormously to the meaning of life. Unfortunate, indeed, is the child—or adult—who is led to believe that sex is a *risqué* or low experience that lies out on the edge of things—a subject to be hushed and covered at every turn. Fortunate is the child whose parent so understands the subject that he may lead the child by gradual steps to a realization of the importance and beauty of sex and who arouses in him a determination to protect and conserve this vital force which unites in him the glorious past and the still more glorious future. There is no better way to attain such a position of wisdom and understanding than by studying the manifestations in those species which represent the steps by which we have attained our present position of eminence in the world of living things.

THE ANATOMY AND PHYSIOLOGY OF THE REPRODUCTIVE SYSTEM

Before one may expect to teach the subject of reproduction to his or her children, he or she should be thoroughly grounded in the elemental principles of anatomy and physiology by virtue of which the miracle of life begins. It is not at all necessary that the layman should know all of the great Latin names for every little part, or that he should hope to understand the chemistry and physics of the whole process, but he does need to know something of the amazing things that take place in the months preceding the birth of a child, and he needs to understand the system well enough to be able to give it the care that hygiene demands. Very badly indeed he needs a vocabulary by means of which he may discuss these matters without the faintest taint of vulgarity or obscenity.

The generative system in either of the two sexes consists of two portions: 1. The sex glands themselves (ovaries in the female, testicles in the male). 2. A system of tubes which carry the sex cells, and later in the female, protect and nourish the developing child. Strange as it will seem to the layman, the organs of the two sexes are really much alike, each organ of the one sex having its exact but poorly developed homologue in the opposite sex.

The sex glands of the male, the *testicles,* consist of a great number of microscopic tubules which are lined with cells which are constantly undergoing cell division after the individual has attained sexual maturity. These cells become the *spermatozoa* or sperm cells, which are tiny little living bodies with long slender tails which whip about and in this way propel the sperm in its search for the egg cell. These sperm cells carry the entire inheritance which a given child will or can get from his father. The spermatozoa may live for several days in the tubes of the male, or may even live for a day or two after they have gained access to the female organs. They begin to be produced when the boy reaches puberty (about fourteen years of age), and continue to be formed until senility has been reached. During the period of sexual maturity they are commonly produced at the rate of millions per day.

In addition to the above function of the testicles, there is another that is nearly or quite as important as the production of the sex cells. Between the tubules which produce the spermatozoa there lie certain cells which are called the *interstitial* cells. They secrete a substance which is absorbed by the blood and is responsible for the development of the secondary sex characteristics of the male. Every one is familiar with the fact that the body of the man differs from that of the woman in other respects than the appearance of the sex organs themselves. The beard of the male, the deeper voice, the heavier bones, the narrowness of the pelvis, the texture of the skin, the scantiness of the sub-cutaneous fat, the lack of development of the breasts are all the results of this secretion. Unfortunate, indeed, is the man who does not have enough of this secretion to cause such a differentiation of his body that he may be immediately recognized as being definitely masculine in appearance. It is because of the loss of this substance that the castrated male (known as a eunuch) loses the characteristics of a manly man. Such individuals are commonly held in contempt by normal members of both sexes.

The *ovaries* of the female serve a purpose in the female exactly comparable to that of the testicles in the male, though there are, of course, differences in the details. The egg cells are already pretty well formed in the ovary at the time of birth, or shortly afterwards. They need to be matured, and stocked with a small supply of food, and then are ready to be extruded from the ovary. At the age of *puberty* (age twelve to thirteen years) the girl begins to produce mature egg cells at the rate of one (occasionally more) per menstrual month (usually twenty-eight days). This is continued until the *menopause* (change of life) is reached. This means that, on the average, less than five hundred egg cells are actually released in a lifetime.

As in the testicle, the ovary contains *interstitial* cells which produce a secretion that is responsible for the secondary sex characteristics of the female. The soft skin, the abundant subcutaneous fat, the development of the breasts, the higher pitched voice, the wider pelvis, and a great many other typically feminine attributes are too familiar to need enumeration. Women, because of loss or atrophy of the ovaries, or because of some other glandular disturbance, occasionally lose much of their femininity and may develop a beard or coarse, man-like features. Such a misfortune is distressing, indeed, to the individual herself, and greatly disfigures her in the eyes of others.

The *testicles* and the *ovaries* are the essential organs of reproduction. Indeed, as we have seen, many of the simpler animals and plants have hardly any other organs of reproduction than just these. Even in somewhat higher animals, as the fish and the frogs, the eggs are simply turned out into the water, and the spermatic fluid is spread over them there. The accessory organs of reproduction in such a case are exceedingly simple, and sex, as we commonly think of it, can hardly be recognized by examination of the exterior of the body. The episode *coitus* which is considered by the thoughtless person to be the whole of the process becomes a trivial part of the program—merely the spreading of the milt of the male over the eggs laid in the water by the female.

As the higher forms of life are studied, it is noted that more and more care is given the fertilized egg. The reptiles and the birds lay large eggs containing abundance of food so that the young may attain considerable size and development before they need to begin to fend for themselves. The mammals give their young even better care, and for weeks and months the female carries the young in her own body, and then, after releasing them, suckles them for another rather long period. Obviously such an arrangement has necessitated an enormous increase in the complexity of the system. The entire body of the female is modified to take care of the fertilized egg, to expel the developed fetus and to nourish the young after it has been born. The body of the male is likewise modified so that it may be able to impregnate the female and protect her and the young during the critical months before and after the birth of the young. Sex as we commonly think of it is highly developed in these animals.

The human species is characterized by the fact that the infant has an unusually long period of gestation, infancy, and dependency. It is this long period of comparative helplessness that allows the child to develop countless possibilities which would have been quite out of the question had he been compelled to look after himself from the first. Likewise it is this which has made necessary the tremendous changes in body structure of the two sexes, and the even more complicated development of the human family life, upon which the happy and efficient functioning of so much in the life of the child depends. There is here a most vital point which is often overlooked by superficial students of sex and its problems. They seem to think that the work of the reproductive organs is finished as soon as the child is born or weaned. Actually this is by no means the case. The child needs a highly stable and secure home until he or she is grown, and even longer if the highest interests of the family and race are to be realized.

Anything that tends to hold the father and mother together in a tight and rugged union until after the child is born and reared is of tremendous advantage to the individual and the race. This is, then, also a function of the reproductive organs. Fortunate indeed is the child whose parents have learned such functions of the reproductive system that they may derive exquisite pleasure and enjoyment therefrom. That child is safe because he will have behind him a father and mother who love each other and are devoted to him. Such a child will usually go much farther than the one from a broken or loveless home. In the human race sex has a function which far transcends mere fertilization of the egg and care of the young for a few days or weeks. The full development of the child calls for a continuing relation to loving parents.

The accessory sex organs of the male consist of the *scrotum*, a baglike sac or pouch, containing the two testicles which produce the spermatozoa or male sex-cells; a long tortuous tube from each of the testicles to the corresponding *seminal vesicles* or reservoirs, where the spermatic fluid and the sperm cells are stored until such time as there may be opportunity for extrusion (ejaculation); the *prostate gland,* which secretes a mucus-like fluid which carries the seminal secretion and makes a medium which will permit the spermatozoa to live and reach their objective; and the *penis,* which is an erectile tube capable of depositing the mixture of spermatic and prostatic secretion into the vault of the *vagina* near the mouth of the *womb.*

The accessory organs of the female are necessarily much more complicated for the reason that they must not only protect the egg cells but must provide a home for the developing child for nine long and eventful months. Essentially they consist of two tubes (*Fallopian tubes* or *oviducts*) which are open at the upper end and receive the egg cells when they are extruded from the ovaries. These tubes open into the *womb,* which is a thick-walled, muscular, hollow organ capable of enormous expansion. The womb in turn empties into the *vagina,* which is for the purpose of receiving the seminal secretion, and later of serving as a passageway for the child at the time of birth. The external female organs are called collectively the *vulva.* The breasts nourish the newly born child until it is old enough to eat other food.

The egg cell, after being released by the ovary, passes into the *Fallopian tube,* where it may or may not be fertilized by coming into contact with sperm cells. In case it does not make such a contact it lies there for a few days and then passes down into the womb and finally to the exterior. If it is fertilized it begins at once to divide rapidly and grows apace, utilizing the food that is stored in the egg cell and probably also some food absorbed from the surrounding tissues. It now migrates down into the womb and attaches itself to the inner wall of the womb (*uterus*) much as would a parasite. After a time a *placenta* is formed. This organ is the point of contact between the mother and the child. The bloods of the two individuals remain separate, both the mother and child having a set of closed vessels in the placenta, but fluids and gases can freely pass from the one to the other through the vessel walls by the process of *osmosis.* The mother furnishes food, water, oxygen, and other requirements; the child gives off waste materials of various sorts to the mother. No nerves pass from the one to the other. Various membranes for the protection of the child are also produced. These membranes and the placenta are delivered after the child is born and are collectively known as the "afterbirth." At the time of birth the walls of the womb contract strongly and expel the child and after a time the "afterbirth."

The life of a new individual begins when the living egg cell of the mother is fertilized by the living sperm cell of the father. Really, then, the human child is approximately nine months old when it is born, and more has happened in the development of the individual during that nine months than will take place in the next nine years. There are many who suppose that life begins in the child at about the time that the mother may feel the movements of the child in the womb. Indeed, it is customary to refer to these movements as the "begin-

ning of life." This phenomenon is usually observed at about the middle of the
pregnancy. Actually, however, the child is alive from the time of the union
of the egg and the sperm, and as a definitive human being has certain recognized human rights.

As soon as it is known that a baby is expected, parents are usually greatly
interested in the speculation as to whether it is a boy or a girl. There is good
reason to believe that the sex of the child is unalterably determined at the
time of fertilization. To date there is no realiable means of controlling the
sex of the offspring, and there is no accurate way of knowing until the child
is born whether it is male or female, though the physician may make shrewd
guesses which will be correct in a high percentage of cases. According to the
most widely accepted theory of sex determination, each cell in the body of the
female contains two determiners for sex (*chromosomes*), while each cell in
the body of the male has but one such determiner. When the egg cells are
produced, each cell contains one of these determiners; when the sperm cells
are made, half of them have one sex determiner and the other half have none.
If, then, the sperm with one sex chromosome meets an egg cell which always
contains one, the fertilized egg cell will have two and is therefore female. If
the sperm cell has no sex chromosome, then the fertilized egg cell will have but
one—the one from the egg cell—and the sex is then male. If this theory is
correct, and there is little doubt about its being correct, it would seem that
the control of the sex of the unborn child by any practical means is probably
quite outside the range of possibility. Many attempts to control sex have
been tried, but none have as yet succeeded.

Even though the sex of the child is determined from the very first, it will
be weeks before the differentiation of the organs is such that the sex might be
recognized, even if the child could be examined closely. By such careful examination it is possible during the third month of fetal life to determine
whether or not the child would have been male or female if it had lived. Previous to this time, the sex organs appear exactly alike, and, even in adult
life, it is possible to find in each sex the exact homologue of the organs of
the opposite sex. In the early months of fetal life the one or the other set of
characteristics begins to be accentuated, and the opposing organs begin to
atrophy.

In case a developmental error is made on the part of Nature it may be
rather difficult to say without careful examination—an examination which
sometimes requires an abdominal operation—whether the full-grown individual is male or female. These unfortunate persons are called "*hermaphro-
dites*" and are looked upon with considerable disdain and pity by their normal
neighbors. Usually they are decidedly more like the one sex or the other,
though, as mentioned above, there are some who present considerable difficulty in diagnosis. These individuals are rarely if ever fertile, either as males
or females, and never are they actually able to function as both father and
mother at the same or different times.

Obviously the matter of reproduction is of the utmost consequence both to society and to the individuals concerned, and for that reason it is extremely important that every person of mature age should understand something of the complex phenomena which take place during the months of pregnancy, the hours of actual confinement, the days of the lying-in period, and the months of lactation. It is, furthermore, most essential that this information shall be highly authoritative. If these relations were well understood, a vast amount of suffering, distress, and danger to the mother and child might be avoided. These matters have been well covered in another part of this book. The race must go on, and there is positively no other way by which it may do so.

There are three proper functions of the reproductive system in the human species: 1. The production of and the bringing together of the sex cells. 2. The production and the protection of the child, whether it be before, during, or after birth. 3. A means whereby a man and wife may express affection for each other, and on that solid foundation build a home which is, in turn, the foundation of society. All of these functions are absolutely legitimate, proper, and respectable when exercised according to the laws, customs, and ethics of the time and domain.

THE TEACHING OF SEX TO THE YOUNG CHILD

We need hardly point out that the process which brings an innocent child into the world and reproduces the species is inherently clean and decent. The parent who attempts to instruct a child in the marvels of sex must thoroughly convert himself to a firm belief in this fact, self-evident though it may seem. The process is right, and the child is pure. If, then, there is anything wrong about it, the difficulty must be in the parent or his understanding of the situation.

It is most unfortunate, for the sake of the child, that we cannot assume that persons about to become parents have become familiar with the fundamental facts concerning the process which has brought the child into existence. Even before marriage they should have talked over these matters and should have sought to learn through legitimate channels the facts about so important a matter. Surely there is no further excuse for hesitancy after marriage. During the months between conception and the birth there are many reasons why intelligent persons will wish to know something of what is going on. Between the time of birth and the asking of the first question there is a period of two to four years, during which time one might be expected to prepare himself or herself for the time when the child will want to know something of vital matters, and yet a large percentage of parents find themselves utterly unprepared for the inevitable time when the intelligent child begins to ask questions. Mothers are shocked when the first question is asked. They seem to think that the child is still a babe in arms. Fathers tell the distressed mothers to explain matters to the children, but usually have no suggestions as to what to tell or how to tell it.

Long before it is time to begin to teach the child by word of mouth about these matters, there are other responsibilities which must be met. Within the first few days of life the genital organs of the baby should be carefully examined for evidence of defects or abnormalities. In case such defects are found they should be corrected when possible, inasmuch as such peculiarities are often responsible for irritations or abnormal stimulations which may greatly complicate the sexual life of the child when he or she is older. The tissues of the infant are still highly plastic, and it frequently happens that corrections made early are surprisingly successful for this reason.

The boy baby should be carefully examined to see if he needs circumcision. If the foreskin can be completely and easily retracted most authorities think that circumcision should not be done, but when there is the least doubt about the matter decision should be made in favor of the operation, which is a trivial one when done within the first week or two of life. When the foreskin is tight or adherent there will accumulate under it secretions which will produce bad odors and cause pain and itching. Such a child is likely to get into the ugly habit of pulling at and handling the genitals and may develop habits which are harmful and unsightly. In case circumcision is not done, the mother or nurse should carefully retract the foreskin each day and see that the organ is thoroughly clean. Many "nervous," restless, and "fidgety" boys can be helped by circumcision, provided there is real reason to think that they need such care.

At an early age boys should also be examined to determine whether or nor the testicles have descended into the scrotum. These essential organs of sex are developed in the abdominal cavity, but at the time of birth or rather soon thereafter they should have descended. If they can be felt in the scrotum or can be gently pressed down into the scrotum there is no need for apprehension. If, on the other hand, they cannot be found, attention should be given to the matter—without causing too much curiosity on the part of the child—and the advice of a physician obtained. If descent does not take place, an operation to transplant the testicle into the scrotum should be performed before the boy reaches puberty. Undescended testicles commonly atrophy, and if both are in this condition sterility may result. The proper development of the testicle is important also from the standpoint of the proper secondary sex characteristics.

The girl baby also should be carefully examined for abnormalities. In not a few instances she may be in need of an operation which is essentially the same as that of circumcision in the male, i.e. the clitoris may be tied down by adhesions. Other defects may be present. In the washing of the female infant, care must be taken. Sometimes the hymen may be ruptured by rough handling. While it is true that the presence of an intact hymen is by no means proof of virginity, or the absence of it proof of sexual experience, there is still a large percentage of people who believe that such is the case, and so care must be taken to prevent an accident which might later put the babe, grown to womanhood, in an embarrassing position. Washing of the parts should be done in such a way that the friction will not cause erotic stimulation and in this way lead the child to the habit of playing with herself.

It is well known that crying babies, male and female, will nearly invariably hush when the genital organs are manipulated. This is an old, old trick of careless nurses and ignorant mothers. Under no circumstances must it be practiced, as it may lead promptly to the practice of masturbation in some form. Masturbation is probably far less harmful than has been supposed. Still, it is certainly an ugly habit, and every reasonable means of preventing it from establishing itself should be taken. It is doubtful if *mothers* have often practised such means of quieting their babies, but others to whom the child may have been entrusted have been less conscientious. The routine care of a child should never be delegated to someone else when it is physically possible for the mother to see to it herself.

During the period when the child is too young to be given definite instruction, much can be done to lay the foundation for sound health and useful habits. The child who learns cleanliness and regularity of body function will be much more likely to respect the purposes of the reproductive system when grown than will a person who as a child was permitted to abuse or neglect the various bodily functions. The strictly normal individual is less likely to develop improper habits or perversions than the one who suffers from various biases or abnormalities. Childhood is the time for health training, and health is the sound base upon which rest normal reactions with regard to sex.

Much of the difficulty in teaching and training children in these matters concerning sex is due to the mistaken idea that children do not manifest interest in such subjects until they are several years old. Sex is far too fundamental a thing to lie dormant for so long a time. The excretory organs are inseparably related to it, and indeed, it has its effect upon the entire body. Regularity in sleep, in eating, and in going to the toilet; pleasant manners and polite speech; love of beauty, truth, and decency; play in the open air; development of a natural attitude toward other children; modesty and respect for one's self are every one of them developed in large measure—if they are well developed at all—before the child is four years old. Every one of these traits is of the greatest value in the development of an admirable sex life. It is hard to see how the child that hears and sees vulgarity and lives as a waif can get a fair start in the understanding of so pure and chaste a subject.

Great care will be needed in teaching the child that the social conventions are necessary without instilling in him or her the idea that the sexual organs are inherently ugly, unclean, or sinful. The nude baby is proudly exhibited to admiring relatives and friends, the nude child of four is to be seen by the family only, and the boy or girl of eight is expected to be careful about such matters even in the bosom of the family. A fine sense of modesty is of the utmost consequence in the social training of the child. On the other hand, there are times, as when medical examinations must be made, when what has been called modesty is really prudery. The development of poise in these fine qualities is of the utmost consequence. It can be taught only when the child has been led to regard the sexual apparatus with respect rather than shame. Dignity and modesty are closely allied here as elsewhere. The child is made to understand that there are some things that are sacred and for that reason not to be cast before swine; there are some things so fine that they must not be permitted to become common. The child is shown that grown-ups, men and women, cover themselves, and that if he or she would be like them he or she must do so as well. Reserve rather than shame, pride in something that is too important to be left lying around, is the motive to be emphasized.

Many of the difficulties attendant to the teaching of sex are immediately solved when the child is taught the proper, the dignified names for the parts of the body. It would be hard to understand how a child could use the vulgar names which are commonly heard without deterioration of dignity and respect. Hardly better are the baby names and the meaningless terms which are often given them in the vain attempt on the part of the mother to save the child from what she supposes to be vulgarity. The child must acquire a dignified vocabulary if he is to keep the subject clean. It is hard to see why it should be more embarrassing to the mother to have the child come to her saying that he wishes to go to the toilet than to have him use some of the other expressions which are equally evident in their meaning under the circumstances. A frank acknowledgment of these things and their meanings is the very basis of future understanding of them. Hypocrisy and prudery have had their day and have made a mess of it.

During this impressionable period of life the attitude of the father and mother toward each other will have a profound effect on the character and sexual behavior of the child in later life. The child who sees his father treat his mother with chivalry and respect is much more likely to treat girls and women in the same way. The little girl who sees in her own mother a beautiful character is unconsciously receiving an education in these matters which is infinitely more effective than all the carefully planned precepts which might be memorized from books or articles on sex education.

But while it is really the generalities which count in the training of the child it is the details which are more perplexing to the parent in charge. This is because the details have a way of demanding immediate attention. What shall the mother or the father tell the child when he asks the highly pertinent and searching questions which have perplexed parents for so long? There is but one thing to tell him. It is the *truth*. By this I do not mean that it is necessary to tell a child of four the *entire* truth, or that it is necessary to give him the *detailed* truth. As a matter of fact, that would be impossible for the good reason that not even the wisest man knows the entire or the detailed truth about these matters. When the child asks a question he does not expect the scientifically complete answer, but in later life he will greatly appreciate the fact that he was told the truth in so far as he was able to understand it at the time.

When the child notices the difference between his or her body and that of the opposite sex it is an easy matter to explain that there are two sorts of people, and two sorts of everything else that is alive. That is so that each little child and each little baby animal may have a father and a mother to care for him and make a home for him. It is pointed out that birds of certain kinds are different in color and appearance, and that there are differences in function which correspond to this difference in appearance. By all means arrange for him to see a bird's nest, if possible, and understand something of what goes on there. He will have observed that fathers and mothers have different purposes in life, and there are marked differences in dress, in habit, and occupation. The whole process is perfectly natural, and when naturally told to a normal child will give rise to no morbid curiosity whatsoever. It is merely an interesting fact about the most interesting thing in the world—life.

A momentous question is that concerning where the baby came from. It is a question that every child should have asked by the time he is four or five years old or even sooner if he is interested. The most ridiculous substitutes for the beautiful truth have been given him—most of them extremely unconvincing. What a pity that mothers have seen fit to tell children that babies— they themselves, indeed—are found in garbage pails, in the straw pile back of the barn, under the leaves in the woods, in a hollow log, in the doctor's satchel, and in other monstrous places. Hardly better is the "made in Germany" story of the stork, except that it is somewhat more dignified. The children of Germany love and respect the stork, but the small children of this country know nothing of such a creature.

Children are invariably tremendously interested in babies and commonly are asking their parents if they may have a baby brother or sister. They see no evil in the possibility, as, indeed, there is none.

The question that is most dreaded is, "How did the baby get in the mother's body?" Here is something that is supposed to be hopelessly vulgar. Well, for those who think it is so we can understand that the problem is difficult. When, however, the father and the mother have loved each other as they should and are legally married, the act that is the expression of that love and the act that enables them to bear beautiful children is not vulgar in any sense. The child— bear in mind that this is a young child—can be told that as a result of the love which the parents bear for each other and for the child the baby began to grow in the body of the mother. An older child will need more information, to be sure, but this is as essentially the truth as the most tediously accurate and scientific account of the union of egg cells and sperms, such as he or she will need at a later stage of development.

The difficulty of explaining the role of the father will fade into nothing at all if the child believes that his father is a great hero who can do no wrong.

When the child has seen his father caressing his mother nothing could be more natural—as indeed nothing is more natural—than that they should desire and have children. It is most unfortunate that so many fathers live and treat their families in such a way that the children may learn to know that their acts are commonly selfish. In such case the teaching of sex will be difficult. In the main, however, small children believe that their fathers are great persons, indeed, and that whatever they do is just right, and in such case nothing could be easier than proper instruction in these matters. The role of the mother is easily taught. As it is perfectly natural for the child to develop in the mother's body, it is perfectly natural that the child should accept the method as the ancient and honored way of life, and that is all there is to it.

After the child is old enough to understand the simple anatomy of the two sexes, it may be explained that the sperm cells of the male are introduced into the body of the mother and there combine with the egg cells somewhat as the pollen of the male plant fertilizes the female. It should then be explained that such transfer of the male to the female must take place only between married persons, else a child may be born when the parents cannot make a home for it. Even a little child can understand that illegitimacy is a pretty serious thing, in as much as every child needs *both* a father and a mother as he grows up. It may easily be explained that the process is one that is perfectly proper when the man and woman are married and much in love with each other, and that it is an act of the utmost intimacy and delicacy.

When the child asks the *details* of birth—as he or she rarely will—care must be taken that he or she is not frightened by morbid details. No small child can understand the forces which come into play in such an event. It is a serious mistake to worry him with the harrowing details in such a case, then. It is enough to know that when the time came, the mother worked hard and was very tired. After such an experience she will need to rest in bed for several days and must be shown every possible deference and affection. She is not *"sick"* in the usual meaning of the word, but is merely *resting* after a tremendously important and vital contribution to the beloved family.

The most important principle in the training of a child in these matters is that the native curiosity of the child should be satisfied, and satisfied with something that can serve as a basis for subsequent teaching. The child must learn that it can depend *absolutely* upon the father and mother as a source of honest and authentic information on this subject, just as he can go to the same source for food, for shelter, and for help of any sort. The child should never be repressed when asking honestly concerning such matters. Once the demand for the truth is filled, the child can then go about his or her normal activities without being bothered with things he or she is too young to understand thoroughly. At this age interest may be keen for a moment, but when satisfied will soon turn to other things more closely related to the development of the child. There is not the least reason for the artificial stimulation of an interest in the subject, but there is good reason for quieting the natural interest by satisfying it. Questions put by the child should be answered when possible, but they need not be provoked. Generalities are sufficient for small children. Mention of pain, danger, or sacrifice should never be made, for the good reason that they cannot be understood by a child of tender years.

In case questions which cannot be answered are asked, the parent must make it clear that the question is perfectly proper if it is honestly asked. If the subject is one that cannot be answered but can be looked up, it is the duty of the parent to tell the child that he will investigate the facts and inform him later. If it is one that cannot be answered, the point should be explained as well as may be and the incident used as an example of the greatness and intricacy of the whole marvelous process. Frequently the ingenuity of the parents will enable them to restate the question so that the child can be satisfied though the direct question was not really answered. Always the teaching and the example set should be on the highest possible plane that the child can understand and appreciate. Parents who understand the process and live the part joyously will have no difficulty. They must not seem to apologize for normal sexual behavior or to make of it some sort of weakness in which they have indulged because they have not had the strength to refrain. Sex is good—in its proper place, of course—and must not be treated as a weakness or in any way sinful when kept in legitimate family circles.

The imagination and resourcefulness of the parent will do better than any "canned" information. It is not necessary that every bit of the information be absolutely scientifically up-to-the-minute provided it is earnestly and truthfully set out as the best that the parent knows on the subject. The development of a sound philosophy of life and living is much more needed than are the latest scientific details.

Whatever is done or taught, the idealism of the child must be preserved. The rôle of the father as hero, provider, and protector; the part of the mother as one who will love and protect whatever may happen, cannot be too strongly emphasized. The child easily understands such teaching and responds eagerly to idealism of this sort. The love of the father and mother for each other and for the child is the means by which the child came into existence and is as essentially the truth as if every detail were explained in full. It is the broad base upon which the family and all modern culture rests. For that reason it should be a real rather than a furtive thing in the every day family life. How reassuring it is when a child sees his parents making love and manifesting close loving attitudes. Such a child is safe. A quarrel between his parents is terribly disturbing to children of every age.

THE SCHOOL CHILD

The school child is no longer under the eye of his parents. He will hear and learn of sex. The pertinent question is not "Will he learn?" but, rather, "Where and of whom will he learn?" It is a foolish parent who thinks that a boy or girl in school will remain ignorant of these matters, and it is, indeed, a trusting parent who is willing to turn the instruction of his son or daughter in these matters over to ignorant companions. The child of this age is getting started to school and is beginning to feel that he knows something of life. Quite naturally he wants to understand things as they are. Fortunately he has not yet reached the age of puberty with its many perplexing problems and disturbing urges which will furnish an additional motive for sex interest.

Except that it will be necessary to give these children more information than was given the pre-school child, the problems are not greatly different from those that have just been discussed, for the good reason that the sexual system is still relatively undeveloped, and the child has only a passing interest in such matters. The teaching is still indirect and should consist of principles rather than details. It is a matter of ideals and of idealism. Questions should be answered fully and frankly—in so far as the child is able to understand or is interested—but disturbing questions are not to be raised in the mind of the child.

This is the time when children are so tremendously interested in nature, and it is easy, indeed, for them to have observed most of the essential phenomena of sex before they have become involved in the complex social phenomena which so muddle the issue in the human race. The parent who understands the fundamentals of sex and life as they are manifested in plants and animals and has the language to transmit such information will have an enormous advantage in the teaching of his children.

An important matter during this period is the teaching of a sense of modesty without at the same time teaching shame. Parents all too often shame their children into a state of mind that is mistaken for modesty. Shame, except for some improper act, is an emotion that should never be utilized in teaching. There is nothing about the reproductive organs for which a child need be ashamed. He learns to cover himself because it is the custom to do so, and because the older persons whom he wishes to emulate do so. There is nothing wrong about the genitals, but rather they are so important that they must be protected. They are so intimately one's real self that one must not go about exposing in a cheap and common way that which is so essentially private. Nice manners prescribe that care must be taken in these matters, and the child soon learns to take this view if he has a good example set before him.

Nearly all normal children have their little love affairs during the first years in school. Since it is so obviously true that one of the most important tasks in later life is the selection of a worthy mate, it is well that even children should be gaining a little proficiency in so vital a matter. Just as the kitten playing with a ball is really learning to catch mice, so these children are practising the greatest of all arts. It is a grave mistake for parents or others to tease children about their love affairs. Such teasing puts the idea into the head of the child that there is something inherently wrong about the whole matter and that he or she has done something that is improper. When, subsequently, a real affair is developing, it will be carefully concealed from the parents, and in this way the parent loses his opportunity to be of service in teaching the child how he or she may select the best companions. Furthermore, the curiosity of the child teaches him to seek the evil which he has been led to believe is in the apparently harmless relation which he or she has with another of the opposite sex. With such stimulation he will all too soon find the evil. The truth insofar as he can understand it is far safer than some silly tale which seeks to give a superficial explanation of the facts of life. "Ye shall know the truth and the truth shall make you free."

Parents who tease their young children about their beaux and seek to deter them from making dangerous alliances should look about them and learn that the best way to insure against these play love affairs going too far is merely to let them run without resistance. Children are far too fickle as a rule to do more than toy with a passion which they are much too young really to understand. Soon it will be forgotten. On the other hand, the parent who attempts to break up such an affair is assuming a grave responsibility. He will be almost sure to intensify it. There is no more certain way to drive a young—or older—couple into each other's arms than for a persistent parent to personify the well-known bull in a china shop and "set his foot down on the whole business." The reason for this is easily seen. We naturally tend to protect our friends when they are attacked, and we invariably learn to love those whom we protect. Not only are the children being set into mischief when they are teased, but the parents are accomplishing exactly the opposite result from that which they desire when they indulge in so low a form of correction —or amusement.

The parent who allows his or her children to assume natural relations with other children of the same or opposite sex need rarely fear that mischief will be done. The child, being still undeveloped sexually, gives no thought to the grosser manifestations of the subject unless they are suggested to him by his elders. When the relation is perfectly natural and the parent has abstained from teasing, the child will be free to talk about the matter, and so the parent may keep himself informed concerning the course of events. In case, then, the child gets on dangerous ground, a frank discussion of the matter is possible and will not be resented if skillfully handled. The parent may be able to point out in a kindly manner the good and bad traits in the favored friends, and in this way may be of real service in the important matter of picking the permanent mate a few years later. God knows the young people need all of the aid they can get in so difficult a project. It is rather evident, too, that many of them have no knowledge whatever about how to go about it—if one may judge by the results.

Boys and girls will frequently play "father and mother" games. Though it may seem far-fetched to some, they are actually gaining much experience which may be of great benefit to them in later life. It is not at all unusual to hear children of this age express themselves as to what they will do when they are men or women, as the case may be. For the most part they will do well if they later come up to these expressed ideals. It is also common to hear children say what they will do when they have children of their own, or what their children will or will not do. The wise parent at such a time may well listen and note. It is possible that he or she may learn something. Under no condition may the children be ridiculed or teased at such a time. Here is manhood and womanhood in the making, and it is mighty serious business.

Much worry has been needlessly suffered by devoted parents who have failed to understand children of this age. Boys and girls are curious. They will naturally examine their bodies, or, if the opportunity presents itself, the body of another of the same or opposite sex. The misguided parent thinks that this is exactly the same as if an adult should do so and gets all excited about it. Frankly, we would be inclined to question the mentality of a child who has not done so. The best way to draw the teeth of such a possible menace is to allow the child to satisfy that fine sense of curiosity which impels him to try to find out how things are made, and, having found out, lets him go on to something else. Two little girls in a closet were caught discussing these matters, and the mother was needlessly alarmed. It was explained to them that such conduct is not considered to be good social form, and no more was said about it. They had satisfied their curiosity, and the episode was ended. It is likely that they rather soon forgot about it. If they had been severely punished, however, they would have had good reason to remember and to wish to continue the experience when the opportunity to do so without being caught presented itself.

Frequently children will get into the habit of playing with or pulling at the genitals. Such children—both boys and girls—may be in need of a thorough examination by a competent physician. It is not unlikely that circumcision or other special corrective measure is needed. If there is no pathologic basis for the habit, the child should be taught that it is bad manners to behave in such a way and that an ugly habit may be formed. With help, rather than scolding, he may soon correct the ugly practice. Parents should remember that no one can break a bad habit except the person who has it, and that the task is one that sometimes requires patience and perseverance beyond that which a child may be expected to have. Little boys and girls are occasionally found to have developed the practice of masturbation. Normal children of this age will rarely go to excess unless they are being stimulated by some older person. If a child of this age masturbates frequently, a careful watch should be made, not so much of the child as of its older associates. The reason for this is evident, as the child is not often sufficiently developed for the habit to have arisen from within.

Children of this age should be interested in many things, and when they are so, one need not worry about their being too much concerned about an instinct which is still far from being mature. All sorts of healthy activities are to be encouraged. Exercise in the open air is far more conducive to good results than excessive poring over books. Regular habits in matters pertaining to health will lay the best possible foundation for a normal sex life in later years. The child should grow in "wisdom and stature" during this time. He or she should develop the body as it was intended to be developed. School interests, play, club work of all sorts, scout exercises, athletic teams, and kindred activities permit little time for those forms of sex activity that might really be dangerous.

Of vast importance during this period and before is the development of self-control. We cannot understand how a subsequent marriage is going to be successful if either partner is unable to control his or her temper or selfish inclinations. Parents are doing the consorts of their children a grave injustice when they permit children to grow up in such a way as to cause them always to consider their own welfare first. This may seem to some as if it were a subject that had nothing whatever to do with the subject of sex, but actually it has everything to do with it. The child that must have his own way, that must have everything that he wants, that has never been taught to give up, that doesn't know how to work, is likely to make a mess of marriage.

The question as to how much direct sex instruction should be given during this period is a rather knotty one. Sex during this period is probably less to the fore than at any time since babyhood, provided the curiosity of the pre-school child has been properly satisfied as discussed in the preceding section. If the child knows in a general way about these matters, he will let it go at that until the problems of adolescence begin to assert themselves. Matters pertaining to sex in its simpler forms should be frankly discussed by the family in the presence of the child. Questions are answered, and basic principles underlying proper conduct are deeply implanted, and that is about all that is necessary. The subject is far less exciting in the open than when it is concealed.

The boy of this age is intensely idealistic. He has his heroes—men of action and high accomplishment. He dreams of hazardous stunts and well-nigh impossible achievements. All too often he is attracted as a moth to the flame by the supposedly brave exploits of the gangster and the gunman. In many cases this is because his own good parents and relatives are so unromantic as to bore him to death. Fathers need more to appreciate the intense desire that their sons have to be able to brag about their dads. The father should attend to his most important business—that of being a "real guy" in the eyes of his children.

Girls are being encouraged to be teachers, stenographers, concert pianists, prima donnas, lawyers, doctors, nurses. As a matter of fact, most of them—fortunately—will become housewives and mothers. Why cannot these objectives be held up also as ideals? Then, when they have a home of their own, they will find in the monotonous routine a purpose toward their ideal. In case, however, they have been taught that they are to have some glamorous career and then find themselves washing dishes for a family, they are nearly sure to despise their task. There are those who suppose that a career as a mother is a narrow experience as compared with that of typing letters for a concern that sells lumber or vacuum cleaners. Some suppose that a mother needs less education than a teacher who does nothing but teach a single subject in a high school. The mother must be a nurse, a physician, a teacher, a legal adviser, a cook, a dietitian, a financial genius, a diplomat, an authority on child psychology, and a hundred other things—at least, she should be. Why cannot this be made a career toward which girls can be pointed with pride?

Psychologists tell us that the child is half educated before he even starts to school. His mother has taught him—very often badly—the mother tongue, his habits, his manners, his attitude toward life, his self-control, his reliability, his respect for truth and right, his religion, his patriotism—and yet the task of a mother is considered too lowly to serve as an ideal! A wife, who has the responsibility of five children, once lamented that she envied a woman of her age who had attained a degree of success in bacteriology. She should be reminded that the other woman grew bacteria in culture tubes, while she was growing men and women in a home. All of this is very important in sex education. Indeed, it is the very heart of the whole thing. The girl who has been brought up to regard her womanhood as a career, the boy who is thoroughly instilled with the principles and practice of manliness, will probably not make great mistakes in their sex lives.

The pre-adolescent age is a period which is immensely important in the orientation of the boy or girl. Orientation is possible at this time for the reason that the strong sex impulses have as yet not taken definite direction because of their relatively immature state of development. A little later they will be so strong that they may take the bit in the mouth and run away. Happy is the adolescent who has been set in such a direction that he or she can permit his or her sex to run away for the good reason that it is running in the direction of the greatest advantage. Those driving men and glorious women who make the world go round are the ones, in large measure, who got their correct bearings in the pre-adolescent period and were able to drive full speed ahead into the business of being someone and of doing important things. Sex is a powerful *driving* force. In which direction, Oh parent, have you set that force driving in your child?

THE PERIOD OF ADOLESCENCE

While a great many sex problems have their origin before the age of puberty and adolescence, the problems which arise at these times are much more urgent and difficult than those of the earlier years. This is the period of anxiety for parents.

This is the time when young people really need help and understanding. It is a time when powerful and utterly new forces are arising in them. New impulses are driving them they know not where. Elated with the new sensation of being comparatively grown up, and intoxicated with the previously unknown freedom which is usually granted them, they go plunging from one extreme to another. While there is some doubt about the matter of their maturity they must do everything possible *to prove that they are grown up,* and so the boys learn to smoke and to swear great and supposedly manly oaths. They affect deep knowledge of women and girls and tell of their conquests with this and that and the other one. They rarely, if ever, drive a car under seventy miles an hour, if one is to believe everything that he hears. It is, of course, obvious to those who understand something of the psychology of the period that they are overcompensating for their all too evident inexperience—whistling to prove that they are unafraid.

The girl usually passes through a "boy-struck" period. She giggles and makes herself conspicuous. Unless carefully controlled or endowed with unusual reserve, she is likely to go in for excessively high heels, extremes in dress, and large use of cosmetics. During this period of unrest she is sadly in need of intelligent and *sympathetic* guidance. Such guidance, however, is likely to be extremely distasteful to her. It will be impossible for parents who have neglected the matter of sex education until this time to pick up the reins of control and go serenely forward. Only those children who have been gradually led up to a realization of the forces at work within themselves will be in a position to appreciate the advice that wise parents can give. How may a mother who has told her daughter that babies slid down rainbows now hope to get control of the situation? Long before the time of adolescence the children have learned that their parents *are* sources of accurate information on the subject, or that they *are not* sources of accurate information. They may be expected to behave accordingly.

In continuation of sex education into the period of adolescence the parent or teacher must know that generalities are no longer sufficient. It is not enough to tell them to behave themselves and be good children. A concrete and detailed instruction in vital matters in which they may be concerned now becomes a necessity. By this we do not mean that every episode in sex life must be carefully diagrammed, but rather that the problems which the boys and girls are likely to meet should be discussed with them in a perfectly natural manner. It will, indeed, be well if the instruction is so natural and so unassumed that the boy or girl is hardly conscious that he has been instructed. Young people of this age should be included in the family conversation about many matters related to the subject of sex. The value of a good example on the part of the parents cannot be overstressed.

Let us assume here that adolescent boys and girls have had their minds thoroughly satisfied concerning the positive and beautiful phases of the subject. They are then ready to have some of the negative phases mentioned. This part of the education must not be made so graphic that it shocks or alarms excessively, but these young people should know about the possibilities of conception out of wedlock, and that under such circumstances the mother and child are sure to suffer severely from the social stigma which such a birth imposes. They should know something of venereal disease, which is perfectly capable of ruining them, their loved ones, and their careers. They should know of the depreciation of character which invariably follows the cheap promiscuity which seems so enticing under certain circumstances. These are not pleasant matters to explain, but children of this age should be treated somewhat as men and women, though they are still boys and girls. Life is coming to be real at this period; it is getting to be rather earnest. Young people will appreciate the confidence that is shown when such matters are frankly discussed, and they will really be grateful, though they may seem not to be so. It is important, of course, that discussion between young and old should be as casual as possible. The parent must not be dictatorial and he or she must be able to speak without embarrassment.

In case the young people have had no proper instruction in matters pertaining to sex during their earlier years; if they have no dignified vocabulary in terms of which these matters may be discussed; if they see in sex only the possibility of sensuous gratification, it will be difficult indeed—or well-nigh impossible—to correct the omission. Still, one can do no less than try. It is unfortunate if one must begin with the negative aspects of the subject, but even so such instruction may be necessary.

It is perfectly possible for boys and girls of the age under discussion to be parents of children. Such being the case, the careful parent can do no less than explain to his children something of the details of the sexual act. Only those who are willfully blind will pretend that it is possible or desirable to keep young people of the age ignorant of so vital a function. If there were any assurance that they might get such information in a relatively truthful form, there would be less need to insist upon parental instruction, but there is absolutely no such assurance. It is doubtful if there is so much misinformation on any other known subject. It is not so much that parents are ignorant, but rather that they "know so much that ain't so." They should be made to understand that sexual relations are of the utmost consequence to the welfare of the individual, the family, and the race, but that they are only for those who are sufficiently mature to bear and rear children, and are married so that they can do so. Unless this can be done in a way that convinces the young people themselves, it had as well not be done at all. Merely to admonish them in abstract terms is of little or no value. The sexual act must not be made an utterly delectable act utterly divorced from all sense of responsibility.

Provided the biology teacher of the high school has an appreciation of the possibilities of his subject, we strongly suggest that at least one course in this subject be taken in high school. Young people are usually safe when they are on familiar ground. It is possible in a biology class to discuss fundamental matters of sex in the most casual manner and in this way to lay an impersonal foundation for a sound understanding of the subject. When home influences and parental instruction then supplement scientific instruction, little concern need be entertained concerning the welfare of youths and maids who have normal poise and self-control.

Of much importance to the youth of this age is an appreciation of the fundamental reasons for the existence of a stable family life. Without the carefully integrated family the human infant or child is placed at a serious disadvantage and may not be able to overcome the handicap. While it is perfectly possible for persons to live in a satisfactory manner without wedlock, it is evident that marriage is fundamentally necessary, and in spite of the fact that many marriages go on the rocks, it is rather certain that men and women are normally better satisfied and happier in that relation than out of it. Marriage should then be held before young people as a probable goal, and careful thought and planning may well be given to the matter. All too frequently boys and girls break out into a scarlet rash as soon as marriage is mentioned. Giggling and protesting, they disclaim any such intentions. As a matter of fact, this behavior is a discredit not so much to these boys and girls as to their parents, for it shows clearly they have not frankly discussed such subjects with their offspring.

The sanctity of marriage may well be taught and illustrated at any age of development, but it is important that it be increasingly emphasized as the child approaches the age when he or she may be expected to enter into such a contract. Unfortunately there are a great many people who cannot understand the reasons why marriage should be more than a mere civil contract. The reason why marriage is more than a civil contract is to be found in the fact that children will probably result from such a union. Conventional marriage is the foundation on which is built the home, and the home is the basis of every one of the other social institutions—the school, the church, the government, industry, and social relations. Without the home it is hard to see how we could get along in any sort of acceptable manner. A community of good homes invariably has good schools, influential churches, thrifty, industrious, intelligent, educated people, and an acceptable government. A community of bad homes is hopelessly in the mire. These are facts that can be made plain to young people, who will consciously or unconsciously adjust themselves accordingly. Happy marriages and healthy homes are not the products of accident, the writers of melodrama to the contrary. They are worked out by persons informed in matters pertaining to real human values.

We shall do well, before we criticize the young people of today, to consider the difficult position in which we place them. They develop sexually earlier than they should and would were it not for the omnipresent sex stimulation which they are constantly receiving. They see moving pictures of the most sophisticated sort; they pick up *risqué* books or hear such books discussed; they hear suggestive songs; they see all sorts of irregularities. At any early age they have been more or less intimately introduced to the urges and passions, but are not permitted to marry until they are well into their twenties, as a rule.

In contrast to this situation is that of our parents, of earlier generations who were not let out into society until they were sixteen or seventeen, and were solidly married, frequently, at the age of eighteen or nineteen. In the early months of the period of courtship they were so awkward and green that they could hardly get into serious mischief, and by the time they were well out of that period marriage was usually consummated. If we are going to bring children up in such a way as to avoid the awkward and green stage, we are under obligation to help them take care of the passions which are aroused but may not be gratified. The awkwardness of the adolescent boy or girl is a protective device of no mean consequence. It is likely that those children who come through this adolescent period slowly and naturally will be better adjusted than those who are hurried through by socially ambitious parents, or who are turned loose on the streets.

It is for this reason that athletics are so important for boys and girls of this age. Many suppose that athletics are for the purpose of developing the physique. They are of much more consequence when they develop character. As a matter of fact, strenuous athletics at this time in life may, and frequently do, actually injure the body when not properly controlled. Play and recreation, rather than highly competitive sports, are needed. The boy who plays tennis, basketball, baseball, or engages in any of the many other wholesome sports, is not in much danger of giving too much thought to the girls. Very often, indeed, he has a fine scorn for the members of the so-called weaker sex because they cannot equal him in the manly sports. He plays until he is tired enough, when he goes to bed, to go promptly to sleep. He has something to think about; he has training rules to keep; he learns to give and take.

Girls will usually be somewhat less interested in athletics, though there are many exceptions. The reaction of girls toward athletics is essentially like that of boys, but there are certain differences which should not be entirely forgotten. There are, for example, the limitations imposed by the regular recurrence of the menstrual period. We do not wish to make invalids of girls, but insist that some consideration be given this matter. This point will be discussed later. The pelvis of the girl is broader and more loosely jointed than that of the boy. This is a relation which is necessary, as the pelvis must be built in such a way as to sacrifice strength for the contingencies of future childbirth. Heavy or excessive muscular exercise, or the carrying of heavy weights can for this reason more seriously injure the girl than the boy. Furthermore, there is an adjustment of the blood supply that is of much consequence. Nature insists that the demands of the reproductive system shall come first. For this reason the blood supply of the pregnant or nursing woman is commandeered for the reproductive organs and the breasts. If a girl is allowed to develop herself too highly in athletic lines she is able, in not a few instances, to train her muscles so that they will make such a drain upon the blood supply as will cheat somewhat the reproductive organs. It is well known that rather poorly developed women often have beautiful babies, while it is also well known that women of the muscular type are often sterile or have puny, poorly nourished (from the breast) babies. An analogy is seen in the fact that beef (muscular) cattle give poor milk and little of it, while the bony Jersey and Guernsey cows give large amounts of rich milk. We strongly believe in athletics for girls, but insist that they should be somewhat less strenuous and competitive. Girls do much better with the types of games that are mostly individual endeavor; boys need the highly coöperative games. This is in line with their probable needs in later life, when men, as a rule, work with others, while a housewife for the most part does her work alone.

Every child of adolescent age should have a hobby. Parents should make the way easy for the development of any special interest that the child may have. Collections of all sorts are made by interested young people: butterflies, beetles, plants, stamps, match-box covers, marbles, buttons, and a thousand and one other things. What a vast amount of mischief can be avoided by such means! The exercises prescribed by the Scout Manual have been of incalculable value in keeping boys and girls in pursuits which permit them to come along without too much attention to the developing forces within them. Of two boys of our acquaintance, one spent his spare time loafing on street corners, while the other was constantly looking for new plants for his herbarium, which already numbered several hundred specimens. It is not hard to guess which was developing best.

The parent who calls the child in from play in order to give him his weekly instruction in sex is entirely out of step. Sex is life. It is just plain wholesome living and doing. Therefore the teaching of this subject must be casual and matter of fact, except under certain conditions, when it must be highly idealistic and romantic. The wise parent will know when to look the other way and likewise when to set up the sanctuary. The best that the adolescent can do is to grow and develop, naturally, normally. When the new-found powers begin to assert themselves, they must be met with frankness and understanding—a sacred trust—a hostage to the future.

The habit of masturbation is likely to be developed during this period. The practice is certainly in bad taste and something of which no one can possibly be proud. Otherwise it is of little consequence unless the boy or girl worries about it or is degraded by it. The best that can be done is to arouse interest in other things, so that it and the memory of it will be forgotten. If masturbation caused only a small part of the ailments of which it has been accused, the human race would be in a bad way, indeed. Forget it.

Boys are frequently alarmed by the occurrence of seminal emissions or discharges of prostatic and seminal secretions while asleep. Mothers finding the stained sheets are sometimes greatly alarmed. It means nothing except that the boy is developing properly and is probably not indulging in masturbation or sexual relations. It is sometimes said that sexual relations are necessary after a certain age is reached, else the organs of the male will atrophy from disuse. Nonsense! Nature is not so dumb as to permit such a misfortune to that system which she so highly cherishes. She has provided the reproductive organs with a safety valve in the form of these seminal emissions. They are perfectly normal, and are indeed an accurate indication of proper and safe development. In the same category are the voluptuous dreams which boys and occasionally girls may experience. Think nothing of them.

Before she is twelve years old the girl should have the phenomenon of menstruation explained to her. Otherwise she is likely to be frightened by it and may be ashamed to say anything about it if she is not accustomed to confide in her mother. Formerly it was the custom of careful mothers to put their daughters to bed for a day or two at each menstrual period and to interdict all activity and bathing during this time. The girl was taught that she was "sick" and that she might expect for the next thirty years to be an invalid once a month and then to pass through a "change of life" that would probably kill her. In all too many instances the girl and woman lived up to the program expected of her. She was taught to be an invalid. Recently we have seen the absurdity of such a method, and now it is customary to go nearly as badly to the opposite extreme. The girl is told to pay no attention to it except to protect her clothing from soilage and to go ahead and do *anything* that she might otherwise do. Some girls can get by with this program just as some got by with the other.

A much more sensible approach is that which takes into consideration the altered condition of the parts but does not emphasize the condition as being morbid. Menstruation is a normal process, but in many respects approaches the pathological. Bleeding, for example, is otherwise always associated with pathology of some grade, as also is pain. The uterus of the menstruating woman is congested, and there are marked changes in the distribution of the blood; the nervous system is often considerably more unstable at such a time, and there are other evidences of altered physiology. Moderate exercise is rarely harmful; exposure to fresh air at such a time will be of no consequence unless there is chilling; bathing in warm water will rarely have a bad effect. It must be borne in mind that chilling of the skin usually tends to increase internal congestion of some sort, and so judgment must be exercised. Certainly the girl should be taught that the menstrual function is essentially physiological and that it should be treated as being such except when there is reason to believe that it is definitely pathological.

Children frequently experience rather intense love affairs. The adolescent is, of course, considerably more inclined to such attacks of "puppy love." On the other hand, some young people become so self-conscious in matters pertaining to sex that they go to the opposite extreme. Either reaction is easily understood and may be regarded as normal. Boys who are so delighted with their developing manhood are likely to become rather contemptuous of girls who have not their virile qualities, and so they sometimes think girls are quite impossible. It is not unlikely, however, that at times they may admire mightily from a distance. Girls who are becoming more careful of many little fine points of life are sometimes inclined to regard boys as being hopelessly uncouth. These reactions are also quite natural and do not presage a continuance of such feelings. As a matter of fact, rather the opposite is true as a rule, inasmuch as overreactions are common. Concerning all of these manifestations we can only say that they are normal, and strictly the affair of the individual concerned. For the rest of us, "Hands Off." The boy or girl should be allowed to develop his or her own individuality provided he or she is not taking a route that leads to deviations from what is considered to be a normal reaction.

Adolescence is a period of much dreaming and idealization. Children at this period are frequently dubbed lazy because of their propensity for dreaming and also because nature is protecting their rapidly growing and developing bodies from injury that might be inflicted by too energetic parents wishing to capitalize on the apparent—but more apparent than real—strength. The spirit of the youngster must not be injured by telling him that he is shiftless and will come to nothing. High ideals and religious motives are characteristic also of this period and may be utilized in helping to hold the young people to trends of action that may be considered safe.

THE MATING PERIOD

There comes a time in the life of every normal youth and maid when he or she is vastly interested in members of the opposite sex. The urge to mate, first in a process of courting and later in a permanent marriage, becomes the dominant factor in the determination of conduct. Older and younger persons may marvel why otherwise sensible persons should appear so foolish, but the young people themselves are intent on having their fling and their fun while they may.

In this country, particularly, the way of the lover is made easy. Young people may choose their own mates almost without help from their elders. Free choice is the inalienable right of every young person. No one is so unpopular as the stern parent who frowns on the dashing young dare-devil who for the moment sends his daughter into a state of ecstasy. In many other countries the young people have little or nothing to say about the matter and must mate according to the wishes or convenience of the parents. We are indeed glad to have this New World freedom, but it does impose a need for responsibility upon the part of the young people themselves. It is for this reason that the young people must be taught the facts of life as they are related to this subject.

Young people should be taught before the mating period is too urgently upon them that it is important indeed to look their companions over pretty carefully before allowing themselves to get too deeply involved. This is what is meant by "falling in love intelligently." We commonly speak of "falling in love" as if it were a sheer accident against which there was no protecting one's self. It is said that "love is blind," but surely this is a time for having the eyes wide open.

How may we hope to teach young people to use more discretion in the vital matter of marriage selection? Who is a suitable mate, anyway? How may one know whether the particular person is going to wear well or not? Obviously these questions are capable of being answered only in the most general of terms. Certainly the following points are extremely important:

1. The prospective mate should come from a family that is free of serious hereditary defects. Inasmuch as this is not a textbook of eugenics we shall not attempt to describe them. Furthermore, the family should be one of intelligence, industry, thrift, and such social standing as will be compatible with the status of the person making the choice.

2. The matter of the health of the individual is very important. The marrying of an invalid is a mistake that is rarely corrected. Physical attractiveness is of some importance, but exceptional beauty need not be required or particularly desired.

3. Similarity of interests and cultural background should by all means be considered. A vivacious wife and a phlegmatic husband are hardly likely to be happy. Likewise a boob, a boor, a clown, or a gigolo will be badly miscast among "in-laws" of the opposite type. Character, industry, thrift, honor, sobriety, and kindred qualities are by no means to be disregarded.

4. Education should be considered. By education we mean the ability to know what should be done in a given set of circumstances and when and how to do it. We have little respect for mere "book-learning" or diplomas in the present connection. Acceptable manners are a part of education, as are cooking, sewing, and the ability to earn funds and use them wisely.

5. It is well to know how the given individual treats the members of his or her family, and how he or she is regarded by the other members of his or her own and the opposite sex.

6. Each party should understand the attitude of the other toward children, toward sex, and toward sexual morality. When such matters are understood it would be very foolish to disregard such information in making the final decision to marry or not to marry.

7. Misgiving is sometimes expressed when the prospective husband is much larger than his mate. It is feared that she may have difficulty in giving birth to his children. This is much less serious than was formerly the case, for the good reason that obstetrical science is now far more proficient. Cæsarean section offers a solution in case trouble should arise. In general, it is better for the couple to be near the same size, but a match need not be called off because of difference of this nature. The small wife of a large man should in all cases see her physician as soon as she finds herself pregnant. If the child appears to be growing too large for safe delivery the physician has several resources which he may use.

8. An accurate inventory of cash on hand, assets, liabilities, the ability to maintain or take care of a home, and a frank understanding of the financial status is essential. By this we do not mean that we would condemn marriage to a person who is financially poor, but we are merely insisting that the situation be understood and soberly considered.

9. It will be much better if the individual has long been known and if the courtship has been long enough and under diverse conditions enough that the wearing qualities have been tested reasonably well before the marriage is actually consummated.

10. In general it will be much better if both of the mates are of the same race and social level. In some instances differences in religion, and even in politics, may cause trouble.

11. Concerning the matter of love for the individual there must be no doubt. One must be willing to make any sacrifice for the loved one, and to prefer him or her above all others. Anything short of a mutual unselfish devotion will almost surely break down in the stress and strain of married life.

It is not expected that many young people will have the discretion soberly to count the debits and credits of the suitor after the love affair has developed, but children who have had such ideals held up to them from an early age will be somewhat less likely to err in so vital a matter when they are older. Young people who understand and appreciate something of the nature of the problems of married life will be much more likely to use judgment. It is too much to expect that children who have had no instruction in sex and character will listen to their elders when they are in the heat of a fervid love affair.

Strangely enough, most parents, when they try to exert an influence upon the choice of mates which their children are making, produce an effect which is just the opposite of that which was desired. An undesirable young man brings daughter home from a function of some sort. The next morning she is questioned, and there is a scene. She is frequently told that he is worthless, good-for-nothing, and altogether impossible. She defends him, of course, and the thing is done because we come quickly to love those whom we defend. There is nothing which will so certainly drive a couple into matrimony as will the idea that the poor dear one is being mistreated and persecuted. It is human nature that we should desire that which we are told we cannot have. An uncouth young man, or a silly girl, can much more easily and certainly be eliminated by inviting him or her into the home and allowing the daughter or son to see him or her in comparison with persons of known value and merit. Many an unhappy marriage has been contracted because the young people have revolted against what they considered an infringement of their sacred right to choose.

Naturally the parent feels that he has some rights in the matter—as indeed he should have, if he has sense to be worthy of the opportunity—and as indeed he does have, if he has made the most of his opportunities in the training of the child. Does not a parent have the right to have some say as to who shall be the other parent of his grandchildren, in whom he will be tremendously interested? Does he not have some rights in saying who shall share the property which he will leave to his child? Does he not have the right to protect his child from what he believes is a disastrous marriage? The answer is that he does have some rights, but that he will have to use all the diplomacy and tact in his possession to get those rights. This is no place for the bungling despot of the home to "lay down the law" or "set his foot down." This is the prerogative of him who has spent two decades or more in preparing a son or daughter for the most important decision that he or she will ever make.

The superior experience of parents *should* make them capable of real aid to the young people, but in a great many cases the judgment of the young is much better. The mother who insists that her son or daughter shall consider social standing above everything else, and the father who demands a fat bank roll, think that they are looking after the welfare of son or daughter, but are really setting up obstacles which will be cleared with difficulty if at all. Loveless, sordid marriages made with an eye on the bank book will rarely be made by the young people themselves, and may be regarded as a legal form of prostitution. On the other hand, young people are rather prone to the "love-at-first-sight" sort of infatuation which may lead them into hasty, ill-considered marriages which rarely turn out well.

A difficult matter in modern courtship is that concerning the payment of expenses. Formerly it was possible for a couple to spend evening after evening in the most delightful companionship without the expenditure of a cent. There were no shows to attend, no gasoline to buy, no sodas, no expensive presents, no boxes of candy, no flowers. Now the matter of expense is one of considerable consequence. As likely as not the girl is earning as much or nearly as much as the man, but the old relic of chivalry demands that the man shall pay the bill and that he shall be ever so generous. Many girls are slipping a coin— or a bill—to the boy-friend sometimes, or are asking him not to spend more than is absolutely necessary, but there are others of the "give-me" type who are bleeding their consorts to the limit and are looking for boys with fat allowances and beautiful cars.

It is most unfortunate that there are expenses to be considered. Sometimes girls have been led to believe that they are under obligation to repay in ways that are destructive to morals and character. So long as the girl was entertaining in her own home, and furnishing lemonade or home-made fudge, she might bid her suitor begone when he made improper proposals; when, however, she has accepted a theater ticket, a soda, and an automobile ride and finds herself miles away from home in her friend's car, the situation is considerably more complicated, and it is not a matter of astonishment that an inexperienced girl who wishes to continue the theater parties, sodas, and rides will sometimes solve the problem in the wrong way. There is also a strong temptation for a sexually aggressive young man to take advantage of the situation. He reasons that he should have something in compensation for the outlay he has made. Being uninstructed in sex ideals, as are most boys, the form of the compensation desired is easily guessed.

Certain organizations in the large cities are giving parties and entertainments which will have the effect of throwing young people together with the express purpose of making it possible for courtship to progress as naturally as possible. Coeducational colleges serve a most useful purpose in this connection. Various church organizations and societies serve the same end. Rooming houses and girls' dormitories usually have some sort of parlor where a degree of privacy may be had. Private homes should give some thought to the matter of providing a place where the daughter may be the hostess and therefore in control of the situation. A midnight lunch from the family ice box will be deeply appreciated by the young chap who has none too much money to spend. It will also put him under a wholesome obligation to be a gentleman, whereas under a different set of circumstances the girl might feel obliged to repay him for favors received.

The matter of privacy is one of some consequence. In this country a young couple expects as their right a degree of privacy which is nearly equal to that which they will enjoy after they are actually married. Whether this is right or wrong, there is apparently little or nothing that can be done about it. To deny it would be to drive them to places where they could get privacy under much less favorable circumstances, or to appear to persecute them, which would have the effect of making them tend to wish to abuse whatever opportunities for privacy they might have. The use of a living room from which other members of the family are not entirely and rigidly excluded would seem to be a proper medium.

Interesting is the fact that the city mother used to worry when she had reason to believe that her daughter was alone with her friend on country roads. All sorts of terrible possibilities arose to worry her, though she felt no such qualms when the couple were together in the city. The country mother, on the other hand, thought nothing of her daughter driving alone with a young man in the country, but was afraid for them to go to the city unless someone went with them. Each mother rather intuitively understood that the young people were most in danger when they were in unfamiliar surroundings. Now that the distinction between city and country has mostly been wiped out, this reaction of mothers is less familiar, but it is still a fact that the young people are most likely to get into trouble when they are treading unfamiliar territory. This is the reason why they should be instructed thoroughly—but not morbidly—in matters pertaining to sex. Just as a democracy must educate the citizens who are the electorate, so must we educate our young people in these matters if we are safely to allow them the privacy that is customary in this country.

Some have supposed that they can control the relation of the two sexes by the use of chaperons. It is true that they can control the more obvious forms of indecency, but that is all. A chaperon thinks that she is saving the virtue of a girl when she compels a couple to use some restraint in their dancing positions. If the possible results were not so serious the idea would be humorous. The couple that wishes to dance in an indecent manner will not be restrained by a chaperon who all too often has been a prim dowager who hasn't the slightest idea what the whole thing is about. We need chaperons, and lots of them, but the chaperons should be *built into the character of the young people themselves;* otherwise they are simply figureheads who believe that there is no mischief simply because they have seen none. The conventional chaperon, of course, serves a useful purpose when she prevents couples who are improper from suggesting such activity to those who otherwise would have had no thought of it.

We must remember that our young people are already tremendously stimulated. We give them dancing lessons early so that they will quickly pass through the awkward age; we show them stimulating and *risqué* motion pictures; we have on our tables books that are written to sell and consequently made as "sexy" as possible; we scoff at conventions and laws which do not happen to suit our tastes; we wink at vice, graft, and illicit liaisons. After stimulating our young people in such manner, we set up economic and cultural standards which will not permit them to marry until they are much older than was the evident biological intention of Nature. According to Nature's standards a couple is ready to marry when fifteen or sixteen years old, but the requirements of conventional society set the time much later. Under such circumstances we marvel that there is no more immorality than there is.

Love between the two sexes is a pure and fine emotion, but those who cast their pearls before swine will soon lose them. For an individual to simulate the expressions of deep affection when such feelings are really not held is to invite an inevitable deterioration of character which will eventually rob that individual of the power of fine and noble emotions of this sort. A girl will soon find herself marked as one who has been pawed over; a boy will soon lose his respect for clean and sweet womanhood. Marriage for the sordid purposes of fortune and social position is an unclean thing which soon soils its nest. He who cheapens so precious an emotion as love will rue it if he has any of the finer sensibilities. He who sincerely and deeply loves another and who has earned the right to legitimate favors is entitled to them, but this presupposes that he would wish to bestow his affection only upon the favored one and has a legal right to do so.

Marriage is of such consequence that it should be carefully considered. The couple expecting to make such a contract should thoroughly discuss every phase of the subject before doing so. All reliable sources of information should be sought, and notes should be compared. Each should frankly tell the other what he or she expects. The desirability or undesirability of having children must be thoroughly threshed out before going ahead. Agreement upon a marriage date that will fit into the menstrual cycle may well be made. Arrangement for the use of contraceptives in the early days of the marriage, and an understanding of such use, is rather important unless the couple is willing to assume the possibility of pregnancy before they are ready for it. If the bride-to-be is anxious that sexual relations not be consummated at once, that point should be understood beforehand—and respected afterwards.

There is nothing finer and more beautiful, nothing more useful, nothing more pure than those prenuptial agreements and arrangements which insure that the couple are really ready to marry and to assume the sacred obligations which marriage entails.

THE HONEYMOON

The honeymoon is the period between the marriage ceremony and the time when the young people shall have become more or less settled into the routine of a married couple. It is frequently used to designate a trip that is taken for the purpose of getting away from prying eyes. It is a period of adjustment to the new regimen and may be wisely or unwisely spent. Not a few marriages are utterly wrecked during this time, and a great many others are so strained as to weaken or damage the prospect of future happiness and usefulness. It is a time of high emotional tension and needs to be rather soberly considered. The obvious purpose of the honeymoon is to grant to the newly married lovers an unusual degree of privacy while they are experimenting with the new status in which they find themselves.

It is unfortunate that there have grown up so many ugly customs about so beautiful a thing as a wedding. Pranks without number are played upon the couple; many of these pranks are in exceedingly bad taste, and not a few are positively indecent, or dangerous.

Wealthy families are inclined to make much of a wedding. There are parties, showers, receptions, and elaborate ceremonies, and finally a long and tiresome honeymoon is planned. A trip to Europe or a tour around the world seems like an ideal wedding present, but is entirely too long and tiresome. On such a trip the lovers are thrown entirely too much into each other's company and may utterly exhaust themselves and their interest in each other. The fatigue of travel and of sight-seeing, added to the strain of adjustment and the enervating effects of excessive sexual exercise, is entirely too much. It would be better if the trip were short and the demands made upon physical and emotional resources were light. A cabin in the woods, or a room at a summer or a winter resort, according to season, is likely to be much better. It is easy also for the pair to lose themselves in a large city, where hotels afford any degree of seclusion that may be desired, and the myriad diversions of the city furnish opportunity for any degree of activity that may be needed.

Families in moderate circumstances often exceed their means in attempting to give their young people a big and elaborate wedding and trip. The worry as to whether the funds will hold out, and the consciousness that the rocket-like celebration is going to end with a thud, make a bad start. Better no honeymoon at all than one that cannot be afforded.

The most important relations of the period, however, are not those which are commonly called the honeymoon. They are those which take place in the very first days and nights of married life. The happiness and even the health of the couple may be seriously crippled by the bungling caresses of one who is not ready for real marriage or is utterly lacking in understanding of the processes involved.

Biologic marriage and conventional marriage have entirely different purposes, but the two are supplementary to each other and are best consummated at approximately the same time. In case the biologic marriage has lagged and one or another of the pair is not ready for the actual union, the process of courtship should continue until the mate—usually the bride—is really ready for sexual relations. Theoretically, legal marriage gives each the right to the body of the other, and many men have been crass enough to insist on those rights as soon as the privacy of the bedroom has been reached. Embarrassed, shocked, frightened, and even sometimes subjected to physical pain, the bride is essentially forced by one who has but a short time before promised to love and cherish her. Under such circumstances she is set against the whole process and, indeed, may never learn to take a normal attitude toward a relation which should be exquisitely pleasurable to both partners. In a short time the husband, being disappointed in the fact that his wife is no longer a lover, may become disgusted and seek mistresses who can take an interest in such things. Modesty is fine and splendid, but a ruined marriage is too big a price to pay for *mock* modesty.

Every prospective bridegroom should understand that, unless he has positive and first-hand assurance to the contrary, the bride may probably wish to delay the climax of the ceremony which has just been performed. Brides without previous sexual experience may be reluctant indeed, in spite of the fact that they are intensely in love with their new husbands. In such case there is nothing for the *gentleman* to do but bide his time and divert himself in the gallant and romantic manner which has so far won her approval that she has been willing to take his name, and share her life with him. The rights which the law gives him are as worthless as dust until they have been ratified by her approval. "Women first" is the code of the gentleman. If this fact could be impressed on the consciousness of bridegrooms most of them would be only too glad to wait until the loved one is ready to invite his amorous advances. Young people, when newly married, are in a highly idealistic and romantic state and are more liberal and unselfish probably than at any other time in their lives. But the young man, being intensely stimulated himself and never having been told that the feeling of the bride may be different, supposes that she as well as he is eager to bring about the consummation of their marriage. If she is so, very well! There is not the least reason for formality in cases where courting has progressed to such a stage. When, however, the bride is reluctant, courtship must be continued, and courtship only.

All or most of these difficulties can be avoided by a frank prenuptial understanding. The couple who are so excessively modest that they cannot discuss this subject had better grow up a little, learn something about themselves, and really get in love before going ahead with a wedding. If the girl seems reluctant, her fiancé can make her happy and reassured if he will promise her that he will consider her wishes in these matters as well after marriage as before. She, in turn, should assure him that she understands the purpose and nature of marriage, and that she will do her best to become interested in that which is so vital to happiness and unity.

In times past there is reason to believe that such an understanding has often not been attained, and that a green, inexperienced, awkward youth and a shy, embarrassed, undeveloped girl were commonly thrown together in utter ignorance of all the arts of conjugal life. Such, indeed, was considered to be the ideal condition, and mothers were prone to boast that their daughters knew absolutely nothing about such matters. It is no wonder that so many marriages went on the rocks. Probably the only reason that so many escaped is that the daughters were rarely so dumb as fond mamma supposed. Young people are much better prepared in this respect for marriage nowadays. There are opportunities to learn; there is a vocabulary in which they may speak to their prospective mates; there are books, pamphlets, and lectures from which they may learn much; and in most instances there is the practice of those intimacies which are the proper prelude to marriage.

Sheer clothing, athletic uniforms, and brief bathing suits have accustomed both sexes to the general appearance of the body of the other sex. It is to be hoped that this has helped greatly to prevent excessive embarrassment in the act of disrobing, and that it also will tend to temper somewhat the excitement of one or both. To one who stands in great reverence of the significance of the marriage relation it seems that a couple intensely in love and entering into a relation of such significance and beauty might find an exquisite delight in coming frankly and gladly together devoid of every covering and artifice. This is no time for silly giggling and undressing in the closet. It is a time for truth, dignity, and that fine sense of self-respect that is proud to proclaim to all the world that this man and this woman are grown up and are taking their places in the long line of those who have lived and loved, and have nourished and cherished the spark of life that has come down without a break since the day of Creation.

The accomplishment of the first act of sexual congress is by no means without its hazards. In case the male organ is of unusual size care will need to be taken, particularly if the wife is small. After some time adjustment will be made and normal relations may be assumed, but until that time the husband may have to practise restraint. The first union will be facilitated considerably if some lubricant is used. Vaseline will serve in this capacity, but a surgical jelly is better. The hymen of the young wife will occasionally present real difficulty: it is so resistant in some instances that considerable pressure may be required to break it. In rare cases it may even require the aid of a physician to remove this obstruction. Occasionally there will be some pain, and there may be slight bleeding as a result of the first union. When such is the case the greatest care must be taken, and the wife should by all means be granted the privilege of being the active party. An aggressive husband essentially attacking a sensitive, frightened, and unprepared wife and hurting her may jeopardize the reasonable hope of a full and happy married life. He must let her be the aggressor while he with infinite patience and tenderness is still the gentle lover subject to her slightest whim.

Concerning the hymen there is need of exact information, else innocent wives may be accused of having had previous sexual experience. At one time the intact hymen was considered an infallible proof of virginity. It is now known that many virgins have lost the hymen as a result of athletic activities, accident, horseback riding, or manipulations incident to bathing. Ignorance of these facts has many times caused the most cruel injustices to be committed.

Many people who should know better suppose that all of these delicate relations can be trusted entirely to the instincts and that for this reason there is no need to discuss them. Nothing could be further from the truth. Nature has furnished us with certain instincts, it is true, but they are the "law of the jungle." It is these instincts which have caused so much trouble in times past for the reason that instinct is utterly disregardful of anything except the desire of the male to consummate sexual relations at every possible opportunity, and to bring about fertilization as quickly as possible. As well go back to the practice of clubbing our wives into unconsciousness and chaining them to the tent pole to keep them from running away. Modern marriage is—or should be—on a different basis. In no other species than man is the pleasure or welfare of the female given more consideration than is necessary to gain her physical acquiescence, but man is more than a beast and should behave accordingly.

Because sexual relations as they are practiced by men and women serve another function than merely that of reproduction they cannot be successfully practised from instinct alone. They are of the nature of an art; they express fine and noble emotions just as do the other arts. Because they constitute an art they must be learned and practised before a high degree of proficiency may be attained. Even after many years a well-matched couple may still be improving in technic and in appreciation of the legitimate pleasures of conjugal love. There are books to be had which give the most detailed description of every phase of the copulative function, but one can hardly expect to learn to play the piano by reading about it. If definite difficulties arise, such information may be of service, but otherwise the couple should be somewhat less sophisticated in the early stages of the honeymoon period. It is only necessary that both remember that *the act is perfectly proper* and that the spirit of love demands that *each shall show the utmost solicitude for the comfort, happiness, and pleasure of the other*. With this as a guide it is hard to suppose that many marriages could go wrong.

THE YOUNG MARRIED COUPLE

Much has been said about the advisability of the wife working after marriage. Until the couple can get a start there can certainly be no objection to the wife's holding her former job or getting another one. It will mean extra hours of work and less leisure now that she has the care of a home or an apartment, but it is all for the good of the cause. It would be a poor wife, indeed, who would not put her shoulder to the family wheel and help to make it turn.

Unfortunately, however, there is more to the matter than just that. It will be hard later for her to give up the outside job and devote herself exclusively to home-making with its comparatively intangible rewards. We need not be surprised that she is loath to give up the independence that comes with a check at the end of the week. There are so many things that are needed and can be had only if the wife as well as the husband earns.

So it is customary to put off, and put off, and put off the real purpose and culmination of marriage—children. If two have trouble making ends meet with two salaries—as two commonly do—how shall three or four or five live on one salary? And so by sex repression, which often eats into the hearts of both, by the use of more or less distasteful contraceptive methods, or sometimes by resort to criminal abortion, the couple more or less successfully cheats Mother Nature of her due. From month to month, with fear and hope combined, the coming of the menses is awaited as if its failure would be a world-wide catastrophe. Years pass, and the couple are still in need of both pay checks. Educated tastes have been developed and seemingly must be pampered; children are forgotten, or are pushed farther and farther into the future. Usually they say that "some day" they want children but hardly see how they can manage it just yet. "Some day" they are going to have beautiful blue-eyed boys and golden-haired girls, but when "some day" comes Nature has all too often become tired of being turned away, and the Gate of Life is closed.

It is hard to criticize a couple who gradually work their way into this predicament. Nothing could seem more logical than that they should have made the decisions as they did. Society as it exists in a civilized community puts a premium on the childless marriage. Just the same, such a ménage is not really a home. After a generation of such homes there would be nothing. The error that young people are so likely to make is to believe that parties, shows, elegant furniture, and sport roadsters can bring more happiness than children. Once they have had the children they would know that nothing can bring the soul-satisfying rapture that a baby brings, but, of course, they haven't had such experience, and quite naturally cannot fully appreciate it. Such marriages are easily broken. With no children, with little property investment as a rule, with both having an income, the slightest friction is likely to cause a serious split. Interesting is the fact that families in which the wife continues to work for years after marriage rarely become well-to-do. If the husband had had to shoulder the responsibility of a growing family he might have waded in and made more of his opportunities. Breezing along, though, with the help of the wife, he has taken it easy and got nowhere.

If the wife works there should be a definite understanding concerning the time when she shall be promoted to the much more important work of real home-making. Marriages when both parties are poor but in good health and willing to work are frequently the very best of marriages. Stories told of the hard times that grandfather and grandmother had in the old days are familiar family lore, and will be a century hence. We frequently see the young wife working to help her husband complete his education, and it makes a most inspiring picture. Likewise, the wife may continue her education after marriage. These are the young people who know what an education is. They will get along.

Health is of the utmost importance to the welfare of the home builders. In the first place, only those who have health are fit to marry. It is foolish indeed for a young person to marry an invalid or semi-invalid—immensely romantic in some instances, and highly idealistic, but nevertheless foolish. It is much like marrying a drunkard to reform him. Better reform him first! Besides, it is most selfish for a sick person to fasten himself or herself upon another person and call it love. Marriage is a big job at the best. It is entirely too much for sick people. When sickness comes after marriage, as of course it is probable that it will eventually come, there is nothing that honor can condone except to see it through, but even so it may and often does utterly wreck the family.

There are several particular health hazards which must be considered by people of this age group. Tuberculosis finds in them its most susceptible victims. The bearing, nursing, and caring for children undermines occasionally the health of the mother, particularly if the children come too close together. Hard work on the part of both in the years when they are so anxious to get a start, accepting extra jobs, taking few vacations, worrying, and falling for the temptation to avoid the expense of doctors' bills when there is real need for professional attention, all take their toll. Nervous breakdown from overwork, pneumonia, organic heart disease, occupational diseases, and other related conditions are prone to attack this group. Health is a matter of much more than personal concern to these people. It involves the welfare of the entire family and for that reason deserves to be considered seriously in this place. What one of us has not heard our fathers and mothers wondering, "What will become of us if one of us should get sick?"

Life, accident, and health insurance have proved themselves of the greatest possible consequence in solving the problems which inevitably arise when health is impaired. It is said that the total amount of life insurance in force in the United States is well over *two hundred and sixty billion dollars*. The effect of such a fund is beyond comprehension. As soon as the family can possibly afford to do so, investment should be made in some form of time-tried insurance. When there are children there is particular need of such protection.

In this place we need no more than mention the importance of a firm economic basis for so important an institution as the family. Unless there is a dependable income, unless the housewife and her husband know how to manage so as to keep within that income and have a little to spare for savings, there is trouble ahead. A savings account, a house to live in, a few life insurance policies and other conservative investments, are essential to the welfare of a home. It may seem a little strange that these should be mentioned in a discussion of sex education, but in the sense that we are using the term they are as much a part of the program of raising a family as is the incident which is commonly regarded as sex. The need of such resources should be understood by children and young people. Everything which helps young people to understand the problems of a family is in a very true sense sex education.

One of the biggest questions which the young couple must decide is that concerning children. Will there be children? And, if so, how many? There are, to be sure, many excellent reasons why a particular couple should not desire children at a given time, and there are even reasons why they should not have them at all. There is, for example, the couple which dares not have children because of some hereditary taint or disease. They act wisely in taking precautions which will prevent conception. On the other hand, it is most unfortunate that they did not find out about such matters before marriage and act accordingly. A given couple may feel that the health of one or the other is such that the burden of parenthood should not be added. This is, of course, a legitimate reason, though many of these persons were ill before marriage, and because of that unfit for marriage. The economic position of the family is often such that children might be endangered by being brought into the home at such a time.

We have no desire to say what should be the size of family which a given couple should seek. Circumstances will need to be consulted. It requires an average of more than three children to the couple for a given stratum of society to maintain itself numerically inasmuch as some die before marriage and others do not marry. Any family of less than four is, then, on the average, falling behind. This is a serious matter or not, according as the group is a useful one or not. Unfortunately, those families which should have no children sometimes have many, and those that might be expected to bear and rear superior children too often have few or none. The loss to society is great, and the loss to the individuals themselves is even greater.

For those couples who cannot for some reason bear children there are infinite possibilities in the adoption of orphans. With care the adopted child that has come from a good family has an even chance with the blood descendant of the same age and physical opportunity. It cannot be shown that adopted children turn out worse than others. They may on the average do better, when they have been carefully selected. A careful physical and mental examination should be made of all children who are being considered for adoption. Couples without children may also satisfy their parental instincts and do a great service by taking up some phase of work which has to do with the welfare of children and young people. It is the only way to stay young and keep sweet. "Suffer little children to come unto Me and forbid them not, for of such is the Kingdom of Heaven" is no idle dogma. It is the essence of life.

The care of the children after they are born is enormously important. It is discussed in succeeding chapters of this work.

There are many problems which are sexual in the sense that the term is usually used. A husband and wife, a man and woman, in vigorous health and living in the intimacy which is properly granted to a married couple, have many opportunities for expressions of love and affection. Shall we deny them the privileges of sexuality except for purposes of reproduction? Certainly not! They will need to learn well the art of love so that they may know the exquisite pleasures of conjugal love. The stability of the marriage will depend largely on this ability, though, of course, there are other factors serving toward this end.

In most cases where there is dissatisfaction with the conjugal relation at this stage in life the cause is to be found in the fact that women are more slowly aroused and require a longer time for gratification than is the case of the man. Husbands are prone to forget that courtship is as necessary after marriage as before. Quickly aroused and quickly satisfied, they are inclined to forget that the partner in everything else should also have her share in the emotions of sex, else she will become disgusted and intolerant of the whole process. Part of the trouble is also due to the fact that a large percentage of women suppose that sex gratification is not for them and that there is something akin to vulgarity in any manifestation of pleasure or interest in it. With the husband as considerate as he should be and the wife convinced of the propriety of legitimate conjugal relations there should be little difficulty in building a sex life that will bind the family together with hoops of steel.

Considerable effort has been made to determine in an accurate way the limits of safe and proper sexual indulgence. The frequency with which the act may be safely performed without injury to health or vigor is not something that can be reduced to formula. It will vary widely in different couples, and it is impossible for an outsider to set out rules. So long as the act is mutually pleasurable, and both the partners are able to go about the usual day's work without unusual fatigue or lassitude, it is evident that no harm is being done. In case either partner feels the strain, moderation must be practised. The average among Americans is probably about two to three times a week. As in the case of everything else, it is better to err on the side of too little than too much. No one would wish to give up the pleasure of eating food, but everyone is disgusted with gluttony. Hardly anything can be so revolting as sexual gluttony. The love embrace is too sacred a thing to be made common.

In practically every family at some time it is considered best that conception should not take place in the immediate future. Improper methods may on one hand fail to control the size of the family, or on the other may cheat the couple of such sexual experience as is essential to health and happiness. The pair that lives in constant fear of pregnancy can hardly be happy and can hardly go about the business and pleasure of living in a way that makes for good family life. There are individuals who by virtue of strong wills, or who by lack of the normal desires, may solve this problem by refraining entirely from intercourse, but the vast majority of couples cannot go along happily on such a regimen. In such case, one or the other of the pair is likely to seek gratification outside of the family, and a whole train of dangerous possibilities is set up forthwith.

Common opinion takes it for granted that sexual appetite is something that cannot be controlled. It is astonishing how many people suppose that a "red-blooded" individual is utterly at the mercy of any sexual passion that may chance to blow. The attitude of irresponsibility for sexual misconduct is a convenient alibi for those who have not the strength of character to stand by their ideals—if any. Such is not a strong and manly attitude, but is a sign of weakness in those who cannot or will not be strong. It isn't smart, or strong, or clever, or evidence of broadmindedness; it is a blow at the very heart of society and the home. A yellow cur can follow any vagrant female who may pass. Indeed a yellow cur *will* do just that.

Marriage is not a lark. There is no more serious business in all the world than that of building a home and rearing children. Prospective husbands and wives had better grow up before undertaking the honorable responsibilities that come to those who assume the social and biological status known as marriage. When happily consummated and honestly lived it is tremendously effective in bringing into being the happiest and most satisfying of all human relationships.

Sex in Middle and Advanced Life

Most men and women experience a considerable shock as they approach and pass the age of forty. They have learned to look upon "fat and forty" as being the zero hour of romance. As young people they have supposed that one so old has lost every good reason for living. To be a solid burgher or thrifty housewife of forty has been supposed to be the end of everything, and now to find one's self at the halfway place in life or a little beyond seems incredible. Actually, however, a large percentage of people are happier after this age than before. Particularly is this true of those who have lived and loved wisely and well. The individual who can adjust his life and thinking to the fact that he is no longer a gay and irresponsible young thing will find many compensations for the fact that he can no longer swim across the lake or beat the young fellows at tennis. The woman who can relax a bit at this time and smile indulgently at the mad struggle for beauty and youth has before her many happy days of comparative quiet and serenity.

Of great importance in this process of adjustment is that which has to do with sex. Ordinarily people of forty and above do not bear children. A few children are born of mothers above this age, but it is a rather risky adventure, as some of the children are hardly up to the standard of their brothers and sisters born at a more vigorous period of life. A small percentage of these children are likely to be defective and are called "exhaustion products." It is also said that an unusual number of these children are of exceptional ability, but the likelihood is rather in the direction first mentioned. Men may continue to be fertile for a long time past the forty mark, but there is some objection to men being fathers after they are much above forty. The possibility that the children will be left orphans in such case is quite obvious.

Are we to suppose, then, that all of the functions of the reproductive apparatus have been filled? Not at all. Usually there are children to be raised. The family still has a purpose. Couples who have enjoyed the embraces of earlier life will still continue to enjoy them and will not need to consider the possibility of pregnancy and additional children with their many responsibilities. With the children from underfoot it is not unusual to see a couple much more attached to each other than when they were so busy. It is, indeed, not unusual to see them almost like two young lovers, or perhaps more often as Darby and Joan contentedly living a life of placid, uneventful domesticity.

It is difficult for younger people to see in this period anything but a tiresome and monotonous existence, and there are many who find themselves at forty or above in an openly rebellious attitude. They want one more fling at "life" and may do foolish things in the effort to get it. The man who has been circumspect and careful about all such matters may get sympathetic for himself and think he has missed a great deal. Somewhat bored with the faithful but unromantic wife, he is prone to yearn for a younger and more vivacious companion. If some degree of affluence has rewarded his labors, he is in a position to indulge himself—and be an easy mark for gold-diggers who really hold him in contempt. Occasionally a woman of forty retains her youth better than her husband and may be tempted to "step out" a bit with a snappy "gigolo" or a neighbor whose "wife doesn't understand him." She yearns for a lover instead of a tired workhorse who prefers his house slippers and shirt sleeves to a "tux" and a ballroom. It is not unlikely that this period offers more urgent temptations than does any other. Certain it is that the opportunities for making a fool of one's self during this time are unexcelled.

Likewise the unmarried person of this age is in danger. The unmarried woman who is approaching the end of what would and should have been the reproductive period of her life sees her youth slipping. Until this time she has usually hoped that the opportunity for family life would come, but she now rapidly resigns herself to the prospect of a lonesome and not unlikely bitter old age. She feels cheated. Life is going without ever having really bloomed or borne fruit. Something of the same feeling is experienced by married couples who have had no children. Fortunate indeed are such childless persons who have attained a vicarious parenthood either by adopting children or by interesting themselves in the children of their friends or in young people. It is easy for unattached persons to be self-centered and in this way to become the typical "old maid." Mothers do not become "old maids" for the good reason that they are more interested in their children than they are in themselves. Because they are interested in other people, other people are interested in them, and everyone has a good time. In case the opportunity for marriage first comes in middle or advanced age, the problem of adjustment will be difficult, to say the least.

It is not uncommon to hear men say that when they are no longer interested in a pretty face or figure they will be ready to die—life will no longer be worth living. The loss of virility in men is looked on as a calamity of the highest degree. Such an attitude reveals an utter lack of understanding of the real meaning of life.

Loss of virility is Nature's way of insuring against "exhaustion products"; it is her way of making sure that fathers will probably live until the work of rearing the child is accomplished; it is her protection for the weakened and wasted organs of the body which in the wear and tear of life have likely become injured to such an extent that ardent wooing and frequent sexual embraces are exhausting. What a fool is the man who seeks rejuvenation by some sort of gland operation or transplantation! Even if gland transplantations were successful, which they are not, little good could come from such meddling. It is like putting a powerful new motor into a rickety old chassis in the expectation of roaring along at eighty m.p.h. Of course something breaks—usually an artery in the brain—and there is real trouble. "New wine in old bottles" has been a dangerous combination for so long that it looks as if the fact might be better appreciated.

The elderly widower gets himself a young wife. How can a young woman be really in love with a man thirty or forty years her senior? For that matter, how can a man of that age who understands things be truly in love with a young woman? Ten years more will find him an old man while she will be just starting. Clashes between the wife and his children—as old as she perhaps—are inevitable. The suspicion that she loves his money rather than him; the fear that she may be stepping out with younger men; the painful effort to entertain her as a young wife deserves to be entertained; the fear that children may be borne at a period in life when children would be a burden; and a dozen other fears real and imaginary, take away every iota of the tranquillity that should be the heritage of him who has lived long. Much wiser indeed is he who chooses a companion who is near his own age.

Respect for gray hairs is a duty of the young. It is even more the duty of those who have the gray hairs. The young people are right when they tell grandma to "be her age." By this we do not mean that men and women of middle age should don the funereal black that used to be the custom, and that they should fold their hands and get ready to die. Quite the contrary! Dyeing the hair, having face-lifting operations, refusing to wear the glasses that they need, nervously driving themselves to act as if they were mere girls, these wretched men and women fool no one and wear themselves out trying to make the stream of life start over at the source. If it could be done there would be some excuse for the effort, but of course they always lose. Almost any young girl can be pretty or even beautiful, but it takes a "heap o' livin'" to make a beautiful old face. The lines of age are simply the character lines that have been developed through years of habitual smiling; or frowning; and constitute real beauty—or ugliness. The beauty of youth is skin deep, but the beauty of age really goes to the bone.

There is nothing which is so capable of building real character as a full understanding and appreciation of sex and its obligations. In times past women have been taught to avoid sex as if it were vulgar and ugly. In consequence, many of them, as soon as they were married, have been careless of their personal appearance and have grown into the slatternly, careless type which is still seen everywhere about us. Some of them have seemed rather to be proud of the fact that they were unattractive. Ugliness has been supposed to be a sign of virtue or of something or other; it has removed them from temptation—most effectively.

The opposite extreme, and one that is just as disgusting, is the woman who never forgets her "sex appeal" and goes to every sort of artificial means to hold her youthful appearance and her "come hither" attitude toward the male sex. Life to many of these women seems to be nothing except a struggle against the onslaughts of age. Hours are spent with hairdressers, skin experts, and beauty doctors of all sorts. Sex to these women has not meant the bearing of children, as a rule. They have emphasized that phase of the program which is merely a preliminary to the real purpose, and in consequence is shallow and superficial. On the other hand, the woman who has loved her mate frankly and honorably, who has borne and reared his and her children, who has sacrificed everything for her loved ones, who has borne pain for them, who has known the pangs of unutterable dread and fear when they were in danger, who has felt her heart bursting with pride of them, who has smiled when she wanted to cry, who has loved and lived, develops in middle and advanced life a beauty which is the beauty of the Madonna.

For those who are at middle age and are capable of reading it, nothing is so valuable as a little book by Aldred Scott Warthin, for forty years professor of pathology at the University of Michigan. The book is entitled *Old Age* and is the life philosophy of Dr. Warthin written when he was old and wise. It is for the intelligent layman and is written in nontechnical language. Unfortunately it is out of print but may be found in many public libraries. Warthin points out that at every age some part of the body is old and worn out and is making way for something else. Even before birth some parts have atrophied and have made way for growing structures. At the time of birth the senile "afterbirth" or placenta is dropped as worn out and no longer needed. It has served its purpose and is cast aside as useless baggage. The thymus of the child is old, or should be, when the child is adolescent; the womb and the ovaries are old at forty-five; the prostate and the testicles are commonly old in the sixties; the body as a whole is old at seventy or shortly thereafter. Those who are religiously inclined—and religion is a great asset at this or any other age—will see in old age and death a further sublimation in which the earthly body is dropped, as was the afterbirth, as being a useless encumbrance to the spirit, which is immortal.

Senility and death are seen by Dr. Warthin as being perfectly natural processes provided they do not come too soon. Death is, indeed, quite as necessary as birth. If there were no deaths there soon could be no births, because the earth would be full and running over with old people living in the past. The aged must make room for those who are younger and more vigorous. Even death is in this view a part of the reproductive act. We must do our best to get our children ready to do the work of the world, and then we must get out of the way so that they can do it. Unjust? Not at all! As young people we took the places of those who were older and as old people ourselves we can expect the same inevitable fate. In the relay race that is life each runner is expected to do his best and then pass the torch to his successor. Having done so, he can perform a last and valuable service by getting out of the way and taking care of himself in such a way as will not divert the attention of the one who is at the time carrying the responsibilities of the race. Everyone who understands the purpose of life knows that "the game is the thing." It's a poor sport that wants to carry the ball every time and unwillingly submits to a substitution when the coach calls him to the bench.

A philosophy of this sort is more than may reasonably be expected of those who are constantly thinking of themselves and are ever and only looking for their own pleasure and advantage. To some it will seem harsh. Those who have children should understand, however, and should be glad to make way for their children—just as they have always made way for their children in other matters. Even this, then, is a part of the reproductive instinct, using the term in its broadest sense. Inasmuch as the end of life must come, it is much better to be philosophical about it and not be like a small boy who has eaten his cake and is crying because he cannot still have it.

The purpose of life is not primarily that we as individuals shall be royally entertained. It is too much to suppose that God, or Nature, or Call-it-what-you-will has created the universe in order that we as as individuals may have full stomachs and sexual gratification. Obviously one of the purposes of life is that the species may be propagated. Another, apparently, is that we may use our wits to control the forces of Nature about us and possibly make something of ourselves. A misunderstanding of the real purpose of preventive and curative medicine and of life itself is responsible for a great deal of trouble and worry. Under our present system, for example, a physician is obliged—and rarely questions the essential wisdom of it—to save and pro-long human life as long as possible. He is honor bound to keep the idiot alive, though the life may be worse than useless. The physician can do no less, and we would not wish him to do otherwise, but the real emphasis should be upon the preservation and creation of those individuals who will be an asset to the community and the race. It is not that we object to saving of the lives of human derelicts, but rather that we wish to emphasize the main ob-jective, the improvement of the general average.

It is commonly said that health is more important than anything else. This is exactly the same sort of false philosophy that is responsible for the des-pondency which comes to those who are attaining advanced age. Health is not, or should not be, an end in itself but merely a means to an end. The earnest parent is anxious to remain well, not so much because he or she is afraid to suffer as that he or she wants to be able to take care of the children until they are able to take care of themselves. When a parent dies the neigh-bors lament not so much the loss of a friend and neighbor as they look with apprehension upon the fact that he or she left little children. The parent who would not jeopardize his own health or safety for the sake of his child is not a real parent but a miserable imitation. And so the aged person who appre-ciates and understands his rôle is much happier and more reconciled to the part which he must play whether he likes it or not.

The individual with this outlook will be buffered against the shock that comes at the age of forty, and the despondency which comes at a later age when it seems that everything is going to pot when actually it is merely the changing of the guard. He will see in his waning sexual powers a reason and a purpose, and will therefore more easily be content that it should be so. He is willing to allow someone else to carry the ball, and is happy if the cause for which he has lived and fought is being advanced by the younger and stronger hands of those who come after.

THE PURPOSE OF MARRIAGE

From the standpoint of society, the real purpose of marriage is the creation of a home into which children may be born legitimately and reared in decency and self-respect. We do not mean by this statement that young people should have in mind only such a purpose in the selection of a mate, but we do mean that they should carefully consider the responsibilities of parenthood before they enter into a relation of such consequence. The fitness of a given individual to be a father or a mother is ultimately more important than the fitness of the same individual to be merely a husband or wife, though both are of the greatest consequence.

The prospective bride or bridegroom should consider the family tree of himself or herself and of the preferred mate. It will be well to consider whether or not a given man is likely to be able to provide for a family, or whether a given girl is of the domestic or maternal type who will enjoy caring for babies. The couple contemplating marriage should frankly discuss the probability of children being born and should come to some agreement in such matters before the ceremony of marriage has been performed. It will be well also if by some means they may attempt to determine whether or not they are probably sexually compatible. In other words, young people should "fall in love intelligently," a phrase which has been much ridiculed by those who believe that love and marriage should never be considered in any other light than that of the moon. Many will protest that we are seeking to take the romance out of marriage. On the contrary, we are really trying to preserve the romance so that it may last and last and last. In our observation the marriages which have been carefully worked out are more likely to be permanently and solidly "romantic" than those which have been consummated in a fever of something or other which passes in the moonlight as true love.

It is the nature of the young of the species to desire the company of the members of the opposite sex. In our eagerness to disclaim everything related to sex we have tried to make ourselves believe that the purposes of such an attraction are entirely or largely idealistic and platonic. Scientific candor forces us to admit, however, that the real purpose of such an attraction is that the species may be reproduced. Nature has no other purpose. If Nature alone were consulted, there would be no such thing as conventional marriage, and as a result there would be no such thing as the civilized home, and, indeed, no such thing as civilization itself. Marriage, by which we mean conventional marriage, has been evolved by man as a means of rising above the chance mating of the animals and as a device for placing about human offspring the care and protection of parents who continue to love each other after the heat of sexual passion has waned.

However much we may disdain the methods of Nature, we cannot divorce ourselves entirely from them. The wise couple will not even attempt to defeat the purposes which Nature has in bringing them together, but will try to sublimate and use those purposes and in this way attain the purposes both of Nature (that there be children) and of convention (that they and their children be properly established in a real home).

Strangely enough, there are persons who, though they are perfectly capable of normal relations as parents, are exceedingly anxious to avoid such responsibilities and privileges. We believe this to be an unnatural attitude for the reason that if it were universalized, it would mean the end of the biological species to which we belong. All animals and plants have the urge to reproduce themselves, and we must agree in such case that the instinct is natural and fundamental. Many species of animals do not, however, breed well when domesticated, and man, the most domesticated of all, responds somewhat in this way. As men and women become more divorced from natural settings and pursuits, as they become more artificialized, more "educated," more "civilized," they tend to have smaller and smaller families. Since death rates of infants and children have now been reduced very greatly, this is clearly a fortunate situation. In very recent years it has become fashionable for our most capable young couples to wish to have a family of rather larger sort than as of a few years ago.

Since the day of creation our ancestors have every one of them been hardy enough to live to the age of sexual maturity. Every one of them has escaped a thousand accidents which, had they had less wit or strength, would have been fatal not only to themselves but to their progeny as well. Every one of them has had the normal instinct to reproduce himself or herself and has been sufficiently comely to be sought and accepted by a member of the opposite sex. If one should believe that man was created some six thousand years ago, the fact that our ancestry goes back to the day of Creation without a break is quite remarkable, but if one believes that man and animal life has existed for millions of years and that during that entire time there has been no break in the continuity which leads to you and me the fact becomes amazing. In the gigantic relay race that is life, a billion, billion ancestors have passed the torch from one to the next in never-ending sequence until the present generation is reached. It is almost unbelievable that men and women should fail to see the significance of, and that they should often seek to avoid taking a place in, so extraordinary a procession.

The real, the primary purpose of marriage, then, is children. That two persons should enjoy the constant society of each other is most fortunate but is really of little concern to anyone but themselves, unless there are children.

When there are children we have the setting for an ideal home. That two persons should quarrel and fight is again of little importance to anyone except themselves, unless there are children. When there are children in such a distraught home there is tragedy. The couple without children is very likely to separate for some trivial reason, and such marriages are often highly unstable. Judges are much more free in granting divorces to childless couples than to those who have dependent children to consider. For a long time the courts have been considering a childless marriage somewhat in the light of a "companionate marriage." If a particular marriage is fruitless from the standpoint of the propagation of the better elements in society it is essentially worthless except as a medium of convenience for two individuals.

When one considers the importance of the relationship which the person to be married is about to assume it makes him wonder why society has been so careless in permitting any Tom, Dick, or Mary who can find a willing mate to enter into such a contract. The parent, in addition to his or her duties as a provider or housewife, must furnish the biological inheritance, must serve as nurse, physician, dentist, teacher, preacher, legal adviser, companion, administrator, and adviser to the child. The parent should be an authority on mental hygiene, infant care, dietetics; he or she should speak the mother tongue with accuracy, beauty, and force; he or she should train the child in proper habits, in obedience, thrift, industry, appreciation of truth, beauty, and virtue. The parent who has usually had not a word of scientific or even practical training in child care and guidance is responsible for the education of the child before he goes to school and all of the time during school except for about six hours a day, five days in the week, and nine months of the year.

In spite of all these facts, society requires of the applicant for a marriage license less than of the applicant for an automobile driver's license. Obviously we must not demand too much of the applicants for a marriage license, but surely it is not unreasonable to demand *something* of them. In most states of the Union, or more likely in all of them, almost anyone can get a marriage license if he is persistent and can find a partner. It is said that in times of old, parents had the power of life and death over their children and could make away with them or sell them into slavery. Atrocious! Nevertheless, parents *still* have the power of life and death over their children. Parents can neglect their young, and frequently do neglect them, so that they die of the results. We have in mind parents who are probably ruining a child by refusing to have him circumcised; another parent will not permit a child's tonsils to be removed, though they need removal badly; another parent denied a child antitoxin and the child died. Other parents are condemning their children to slavery to vicious habits, or to physical defects that could be corrected, or to modes of living that will make their lives miserable. The parent *still has the power of life and death over his children,* and for this reason should be a person who can and will administer such power wisely.

In consideration of the great importance to society and to the individual it seems as if the schools would have worked out a method long before this time of imparting instruction that would really "help solve the problems of life." Children are taught nearly everything except what might be expected to help them support or care for a home and a family. In recent years girl are being taught domestic science but many such courses are quite impractical. Biology courses can, and occasionally do, give a valuable insight into the problems of life. As a rule, however, they are as barren of human living relations as is the Sahara.

The family is the real unit of society; the home is the place where the unit lives, and marriage is the bond which holds the family together until the task is really finished. A community of good homes is one with good schools and churches, flourishing business enterprises, and loyal community interest. The teachers have little trouble at school; and policemen patrol the district only to protect it from outsiders; there are no riots, no antisocial manifestations, no need of the strong arm of the law. A community of vicious or wretched homes, on the contrary, is a constant menace to every good thing. All the policemen, all the teachers, all the jails, all the hospitals, all the correctional institutions in the world will not be able to undo the ills that are bred in those ugly homes. It is impossible to purify a stream by planting flowers along its banks while we leave the source foul. Society can never rise higher than its source—the family in the home.

When the home is inadequate, society is compelled in various ways to try to assume the relations which should have been assumed by the parents. But so often the parents will not, cannot, or at least do not accept their responsibilities, and in such cases organized society can do no less than to attempt to palliate the evil. We go to great expense to stand *in loco parentis* for these children who are obviously unfit for the problems to be met in modern life. There is nothing else to do about it. We have permitted these people to be born, now we must take care of them. It seems that at present they are rather rapidly increasing, and society is assuming more and more responsibility for them. All of which costs money and constantly more money.

The ultimate purpose of marriage is superior children. Legal marriage gives these children a name; it gives them property rights; it gives them citizenship; it establishes their legal status; it places the protection of the state about their home where they may be born and reared in security. In addition to these legal bonds there should be other bonds which hold father, mother, and child in a tight and compact unit. Any relation which will strengthen that bond is of the greatest possible consequence, while any relation which endangers the bond is pregnant with dire results for the individual and for society at large.

An ideal family is like nothing so much as a beautiful flower. There is present in each a male or father element and a female or mother element. Beautiful in design, arrangement, color, and fragrance, the parts of the flower act together as a unit for the production and preservation of seeds—children

—until they have attained such a degree of maturity that they may be safely entrusted to the dangers of the outside environment. By such means the perpetuity of the species is insured so long as the flower shall continue to exercise its primary function—the production of seeds—the rearing of children.

ABNORMALITIES OF SEXUAL FUNCTION

In spite of the teaching which we have received to the contrary, the individual with normal emotions and sensibilities regards his (or her) sex as the core of his (or her) personality; he looks upon this thing as being the most intimately personal of all his attributes. For this reason any deviation of sex from normal as seen in others or as experienced in one's own self is sure to make a profound impression and to arouse most unpleasant emotions.

MASTURBATION

Masturbation is admittedly an ugly habit. Millions of people claim to believe that it causes insanity, feeble-mindedness, epilepsy, loss of virility, pimples, specks before the eyes, and a dozen other symptoms which are more or less terrible. As a matter of fact, it does nothing of the sort. A great many wild animals practice some form or another of self-sexual stimulation (auto-eroticism). At some time in life nearly all men and boys have practised this form of self-gratification, and likewise a great many women and girls. If it were really a cause of insanity there would be mighty few sane persons. It is likely that the reason so many people so vehemently deny ever having practised masturbation is because they really have done so and are so thoroughly ashamed of it.

The bad effects of masturbation are the indirect results of the act and of the attempt on the part of the elders to stamp out the practice. Children are shamed, they are whipped, they are spied upon, they are threatened with insanity and all sorts of dire consequences, they are led to believe that they are lower than the dirt, and, as a result of these clumsy attempts at correction, they really are injured. The constant reminder of these awful consequences keeps the child thinking about what it is much better to forget.

When children are taught early that the reproductive organs are clean and wholesome; that sex is something that has a great and beautiful usefulness; that it is something to be kept unspoiled for the future, and that it serves a purpose that is essentially sacred; when children are kept busy with wholesome play, work and planning, and when they are loved and understood in matters such as these, there will possibly be a little masturbation, but inasmuch as that little will be speedily forgotten there will be no harm done. Be sure the children are healthily tired when they go to bed. Be sure that there is no need of circumcision, or if there is that it is corrected. Be sure the organs are clean so that they will not be irritated by foul secretions. Be sure that tight underwear does not demand constant pulling at the clothing.

Excessive masturbation is, of course, injurious in itself, but is rarely seen except in the mentally defective or in those who are driven too much into themselves. It is much more likely to be the *product of* rather than the cause of mental deficiency.

Persons who are extremely restless because of urgent sexual desire may possibly be more injured by the racking and the loss of sleep than by the act that will permit them to obtain relief. Husbands or wives who make excessive demands on their mates might well practice masturbation rather than wreck their home life by insisting upon their conjugal rights when the partner is sleepy, tired or for any reason unwilling to cooperate. As the potent male rather regularly has seminal emissions if he has no other sexual outlet, it is evident that masturbation becomes merely a waking instead of a dreaming activity. Physiologically, its effect, when not in excess, is no greater than emissions, which are obviously merely an overflow. Psychologically, the effect is nil, bad, or extremely bad, according as no, some, or much attention is paid to it.

EXCESSIVE SEXUALITY

A dangerous form of sexual abnormality is that which puts excessive emphasis on the subject. The male of this type is sometimes referred to as being a satyr. The damage which such a person can do is incalculable. He spreads veneral disease, he seduces wives and maids, he becomes the father of illegitimate children, he may commit rape or other crimes of sexual violence. No woman or girl is safe while he is about.

When the female displays excessive sexuality she is known as a nymphomaniac. The nymphomaniac is not to be confused with the normal individual who quite properly desires a pleasurable relation that is legitimate. The term would, of course, have different meanings in different communities and in different times, inasmuch as in some places and times any woman desiring sexual relations would be considered such a person. In case the individual seems utterly unable to control the urge and exposes herself in a wanton manner she should be subjected to thorough medical examination. It is possible that there is local irritation of the genital organs or some internal glandular disturbance that may be corrected. Proper sex education of little girls will probably be of aid in preventing cases which are not on a pathologic basis. Dissatisfaction with existing marriage relations may be a cause that can occasionally be corrected. Incarceration may become necessary when other means fail.

SEXUAL FRIGIDITY

At the opposite extreme are those women, many of them married, who either have no desire for sexual experience, or are even definitely averse to it. In times past this has frequently been accounted as a virtue, but with a fuller understanding of the subject it is recognized both as a personal tragedy and a cause of serious difficulties in the family.

There are many causes of this condition, which is commonly called *frigidity*. In the first place, the instruction which many girls receive from their mothers is such as would produce in them an intense distrust of the male of the species, and would repulse any normal instinct with regard to sex. The mother often deliberately teaches the daughter to take this attitude, doubtless thinking that she is protecting the girl from temptation. She does not realize that she may be preparing the daughter for an unhappy marriage. The girl whose father has been crude and repellent is quite likely to develop in an unnatural way as a result of the harsh treatment he has shown his wife and children.

Probably the commonest cause of frigidity is lack of preparation for marriage on the part of inexperienced girls. Awkward bridegrooms thinking that inasmuch as marriage has taken place there were no further reasons for gentlemanly restraint, have frightened, shocked, shamed, and even injured their brides at a time when the destiny of the marriage was in the balance. With such a start, and with the same act repeated as often as the new husband is able or may wish, the wife is set strongly against the whole program and is likely to develop into a woman who has the most intense disgust for anything of a sexual nature. It is extremely important that wooing should continue until the conventionally married couple are really ready for biological marriage. When this is done and patience is practised—when the bride is shown the same deference as the fiancée—there will be very few women who will fail to develop a strong desire for the conjugal embrace.

Another common cause of frigidity is fear of conception. Wives may have ever so many excellent reasons why they do not desire children at a given time. Frequently most or all of the responsibility for the prevention of conception is placed upon them. They dread the long months of pregnancy. Frequently there have already been born more children than is best for the welfare of the family or the mother. Under such circumstances the wife is under the constant dread of another conception and as a result wishes to avoid every possibility of such a happening. In a similar relation is the woman who has reason to believe that her husband is unfaithful to her. She resents the fact and fears the possibility of veneral disease which he may have contracted.

Sometimes religion, sometimes training, or lack of it, sometimes abnormality of the organs, sometimes a disproportion between the organs of the two mates, sometimes psychological incompatibility between the two may be responsible. Whatever the cause, it is pretty certain that a couple will be unhappy if the wife is frigid. If there are children the couple may hang together but furnish the children a decidedly bad environment; if there are no children divorce or separation is nearly inevitable. Not only does a satisfactory relation pay large dividends in personal enjoyment, but it enables couples to form a strong and stable marriage which will insure that their children have a good home until they are old enough to take care of themselves. Body odor, sweaty or dirty skin, untidy garments, beds and bed-clothing may easily cause disgust in a sensitive person; vulgar language, un-couth behavior or untoward behavior may cause revulsion on the part of a person who is fastidious in such matters.

SEXUAL COMPLEXES

An interesting relation is that which is known as the Oedipus complex. It is seen when there is an unusual attachment between mother and son. The Electra complex is the relation when a daughter has an excessive love for her father. This does not mean an improper relation. As a matter of fact, these children are often cited as being particularly praiseworthy. These ex-cessive attachments however may do serious harm to the exemplary young men and women who are so unfortunate as to get caught in their mesh. Par-ents—particularly parents of a single child—should watch for this trap into which an adoring child may be lured. Particularly if the father lives alone with the daughter or the mother with a son there is danger. Likewise there is danger if the child resembles in a striking way the appearance and character of a dead parent.

Much has been said concerning repressions of various sorts, and of sexual repressions in particular. Some have seen fit to follow blindly the teachings of Freud and to see in every sort of dream, in every sort of twist in character, and in nearly every sort of mental deviation a tangle of repressions which are basically sexual. There is no doubt that there is much truth in the theory which has been developed, but it is quite certain that the whole thing has some-times been grossly overdrawn. Some have even advised that one should not attempt to control or repress the impulses that arise for the reason that terrible complexes may develop if such is done. This position is, of course, quite impossible since society could not exist if everyone simply followed any urge that he might feel. On the other hand, it is a fact that spinsters, bachelors, and persons who have been disappointed in love or have strongly loved some-one under conditions which made it necessary to conceal the feeling are very subject to all sorts of disturbances which may seriously undermine the health of the body and mind.

Extremely important is the matter of suggestion or of direct teaching of irregular practices. A child who has wrong ideas about such matters can ruin a school or a neighborhood. Children who have had developed a vacuum in their minds regarding sex are easily led into almost any sort of abuse of the sexual apparatus, and serious damage may be done in a short space of time. Children who have had adequate sex instruction will be far less attracted to perverted persons and also much less likely to follow improper suggestions. As in every other instance, we can best overcome evil with good. *Disgusting practices are in many instances more directly to be charged to the parents who failed to instruct the child in healthy ways than they are to be held*

*against the unfortunate victim of distorted perspective who has taught the
unsophisticated child in these matters.*

THE HYGIENE OF THE REPRODUCTIVE SYSTEM

A fine watch does best when it is meddled with least. The same is true of
any complicated mechanism and in particular of the generative apparatus.
A policy of "hands off" is hard to beat in this connection. There are, to be
sure, elemental points in the care of the organs which should be understood
by everyone, but further than this the layman should not go. There has
been so much ignorance and misinformation concerning the sexual apparatus
that the layman may hardly trust anything that he has learned from the
usual source. When there is reason to believe that something is really wrong,
the family physician or a specialist whom he may designate should be consulted at once. It surely is needless to say that the physician should be
furnished with a full and frank history of the ailment and its possible causes.
Furthermore, he must be permitted to make such examinations and to ask
such questions of the parents as he may think necessary. Some of his questions will seem impertinent but it is exactly such questions as may bring
out the basic difficulty.

CLEANLINESS

The first principle to be considered in the hygiene of the reproductive
system is cleanliness. By this we do not mean to imply that lack of cleanliness will often jeopardize the physical health of the individual. Actually
there is more danger that meddlesome methods of attaining cleanliness will
cause disease than that lack of cleanliness will cause it. This is particularly
true in the case of the female. But there is more to this matter of hygiene
than mere maintenance of health. The reproductive organs must be clean if
they are to be held in high regard; they must be free of odor; they must be
wholesome; they must not offend. They are so exceedingly important to the
welfare of the race, the self-respect of the individual, and the happiness of
family, and yet they are so likely to be regarded as being vulgar by those who
do not understand that there must not be any doubt about their basic
wholesomeness.

Odor is undoubtedly of first consideration. The fact that we wear clothing
complicates the matter for the good reason that the clothing does not permit
the free ventilation that will carry away odors before they become concentrated
and will permit the rapid evaporation of perspiration. Clothing should be as
light and as well ventilated as comfort will permit. Great improvement in
underwear has been made in recent years. Undergarments should be changed
as often as one's finances will permit and should of course never be worn
after they are definitely soiled. Night clothing should entirely replace the
underwear that has been worn through the day. This will give opportunity
for airing and drying of the various garments which would be most likely
to offend.

Frequent washing of the external genitalia is of course extremely important. It is the *external* organs that need washing and not the internal. Much harm has undoubtedly been done by the use of antiseptic or even cleansing douches as many women use them. In the first place they are not necessary from the standpoint of preventing odors for the good reason that the odors of the vagina proper are practically never concentrated enough to cause trouble if the external organs are clean. The normal vagina nearly always contains great numbers of germs which are known collectively as "Doderlein's bacilli." These germs are not only harmless, but actually beneficial, because they prevent the growth of other germs which can really cause trouble. Incidentally these germs are closely related to, or by some are considered to be identified with, the germs that are deliberately put into acidophilus milk which is much used for restoring healthy conditions in the bowels. There is not a bit of doubt that the presence of these acid producing organisms is of positive value in the vagina. If they are frequently washed away with cleansing douches or inhibited with antiseptics, abnormal conditions may develop in the vagina, and real trouble may ensue. Furthermore, strong antiseptics frequently irritate the mucous membrane and make it more susceptible to invasion by other bacteria. Not a few of the commonly used douches are definitely irritating or even poisonous when used in too concentrated form or when used frequently. This is particularly true of bichloride of mercury and lysol.

Sometimes, particularly in the male, it is impossible to hold down odors merely by washing the external genitalia. In some individuals the foreskin is so tight about the end of the penis that it cannot be retracted and the groove beneath it cleaned of the white secretion—known as smegma—which accumulates there. This secretion is of an oily nature and easily becomes rancid, producing exceedingly bad odors and also irritation of the mucous membrane. At the time of birth every male child should be carefully examined to determine whether or not he is in need of circumcision which consists in removing the foreskin. When done in the early days of life the operation is a trivial one. Later it is somewhat more serious, but never dangerous when performed by a competent surgeon. Even those individuals who are not in need of circumcision should retract the foreskin and clean the groove beneath it carefully at least once a day. A child in need of circumcision is often made nervous by the irritation of the rancid secretions and will be constantly twisting, squirming, and pulling at himself. He may also develop the habit of masturbation as a result of the irritation which induces him to handle his penis. We do not advocate that all boys and men should be circumcised, but are emphatic in recommending such treatment when there is difficulty in keeping the parts clean otherwise. Girls are also occasionally in need of circumcision, or what is essentially the same thing.

Occasionally discharges of various sorts from the genital organs will greatly complicate the habit of cleanliness. In *every* case in either sex the cause of any discharge should be ascertained if possible. The family physician or a reliable specialist should be consulted, *always. Never* should patent medicines or home remedies be used as a substitute for careful examination and treatment by a physician. *Never* must the patient go to an advertising physician or to one who is known to be, or suspected of being a quack. In case the discharge can be cured and the cause removed the problem is solved. When the condition cannot be corrected, the greatest of care will be needed to prevent offensive odors and a disgusting local condition.

MENSTRUATION

The peculiar demands of menstruation call for attention in a discussion of hygiene. There is first to be considered the necessity of caring for the actual physiological needs. During this period the pelvic organs of the female are considerably congested, and for this reason are more subject to infection and circulatory disturbances. It is for this reason that excessively long hours of standing on the feet, dancing, strenuous athletics, and similar activities are not advisable for many women. Likewise sexual excitement will intensify the effect, and may cause trouble. Bathing was formerly interdicted, but is now permitted in most cases if the water is warm. There is, of course, additional need of cleanliness at such a time, and local bathing is always perfectly safe. There are many women and girls who can even swim in cold water while menstruating, but such chilling of the skin is likely to drive the blood inward and increase the internal congestion or cause severe cramping.

In case the menstrual periods should cease in a girl or woman who is probably not pregnant, careful physical examination should be made to determine the cause. In earlier times this cessation was supposed to cause tuberculosis. Now we understand that in most such cases tuberculosis is already present and the checking of this drain is a means by which Nature seeks to conserve the patient's strength. Patients with anemia of any sort or those with nervous disturbances are also likely to cease menstruating until they are restored to their normal condition. Of great importance is the mental attitude of the woman toward her menstrual periods, and toward the "change of life," at which time the periods gradually cease from natural causes. In times past girls were literally taught to make invalids of themselves, and women were led to believe that "the change" was something greatly to be dreaded and a time of danger. We understand now that menstruation is a perfectly normal process, and that the menopause need cause little apprehension if it is approached with understanding and poise. The fact that women are now so much less embarrassed in visiting a physician about such matters has opened a way of escape from many of the dangers and discomforts. The frank consideration of all subjects relative to sex and the far more natural attitude toward them has in large measure taken them out of the limbo to which they were formerly assigned.

With so much advertising of absorbent pads and other aids to feminine hygiene it is hardly necessary to describe in detail the means by which women may avoid the soiling of their clothing with the menstrual discharges. As stated elsewhere, young girls should have these matters explained before they are twelve years of age, or by the time they are ten or eleven if they are somewhat precocious in their development. It is important that the girl be taught so that she will not be frightened by the first appearance but will come to her mother for aid and advice. This is, of course, an excellent opportunity for the mother to explain something of the nature and purpose of the genital organs and to impress the girl with the value of the process of which the menstrual cycle is a part.

In recent years there has been much discussion of the use of a vaginal tampon as a means of controlling menstrual bleeding. Medical opinion is now pretty well agreed that the method is safe provided the tampons are of proper size and are removed as may be needed. When—as in virgins—the opening in the hymen is small, there is difficulty in inserting and particularly in removing the tampon. The objection to this method of feminine hygiene is for the most part a traditional objection to putting anything into the virgin vagina.

DISEASES OF THE GENITAL ORGANS

There are various serious diseases of the genital organs which need to be understood so that they may be detected at the earliest possible moment. We shall not describe the venereal diseases in this place, as they will be discussed in a later chapter. Various other chronic inflammations and injuries resulting from childbirth or injury usually manifest themselves by symptoms or pain of some sort. Of greatest importance are the various forms of cancer which may be found. Unfortunately cancers are not painful in their earlier stages. To be sure, they are terribly painful later, and this fact may mislead persons who are really in danger and will not believe that they are so because they are not in pain.

At the present time about one woman in seven above the age of forty years is dying of cancer of one kind or another. About one third of these cancers are of the womb, usually the mouth of the womb. We shall not attempt to give such a description as will enable the layman to make an unerring diagnosis of cancer of the womb, but merely call attention to the fact that any sort of unnatural bleeding from the privates should be investigated thoroughly. Excessive bleeding, bleeding after the change of life, continuous bleeding, or the passing of *clotted* blood, constitute "unnatural" bleeding. These signs do not mean that a given person surely has cancer, but they do mean that there is *something* wrong, and that a *thorough examination is needed*. The physician should be required to prove if at all possible that it is *not* cancer before the investigation is ended. Once the diagnosis of cancer is made, treatment in the hands of a reliable surgeon or radiologist is the only hope. It is believed that unrepaired tears of the mouth of the womb may be the cause of cancer in many instances, since they cause long continued irritation. The wearing of a pessary for long periods of time may also serve in this way.

Another third of all deaths from cancer among women is from cancer of the breast. These growths are always small before they are large, always localized before they are generalized, and always painless before they are painful. The growth usually manifests itself as a lump or nodule in the breast, or sometimes as a thick place in the skin reminding one of a piece of bacon rind. It is usually irregular in shape, attached to the skin and deeper tissues, and solitary in number in the earlier stages at least. As the breast is moved the nodules cause dimpling. If near the nipple, they commonly cause the nipple to be drawn in. The chances for recovery are good if the diagnosis is made early and the appropriate treatment begun at once. If surgical treatment is delayed, the operation is much more severe, and there is less chance of cure. Rarely cancer of the breast is seen in the male.

Cancer of the prostate and bladder are fairly common in the male. The earliest symptom is usually blood in the urine or difficulty in emptying the bladder. These symptoms should call for an immediate examination to determine the cause.

The reproductive system of the female is much more complicated than that of the male and is for this reason more subject to disease and injury. It furthermore is under far greater stress in the performance of its function of reproduction. For this reason care must be taken to avoid as many as possible of the dangers which beset the sexual life. In the first place, women— and men, too, for that matter—should not marry unless they are reasonably sure that they are free from disease and deformity. Women who have suffered from rickets as children should make sure that the pelvic opening is large enough to permit the passage of a child at the time of birth. In recent years it has been possible for such women to bear children by submitting to Cæsarean section, but even in such cases it is better if the obstetrician knows beforehand that the child cannot pass through the birth canal. Women who have reason to believe that they are suffering from active or recently arrested tuberculosis should refrain from childbearing both for their own sake and for the sake of the child.

We believe there is no legitimate excuse for an intelligent woman to go into maternity without informing herself thoroughly concerning the risks and the means of reducing those risks to the minimum. Certainly there is no excuse for delay after she finds herself actually pregnant. She should consult her family physician or the specialist of her choice as soon as she becomes aware of her condition. If the pregnancy is the first, there is additional reason for such professional care. Likewise the women beyond the age usual for childbearing and those who have reason to believe that they may have weak hearts and kidneys should take extra precaution. All pregnant women should have their blood type known. In case the wife is RH negative while her husband is RH positive there is particular reason to know and be prepared to cope with the situation. With modern care the condition is usually handled with success, without such care the results are often disastrous to the child.

SEXUAL INTERCOURSE IN PREGNANCY

Many couples wonder if sexual intercourse may be indulged in during the period of pregnancy. This will depend upon several factors. Certainly it should not if there is a feeling that the act is degrading during this time. Likewise it may only be practised when both mates desire it. There is good reason from the standpoint of the possibility of infection for refraining during the last few weeks of the pregnancy. In case the wife seems to have been injured by marital relations on previous occasions, or if she is one who is easily aborted, continence is the only safe rule. In those instances—and they are many—in which the wife desires the relation at this time and does not seem to be injured by it there is no real objection. The fear that the child may be injured is quite without foundation except in those women who are easily aborted. Unfortunately we must take into consideration the fact that many husbands might seek other mistresses if they were required to refrain from sexual relations at home. The danger of venereal disease in such case is probably greater than the danger of injury to the wife as a result of intercourse, provided the wife is not definitely pathological.

CONTRACEPTIVES

Strange as it may seem at first thought, there is often more danger in attempting to prevent conception than in going through with the pregnancy. Several of the contraceptive measures are definitely hazardous. Contraceptive devices and their dangers may be roughly classified as follows:

1. *Antiseptic douches used after the sexual act.*

If these douches are irritating or poisonous, or if they disturb the normal bacterial growth of the vagina, we are sure that they may do harm. Bichloride of mercury and lysol are particularly to be feared. All such means are frequently ineffective.

2. *Vaginal suppositories or injections containing organic acids or substances which kill or render immotile the spermatozoa.*

These are probably not often dangerous. They are frequently put up in a cocoa-butter base, and there is some objection to oily applications to mucous membranes. These methods are by no means surely effective.

3. *Pessaries of some sort are much used.*

Pessaries that are left in position for long periods of time are always irritating and may cause serious trouble. They may cause infection, or the chronic irritation resulting from their use may possibly lead to cancer. Those that are inserted at the time are a nuisance and likely to be regarded with considerable distaste.

4. *Rubber devices to hold the semen from contact with the womb.*

These devices considerably diminish normal sensation and are unpleasant to use. They are likely to cause dissatisfaction and incompleteness of the act, which may in turn have a bad effect upon the nervous system. They are recommended to prevent venereal disease.

5. Recently a stiff creme like substance has been devised which is said to stick to the cervix and effectively to occlude it for several hours during which time a chemical kills the spermatozoa. The method is safe and probably rather highly effective in preventing conception.

6. *Incomplete act of coitus.*

This method of preventing conception is nearly sure to cause dissatisfaction with the marital state if it is used habitually. The method is not very effectual in many instances.

7. *Sterilization by surgical means.*

In the instance of those who have very good reasons for not having children, or of those who are adjudged by society as being unfit for propagation, this method is excellent. Sterilization does not unsex the individual. He or she can still indulge in sexual relations with pleasure.

8. *Continence.*

The prevention of conception by refraining from the sexual act is recommended for all *unmarried lovers.* It is, however, a somewhat dangerous means in the instance of married couples unless there is mutual agreement concerning it. Most couples practice continence or some of the less drastic forms of contraception during the period in the menstrual cycle when conception is most likely to occur. These methods have much to commend them.

9. *Rhythm Method.*

By this method sexual contact is avoided during the period in each month that the wife is in a condition to become pregnant. When menstruation is regular this period for the release of the ovum is about fourteen days before the beginning of the next menstrual flow. The full discussion of the subject is complex. For a short treatise see the discussion on the rhythm of menstruation—page 51.

10. *A combination of methods as recommended by a physician.*

Every couple desiring to practice contraceptive methods should consult a reliable physician. The methods available are many, and will need to be selected according to the requirements of the particular couple at a particular time. It is impossible to give details in a book of this sort because all methods must be chosen to suit the persons concerned.

ABORTION

In many instances when contraceptive measures have failed, criminal abortion is practised. This is always a more or less dangerous procedure. When done even under the most careful conditions it is still dangerous, because Nature protests strongly against such practices. In addition to the physical danger there is also the mental side to be considered. Maternal nature receives a severe shock even when physicians undertake the deliberate death of the child which by all rules should be the joy of the mother's heart. When abortion is done by ignorant persons under urgent necessity of concealing the act and not quite free to call the physician as needed it is exceedingly dangerous and often ends fatally for the mother as well as the child.

SEXUAL STIMULATION

The health of the reproductive system can be injured also by various attempts to stimulate the sexual function. The elderly or weakly man attempts to boost his waning powers by some sort or other of gland therapy. The eating of the testicles of castrated animals, the taking of tablets purported to contain dried testicle of slaughtered animals, the transplantation of monkey, or even human, glands is familiar pseudoscience of recent years. The effects are transient if they exist at all, and it is quite likely that they are entirely psychological. Even if there were a definite increase in sexual power, it is likely that the operation would be dangerous to the degree that it was effective. Old men's bodies are not able to stand the strain of highly active glands. Elderly men should not be parents and should be potent only when the physiological mechanism for such a purpose is functional of its own accord. The use of drugs which are supposed to stimulate sexual desire is another dangerous mirage. Cantharides (Spanish fly) is particularly dangerous and must never be used for this purpose, as it is an intense kidney irritant. Furthermore, it is not able to do the things which popular tradition claims for it.

Of the utmost importance in sexual hygiene is temperance in the exercise of the various functions. It is doubtful if there is a more disgusting creature than the sexual glutton. On the other hand, the individual who does not permit, or cannot enjoy, the reasonable use of the reproductive system, misses one of the biggest things in life. The man or woman who has short-circuited the reproductive act and so has escaped the responsibilities of parenthood has cheated himself of the high points of existence. One must come to understand that sex is the foundation of marriage but by no means the whole thing. Happily married couples think of sex only a small portion of the time, while dissatisfied couples brood over it constantly. Properly understood and exercised the sex life of a married couple is a source of tremendous enjoyment and profit. It is a relation that is unselfish, clean and good.

CHAPTER VI

Care of Mothers before and after Childbirth
J. P. GREENHILL, M.D.

INTRODUCTION

WOMEN USED TO KEEP *secret, even from their husbands, the fact that they were going to have a baby. As the time approached when the child was to be born, she would notify the physician. In many instances, however, even this did not occur, but the doctor was called posthaste at the moment of childbirth. Then, in the home, with the aid of a neighbor or a relative, the child would be brought into the community.*

The advances of scientific medicine have greatly changed our points of view in relationship to what is proper in childbirth. Nowadays the intelligent woman may consult her physician even before trying to have a child. She finds out whether or not her health is such as to permit her to have a child without seriously injuring herself and without danger to the prospective child. When the physician's examination has revealed that her condition is satisfactory she may proceed.

Nowadays the intelligent woman consults her physician also as soon as she realizes that she is pregnant. He then examines her again to make certain of the diagnosis. This he confirms by various tests in the laboratory as well as by physical examination of the patient herself. During this period her life must be regulated according to her condition. It is important to control her diet, her exercise, her rest, her work, and every other factor of her existence. Examinations are regularly made of her excretions in order to determine whether or not the organs are functioning satisfactorily.

Such prenatal care in childbirth is of the utmost importance for lowering the death rates associated with this condition, and also for bringing into the world healthy and normal children.

M. F.

Because of ignorance, negligence, territorial inaccessibility, financial distress, or other reasons, thousands of women in this country fail to be examined by a physician while they are pregnant. These women do not call in expert aid until the child is actually ready to be born. Since most of the mishaps from childbirth may be prevented by proper care before the baby arrives and by skillful management of confinement, every woman who is to have a baby should visit a doctor long before the expected date of confinement. Not only will the lives of hundreds of mothers be saved, but countless other women will be spared temporary or permanent invalidism. Furthermore many thousand babies will be born alive who would certainly perish in the absence of proper supervision. The care which a woman receives before the baby arrives is known as antepartum or prenatal care. In contradistinction to this is the care after the child is born, and this is spoken of as postpartum or postnatal care.

Really a confinement case begins at the time of conception. Hence the woman should consult a physician as soon as she believes she is going to have a baby. The ideal arrangement would be for a woman to have a thorough examination before she decides to have a child, because not infrequently abnormalities are found which, unless corrected, may make childbearing a hazardous undertaking. Occasionally a disturbance is found such as serious heart, kidney, or lung trouble, which absolutely precludes pregnancy. A woman should know this before she conceives. She should seek a physician who has a sympathetic nature and one in whom she can have utmost confidence. Faith in the doctor is important to allay the fears which young prospective mothers frequently have. Advice should be sought from the physician and not from well-meaning but misinformed friends and relatives, many of whom instill fear rather than dispel it.

If a woman cannot afford the services of a specialist in obstetrics or an experienced general practitioner, she should visit one of the numerous prenatal clinics to be found in every large city and in many small ones.

SIGNS OF PREGNANCY

A woman may suspect she is to become a mother in a number of ways. The most important sign is absence of the monthly flow, especially in a young woman who has usually had regular monthly periods. A second significant sign is morning sickness or nausea and vomiting. Frequently the breasts feel full, they are tender to the touch, and they have peculiar sensations such as tingling or throbbing. The skin around the nipples becomes darker in color, especially in brunettes. Another sign is a desire to pass urine at frequent intervals. Not one of these symptoms by itself indicates pregnancy, but a combination of two or more is presumptive evidence that a baby may be expected. A physician can nearly always detect a pregnancy as early as six weeks after the last monthly flow. If he is in doubt he can have the woman's urine subjected to biologic tests which correctly indicate the presence of a pregnancy in about 96 per cent of all cases. A woman does not usually feel the baby move around until the sixteenth or eighteenth week of the baby's development. At this time the abdomen is usually enlarged sufficiently to verify the suspicion of a pregnancy, and a physician can feel the baby and hear its heart beat. After the fifth month a baby or at least parts of it may be shown on X-ray pictures.

VISIT TO PHYSICIAN

When an expectant mother visits the doctor the first time, he will take a complete history and make a thorough examination. This includes external and internal investigation of the organs directly associated with childbearing; also an examination of the teeth, thyroid, breasts, nipples, and other organs. The blood pressure and temperature will be taken, the urine examined, the weight recorded, the blood studied for anemia, syphilis and the Rh factor. A knowledge of this factor is important in case a blood transfusion is necessary and also because a very small percentage of babies suffer when there is a difference in the Rh factor in the husband and wife.

A woman should visit her doctor at least once every three weeks during the first seven months of pregnancy and once every two weeks thereafter. If abnormalities exist, the patient may have to see her physician more often. At each visit she should bring to the physician a three- or four-ounce bottle of urine. The bottle should be carefully washed before it is used, because its former contents may be the cause of false tests. Once a week it is advisable to measure the amount of urine passed in twenty-four hours. If there is a considerable reduction in the amount usually passed and the patient has been drinking the customary amount of fluids, this fact should be reported to the physician. It may indicate a disturbance of the kidneys. A label should be attached to the bottle giving the patient's name, the date the specimen is collected, and in certain instances the amount of urine passed in twenty-four hours. If a specimen of urine is to be mailed to a doctor, a teaspoonful of chloroform should be added to the specimen before it is sent.

SERIOUS SYMPTOMS DURING PREGNANCY

During each visit the doctor will ask the patient certain questions and listen to any questions or complaints. He will usually inquire about the following symptoms: nausea, vomiting, swelling of the hands, feet, or face, headaches, constipation, dizziness, pain in the abdomen or legs, spots before the eyes or other visual disturbances, bleeding from the vagina, movements of the baby, shortness of breath, nervousness, and other symptoms. He will observe the patient's blood pressure, the pulse rate, abnormal swellings, excessive gain or loss in weight, and the results of the examination of the urine. It is not necessary to be examined internally at each visit, but at least one examination should be made in addition to the first one, and this preferably about four weeks before the expected date of confinement.

ESTIMATING THE DATE OF BIRTH

It is impossible to predict accurately the day when a baby is to arrive. However, the approximate date can be estimated in a number of ways.

1. Add seven days to the first day of the last monthly flow and subtract three months. Thus if the last menstrual period began July 10th, add seven days, giving July 17th, and subtract three months, which gives April 17th as the approximate day labor may be expected. In most cases the confinement will take place within a few days before or after this calculated date.

2. A woman having her first baby may add twenty-two weeks to the day she first feels the baby move. A woman who has already borne children should add twenty-four weeks because she usually recognizes movements of the baby about two weeks earlier than women pregnant for the first time.

3. If the exact day of conception is known, 266 days added to this will give the approximate date of confinement.

4. By repeated examinations, a physician can often tell within a few days when a baby will be born.

THE DIET

The child in the womb depends on its mother for its supply of food. The nourishment is not given to the child directly, because there is no direct connection between the mother and her child. The latter lies in a sac filled with fluid which permits the child to move about freely. In one part of this sac is an organ known as the placenta or afterbirth. This is made up of myriads of small projections known as villi, in each of which is a small blood vessel. These villi dip into a collection of the mother's blood, and it is the coverings of these villi which extract from the mother's blood the food which the child requires. The nourishment which the villi take up is transported from the small blood vessels in the villi to large blood vessels which pass through a tube connecting the afterbirth with the child. This tube is known as the umbilical cord, and it usually contains one vein and two arteries. The vein carries fresh blood containing nourishment to the child, whereas the arteries carry blood containing waste products from the baby to the afterbirth. This impure blood is transmitted from the afterbirth to the mother's blood, and the mother purifies this blood in the same way she cleanses her own blood, namely, by eliminating the waste products through her bowels, kidneys, lungs, and skin.

Since the connection between the mother and the child is as intimate as just mentioned, it is obvious that the child's development depends to a large extent upon the mother's nutrition. The child's growth is not entirely dependent on the mother's food intake, because if the diet is lacking in certain substances which the child requires, these substances in many instances will be extracted from the mother's tissues, usually to her detriment. Hence it is important that the mother's diet contain both the proper quantity and quality of food each day to supply all the demands of the fetus.

Not only is the mother's nutrition important for the baby, but it is important also for her own benefit. In order to avoid trouble there should be certain additions and restrictions to the diet the expectant mother has usually followed. As a general rule it may be said that the expectant mother should eat a well-rounded diet, just as she eats in the non-pregnant state, except that she should drink plenty of milk, eat more fresh fruits and vegetables, and less condiments. She should use a minimum of table salt. A woman should not make the serious mistake of overeating because she believes she must eat for two individuals. The excess food is not transferred to the baby but is stored in the mother. This may lead to serious consequences. However, women should not starve themselves in an attempt to keep down the weight of the baby, because the weight of a newborn baby is not dependent entirely or even in great part on the amount of food its mother eats. Heredity is a much more important factor than diet.

A proper diet during pregnancy contains the following:

1. *Water*, which serves many functions. At least eight or ten glasses of liquids a day in one form or another should be taken.

2. *Proteins*, which build and repair the tissues of the body. These are found chiefly in meat, eggs, milk and milk products, and such vegetables as peas and beans.

3. *Fats*, which furnish fuel for heat and energy. These are found in cream, butter, cheese, oils, and fat meats.

4. *Carbohydrates* or *starches*, which also supply fuel. They are found chiefly in sweets, sugar, bread, potatoes, cereals, milk, and rice.

5. *Minerals*, which are the most important substances for the growth of the bones and teeth. They also increase resistance to disease, and they keep the blood in good condition. They are found especially in milk, certain fruits, and most vegetables. If vegetables are cooked, the water should not be thrown away but should be used for soup. The chief minerals necessary during pregnancy are calcium, phosphorus and iron.

6. *Vitamins*, which regulate the growth of the body and in some instances prevent miscarriages. They are found in milk, eggs, meat, whole wheat, fruits, vegetables, cod-liver oil, viosterol, and halibut-liver oil. In the winter months cod-liver oil takes the place of sunshine.

7. *Iodine* in certain regions of the country is necessary to prevent the development of a goiter in the mother and the child. It is found chiefly in such sea food as oysters and salmon. Iodized salt or iodine tablets may be used, but only under the direction of a physician.

It will be observed that milk is the ideal food because it contains water, proteins, fat (in the cream), sugar, minerals, and vitamins. It is easily digested in all its forms (sweet, sour, or buttermilk). At least a quart of milk should therefore be taken every day not only throughout pregnancy but also after the baby comes as long as the baby is nursed at the breast.

Some pregnant women have a strong desire for unusual foods out of season or odd things. Chief among these are pickles, highly seasoned foods, and chalk (calcium). This perversion of appetite is known as "pica," and unless these foods disagree with the mother, they may be indulged in.

It is best for the expectant mother to restrict the use of alcohol and to limit the number of cigarettes smoked to ten a day.

SPECIAL DIETS

During the first three months of pregnancy at least 50 per cent of all women suffer from nausea or vomiting or both. These women should not attempt to eat the usual three meals a day but should take small amounts of solid food, especially starches and sweets, every two or two and a half hours. If part or all of the food is vomited, more solid food should be eaten immediately. Water should not be taken with these meals but between them. The following diet may prove useful:

Before getting out of bed:
  Crackers or dry toast.

One half-hour later breakfast consisting of the following:
  Orange, grapefruit, stewed prunes or apricots.
  Cereal with cream and sugar.
  One soft-boiled egg.
  Thin buttered toast (with unsalted butter).
  Milk, cocoa, weak tea or coffee with sugar.

10:00 a.m.:
  Glass of milk with crackers (graham, nabisco, oatmeal, etc.).

Lunch:
  Cup of cream of celery, asparagus, spinach or potato soup.
  Soup crackers.
  Salad of lettuce, tomato, endive, etc., with sugar and a small amount of lemon
     juice.
  Whole-wheat bread, or toast, buttered.
  Ice cream, water ice, or custard.

4:00 p.m.:
  Milk, cocoa, chocolate or weak tea.
  Small piece of cake, crackers, or wafers.

Dinner:
  Cup of bouillon or vegetable soup, especially tomato.
  Soup crackers.
  Small lamb chop, broiled steak, or veal chop, well done.
  Baked potato, mashed potatoes, or carrots.
  Thin bread, or toast, buttered.
  Lettuce or tomato salad.
  Ice cream or water ice.

At bedtime:
  Glass of hot milk, chocolate or malted milk.
  Graham or oatmeal crackers.

The nausea and vomiting usually cease spontaneously after the fourth month, and from this time on the following diet is recommended:

Breakfast:

Fruit, such as orange, grapefruit, stewed prunes, or baked apple.
Cereal with cream and sugar.
One boiled or poached egg.
Two slices of crisp bacon.
Buttered toast, roll, or corn muffin.
Cup of cocoa, chocolate, weak tea, or coffee, with sugar and cream.

10:00 a.m.:

Glass of milk.
Fresh fruit or fruit juice.

Lunch:

Cream of celery, tomato, or asparagus soup.
Crackers or wafers.
Baked potato with butter.
Lettuce or tomato salad with sugar and small amount of lemon juice.
Ice cream or blanc mange.

4:00 p.m.:

American or cream cheese sandwich.
Glass of milk or malted milk.

Dinner:

Celery, pea, spinach, or corn soup.
Salt wafers.
Small lamb chop, steak, or equivalent in fish.
Mashed or baked potato, carrots, peas, beet tops, or spinach.
Lettuce, tomato, endive salad with sugar and lemon.
Cheese and crackers or toast; nuts.
Ice cream, jelly roll, plain cake or fruit.
Cup of weak tea or coffee with cream and sugar.

At bedtime:

Glass of hot milk or malted milk.
Crackers.

If a woman finds that certain foods disagree with her, she should eliminate them from her diet for a while. If the distressing symptoms reappear when she resumes eating them, these foods should not be eaten for the remainder of the pregnancy. In general it is advisable to avoid highly seasoned, spiced, greasy, fried, or fatty foods, rich pies, pastries, and other desserts, too many sweets, strong condiments, alcohol, and strong coffee and tea. A woman who is underweight when she becomes pregnant may eat more than one who is overweight.

Most of the water should be taken on arising in the morning, between meals, and before retiring at night. On the day the twenty-four-hour specimen of urine is measured, the amount of water taken should also be recorded, and both of these figures should be given to the doctor.

CARE OF THE BOWELS

A pregnant woman should have at least one bowel movement every day, in order to eliminate not only her own waste products but also those of the baby in the womb. If the bowels are not emptied daily, poisons accumulate in the system, and an extra load is placed on the kidneys, which already have a great deal of important work to do during pregnancy. As a general rule, women have a strong tendency to be constipated while carrying a baby. Constipation is still more likely to occur in women who do not drink enough fluids and do not eat the proper kinds of food, and in those whose bowels did not move regularly before pregnancy supervened.

In order to prevent constipation as much as possible and also to overcome it when present, the following rules should be observed:

1. An abundance of water should be taken upon arising, during the day, and before going to bed.

2. Every day an attempt should be made to have a bowel movement at exactly the same hour. The best time for this is after breakfast, and one should have patience. However, there should not be too much straining. A glycerine suppository inserted into the rectum may stimulate the bowels to move.

3. The diet should contain a large amount of fresh fruits and vegetables. The fruits should include apples, apricots, cherries, figs, grapes, ripe olives, oranges, peaches, pears, pineapple, plums and prunes, raspberries and strawberries. The vegetables should include asparagus, beans, cabbage, carrots, celery, corn, lettuce, onions, peas, spinach, tomatoes, and watercress. Other foods which may help are bran, cereals, and bread. Tea should be avoided if there is marked constipation.

4. In some cases it may be necessary to inject four to six ounces of warm olive oil into the rectum before retiring. This is to remain overnight, and its purpose is to soften the stool, protect the lining of the rectum, and prevent or remove a spasm of the bowel.

5. If the above measures do not prevent or relieve constipation, drugs must be used. In nearly every case such simple substances as metamucil (every other night), or milk of magnesia (one tablespoon every night), or occasionally phenolphthalein in the form of "Phenolax" or "Ex-lax" (2 tablets at night), usually suffice. In more stubborn cases it may be necessary to take a teaspoonful of fluid extract of cascara sagrada each night. An enema should be the last resort, and the fewer that are taken throughout pregnancy the better. The simplest enemas consist of weak salt solution or a very weak soapsuds solution.

CARE OF THE KIDNEYS IN PREGNANCY

The kidneys have an extra amount of work to do during pregnancy, and they frequently give rise to serious disturbances. If a woman knows she has or has had kidney trouble she should visit a physician before she plans to have a baby and let him tell her whether it is safe for her to bear a child. Women who have serious kidney disturbances, such as chronic nephritis, should not attempt to have children, because the kidney trouble will nearly always be aggravated, and the baby in many instances will not be born alive. However, if a woman has only a mild degree of nephritis she may go through a pregnancy without complications provided she is carefully watched by a competent physician.

Women with normal kidneys should have a specimen of urine examined at least once every three weeks, and more frequent examinations toward the end of pregnancy. However, women with kidney disturbances should have their urine examined at least once a week, and they should measure their urinary output every day. At least three pints of urine should be passed daily, and if the amount decreases the doctor should be informed.

If swelling of the feet, ankles, hands, or face is noticed, the doctor should be notified. Frequently these swellings indicate some abnormality in the function of the kidneys.

Chronic nephritis is not the only kind of kidney trouble which occurs during pregnancy. There may be a condition known as pyelitis, in which part of the kidney is inflamed and the urine contains pus and bacteria. Examination of the urine will also reveal whether diabetes or a tendency to diabetes is present.

CLOTHING IN PREGNANCY

The manner in which an expectant mother dresses herself is important. Comfort should not be sacrificed for the sake of appearances. In cold weather sufficient clothing should be worn to keep warm, whereas during the hot months the clothing should be light. In some regions it is important to be prepared for sudden changes in the weather in order to avoid chilling. Most of the clothing should be simple and should be washed frequently. None of it should hinder free movements of breathing or of the arms and legs. There must be no circular constrictions anywhere; hence it is important to give up using round garters, belts, tight corsets, or tight skirt bands. Side elastics attached to a maternity corset are the proper type of garter.

Underclothing should always be worn, the kind and amount depending upon the weather. It may consist of one or two pieces, but it is best that the drawers be closed. The under-garments should be changed every day or as often as possible, because they absorb the waste matter eliminated by the skin. All clothing should be well aired at night.

Up to the end of the third and sometimes the fourth month the usual type of corset may generally be worn. After this time the customary type of corset compresses the abdomen and may lead to harm. Hence after the fourth month it is often necessary to wear some type of maternity corset, the chief purpose of which is to support the growing womb. It is more important for a woman who has already had one or more children to use a maternity corset than for a woman who is to have her first baby. The reason for this is that most women who have given birth have some weakness of the abdominal wall, and this requires support. Women who have a flabby abdominal wall must wear a proper maternity corset constantly, or they will have a good deal of discomfort, especially backache. On the other hand, many women carrying their first baby may be comfortable throughout pregnancy without a corset.

Most women must wear a support for the breasts, or the latter will be painful. This support should not be tightly applied, but should elevate the breasts.

Proper shoes are essential. The usual narrow, high-heeled shoes not only cause pain but are actually harmful. During the latter months of pregnancy the feet spread and enlarge somewhat, hence slightly larger shoes must be worn. Furthermore, as the abdomen continues to grow, there is a tendency to pull the body forward. To overcome this, the woman instinctively throws her shoulders back. If the woman wears high heels, the body is pushed still farther forward, and to save herself from falling she must throw her head and shoulders much farther backward. This causes a good deal of backache, discomfort in the lower part of the abdomen, and fatigue. The proper shoe for a pregnant woman is one which is sufficiently wide and has low broad heels somewhat on the style of the Cuban heel, or one still lower and wider. Rubber heels lessen the amount of jarring while walking.

It is natural for women to want to prevent the ungainly shape and "high stomach" which some of them have after giving birth to a child. Most of this is due to relaxation of the skin and the rest of the abdominal wall and to markings on the skin known as striæ gravidarum. Much can be done to prevent these by wearing a proper maternity corset, avoiding constricting bands, wearing proper shoes, and massaging the abdominal wall with mineral oil or olive oil every day during pregnancy. Beginning a few weeks after the baby comes, this should be continued, and likewise systematic body exercises. Regular bowel movements are essential to prevent this also. However, it must be borne in mind that in women with an inherited predisposition to flabbiness, little can be done to prevent a "high stomach" or striæ gravidarum.

EXERCISE IN PREGNANCY

A woman who expects a baby should take a certain amount of exercise daily, unless there are special reasons for not doing so. The benefits derived from exercise are improvement in the circulation of the blood, better appetite and digestion of food, better elimination of waste products of the body, more restful sleep, and an opportunity to divert the mind from household responsibilities.

The amount and kind of exercise for an expectant mother depend to a certain extent on the individual woman. One thing is certain, however: the expectant mother should never exercise to the point of fatigue. She should stop as soon as she begins to feel tired. The nearer the day of confinement, the more readily does fatigue set in. Women who are accustomed to participate in strenuous sports can tolerate more than women who lead an indoor and sedentary life. Women who have many household duties to perform do not need as much exercise as women who do not have such duties.

WALKING

Practically the only active exercise available for expectant mothers is walking and this should be outdoors, except during inclement weather. For this purpose, broad, low-heeled shoes with wide toes should be used, because high-heeled shoes may cause backache and missteps. It is best to walk during the hours of sunlight, because the sun's rays are beneficial. They help the body utilize the minerals in the food. However, during the summer months the expectant mother should be cautious about taking a walk in the hot sun. While walking, it is advisable to proceed leisurely and to avoid crowds. Long tramps are too strenuous for most women. About two or three miles is a fair average daily walk.

If even a short walk produces a tired feeling, the expectant mother should not walk much but should rest in the open air. While resting, the mind may be occupied with reading, knitting, or chatting. At least two hours each day should be spent outdoors. This time is best divided into two periods, one in the morning and the other in the afternoon. When the weather is unusually bad, a walk should be taken at home, either on an open porch or in a room with all the windows wide open. In winter, warm clothes should be worn for this, just as if one were on the street. It is needless to emphasize that the home should be well aired at all times, night as well as day. It is advisable to take five or six deep breaths night and morning before an open window. Likewise, while walking outdoors, deep breathing should be practised for short periods each day.

VIOLENT EXERCISE

Violent exercise in any form should be avoided. This includes running, tennis, golf, swimming, cycling, skating, and horseback riding. Dancing should be indulged in only occasionally and for short periods of time; but the prospective mother should never dance in a crowded room.

TRAVEL

Driving an automobile should be given up during the last two months of pregnancy. However, most women may safely undertake long journeys by train, automobile, boat or airplane without mishap. The chief drawback is that should trouble arise during the journey or at the destination, skilled obstetric care may not be available.

Women who have lost babies before full term should avoid traveling whenever possible and should undertake a journey only after consultation with a physician. The dangerous period of travel is that time in each month when menstruation would ordinarily occur. At this time more than any other, over-exertion of any kind may produce premature birth of the baby. When railroad travel is imperative for a woman who has had miscarriages, the smoothest road and the most comfortable accommodations should be chosen and she should recline as much as possible during the journey.

HOUSEWORK

A certain amount of housework is not only permissible but is desirable. Here also the expectant mother should never proceed to the point of fatigue. Only light work should be done. If there is a young child at home, the expectant mother should not lift and carry him around any more than is absolutely necessary. By observing these precautions many backaches and much fatigue will be avoided.

When an expectant mother has much housework to do and finds that the additional walking outdoors makes her tire quickly, she should take only a short walk and spend most of the outdoor allotment of time sitting and resting, especially when the sun is shining. This will insure not only physical but also mental relaxation.

REST AND RECREATION

The prospective mother should learn to rest frequently, especially if she does housework. Most women, and more particularly those who tire easily, will find an afternoon nap of an hour or more of great help. Even if one does not actually sleep, complete relaxation in a reclining position will prove refreshing. To obtain the full benefit of such relaxation, it is essential to undress and go to bed. Where there are young children in the home, the mother may take her siesta when the children take theirs. If exercise is taken during the day, there need be no fear that an afternoon nap will prevent sleeping at night.

It may not be amiss to add a word about modesty. Not infrequently women refuse to leave their home, even for a short walk, during the last few weeks or months of pregnancy because they are sensitive about their appearance. This attitude is entirely unwarranted. Women should be proud that they are to become mothers, for there are women, and unfortunately they are numerous, who would give a part of their lives for the ability to give birth to babies but who cannot have children.

Places of amusement may be visited, but those that are poorly ventilated or overheated should be avoided.

Massage during pregnancy is rarely necessary and is permissible only on the advice of a physician. Women who must remain in bed for a few weeks during pregnancy usually need massage.

BATHING

Many people firmly believe that bathing during pregnancy is harmful. This is a pernicious belief. The skin should be kept clean at all times, but more especially during pregnancy, because the activity of the skin is greater than usual at this time. This is due to the increased elimination and excretion of the body during pregnancy, and the skin constitutes an important organ for these purposes. The expectant mother must eliminate not only her own waste products but also those of the child within the womb.

The skin contains myriads of openings called pores, which lead to sweat glands. By means of these pores certain excretory products of the body are eliminated. If these pores become clogged, proper elimination is prevented, and the expectant mother suffers in consequence.

The water and waste products that cannot be thrown off by the sweat glands remain in the blood until the kidneys, the bowels, and the lungs do the work. An unpleasant odor usually develops. To keep the pores open, to remove the accumulation of degenerated skin, dirt, grease, and dried perspiration, and to keep the skin functioning, it is necessary to wash the entire body with soap and water, and this must be done daily.

KIND OF BATH TO TAKE

The kind of bath is important. One may take a shower, sponge, or tub bath, but the water should be neither too hot nor too cold. Very hot baths cause fatigue. The water should preferably be at a temperature between 85 and 90 degrees F. Even the woman who is accustomed to a cold bath each morning should increase the temperature of the water during pregnancy; for while a cold bath is stimulating, it is not as efficacious as a warm bath for actually cleansing the skin. However, women who are accustomed to a cold shower or tub bath may take such a cold bath in the morning and leave the cleansing bath for the evening.

Since the object of a bath is not only to cleanse the skin but also to stimulate the circulation, it is advisable to rub the whole body with a rough towel fairly vigorously.

WARM BATH DAILY

It does not matter much whether the daily warm bath is taken in the morning or in the evening before retiring. However, for women who do not sleep well, it is best to take the warm bath at night, because it is soothing and will promote sleep. If the warm bath is taken in the morning or during the day, at least an hour should elapse before one goes outdoors. If the bath is taken in the afternoon, at least two hours should have passed after the midday meal.

Sponge baths and shower baths may be taken up to the time of actual confinement, but tub baths are customarily forbidden during the last four weeks of pregnancy because of the rare possibility of the bath water gaining access to the pelvic organs and causing infection in women who have already borne children. When taking tub baths, women should be especially cautious to avoid slipping or falling while getting in and out of the tub.

The following types of bathing should be avoided by most women: cold tub baths, cold plunges, cold showers (except for those who are accustomed to such baths), ocean bathing, and Turkish and Russian baths. Hot sitz baths should be taken only on the recommendation of a physician. Sweat baths should also be shunned except on the physician's recommendation, because they usually prove to be too exhausting and rarely do normal women any good.

CARE OF THE BREASTS

Special attention should be paid to cleansing the breasts and nipples. Care must be exercised to avoid compression of and injury to the breasts; this holds true not only during pregnancy but also during the entire life of the woman, from early infancy. Certainly beginning with puberty, the breasts should be protected from excessive pressure and from injury.

During pregnancy a breast supporter should be used, especially if the breasts are large. The skin of the breasts should be washed with soap and water daily just as the rest of the body. Special precautions should be taken to remove the scales that frequently cover the nipples. These scales are due to drying of the discharge which normally exudes from the nipples during the pregnancy. The nipples may be anointed daily with cocoa butter, cold cream, or lanolin. Astringents, such as alcohol, should not be used because they harden the nipples, thereby favoring the formation of cracks, which may becomes avenues of infection.

If the nipples are flat, they may be drawn out for a few minutes each day during the last few weeks of pregnancy; but this must be done with the utmost gentleness and after demonstration by a physician or nurse.

CARE OF THE GENITAL ORGANS

The genital organs likewise require some special attention. During pregnancy there is increased secretion, but this does not require removal. On the contrary, this increased secretion is a helpful measure and should not be disturbed. If, however, the discharge is profuse or has a disagreeable odor, the doctor should be told about it. Douches should never be taken without consulting the doctor.

SEXUAL INTERCOURSE

Sexual intercourse should be restricted as much as possible during pregnancy and entirely eliminated during the last six weeks, because of the danger of rupturing the bag of waters and of serious infection. Women who have a tendency to abort, who have bled during the pregnancy or who have had premature labors should indulge in as little intercourse as possible throughout the entire pregnancy. The times when intercourse is absolutely forbidden are the days in each month when the menstrual period would have occurred if the woman were not pregnant. It is at these times that the greatest danger of a miscarriage exists.

CARE OF THE HAIR

The hair should be washed once a week, using a mild soap for this purpose. The lather should be worked into the scalp before rinsing. The scalp should be massaged and the hair brushed daily. If the hair is dry or there is dandruff, olive oil should be rubbed into the hair and scalp. There is no harm in having a permanent wave but this should not be done in the last four weeks of pregnancy.

CARE OF THE TEETH

It is important for every expectant mother to have her teeth examined and cleaned at least twice during her pregnancy. If the dentist finds defects which he can remedy, it is perfectly safe for him to correct the abnormalities. But he should not do more than is absolutely necessary. He may fill, clean, and pull teeth, but not attempt work which requires a long time and causes a good deal of discomfort unless it cannot be postponed until after delivery.

In some pregnant women the teeth decay and loosen. Sometimes, but not often this abnormal process may be corrected by eating an abundance of calcium (chiefly in the form of milk), phosphorus (chiefly in the form of eggs), cod-liver oil, haliver oil, viosterol, fresh fruits, vegetables, butter, and whole-grain cereals. Likewise an abundance of sunshine is essential in order to enable the body to utilize the calcium and phosphorus which are eaten. The teeth should, of course, be carefully brushed at least twice a day and dental floss used to remove particles of food lodged between the teeth. If the gums have a tendency to bleed they should be vigorously massaged with the fingers two or three times a day.

THE MIND

The expectant mother should try to lead a quiet, cheerful life and avoid mental as well as physical upheavals. There is usually nothing to fear about pregnancy and labor, and the best proof of this is that millions of women constantly go through these physiologic processes without harm, all over the world. It is best to avoid contact with friends or relatives who relate tales about difficult obstetric cases they know. If a woman has any fears she should speak to her doctor about them. He will usually be able to prove there is no basis for them, and if there is good cause for the fears the physician will be able to correct or overcome the cause. Reading cheerful books helps a great deal.

SIGNS OF TROUBLE

There are certain signs and symptoms which arise during pregnancy and which may be forerunners of trouble unless attention is paid to them. The following is a list of them, and when any of them are present they should be called to the attention of the physician without delay:

1. Persistent vomiting of most of the food eaten.
2. Stubborn constipation.
3. Frequent or persistent headaches, especially if associated with dizziness and marked constipation.
4. Swelling of the feet, ankles, hands, eyelids, or face.
5. Rapid gain in weight.
6. Diminished output of urine.

7. Blurred or double vision, or spots before the eyes.

8. Shortness of breath or inability to sleep unless the head is elevated on a few pillows.

9. Vomiting after the fifth month.

10. Frequent fainting spells.

11. Any infection or fever.

12. Failure to feel the baby after it has been definitely felt for a while.

13. Escape of bloody or watery discharge from the vagina with or without cramps in the lower part of the abdomen. During the early months of pregnancy these are symptoms of a threatened or beginning miscarriage or abortion. Should they occur, someone should notify the doctor and the patient should get into bed. Her feet or the foot of the bed should be elevated. The patient should not become excited, because nothing serious can happen during the first few hours, and a doctor can surely reach her during this time. It may happen that the fetus and afterbirth are expelled spontaneously. All tissue, including blood clots, which is passed, should be saved in a towel or in a jar so the doctor may see whether all the parts came away. This is important, because if part or all of the afterbirth is left in the womb, it may have to be removed with instruments.

MINOR AILMENTS DURING PREGNANCY

HEARTBURN AND BELCHING

Many women are greatly disturbed by frequent attacks of heartburn or belching or both. In spite of its name, heartburn has nothing to do with the heart. It is a peculiar burning sensation in the chest and throat, accompanied by the presence of a bitter fluid which escapes from the stomach into the throat. Sometimes heartburn may be prevented by drinking a glass of milk and cream mixture a few minutes before meal time. The fat in the cream and milk prevents the secretion of acid in the stomach. However, when heartburn is actually present, fats will not help. In fact, they may even aggravate the condition. The best remedies for heartburn are a half-teaspoonful of baking soda (sodium bicarbonate) in a half-glass of water, a teaspoonful of milk of magnesia, or two or three soda-mint tablets. These substances neutralize the acid which causes the heartburn. However, the amount of sodium bicarbonate and other alkalis taken during pregnancy must be strictly limited because an excessive intake of sodium may lead to high blood pressure, swelling of parts of the body and other serious disturbances.

FAINTING AND DIZZINESS

It is not uncommon for pregnant women, especially those who are anemic, to have attacks of fainting or dizziness. The condition is not serious; hence, there is no cause for alarm or worry. If a woman feels faint she should immediately lie down on a couch or bed. If she is in a place where there is no bed or couch, she should gently slip down to the floor and lie flat. The faintness will pass away in a few minutes. If the attacks are frequent, it is a good thing to keep spirits of ammonia or smelling salts in the house within easy reach or in the purse. If a woman becomes dizzy she should sit down and lower her head to her knees in order to permit more blood to reach the brain.

VARICOSE VEINS

Varicose veins are much more common in women who have had children and there is a large hereditary factor in most of these women. Women who have varicose veins on the legs and thighs should keep the legs up on a chair or a stool while they are sitting. They can read, sew, or fulfill most sedentary occupations with their legs elevated. This relieves the distended veins of the extra load of blood they must carry when the patient is standing or sitting with her feet lowered in the usual position. Care must be exercised not to injure varicose veins, because they may bleed or become infected. In cases where the veins are unusually large, a rubber stocking or elastic bandage must be worn. This should be long enough to extend above the highest visible varicose vein and should be put on the leg in the morning before the woman gets out of bed. Occasionally treatment in the form of injection of medicine or an operation is necessary during pregnancy. The results of this type of treatment are good.

HEMORRHOIDS OR PILES

Many pregnant women are troubled by piles. The usual symptom is bleeding from the rectum while having a bowel movement but pain may be present. Piles are a special form of varicose veins, and they are always made worse by chronic constipation and straining at stool. They are much more common in women who have had children than in those who are pregnant for the first time. It is important to eat the proper kinds of food and to go to the toilet at the same time every day because hemorrhoids are always aggravated by constipation and straining during bowel movements. In addition, a tablespoonful of metamucil should be taken by mouth morning and evening. If the piles are much swollen, ice or witch hazel compresses will help. If the hemorrhoids do not readily go back into the rectum, they should be pushed back with a lubricated finger, because there is danger of obstruction and infection of these veins. If they cannot be pushed back or if they bleed frequently the doctor should be notified.

CRAMPS IN THE LEGS

Cramps or muscular contractions occur rather frequently, especially in the second half of pregnancy, and particularly during the night; they are most likely a sign of neuritis. They may be relieved by changing position, by rubbing the cramped part, by applying heat or cold, by bending the foot at the ankle, and by standing on a cold slab such as the floor of the bathroom. Medically, the cramps can usually be prevented by taking a 5 or 10 mg. tablet of thiamine hydrochloride daily.

PREVENTION OF GOITER

In all pregnant women the function of the thyroid gland is increased, and, because of this, slightly more iodine is needed during pregnancy than otherwise. If insufficient iodine is eaten, the thyroid gland of both mother and baby may enlarge. In most parts of the country there is ample iodine in the drinking water and in the vegetables and grain grown in these regions. However, in certain localities like the Great Lakes region there is a lack of iodine, and the expectant mothers in these places must take iodine in some form such as iodine tablets, iodized salt, or Lugol's solution. However, none of these should ever be taken without orders and strict supervision by a physician, because harm may result.

PREPARATIONS FOR CONFINEMENT

The large proportion of women in cities have their babies in a hospital because of the numerous advantages gained thereby. The doctor or the patient may make the necessary arrangements. Since premature delivery is not uncommon, it is a good plan to have certain articles packed in a suitcase a few weeks before the expected date of confinement. These articles should consist of two nightgowns, a bathrobe, two pairs of stockings, a pair of slippers, a few handkerchiefs, a toothbrush and toothpaste or powder, and a comb and brush. In most hospitals the baby's clothes are supplied by the hospital until the child is ready to leave. Hence the day before the patient expects to depart from the hospital, the husband or someone else should take to the hospital for the baby a shirt, a nightgown or robe, safety pins, a few diapers, a sweater, a cap, and two blankets. Of course these are only a few of the things which the expectant mother should have bought a few weeks before the baby arrives. Since newborn babies quickly outgrow the clothes, not much is needed at the time of birth. Nowadays clothes for the baby are made to be comfortable for the child and easy to put on and take off. They should be of light texture, particularly, because in steam-heated apartments babies are generally burdened with too many clothes.

The following is a list of clothes necessary for a baby:

Shirts. Four shirts are usually sufficient. They should be infant size No. 2 for they will soon be outgrown. For summer, cotton mesh should be used and for winter, cotton and wool. The shirts should have long sleeves and high necks, they should open in the front and they should reach down below the hips.

Dresses. Two dresses are ample because they are worn only occasionally. They should consist of nainsook or dimity and should open all the way down the back.

Kimonos. Four kimonos should be purchased because they are used more than dresses. They should consist of cotton and wool, flannelette or cashmere.

Nightgowns. Six nightgowns are usually necessary. They should be made of soft flannel or stockinet. Most of the nightgowns have drawstrings in the sleeves and at the bottom in order to keep the baby warm should it become uncovered during the night.

Diapers. At least four dozen diapers should be obtained. The old type of bird's eye diaper (22 by 22 inches) is still generally used, but there are newer varieties. All diapers should be soft, absorbent and of loosely woven material such as bird's eye, stockinet or cotton flannel. Some diapers are made to throw away after they are used once. In many large cities there are laundries which for a fee deliver clean, sterilized diapers every day and take back the soiled ones. The laundries provide diaper containers.

Bootees. Two pairs of bootees are sufficient. They should be long enough to extend over the knee. Stockings are not to be used.

Sweaters. Two sweaters either knitted or made of cashmere are necessary. They should be open down the front, so there will not be any need to slip them on over the baby's head.

Cap. One cap will suffice.

In addition to the foregoing list of clothes for the baby, other articles may be secured. For the baby's nursery the following will be necessary:

1. A bed or large basket with a suitable mattress.
2. Four sheets made of cotton knit.
3. Two large rubber sheets to be placed between the mattress and cotton sheet.
4. Six pads made of Turkish toweling each about 20 by 20 inches.
5. One rubberized pad, about 20 by 20 inches, to be placed under the Turkish toweling pads.
6. Two woolen blankets.
7. A bath table for bathing and dressing the baby. Most of these are collapsible.
8. Scales which may be purchased or rented. They should be of the balance or beam type and not of the spring type.
9. A clothes horse for hanging and drying the baby's clothes.
10. A baby's toilet tray on which should be placed a rectal thermometer, a bath thermometer, Pyrex nursing bottles, safety pins, and covered jars containing rubber nipples, bottle caps, cotton balls, toothpick swabs, a bottle brush, albolene and soap.
11. Towels and wash cloths.

WHEN TO CALL THE DOCTOR FOR CONFINEMENT

Labor is the term applied to the process of giving birth, and there are usually three signs by which the beginning of labor may be known:

1. Rhythmic contractions of the womb which the woman experiences as abdominal cramps. These may be felt by placing the hand on the abdomen, because the latter becomes hard during a contraction and relaxes when the cramp subsides. At first these cramps or labor pains are irregular in frequency and intensity, and they begin in the back and radiate to the front. Later they become more frequent, more regular, stronger, and located in the abdomen. "False pains" are weak contractions which occur a few days or a few weeks before actual confinement. They may be distinguished from true labor pains by

the fact that they do not increase in frequency, intensity, or duration, and they subside after a while.

2. The escape from the vagina of water which is not urine. This is due to rupture of the bag of waters in which the baby lies. Labor pains usually do not begin for a few hours after this starts, but it is advisable for the patient to remain in bed while waiting for the pains to begin. Better still, she should go to the hospital after notifying the doctor.

3. A thick, mucous, bloody discharge from the vagina, known as the "show."

Only one of these signs is usually present at first, and it is sufficient to warrant notifying the doctor. Then the hospital should be informed that the patient is on the way. Abnormal symptoms may sometimes arise just about the time of confinement, and the doctor must be told about them without delay. These symptoms include bleeding from the vagina, a sudden fainting attack, severe persistent cramps in the abdomen, vomiting, disturbances in vision, and muscular twitchings. It is a good thing to keep the telephone numbers of the doctor, his assistant if he has one, and the hospital, in a place where they can be obtained without delay.

What to Do if the Baby Is Born at Home before the Patient Can Go to the Hospital

The average duration of the first labor is about thirteen hours, and the length of labor after the first one is about eight hours. Hence there is no need to be panic-stricken when labor begins. With few exceptions there is always ample time to get to the hospital. Occasionally, however, for one reason or another, especially in the case of a woman who has had a few quick labors, the entire duration of labor may be so short that the baby is born at home. When it is obvious that the child will be born in the home, the patient's physician should be informed of what is happening. If he cannot be reached, his assistant or another physician should be called to act in the emergency. A kettle of water should be placed on a stove to boil, and a small pair of scissors and two pieces of tape or string dropped into the water.

The cleanest room should be chosen for the patient, and there should be sufficient warmth, especially for the sake of the baby. The expectant mother should, of course, remain in bed. If a baby can be born in such a short time, the process is nearly always normal and easy. As soon as the baby is born, if it cries spontaneously, nothing need be done except to wrap a warm, clean towel around its body to keep it warm. There is usually no harm in leaving the child in bed just as it is, provided it is breathing normally and its color is pink. If the doctor is informed of what happened at home he will usually be able to arrive in time to clean his hands properly to tie the cord and see that the afterbirth is delivered.

If the baby does not breathe or cry immediately after birth, someone should thoroughly wash his or her hands and fore-arms with soap and water and then with alcohol and should rub the baby's back up and down with two or three fingers. If this does not produce crying, the baby should be held up by its feet, and its buttocks gently spanked a number of times. This usually causes the baby to cry. Then it should be kept covered with a clean warm towel.

If the afterbirth should be expelled before the doctor arrives, someone should thoroughly scrub his or her hands with soap and water, and with the two pieces of boiled tape or string, tie the umbilical cord in two places. The first should be about one inch from the baby's body and the other about one inch farther away. Before tying the two tapes, iodine on a cotton applicator should be applied on the part of the cord where the strings are to be tied, and the strings should be saturated with iodine. Great care should be exercised that none of the iodine touches the baby's body, because it may produce a burn. The cord should then be cut between the two pieces of string with the scissors which is in the kettle of boiling water. More iodine should be applied to the cut edge of the cord which is attached to the baby. It is important to be sure there is no bleeding from this end of the cord. If there is bleeding, another piece of string should be applied tightly.

The afterbirth and the sac should not be thrown away but should be saved for the doctor to see. It is important to know whether all of the afterbirth and the sac came away intact. If a piece is left behind, it usually causes hemorrhage and frequently infection unless it is removed immediately.

THE PUERPERIUM

The puerperium is the time interval that extends from the birth of the baby until the organs of reproduction return to their normal condition. This interval usually lasts from six to eight weeks.

For the first three days after the delivery it is a good policy to disconnect the telephone and to have only the husband, the patient's parents, and the husband's parents as visitors. After this only two visitors a day, other than the husband, are sufficient and best. The fewer visitors and telephone conversations the patient has during the first week, the stronger and more rested she will be. If a baby is born at home it is difficult to restrict visitors, but someone should be delegated to act the firm and stern policeman. Certainly no one who has a cold or infection of any kind should be permitted to visit the mother of a newborn child or be allowed in the baby's room. In hospitals there is an excellent rule which forbids children less than fourteen years of age from visiting the mother of a newborn baby. Young children are prone to carry infections, and, of course, the sight of her other children will usually upset the mother and make her homesick.

The discomfort that most women feel passes a few hours after the baby is born. Women who have had children before may have "afterpains," or painful contractions of the uterus, for twenty-four to forty-eight hours, but these are relieved easily by mild drugs. Women who have just given birth to their first child seldom have afterpains. Many women who have stitches on the outside of the vagina suffer a good deal of pain. In addition to the use of medicines for the relief of the pain, a helpful procedure is a hot tub bath once or twice a day after childbirth. For generations tub baths within the first few days or even weeks have been taboo, but there is no harm in indulging in them and they afford great relief from pain.

On the third or fourth day most women complain of pain and swelling of the breasts. This is caused by the onset of the flow of milk. The discomfort is seldom troublesome and generally disappears after twenty-four to forty-eight hours when the baby, by its sucking action, has regulated the amount of milk in the breasts. Babies are generally put to the breast only twice during the first twenty-four hours, and after this they nurse every four hours, except during the night. Breast nursing is beneficial to the mother as well as to the newborn baby. The genital organs return to normal more quickly in women who nurse their babies.

Today patients are permitted much more freedom than was the custom in previous years. We generally permit our patients to get out of bed and even walk the day the baby is born, but surely the next day unless there is a strong reason against this activity. Most mothers return to their homes when the baby is seven to ten days old. For this reason many hospitals have a flat rate for obstetric cases, which includes not only the delivery of the baby but also hospital care for seven or ten days.

If a patient had some disturbance during pregnancy, she will need special aftercare. Thus, if a woman had high blood pressure, she will have to have repeated blood-pressure readings. If she had a kidney infection, her urine will have to be examined every day. These women must be watched not only during their hospital stay but for months and perhaps years afterward. Such follow-up care is important for the patient's future health and certainly for a decision about having more children.

POSTPARTUM CARE

Postpartum means after delivery. When a patient leaves the hospital she is advised not to walk the steps leading to her apartment if one or two strong-armed men can carry her. If she must walk, it is advisable for her to walk slowly and to rest frequently. Since there is considerable excitement incident to dressing the baby, packing suitcases, saying good-bye to the nurses, riding home, meeting neighbors, and so on, in the process of getting home, it is advisable that the patient go to bed as soon as she reaches home and remain there until the following morning. It is best for her to leave the hospital in the afternoon because of the advantage of traveling during the day and because by the time home is reached there are not many waking hours left. Once in the home, the patient should not go into the street until the baby is almost three weeks old.

Probably the most important factor necessary to safeguard a happy household with a newborn baby is a mentally calm and unperturbed mother. This is determined to the largest extent by the health of the baby. As was previously said, the day of departure from the hospital is one of excitement. As a result the baby not infrequently loses weight on that day. After the first day at home the mother must learn to be more or less callous to disturbing influences. Certainly petty inconveniences should not be permitted to interfere with her peace of mind. If there is a nurse at home, she, of course, assumes much of the responsibility in the care of the child. Tranquillity of mind and regularity in feeding the infant will usually guarantee a thriving baby.

During the puerperium the mother should have an abundance of sleep and, in addition, should rest in a reclining position for definite periods of time in the morning and in the afternoon. While resting, it is advisable for her to lie on her abdomen for fifteen to twenty minutes, just as we ask our patients to do when they are in the hospital.

During the first week at home visitors should be restricted to two a day besides the immediate family. Tact is necessary to avoid talkative visitors or to limit their stay. Likewise, telephone calls should be limited in number and length, especially if at the other end of the wire there is a garrulous individual or one who wants to impart information concerning dreadful occurrences. Visitors who have colds or infections should not be seen and definitely must not be admitted to the baby's room.

If the mother herself has a cold, she should cover her mouth and nose with a handkerchief or a mouthpiece when nursing or bathing the baby. No medicine sould be taken by the mother or given to the baby without the sanction of a physician. Some drugs reach the baby through the breast milk.

If there are three- or four-year-old children in the home, the development of jealousy in them should be looked for and averted. Sometimes they resent the attention showered on a new arrival. Showing the baby off before relatives and friends may aggravate such a tendency.

When nursing the baby one may sit up or recline. An extremely important thing to avoid is constant observation of the baby while it is at the breast; for this not only strains the mother's eyes and produces headaches, but strains the muscles of the neck and back, which likewise become the seat of pain.

For the woman with a lax abdominal wall a supporting garment is most helpful. Showers or tub baths should be taken daily during this time. Exercise, especially walking, is advisable after the third week; but strenuous exercise, such as playing golf or tennis, swimming, skating, or even driving a car, should be avoided during the puerperal period. Social functions during these weeks should likewise be reduced to a minimum.

Systematic exercises should be started after arriving home. During the first three or four days they should be done for only five minutes, but gradually more and more time should be devoted to them.

RETURN OF MENSTRUATION

The return of menstruation varies in different individuals. In those who do not nurse their babies the flow usually returns at the end of six weeks, while in those who do breast-feed their babies the first menstrual period appears any time after the third month. In some, however, the menses do not return until the baby is weaned. The first period is usually profuse, sometimes enough to cause alarm. At the time of the first period it is best for the woman to keep off her feet as much as possible; but if the flow is too profuse, the advice of a physician should be sought. In fact, if the mother has any doubt concerning herself or the baby she should consult her physician rather than take the advice offered by well-meaning but often misinformed friends and relatives. Cracked or bleeding nipples or painful breasts particularly call for immediate notification of the physician.

It is customary for a patient to return to her physician at the end of the puerperal period; namely, six to eight weeks after the birth of the baby. At this time the physician will determine, by an abdominal and vaginal examination, whether the reproductive organs have returned to their normal state. Generally this checkup is designated as the "final" examination. This is unfortunate, because the patient regards it as the final contact with her physician until a new pregnancy begins or some disturbance arises. Since some women have complications or abnormalities, or they develop after childbirth, it is advisable for women to see their obstetricians when the baby is six months old, and again when it is a year old. All women should be examined once a year, even if they feel entirely well.

WEANING THE BABY

The time when a baby is to be weaned varies considerably. Women who have an abundant supply of breast milk should nurse their baby for eight or nine months. However, few women have a supply of milk which will last as long as this. Women with ample breast milk should not wean the baby during the first few months without an urgent reason. Breast feeding is helpful for the mother as well as for her child, because it helps to restore her organs more quickly and more completely than otherwise. A doctor's advice should be sought before a woman with a good supply of milk decides to discontinue breast feedings.

SUPERSTITIONS AND MISCONCEPTIONS ABOUT CHILDBIRTH

From the dawn of history there have been innumerable superstitions associated with childbirth. The ancients held such peculiar notions about reproduction that laymen of today who are familiar with these ideas consider them ludicrous. However, the vast majority of the laity who today scoff at the credulity of the uncivilized and the semicivilized hold fast to enough erroneous beliefs about childbirth to make physicians laugh at them in turn.

There is an almost universal belief among the laity in so-called maternal impressions. This expression signifies that a child in the womb may be marked in some obscure way by what the mother thinks, feels, or sees during pregnancy, especially if the experience is disagreeable or shocking. This belief is one of the oldest in history. Not only was it prevalent among the uncivilized peoples, but many of our most prominent literary celebrities used it as a theme for their writtings. Among the latter may be mentioned Goethe, Scott, Dickens, and O. W. Holmes. When a child is born with a birthmark, those who believe in maternal impressions make an effort to detect a special form in the birthmark and link it up with some frightful occurrence which the mother experienced during the last few months of pregnancy. However, there is absolutely no support for the belief in maternal impressions. In the first place birthmarks and other defects are usually accidental aberrations in the growth of the child. These abnormalities begin to manifest themselves when the fetus has been in the uterus only a few weeks, because the child is almost completely formed by the time it reaches its eighth week of development. Hence nothing which happens to the mother in the latter part of gestation can possibly affect the child in the womb. Secondly, there is no direct contact between the mother and the baby in the womb, by way of either the nerves or the blood. The nerves connect the mother with the womb but not with the baby; hence the worst thing which can occur is stimulation of the uterus, with subsequent interruption of pregnancy. Even this occurrence is uncommon. The baby receives nourishment from the mother, but only because the afterbirth extracts the necessary ingredients from the mother's blood. Thirdly, in most instances, where the child presents defects, the mother was never frightened or upset in any way. In spite of the horrors to which women abroad were subjected during World War I and II, there were no more "marked" babies than are usually born.

Another common belief is that a baby born during the seventh month of its intrauterine existence can live, whereas one delivered during the eighth month cannot. This is incorrect. The truth is that the longer a baby remains in the womb before it is born, the more advanced is its development, and hence the greater its chances for survival. The few exceptions do not disprove this rule.

There are many misconceptions concerning the determination of the sex of a child before birth. It is commonly held that if a baby's heart tones are more than 140 per minute the baby is a girl, whereas if the heart rate is less than 140 the child is a boy. This belief is based on the fact that large babies usually have slower heart rates than smaller ones, and since boys are generally larger than girls it is assumed that slow heartbeats indicate boys. The truthful physician will tell his patients that he guesses the sex of babies incorrectly almost as often as he guesses it correctly. Normally about 105 boys are born to every 100 girls, and this ratio holds true regardless of seasonal variations and geographical divisions. Hence, if a physician guesses boys more often than girls, over a long period of time, his correct guesses will be slightly greater than his incorrect ones. Among premature babies the proportion of males is higher than

105 to 100, and among fetuses which are expelled during the early months of pregnancy the males are still more predominant. There is as yet no satisfactory explanation for this phenomenon.

Some people believe that the sex of a baby depends on the time in the menstrual cycle when conception takes place. This is wrong. In human beings the sex is determined at the time the female egg is fertilized by the male spermatozoön or sex cell. It is the latter which determines whether a child is to be a male or a female. There are two types of spermatozoa, one of which produces males and one of which is responsible for females.

Some individuals believe that a woman who has only one ovary is capable of having only male or only female children. This belief is not true, because women with only one ovary may give birth to babies of either sex. Likewise these women have a menstrual flow every month, and not every second month. In other words, women with one ovary are just as capable from a reproductive point of view as women with two ovaries.

There is an almost unanimous belief that a woman who has a Cesarean section must have all her subsequent babies delivered in the same way. This is erroneous, because many women have babies through the natural passages after having had a Cesarean section. Of course, if the first operation was performed because a woman has small pelvic bones, the operation will have to be repeated for each baby unless the babies are unusually small. On the other hand, if abdominal delivery was resorted to because of such complications as hemorrhage, convulsions, etc., and this complication is absent during subsequent pregnancies, delivery may often be accomplished in the natural way. However, if natural delivery is awaited after the old type of Cesarean section, there is a distinct risk of rupture of the uterus. This hazard is slight after the new type of abdominal delivery.

Another misbelief is that a Cesarean section cannot be performed until a woman is in actual labor. However, this operation may be done at any time during pregnancy, even weeks and months before the time of the calculated confinement. Likewise it may be performed at any time during labor, but the longer a woman is permitted to have labor pains before the operation is resorted to, especially if the bag of waters has ruptured, the greater the risk of infection.

Some individuals are of the opinion that a woman can have only two Cesarean sections. The truth is that there is no limit to the number of these operations a woman may have. In fact, there is a case on record of a woman who had ten babies by Cesarean operation. Fortunately this is a unique case. Because every abdominal operation carries with it some risk, usually most physicians sterilize a woman after her third Cesarean operation, and even after the second one if this is desired by the patient and her husband. Sterilization as performed today does not prolong a Cesarean operation greatly and does not increase the risk of the operation. Even if the womb is removed after delivery of the child, there is no increased hazard. The womb is seldom removed unless it is diseased. In rare instances however, it is taken out at the time of a Cesarean section as a means of preventing conception in seriously ill women.

Contrary to a common notion, sterilization as now performed has absolutely no deleterious effect on a woman in after life. If she were not told that she can no longer have babies she would not know she was sterilized. All her normal functions, including menstruation, continue except the ability to conceive. It is only when the ovaries or the uterus is removed by operation or their function is destroyed by radium or the X-rays that the menstrual flow ceases and the symptoms of the change of life set in.

A fairly common misconception is that which maintains a woman is incapable of becoming pregnant as long as she nurses a baby. Many women have had an opportunity to learn otherwise. Conception is possible at this time regardless of whether a woman menstruates or not. Most women begin to menstruate within a few months after their babies are born. Those who do not nurse their babies usually have the first flow at the end of about six weeks, whereas those who nurse do not begin to menstruate until a few months later. Strange as it may seem, pregnancy is possible not only during the period of nursing but also before a young girl of twelve or thirteen years begins to menstruate, and also at the end of the reproductive career for a year or more after a woman ceases to menstruate because of the change of life. In other words, even though there is no monthly flow, the ovaries may produce and expel ova or eggs which are capable of being fertilized.

A common belief not only among the public but also among some physicians is that the size of the baby at birth is dependent for the most part upon the amount of food the mother eats during gestation. While this appears to be logical, it has not been proved. There is no constant ratio between the gain in weight in the mother and the size of the baby. The size of babies depends chiefly on heredity but also in some cases upon abnormal conditions in the mother. For example, women with kidney trouble usually have puny babies, and mothers with diabetes frequently have abnormally large offspring. Physicians carefully control the weight of obstetric patients because an excessive gain is primarily deleterious for the mother and only secondarily for the baby.

Since the baby is in reality a parasite, it takes all the nourishment it needs from its mother's blood. If the mother's food does not contain all the ingredients a baby requires, the child will obtain these substances at the expense of the mother's tissues. Hence it is important for a pregnant woman to take not only the proper amount of food but also the right kinds of food, minerals, vitamins, etc. While this is true, there is no reason for women to believe in the false notion that a pregnant woman should eat for two individuals, herself and her baby. It is unnecessary for an expectant mother to eat more than usual, because her body metabolizes the food she eats in a much more economical way than in the nonpregnant state.

Of lesser extent is the belief that one can tell the sex of a baby from the shape of the mother's abdomen. Thus a high prominence is said to indicate a boy, whereas a more even distribution to the sides and to the back is said to be indicative of a girl. These notions have absolutely no truth in them. Likewise there is no basis for the belief that if a woman extends her arms upward to reach for objects the baby will be born with a loop or cord around its neck. In the first place, stretching cannot result in lassoing the child around the neck because the baby moves about freely in a spacious sac of fluid. Secondly the finding of one or more loops of cord around a baby's neck at birth is fairly frequent and usually has no significance at all. Only rarely does a loop of cord wound around a child's neck produce trouble.

It is frequently said that a child will be lucky if it is born with a caul or veil, that is, with the sac in which it lies throughout pregnancy. Maybe so—but it has never been proved.

Many women and physicians believe that a tight binder applied to the woman's abdomen after childbirth will result in the restoration of a normal figure. Unfortunately this is not true. No matter how snug a binder or bandage is applied, it cannot restore tonicity of weak abdominal muscles. On the other hand a tightly applied abdominal binder may result in harm. A loosely applied binder helps to steady the enlarged uterus when the patient moves around in bed, it relieves the feeling of emptiness in the abdomen, and it allays the minds of those women who believe that the binder will restore their anteconceptional figure.

CHAPTER VII

Care and Feeding of the Child
PHILIP C. JEANS, M.D.
Revised by M. F.

INTRODUCTION

INVESTIGATIONS INDICATE *that the boys and girls entering college these days are on an average two inches taller and from seven to ten pounds heavier than their parents and grandparents who entered these same institutions at the same ages in the previous two generations. The fact is significant because it shows what preventive medicine and hygiene have done to build better bodies. In an earlier day children just "growed" like Topsy in* Uncle Tom's Cabin. *Nowadays the diets are regulated, as well as the hours of sleep, the hours of exposure to sunshine and fresh air, the clothing, and all of the other factors of the child's hygiene.*

The reason for such regulation lies, of course, in the change in the habits of civilized man. In a previous generation, children were raised largely in rural populations where they had plenty of sunshine and fresh air, plenty of fresh vegetables and milk, and all of the circumstances combined to promote the growth of a healthy little animal. As human beings moved into great collections of humanity in cities, the sunlight and fresh air began to be shut out. Because of the difficulties of transportation, it became necessary to depend largely on food from cans and on materials transported over many hundreds of miles before they were used by the consumer. The more food and milk are handled, the more likelihood is there of contamination from the hands of those who bring them to their final market.

DEVELOPMENT OF THE INFANT

In order to know whether a baby is normal and developing as he should, it is necessary to have certain standards for judgment. In setting up any such standards, it must be remembered that individual babies will vary somewhat from the average. To say that a baby should weigh seven pounds at birth is stating an approximately average value which everyone knows is strictly true for only a few babies. Babies at birth may weigh six, eight, or nine pounds and be perfectly normal. Extreme variations from the average are of significance. A baby weighing five pounds or less at birth must be classed as a delicate or premature baby requiring special care. Similarly moderate variations from the average in all of the other criteria of growth and development are not to be taken seriously in themselves. The weight or development at any particular period is not of as great significance as the progress which the baby makes from time to time. The infant should show constant and steady progress as indicated by the various standards.

A baby of average weight at birth should double the birth weight by five to six months and treble it by one year. These are average values. A baby who is well fed with ample food will grow faster than this. If the diet has been a balanced one, it is probable that the larger baby is physically superior. The baby may be expected to gain six to eight ounces a week in the first six months and four to six ounces a week during the second six months. After this time the weight gain is much less.

The body length of the baby is also a criterion of growth, but it is not always used in routine evaluation of progress, because of the greater extremes of food quality and quantity required to affect growth in length.

The head grows rapidly in size during the first year, increasing two and one-half inches in circumference in this period. The bones of the skull are relatively soft and may be moulded easily by permitting the baby to lie in the same position. Many infants' heads have become permanently misshapen because the mother did not take care to see that the baby's position was changed frequently. A good practice is to turn the baby on the left side after one feeding and on the right side after the next one. The soft spots or fontanels of the skull represent areas which have not yet calcified. The small one at the back of the head is usually hard by three months. The large one in front should close by eighteen months, but in many vigorous, well-nourished babies, the anterior fontanel has disappeared by one year of age.

The first or deciduous teeth are twenty in number. These begin to erupt at about six months of age and should be completely erupted by two and one-half years. They tend to erupt by pairs, the lower central incisors coming first, then the two upper centrals, followed by the upper lateral incisors. These six incisor teeth should be erupted by one year of age. Moderate variations in the time of eruption of teeth may indicate nothing abnormal.

The muscular movements soon after birth are few, but activity increases rapidly, although in the beginning the movements seem purposeless. By three months the neck muscles are strong enough to support the head. At three months the infant will attempt to grasp objects although with poor muscular control. The grasp becomes accurate at five to seven months. Vigorous well-nourished babies sit alone at six months with occasional falls: they usually sit securely at eight months. Although babies may stand awkwardly earlier, they usually are able to stand well when supported at nine months. The usual time of first walking is sometime between twelve and fifteen months. Between the ages of sitting and walking, most babies accomplish progression over the floor by creeping or otherwise, although a few normal babies do not.

Babies are able to laugh and coo sometimes at two months, sometimes not until several months later. They do not say understandable words until the latter part of the first year. By the end of one year usually several simple words are in the vocabulary. By two years simple short sentences are used. Many entirely normal children are late in talking. In a few instances this delay is of several years, often it seems because a child has felt no necessity for speech, in that all desires are anticipated. Parents should not use baby talk to children, as they learn only that kind of speech which they hear.

The infant's vision seems very imperfect in the beginning. It is not until five or six weeks of age that he pays attention to objects held in front of him. He does not follow with his eyes until he is three to four months old, at which time, or soon thereafter, he makes combined purposeful movements of head and eyes and recognizes people and objects familiar to him. At about this time, or a little earlier, he will turn his head toward a sound and be able to recognize voices.

The mental development of the infant in the first year or two is judged largely by the criteria of physical development which have been discussed. A baby may be slow in sitting, standing, and walking, for the reason that he has been ill or has been poorly fed; or it may be because he is mentally backward. With good food and in the absence of illness, mental backwardness should be suspected when purposeful motor behavior of all types is abnormally delayed or when the infant is inattentive to familiar sights and sounds.

PHYSICAL CARE AND HYGIENE

The baby should always have his own bed. Whenever possible he should have a room exclusively for his own use. The room which he occupies should be well ventilated or the air changed frequently. During his waking or play hours the temperature should be in the neighborhood of 70 degrees F. During sleep time the temperature can be 10 to 30 degrees lower than this, depending upon the age, size and vigor of the baby. When the room is kept cold for sleep it is advisable to have available a warm room to which he can be taken when necessary. When properly supervised and protected, a baby can spend much of his time out of doors after two weeks in summer or after three months in winter. Common sense must be used in putting the baby out of doors, particularly in winter. One criterion for the winter is the baby's reaction to cold; if his face becomes pale and blue and his hands and feet cold, he should not be left outside. The baby must be provided steady warmth and fresh air; if this cannot be done out of doors, the baby must be kept indoors. In the summer babies placed out of doors in the shade usually present no special problem. Several precautions are necessary, however, for sun bathing. Sunstroke from excessive heat is possible. The eyes should be protected from direct sunlight. In the beginning only a limited area of the skin should be exposed; usually the feet are exposed first and the area gradually increased. The first exposure should be not more than 5 minutes. Exposure time is increased gradually until the skin is tanned.

In the first weeks after birth the infant will sleep practically all of the time except when he is bathed and fed. At two to three months he sleeps fourteen to sixteen hours daily, and lies quietly for possibly two hours more. At six months the average baby sleeps about fourteen hours and at one year very little less than this. After eighteen months one expects a twelve-hour sleep at night with an additional daytime nap. Although sleep requirements are stated rather definitely here, there are found to be individual differences in sleep needs. The criterion as to adequacy of sleep should be the health status of the infant or child. One who is getting enough sleep should have a good color and show no undue fatigue, should be bright-eyed, happy and not irritable. If no undesirable symptoms are evident and yet the amount of sleep is minimum for the age, the chances are that the sleeping time is adequate.

The daily bath should be given before one of the morning feedings. After the cord comes off, this should be a tub bath. The room should be warm, not hot, and without drafts. The temperature of the bath water is best at about 100 degrees F. for the young baby, gradually decreased to 90 degrees F. at one year. Unnecessary exposure is to be avoided, especially for the young or delicate infant. Avoidance of exposure may be accomplished by lifting the baby directly from the tub onto a large bath towel. Whether the baby is dried on the mother's lap or on a table matters little, although usually the procedure is more quickly performed on a table. The use of talcum powder is not a corrective for poor drying. Babies would be fully as well off without this accessory. In very hot weather it is often advantageous to give the baby one or more sponge baths in addition to the morning tub bath. Routine care concerning the eyes, ears, nose, mouth, and other details of body cleanliness, is given at the time of the morning bath. The only care needed for the eyes is possibly the cleaning of the inner corners. In cleaning the ears there is no need and some danger in entering farther than the tip of the canal. Nothing should be inserted into the nose. Any crusts or secretions in the lower part of the nostrils may be removed with absorbent cotton. The mouth ordinarily needs no attention until the teeth appear. Then all that is required is to keep the teeth clean. While the teeth are few, this can be done easily with cotton on a toothpick, perhaps with the aid of a toothpaste (not powder). While the baby is young the hair and scalp are washed daily at the time of the bath. This is done with soap and water, as for the remainder of the body. In case there is a "milk crust" on the scalp, some simple oily preparation, such as mineral oil or vaseline, may be placed on the scalp at night and the scalp washed as usual in the morning. At the time of the bath also the genitalia should receive attention. Boys are prone to have adhesions of the foreskin to the glans, and a material known as smegma accumulates back of the glans. If the foreskin is retracted each day and a small amount of oil applied, the part is kept desirably clean and adhesions are prevented. If the foreskin retracts with difficulty, a physician should be consulted in order that the difficulty may be corrected. Smegma accumulates also in the vulva of girls and this part should be cleansed daily. Cleaning is desirable only of the visible parts.

Very young babies often have a small amount of milk in their breasts. The only importance in this fact is that it be recognized as normal, and all that is required is to let the breasts alone.

It is desirable that the baby's buttocks be washed with soap and water after each stool. Occasionally the buttocks become reddened or even excoriated. This is due to one of two causes. One of these is the strong acid present in diarrheal stools; the other the formation of ammonia from the urine as it remains for a period in the diaper. In either case it is useful to keep the baby's skin protected with some simple ointment. When due to diarrhea the trouble will cease as soon as the diarrhea is controlled. Since the ammonia is formed by the growth of certain bacteria in the urine as it is kept warm next the body, and since it is not possible always to change a diaper immediately it is wet, the management of choice is to place some antiseptic in the diaper which will prevent bacterial growth. Several effective antiseptics are available. Those belonging to the safest and least harmful group are known best by their proprietary names. A good example is Diaparene chloride. For use, one commercial tablet (0.09 gram) of Diaparene is crushed and dissolved in 2 quarts of water, making an amount of solution that will take care of 6 diapers. The solution is used in the final stage of laundering the diapers, after they have been freed from soap and wrung out. The diapers should be allowed to soak in the solution for at least 3 minutes, then wrung out and dried without further rinsing.

In the care of the diaper much has been said against the use of laundry soaps and washing powders, because it was felt that these were instrumental in causing ammonia formation and excoriations. Since these are not the cause of such difficulties, diapers may be washed in the same manner as all other clothes, and then should be well rinsed.

A substance called Silicare is useful in controlling the inflammation of diaper rash.

CLOTHING

Lists of clothing for babies and children can be found in many books; probably no two lists are alike. Customs in clothing change. Clothing lists of a few years ago are outmoded now to some extent. The gertrude and petticoat of former lists have now disappeared. Selection of clothes for a baby should be guided by experience and common sense. The baby should be clothed for comfort and health and not primarily for the gratification of the mother. The clothes should be simple and easy to use. Most of the clothes for the young baby are outgrown by six months. After this age, when the baby is more active, a different type of clothing is used.

A list of clothes for a young baby could include diapers, shirts, night gowns and possibly sweaters. Small blankets also should be added to the list. Stockings and dresses could be added, depending on circumstances.

Shirts can be long sleeved or short sleeved, depending on the temperature. On very hot days no shirt is worn. Night gowns for the young baby should be long enough to reach well below the feet; in such case usually stockings are unnecessary. In very hot weather no gown is needed.

It is obvious that wide variation exists in the choice of clothing. The chief objective is comfort of the baby. He should be dressed warmly enough in cold weather and lightly in hot weather. Too often babies are dressed too warmly; they perspire and become restless. If they should kick off the bed covering, they may become chilled.

CRYING

A certain amount of crying daily serves a useful purpose. It is a form of exercise and constitutes a large part of the exercise a young baby gets. Also, in the very young, crying helps to expand the lungs and keep them expanded, overcoming the state of collapse which is normal before birth. However, crying is sometimes excessive. Such crying is usually due to discomfort, which may be from hunger, extremes of temperature, colic or other pain. Although babies cry from fright and anger, these are not causes of habitual crying. It must be admitted also that babies cry sometimes in order to get the attention which they find that crying brings them.

EXERCISE

Exercise is essential for good development. In the early weeks, when the infant is relatively helpless, sufficient exercise is obtained by the usual carrying around of the baby by the mother, although some mothers have been taught to leave their babies too much alone for fear of spoiling them. As muscular development progresses the baby gets his exercise by kicking and other movements while lying unrestricted on his bed. Later he sits, plays, creeps, and walks. After the first few weeks, if permitted, the baby usually will obtain sufficient exercise for himself, but care must be taken that he is at liberty to do so. In addition to permitting the baby to exercise himself while lying unrestricted on the bed, certain formal exercises may be given. After 5 months the baby may be pulled to a sitting position by his hands; while holding his feet gentle resistance can be given to his kicking movements; his straightened legs can be bent upward at the hips until the thighs are on the abdomen. For the runabout child, two hours' exercise in the open air, preferably playing with other children, may be regarded as an average daily requirement.

TRAINING

The training of children begins in early infancy. Babies are born without habits, and those which they get are either accidentally acquired or are taught to them. In infancy small things lead to habit formation. Regularity in feeding and in everything done for the baby is conducive to good habits. The baby should become accustomed to going to sleep without the presence of the mother, and certainly he should not be rocked to sleep. He should become accustomed to sleeping without a light at night and if he should awaken at an unusual time and cries, he should be allowed to "cry it out," if it is reasonably certain nothing serious is wrong. The age at which babies can be trained to the toilet is early in proportion to the amount of teaching energy spent in this direction. At three to four months of age, sometimes sooner, the bowel movements tend to occur at rather regular times each day, viz., immediately after the morning bottle. It is a good plan to place the baby over a small vessel regularly at this time after he is mature enough to be held comfortably in this position. In this early period of training the baby should not be held over the vessel for long and no special measure should be used to induce a movement. Although encouragement in developing a regular habit is useful, the baby should not be expected to be reliable for many months. Reliability as to wetting is even slower in development. A good degree of reliability by day may be expected by 18 months and many children have dry beds by 2 to 2½ years.

Thumb sucking of a happy, well fed baby can be disregarded, so long as it occurs only in the period of infancy. Most babies suck their thumbs for a while and then cease as they find other satisfying things to do. Persistent thumb sucking may be associated with malocclusion of the teeth. Moderate thumb sucking in early infancy is normal. Persistent thumb sucking usually represents a feeling of insecurity or other emotional disturbance. In management, preference should be given to efforts at proper education using rewards for compliance rather than to mechanical devices for the thumb.

NUTRITION OF THE INFANT

INTRODUCTORY DISCUSSION

Nutrition deals with the food we eat and the structures which the body makes of it. A diet which is adequate to maintain the body in good nutritional health must include the essential food materials. These essentials are protein, carbohydrate, fat, mineral salts and water.

The body needs all of these various food materials at all ages of life, although the amount and the form in which they may be offered vary according to the age. The infant, the child, and the adult need exactly the same essential food elements. The foods chosen to supply them must be adapted to the digestive capacity and the relative need of the individual. Many foods as prepared for the adult are not in a suitable state for digestion by the infant. Because milk is so easily digested by the infant and because it is so nearly a perfect food, it is commonly the basis on which the infant's diet is constructed.

In the life processes of the body, certain materials are constantly being broken down to simpler ones; the process is comparable in some respects to the burning of fuel in a furnace. This combustion takes place even when the body is in complete repose, and it is increased by activity in proportion to the degree of muscular exertion. In the process of combustion, heat is liberated. This is what keeps the body warm. Heat produced in this manner can be measured. The measurements are made in heat units or calories. A known amount of food will give rise to a definite amount of heat, which can be calculated. Thus it is that food is often measured in terms of calories. If insufficient food were furnished, the body would consume itself to the point where life would be impossible. It is necessary therefore to supply energy (food capable of producing energy) to the body for the purpose of maintaining life. In order that the infant may grow and develop properly, it is necessary to supply energy in addition to that which will only maintain life. Growth takes place only when food is supplied in excess of the amount needed to replace that which is burned to maintain the body. The infant's need for energy is relatively (per unit of body weight) far greater than that of the older child or adult and the effects of an inadequate supply show themselves more quickly. Between 85 and 90 per cent of the infant's energy needs are supplied by fats and carbohydrates, this being the chief function of these two food materials. The remainder of the energy is derived from protein.

Protein is an essential part of all cells; without it, life would be impossible. Plants can form protein from substances which they are able to obtain from the soil and the air. Man and the animals cannot do this but must have the constituents of protein supplied to them either from plants or from other animals. For existence a certain amount of protein must be supplied in the diet, and for body increase (growth) an increased amount is necessary. Since no other food material can replace it, protein is an essential part of the diet. A sufficient amount may readily be supplied by the milk of the infant's diet provided the amount of milk offered is adequate. A moderate deficiency of protein causes slow growth and feeble musculature. Gross deficiencies will eventually lead to death. Proteins from different sources differ in their chemical structure. When a protein has all the components necessary to build the kind of protein needed by the body it is called a "complete" protein. Milk protein may be considered as complete. It is characteristic of the vegetable proteins that they are not complete and as a consequence are not as adequate for producing good growth as are the proteins from animal sources.

The food materials that have been discussed (fat, carbohydrate and protein) are present in the food in relatively large amounts. Other food essentials are present only in small or even minute amounts. The latter group includes both the minerals and the vitamins that are necessary for growth and the maintenance of health. The materials that have been grouped under the general term of vitamins differ widely from one another, yet some similarity exists in that they all are organic substances similar to enzymes and hormones. Formerly they were designated exclusively by letters of the alphabet, but as their structure becomes known their chemical names are used.

Vitamin A is necessary for growth, for a normal state of the skin and the various mucous membranes, for ability to see in a dim light and for certain other functions. While some vitamin A is present in milk fat, egg yolk and in the glandular organs (such as liver) of animals, the largest part of the vitamin A of the diet is in the form of the yellow pigment carotene, which is of vegetable origin and which is changed into vitamin A in the body. Any diet of the infant or child that is considered good from all other points of view contains also adequate amounts of vitamin A or carotene. Additional vitamin A from sources such as cod liver oil, although unnecessary, serves as a safeguard against possible deficiency. A large excess of vitamin A is toxic.

The vitamin B complex is composed of a group of vitamins which tend to occur together, although the relative proportions of each vary in the different foods. Deficiencies of a single member of the group are thus improbable, although deficiencies of one vitamin may predominate. Thus, beriberi is chiefly a thiamine deficiency disease, pellagra results from a shortage of niacin, and a shortage of riboflavin causes sores about the corners of the mouth and disturbances of twilight vision. The B complex occurs in the embryos of seeds, in meat, milk, eggs, fruits and vegetables.

The amount of the B vitamins in human milk depends in a large measure upon the amount in the diet of the mother. The diet of many mothers is so incomplete that the B in the milk is often dangerously low. For this as well as other reasons the diet of the infant is advantageously supplemented at an early age with B containing foods. Although a deficiency of B leads to a loss of appetite, not all babies have their appetites improved by addition to the diet of vitamin B preparations, for the reason that other causes for poor appetite are also common. If fruits, vegetables and egg yolk are included in the infant's diet at an early age it is rarely necessary to give special vitamin B preparations.

Vitamin C also is present in fruits and vegetables. For the young infant either orange juice or tomato juice is relied upon as an adequate source, and the diet should be supplemented early with one of these foods. Deficiency of vitamin C in the diet leads to the disease scurvy. As with vitamin B, the amount of vitamin C in human milk depends on the amount in the diet of the mother. When the mother's diet is good, her milk contains enough vitamin C to meet the needs of the baby. Even so, it is good practice to have the baby accustomed early to orange juice in preparation for the time when he is no longer breast fed. The amount of C in fresh cow's milk may be sufficient to protect the artificially fed infant, but this never should be relied upon, as vitamin C disappears rather rapidly from milk with the lapse of time and especially when milk is pasteurized or kept hot for longer than a few minutes. It is not advisable to feed to an infant fresh cow's milk unless it has undergone some heat treatment. It is a good general rule, therefore, to supplement the diet of every infant with vitamin-C-containing foods, such as orange or tomato juice. If necessary, pure vitamin C (ascorbic acid) can be given as a medicinal preparation.

Vitamin D is essential to the body for the proper use of calcium and phosphorus with which to build bone and teeth. A deficiency of this vitamin in infancy leads to rickets, a condition in which the bones become soft and often crooked. Vitamin D is present in any common food in very large amounts. A well-known and moderately concentrated commercial source is cod-liver oil. Other fish liver oils (percomorph) supply vitamin D in greater concentration. Fat-like substances (sterols) which are normally present in the body may be converted into vitamin D by the action of ultraviolet energy. The common source of ultraviolet energy is sunshine, which explains the infrequency of rickets in the summer and its prevalence in the winter and spring. The very short energy waves which are classed as ultraviolet are easily filtered out of sunshine by clouds and dust, and they do not pass through ordinary window glass. Special lamps have been devised for the production of ultraviolet energy, some of which give off this energy in an amount considerably greater than that obtained from sunshine. Ultraviolet energy converts certain sterols into vitamin D wherever it may come into contact with them, whether it be in the body, in food material, or in some concentrated state. Ergosterol and dihydrocholesterol are the two sterols used for manufacturing vitamin D by irradiation. These two forms of vitamin D can be prepared in a pure crystalline state; they are highly potent in minute amount and are diluted in a solvent for distribution, sometimes in oil, sometimes in a water dispersible solvent. In many communities milk fortified with vitamin D is available. All evaporated milk is fortified. The standard amount used for fortification of milk is 400 units to the quart, or in the case of evaporated milk 400 units to the reconstituted quart. A supplement of vitamin D is highly desirable throughout the growth period, particularly in infancy. Many preparations of vitamin D are available. So far as effectiveness is concerned, little choice exists among them. An appropriate amount of vitamin D is 300 to 400 units a day. When nutritionally adequate amounts of fortified milk are taken, no additional supplement of vitamin D is needed.

Vitamin E is unimportant for the infant because of its wide distribution and the improbability of any infant's receiving an inadequate supply.

Vitamin K may be given to the infant at birth when there is bleeding because of a disturbance of the clotting mechanism.

Under usual circumstances it may be considered that all of the mineral salts necessary to the body, with the exception of iron, are supplied by the milk of the diet. Normally the infant is born with a store of iron which will serve his iron needs for several months. Certainly not later than six months after birth, and preferably sooner, iron or iron-containing foods should be added to the diet. The addition may be by means of egg yolk, strained meats, ground boiled liver, vegetables and fruits, or if desired by iron salts used as a medicine. Babies born prematurely do not have the usual iron stores at birth, and babies who are ill during the early months may have their iron stores exhausted sooner than the normal expectation. Calcium and phosphorus are essential minerals which are supplied by milk in relative abundance, but are markedly deficient, as compared to milk, in all other foodstuffs. This is important when in later infancy the baby refuses milk.

Water is essential for the storage and combustion of food, for the excretion of waste products, and for many other life processes. The baby's needs for water are relatively much greater than those of the adult, and he shows the harmful effects of deprivation or loss much more quickly and more seriously. This fact becomes important in certain illnesses, such as diarrhea with marked water loss in the stools, and vomiting with failure of water retention. Sometimes a baby becomes so dehydrated (dry) that its life is threatened for this reason alone. In health and with a good diet the amount of water ingested usually need be no cause for special concern since the infant's diet normally contains such a high proportion of water. Water, in addition to the regular diet, may be indicated in hot weather or in case of sweating from any cause. Because of the difficulty of determining when a baby is thirsty, water can be offered regularly at suitable intervals as a routine measure, but frequently it will be found that the baby will refuse it.

DIGESTION

It is common knowledge that the digestive capacity of the infant is limited. Many foods served to adults would cause digestive disturbances if fed to an infant. The basic food of an infant's diet is milk. The stomach of the newborn baby seems to have acid and digestive juices adequate to digest human milk without difficulty. Unmodified cow's milk tends to cause more or less digestive difficulty in the early months of infancy. The common modification of cow's milk, such as boiling, acidification, or dilution, makes it better adapted to the digestive capacity of the infant.

The young infant has relatively little capacity to digest starchy foods. Babies who are fed cereals or other starches in the early weeks usually have no difficulty from them, as the undigested part of the starch merely passes through as a harmless foreign body. Only occasionally are fermentative processes set up with their consequent distress.

Other foods commonly offered to infants (fruit juices, fruits, sieved vegetables, cod-liver oil) usually cause no digestive difficulties, although sometimes the coarser parts of some of these foods are not digested and are passed in the stools.

The emptying time of the infant's stomach is of some importance. The stomach usually is empty in from two to three hours after a feeding of human milk; and two and one half to three and one half hours are required for cow's milk in the usual modifications. It is inadvisable to feed babies at such short intervals that the stomach at feeding time still contains some food from the last feeding. Too frequent feeding leads to digestive disturbances. Illness from any cause tends to delay the emptying of the stomach and to affect the digestive capacity sufficiently to cause digestive symptoms. Sometimes when the digestive symptoms (vomiting or diarrhea) are prominent and the responsible illness somewhat obscure, the illness is attributed erroneously to the digestive tract.

STOOLS

The first passages from the bowel after birth are dark green. As soon as food is given, the character of the stool begins to change and usually by the fifth day it has assumed the type characteristic of infancy. When the baby is breast fed the stools are usually passed two to five times daily; they are soft, bright yellow, acid in reaction, and have a slightly sour cheesy odor. The stools from cow's milk are less frequent (one to three daily), somewhat firmer, a less brilliant yellow, and with a more disagreeable odor than those from human milk.

When milk is the principal food, the color of the stool depends in a large measure upon the speed of passage through the bowel. If the passage is rapid, as in cases of diarrhea, the bowel movements do not have time to turn from their normal green to a yellow color, and the stools then are green. If the rate of movement of the intestinal contents is very slow, the stools may become gray or white in color. These various colors are of no significance except as indicators of the speed of movement of intestinal contents. If for any reason the baby is deprived of food, the stool color becomes brownish and increasingly dark and finally dark green, depending upon the degree of starvation.

Probably much more attention is paid to curds in the stools than their importance deserves. The curds most frequently observed are composed of soaps which have been derived from the fat of the food. A moderate amount of these curds may be considered normal for the baby receiving human milk. Usually with cow's-milk feeding, the intestinal contents are moved along more slowly, and soaps are drier from absorption of water and are pressed more firmly together so that they do not appear as curds. Anything which causes diarrhea or increases the frequency of stools allows the passage of soaps in the form of small masses or curds, so that usually their presence has no greater significance than an indication of more rapid movement of intestinal contents.

The significance of mucus in the stools is also commonly misconstrued. Mucus appears in the stools when the intestinal tract is irritated for any reason. Diarrhea is commonly associated with irritation and consequently with increased mucus. Most cathartics are irritative and are productive of increased mucus, and the common idea of continued catharsis for the purpose of getting rid of mucus is absurd, for the reason that the greater the amount of catharsis, the greater the amount of mucus.

BREAST FEEDING

It seems unnecessary to present arguments that every mother who can should nurse her infant, and most mothers can, at least for the first few months. It is in these early months that natural feeding is of greatest importance. Despite the fact that human milk is such an excellent food, it must be recognized that the milk varies in quality with the diet and habits of the mother. For example, the various vitamins cannot be present in the milk unless they have been taken in adequate quantities by the mother. In order that her milk be at its best and serve well its intended purpose, the mother must observe the common rules of good hygiene and diet. These rules are fully as necessary for her own health as for that of the baby. Mothers frequently develop cavities in their teeth during lactation, because they secrete more calcium in the milk than they ingest. It is desirable also that the mother have sufficient sleep and moderate exercise but never to the point of fatigue. Worry and other nervous states often have a harmful effect which may be reflected in the quality of the milk.

The diet of the mother may be quite varied, and any food is permissible unless it causes digestive disturbance. The avoidance of acid foods is a fallacy. Examples of a well-balanced diet for the pregnant and nursing mother are given in the preceding chapter.

Sometimes it is found that the mother is unable to secrete adequate quantities of milk. If the mother's diet already is good, the milk supply cannot be increased by increasing the diet, although the milk may be increased by improving the diet when this has not been satisfactory. The best stimulus to maintaining or increasing the milk is regular and thorough emptying of the breast. When milk accumulates in the breast because of incomplete emptying, parts of the breast tend to become hard and painful from the pressure of the retained milk. This condition is often called caked breasts. The surest way to decrease the milk is to permit the breasts to become and remain caked.

There are very few good reasons for the mother not to nurse her baby. She should not nurse it if she has tuberculosis or a serious chronic illness. Nursing should be suspended temporarily during a severe acute illness. Menstruation is not a good reason for weaning, even though the baby may be uncomfortable for a day or two. Should the mother become pregnant the baby should be weaned gradually to avoid overtaxing the mother. Medication taken by the mother need not constitute a reason for weaning, for no drugs given in customary doses are secreted in the milk in harmful amounts.

TECHNIC OF NURSING

It is customary to place the baby to the breast six to twelve hours after birth and every six hours during the next twenty-four hours and every four hours thereafter. During these first few days little is obtained by the baby, but the nursing helps to stimulate the flow of milk. Water or 5 per cent sugar solution is offered every four hours. The milk usually is secreted after the third or fourth day. The nursing interval then should be either three or four hours, depending upon the quantity of milk available. More milk is obtained with the shorter interval, and this is usually the better choice in the beginning. The baby should be nursed at one breast at one nursing and the other breast at the next. If the milk supply is not fully adequate, the baby can be fed briefly from the second breast. The average time at the breast is about fifteen minutes. More than half of the milk is obtained in the first five minutes, and the greater portion of the remainder in the next five minutes. Usually something is wrong when the baby nurses longer than twenty minutes.

All babies swallow some air with the milk. This may be a cause of vomiting or of discomfort. It is desirable therefore to hold the baby upright after each nursing and to pat him gently on the back until eructation of the air occurs.

The care of the mother's nipples is important. They should be bathed before and after each feeding. A fissuring of the nipples may occur. This is always painful and sometimes leads to breast abscess. Fissuring of the nipples has the same cause as chapped hands, and can be prevented in the same manner, viz., keep them as dry as possible as far as milk is concerned, and if necessary keep them greased with some simple ointment such as vaseline or cold cream.

DIFFICULTIES

The difficulties encountered in breast feeding are few. Some babies are overfed. This may be evidenced by a large weight gain and intestinal discomfort often of a colicky nature. There may be unusual regurgitation of food and increased frequency of stools. Since most of these symptoms may be produced by other causes as well, it is desirable to make certain of the diagnosis by weighing the baby before and after nursing. The remedy for overfeeding is simple. The baby should be placed on a four-hour schedule. Usually this is sufficient. If it is not, the time at the breast should be shortened. Another measure is to give the baby water immediately before nursing so as to satisfy his hunger sooner.

Relatively large numbers of babies are underfed. This often happens in milder degrees without the mother being aware of it. The chief symptom is a slow or negative weight gain. There may be evidence of hunger, or intestinal discomfort, colic and regurgitation from swallowed air. Air swallowing tends to be greater in underfed babies. Weighing before and after nursing to determine the amount of milk taken will disclose the difficulty. The remedy in underfeeding is to give food in addition to the breast milk, and not to wean the baby. A suitable formula prepared from cow's milk should be given after each breast feeding. In some instances enough human milk may be obtained by feeding the baby at both breasts each nursing.

Whenever the baby becomes ill from any cause, he is likely to have gastro-intestinal symptoms, even though no primary disease exists in the intestinal tract. Thus, one should not be too ready to blame these intestinal symptoms upon the milk and to overlook the real causative factor. So often when the milk "disagrees," the difficulty is entirely unrelated to the milk.

WEANING

In general it is the choice of wisdom to wean the baby from the breast at the age of six to nine months. This may be done gradually by substituting an increasing number of bottle or cup feedings. If the baby has reached the weaning age without being accustomed to a bottle or cup, it often happens that he will refuse it as long as he can get the breast. Thus abrupt weaning is necessary at times. In the case of abrupt weaning, when the baby is un-accustomed to cow's milk, it is usually preferable to have the formula slightly weaker for a few days than it would be normally for the baby's age. Weaning in the summer is still feared by many mothers. There need be no such fear if the milk formula and other foods are appropriate for the baby and are properly prepared.

ARTIFICIAL FEEDING

Human and cow's milk are similar in many respects. They have the same constituents, but the proportions are different. It is chiefly because of these differences in proportion that digestive difficulties occur when unmodified cow's milk is fed to young infants. The milk of all cows is the same except for the quantity of fat. For infant feeding it is generally advisable to use milk of medium or low fat content. Holstein milk or milk from a mixed herd is preferable. Milk from Jersey or Guernsey cows should be partially skimmed.

Milk is easily contaminated in the milking and handling and is an excel-lent food for the growth of bacteria. All harmful bacteria and most of the others are killed by pasteurization. Boiling milk for several minutes also kills the bacteria and in addition alters the milk in such a way that the casein forms a finer curd and is thereby more easily digested by the infant. For this reason it is generally preferable to use boiled milk, and when this is done pasteurization is unnecessary.

Evaporated milk is ordinary fresh cow's milk which has been concentrated to slightly less than half of its volume by the evaporation of the water. It is then sealed in cans and sterilized. It has been shown to be an excellent, safe, and convenient food for the artificial feeding of infants. For use it may be diluted back to its original volume with water and used in the same manner as fresh milk. The sweetened varieties of evaporated milk (condensed milk) are not suitable for the routine feeding of infants, as the protein content of such milk when diluted for use is so low that it does not permit proper growth of muscle tissue.

Dried milk is milk which has had practically all of its water removed. It is useful in infant feeding, although usually more expensive than fresh or evaporated milk. Some dried milks are prepared from skimmed milk instead of from whole milk. Dried milk is used frequently in communities which cannot obtain fresh milk and for other special reasons. To obtain a product similar to whole milk it is necessary to add one part by weight of the dried whole milk to seven parts of water.

SUGARS AND CARBOHYDRATES

Milk alone is not a suitably balanced food in early infancy without the addition of sugar, and when the milk has been modified by dilution sugar is necessary to satisfy the energy requirements of the infant. Thus some variety of sugar is usually used in the milk formula. The sugars commonly used are lactose (milk sugar), cane sugar (table sugar), and derivatives of starch (dextrin, maltose, dextrose, and mixtures of these). All of these serve the baby equally well after they have been absorbed from the intestinal tract. The choice of sugar is based upon its cost and upon its behavior in the intestinal tract of the infant. Certain sugars are more laxative than others. For example, lactose is absorbed relatively slowly and usually passes far down the intestinal tract before complete absorption. This long presence in the tract has a laxative effect. At the other extreme is dextrose, which is absorbed quickly and consequently is a good sugar to use in cases of diarrhea. Corn syrup is a mixture of dextrin, maltose and dextrose and has found favor because it is inexpensive as well as useful, although it is less convenient to handle than the dry sugars. Dry dextrin-maltose mixtures are extensively employed.

DILUENTS

One of the chief objects in the modification of cow's milk to make it more suitable for young infants is to alter the casein in such a manner that it forms a fine curd in the stomach. This object is very commonly achieved by dilution with water. Sometimes cereal water, usually barley water, is used for this purpose. Such diluents do no harm but provide little food value. Limewater, so commonly used in the past, is now seldom employed as a diluent.

SYNTHETIC FOOD MIXTURES

Several manufacturers have prepared mixtures of milk and sugar in proportions thought to be suitable for infant feeding, and these may be obtained in a dry or liquid form. All that is required for use is the addition of water in specified proportions. All of these mixtures are relatively expensive. In most instances an attempt has been made to make these synthetic foods similar to human milk. Because of their low protein content, many such milks are not well suited to the rapidly growing infant. Malted milk and sweetened condensed milk are examples of milk and sugar mixtures which are quite ill suited for infant feeding, because of their high sugar content.

FORMULAS FOR WELL BABIES

Milk satisfies the need of the infant for most of the nutritional essentials when at least 1½ ounces for each pound of weight is given each twenty-four hours. By the time the baby is taking a quart of milk a day, other foods may be added to supplement the diet in such a way that more milk is unnecessary.

The amount of sugar added to meet the total food requirement is usually one ounce daily during the first two months and one and a half ounces during the succeeding four months. More or less than this may be indicated under special circumstances.

The amount of diluent (water) used should be sufficient to bring the total volume to that which the baby will take conveniently in twenty-four hours. In general it may be stated that a young baby should take at a single feeding two to three ounces more than his age in months. Seldom is it desirable to give more than seven ounces at a feeding at any age, for by the time the baby is receiving seven ounces he is taking also foods other than milk.

As an example, a baby four months of age weighing 14 pounds might do well with a formula containing twenty-four ounces of milk, one and one half ounces of sugar, and water sufficient to make five feedings of six and one half ounces each, or six feedings of six ounces each, as seems best suited to the individual baby.

During the first two weeks after birth the milk dilution usually should be a little greater than that which has been specified until the baby becomes accustomed to the cow's-milk feeding. The original mixture should never be less than half milk, and this should be used for only a few days. It is frequently customary to start with two thirds milk and one third water.

A feeding schedule which will be found suitable for the majority of well babies is as follows:

Age Months	Weight Pounds	Milk Ounces	Water Ounces	Sugar Ounces	Feedings Number	Ounces
½	7	11	7	1	6–7	2½–3
1	8	14	10	1	6–7	3½–4
2	10	18	12	1¼	5–6	5–6
3	12	21	9	1½	5–6	5–6
4	14	25	10	1¾	5–6	6–7
6	16–17	28	7	2	5	7
8	18–20	32	8	1½	5	7
12	22	32	—	—	4	8

If corn syrup is used as the sugar, an equal volume of water is omitted.

Sugar Equivalents

1 ounce by weight of cane sugar = 2 level tablespoons.
1 ounce by weight of lactose = 4 level tablespoons.
1 ounce by weight dried malt sugar = 4 level tablespoons.
1 ounce by volume of corn syrup = 2 level tablespoons and contains 1 ounce of sugar.

It must be remembered that the formulas and schedules given are calculated for the average baby and that adjustments frequently will be necessary for any individual baby. A baby who is hungry, not gaining as he should, and who is having no digestive difficulties should have more food than is indicated in the schedule. Often minor adjustments in the quantity or type of sugar will make the difference between constipation and loose stools. For these and many other reasons it is highly advisable to have the infant's feeding under the supervision of one who is expert in such matters.

FORMULAS WITH UNDILUTED MILK

Cow's milk may be altered in other ways than by dilution so that it is readily utilized by the infant. One of the methods of accomplishing this is by the addition of an acid in carefully regulated quantities to milk which has been previously boiled. Lactic acid (the acid of naturally soured milk) and citric acid (the acid of citrous fruits) have been used extensively for this purpose. Milk which has been soured by bacterial growth under laboratory control is excellent when it is available. The feeding of undiluted acid milk permits a greater food intake and thus a more rapid growth is brought about. These babies exceed the averages in height and weight. In the light of some of our more recent knowledge this would seem to be an advantage. The following table gives an approximate feeding schedule for the average well infant using undiluted acidified milk:

Age	Milk oz.	Sugar oz. (wt.)	Feedings oz.
1 wk.	12	½	6 x 2
2 wk.	15	1	6 x 2½
1 mo.	18	1½	6 x 3
2 mo.	25	2	5 x 5
4 mo.	30	2	5 x 6
6 to 10 mo.	35	2	5 x 7

If corn syrup is used as the sugar, an equal volume of milk is omitted.

THE PREPARATION OF FORMULAS

Sweet Milk Dilutions

The milk, sugar, and water should be mixed and then boiled from one to three minutes with constant stirring. It should be poured immediately into boiled nursing bottles, stoppered and cooled rapidly, and placed on ice until ready for use.

Lactic Acid or Citric Acid Milk

The milk and sugar should be mixed and boiled for two minutes while stirring. It should be cooled rapidly; when quite cold the acid is added slowly while constantly stirring. It should then be poured into nursing bottles, stoppered, and placed on ice.

The amount of citric acid required is usually two grams to the quart of milk. Citric acid is purchased as a powder, of which one teaspoonful weighs approximately two grams. It is dissolved in a small quantity of water and the solution stirred into the milk.

Lactic acid is purchased as an 85 per cent solution. One teaspoonful or one hundred and twenty drops is required for each quart of milk.

Sometimes orange juice is added to the milk. The amount required to bring a quart of milk to the proper acidity is about two ounces.

The amount of lemon juice required is about two-thirds of an ounce.

Evaporated Milk

Evaporated milk is sterile and further heat treatment is unnecessary. For the preparation of a formula the mixture of water and sugar is boiled and added to the evaporated milk. To prepare an acidified formula only two-thirds as much acid is required as for fresh milk.

CHOICE AND CARE OF BOTTLES AND NIPPLES

It is preferable to have as many nursing bottles and nipples as there are feedings in the day. Both the bottles and the nipples should be of such a type that they can be readily and thoroughly cleaned. The bottles and nipples should be washed with soap and water and boiled for five minutes. The bottles are then ready for filling and the nipples for clean storage.

Any funnels, spoons, pans, etc., used in the preparation of the formula should be boiled each time before use. If possible it is advisable to have one set of utensils for use in the preparation of the baby's formula only.

TECHNIC OF FEEDING

For feeding, the milk should be warmed to body temperature by placing the bottle in a vessel of hot water. Care should be taken not to heat acidified mixtures much above body temperatures for the reason that the curd is likely to clot and settle out. The size of the hole in the nipple should be such that when the bottle is inverted the milk drops out rapidly but does not flow in a steady stream. The baby should be fed in arms and in a position in which the shoulders are higher than the buttocks. Any milk refused should be discarded. After feeding and before being put to bed the baby should be held in a position which will permit regurgitation of any swallowed air. Gentle patting on the back will assist in eructation of the air.

ADDITIONS TO THE MILK DIET

Neither human nor cow's milk is a perfect food. Babies fed exclusively on either for a long period will develop certain nutritional diseases. Iron and vitamins C and D and possibly some of the B vitamins are likely to be deficient. Foods which supplement the milk diet in these respects should be given early.

Orange juice should be started early in the first month. Two tablespoons of orange juice should be diluted with an equal quantity of water and given once daily. This amount is gradually increased to the juice of half an orange at three months of age and then to that of an entire orange daily. In some instances it is advisable to substitute tomato juice for orange juice. When this is done a somewhat greater quantity of tomato juice should be used.

Vitamin D should be started early in infancy. If cod liver oil is used, the amount in the beginning can be one half teaspoonful daily and gradually increased until one teaspoonful is given. One teaspoonful daily of a high-grade cod-liver oil will be found sufficient for most babies. It is probable that the baby needs cod-liver oil in the summer as well as in the winter, for during the hot summer months it is not always possible to give him sufficient sunshine. Iron in some form should be given the baby before he is six months of age. Although it may be given in the form of medicinal iron, it is usually preferable to administer it in some iron-containing food. Egg yolk, green vegetables and fruits are the foods commonly chosen for infants. They are offered to babies at increasingly earlier ages and are of value not only for their iron, but also for their content of B and other vitamins and minerals.

It is customary to give various cereals to infants beginning at about 3 months. Cereal is entirely satisfactory as an infant food, although it is probably not as important as are the fruits and vegetables and egg yolk. Consequently it seems more advisable to have the infant well established on these other foods before cereal is started, unless a fortified proprietary cereal food is used.

CARE OF THE SICK INFANT

The illnesses of an infant are usually of an acute rather than of a chronic nature, and the general care is very similar for all illnesses. The infant should be allowed to lie quietly in bed, and the feedings, treatments, etc., should be spaced at as long intervals as possible. There is often a strong tendency to keep doing things to and for the patient, with the result that little of the much needed rest is obtained, and the baby becomes exhausted. Excitement should be avoided and unnecessary entertainment reduced to a minimum.

An effort should be made to have the air of the sick-room fresh at all times, but this does not mean that it need be raw, cold winter air. No illness of infancy requires any special type of clothing. The clothing should be that to which the infant is accustomed during sleep in health. Except in the case of premature and very delicate infants, the patient should have a cleansing bath (at least one) daily. There is no acute illness in which bathing is harmful. The feeding of the sick infant is discussed subsequently.

Infants have higher body temperature from the same or less important causes than do adults. A temperature of 104 or 105 degrees in an infant does not demand any measures for relief unless it is of considerable duration or unless it is associated with such nervous symptoms as restlessness and inability to sleep.

A common and effective method of reducing high temperature is bathing. A bath of the type designated as a sponge bath is satisfactory.

At times definite indications for the use of drugs are encountered in infancy, but in general, drug treatment plays a relatively minor rôle. The measures which assume greater importance are diet, hygiene, and general nursing care.

COMMON ILLNESSES AND ABNORMALITIES
JAUNDICE IN THE NEWBORN

Icterus or jaundice occurs in newly born babies with considerable frequency and in the vast majority of instances is without significance for the health of the infant. When jaundice is present the white part of the eyeball is yellow, and in the more marked cases the skin also has a definitely yellow color. It appears in the first two or three days after birth, and its persistence varies from a few days to several weeks. No treatment is indicated for this common form of jaundice.

HERNIA OR "RUPTURE"

The most frequently encountered hernia in infancy is at the navel or umbilicus. At this point the usual finding is a weak place in the abdominal wall, which upon finger pressure is felt as a hole, usually smaller than the end of the finger. With the intra-abdominal pressure produced by crying a protrusion is to be observed at the site of the hernia. Umbilical hernia usually causes no discomfort or other difficulty. With the wearing of some device which effectively prevents protrusion of the hernia, the defect nearly always disappears in the course of some months. The simplest method of controlling the hernia is to cover it with a tightly drawn strip of adhesive tape. No device should be used which keeps the defect open by pushing inward through it.

The inguinal hernia occurs with considerably less frequency. In this condition the protrusion is on one or both sides of the lower abdomen (the groin) immediately above and to either side of the genitalia. The general principles of management are the same as for umbilical hernia. Adhesive tape cannot be applied effectively, and the simplest truss is made from a skein of yarn.

COMMON COLDS

The symptoms of the common cold are well known to everyone, and it is unnecessary to enumerate them. Some of the consequences of this infection are very important for the infant. An infant cannot suckle satisfactorily when the nose is obstructed. Difficulty will be encountered in the feeding, with the possible result of marked underfeeding. In infancy some vomiting and looseness of the stools frequently accompany a cold. In general, colds affect infants much more seriously than older persons, not only by producing more marked symptoms, but also by having a greater frequency of complications. Secondary inflammations in the ears, bronchi, and lungs are not infrequent.

In the endeavor to prevent colds it is important to realize that they are infectious and contagious. They are readily contracted from others. Exposure to drafts and low temperatures can be of no significance unless infectious material is present also. The difference between those who are subject to frequent colds and those who seem relatively immune is not known with exactness, but in general those who have good hygienic care, receive a complete diet, and are in a good state of nutrition, have fewer colds than those who are lacking in these factors.

A measure important in the management of a cold in an infant is an endeavor to keep the nose open sufficiently for breathing and for drainage. Oil preparations, particularly those containing such substances as camphor or menthol, should not be used in infancy. Frequently physicians prescribe a drug, such as a solution of ephedrin or neosynephrin, to be sprayed or dropped into the nose for the purpose of reducing the swelling and thus producing a larger breathing space. Often free drainage from the nose is a great aid in the prevention of a complicating ear infection.

OTITIS MEDIA

Otitis media is inflammation within the cavity of the ear immediately behind the eardrum. This cavity is connected directly with the throat by what is called the eustachian tube. Thus infections in the nose and throat have a more or less direct path to the ear. It is the rule in infants that otitis media produces a relatively high fever, pain, restlessness, and often general constitutional symptoms among which may be vomiting and diarrhea. A few babies sometimes have otitis media with only a part of these symptoms or even none of them, and the otitis is diagnosed only by examination of the ears.

Otitis media occurs in varying degrees of severity and may be seen first by the physician in different stages of development or subsidence. The treatment to be instituted depends upon these various factors. With a severe inflammation and bulging of the eardrum, the drum should be incised to permit drainage of the pus lying within. In cases of moderate or early inflammation the proper treatment may be to let it alone and observe its progress.

If there seems to be pain, the physician often advises the dropping into the ears of certain pain relieving preparations. Often also one of the antibiotic or sulfa drugs may be prescribed.

The bony cavity of the mastoid connects directly with the middle ear and consequently is inflamed in every case of otitis media. In most instances the products of inflammation drain by way of the middle ear, and the mastoid inflammation subsides along with that of the ear. In a few instances the mastoid inflammation causes sufficient swelling about the opening into the ear that drainage is not possible. The mastoid inflammation then assumes increased importance and is designated mastoiditis. In many of these cases it becomes necessary to make a surgical opening into the mastoid from the exterior. Mastoiditis is even more likely than otitis media to produce constitutional symptoms, and sometimes in infancy the resulting vomiting and diarrhea constitute a grave menace to life. Often the gastro-intestinal symptoms completely overshadow the slight or even negative external evidences of mastoiditis.

CROUP

The term croup has been used to designate inflammations in the larynx which give rise to difficulty in breathing. The term "membranous croup," now being used decreasingly in the interest of more exact diagnosis, has been applied to the obstruction of the larynx produced by inflammations associated with exudates in a form resembling membrane. Membranous croup is practically synonymous with diphtheria of the larynx.

The less serious form of croup, and the form which is usually implied in the term croup, is known also as spasmodic or catarrhal croup. In this condition a relatively mild inflammation of the larynx leads reflexly to a spasm of the muscles of the larynx. During a period of spasm the opening through the larynx is almost completely closed, and air is drawn into the lungs with considerable difficulty and with a plainly audible noise. No difficulty exists in expiration. The attacks of spasm, which are often alarming but rarely serious, tend to recur for a period of about three days, when the inflammation and its symptoms usually subside. The attacks are more frequent at night, the days often being entirely free from them.

The attacks may be relieved by breathing air containing warm-water vapor (steam), and for this purpose croup kettles have been devised. A less troublesome, effective method is the administration of certain antispasmodic drugs, with which the attacks may be forestalled and prevented as well as relieved. In using croup kettles be sure to avoid turning them over and burning the child.

PNEUMONIA

Pneumonia may be primary or secondary. By secondary is meant that the pneumonia occurs as a complication or an extension of some other disease, such as a common cold, bronchitis, measles, influenza, etc. Primary pneumonia occurs in a manner similar to other contagious diseases, being contracted from one who has the disease or a carrier, and not ordinarily secondary to or complicating some other disease. In many respects the general nature of the illness is much the same in these two types of pneumonia. Both types of pneumonia are serious, but the primary type is much less so.

The fear of pneumonia has been removed to a great extent by the use of sulfonamide drugs and the antibiotics, and the course is greatly shortened. The treatment in infancy is much the same in the two types of pneumonia. In addition to the treatment mentioned, other treatment is given according to the symptoms present. Sedatives are indicated for severe and constant cough; bathing for high fever accompanied by nervous symptoms; oxygen for breathing if the baby should become blue; stimulation in case of failing vital functions. Babies with secondary pneumonia, babies with any considerable degree of bronchitis, and delicate infants should not be placed in cold air, but should be given warm moist fresh air. Babies with pneumonia should have their position changed frequently. Pneumonia is one illness in which it is of advantage to hold the infant in arms, because of the frequent change of position that this causes. The administration of considerable amounts of water or fluid is especially advantageous in pneumonia.

THRUSH

Thrush is the result of the growth of a specific fungus on the mucous membrane of the mouth. The fungus in its growth forms small slightly elevated white plaques which are difficult to remove. Thrush, as it usually occurs, causes no symptoms. The treatment consists of local applications made gently by means of cotton on the end of an applicator. Roughness in treatment tends to spread the infection. The preparation to be used as a local application depends upon the preference of the individual physician. Several preparations are about equally effective.

INTUSSUSCEPTION

Intussusception is a condition almost exclusively of infancy, in which one part of the bowel enters and becomes infolded in the part of the bowel in immediate contiguity to it. The blood supply of the invaginated bowel becomes cut off and in the course of a short time that part of the bowel dies and becomes gangrenous. The condition is characterized by an abrupt onset, associated with vomiting, sharp pain, and increasing prostration. At the onset there may be one or two small bowel movements, usually with some evidences of blood. After this time nothing is passed by the bowel. If an enema is returned it will usually contain blood.

Intussusception demands immediate operation for its relief. Early operation has a low mortality, while delay increases the seriousness of the condition.

RECTAL PROLAPSE

Rectal or anal prolapse is a protrusion of the mucous membrane of the anus or anus and lower rectum which occurs usually only at stool. It is possible for this to occur occasionally in a normal infant when the stool is large and hard and is passed with much straining. However, it is more frequent in babies who are poorly nourished and as a consequence have relaxed muscles about the anus. In these prolapse may occur either with constipation or with diarrhea; occasionally when the prolapse has recurred over a long period, it may occur with more or less normal stools.

Three factors should be considered in the treatment. The prolapse should be replaced whenever it occurs and some means should be used in an endeavor to hold it in at all times. For this purpose the buttocks can be strapped tightly together with adhesive tape or a pad should be worn which makes pressure at the anus. If either constipation or diarrhea is present it should be corrected by appropriate means. The stools should be made of such a consistency that they are passed with a minimum of effort and without straining. The general nutrition should be improved, thus improving general muscular tone. It is seldom that the proper application of these measures fails to be effective.

PYELITIS

Pyelitis is an inflammation of the pelvis of the kidney. It may occur at any age, but is much more common in infants and young children, and more frequent in girls than in boys. The infection may ascend the urinary tract to the kidney from the exterior, or perhaps more frequently the bacteria causing the inflammation are carried to the kidney by the blood. The bacteria most often responsible are normal inhabitants of the intestinal tract. The intestinal wall seems more permeable to these bacteria in the presence of diarrhea or marked constipation. In infancy the tendency to intestinal disturbances as a result of colds and respiratory infections increases the frequency of pyelitis during the existence of these head infections.

The symptoms of pyelitis in infancy are usually general rather than local. Fever is the most constant symptom, and this tends to be very irregular. Sometimes fever is the only definite symptom, or perhaps fever and irritability. Because of the lack of localizing symptoms, the diagnosis is not made except by examination of the urine. The urine shows evidence of inflammation, chiefly pus cells and bacteria.

These urinary infections usually respond promptly to treatment with sulfonamides or antibiotics. In the few instances in which the inflammation recurs frequently or becomes chronic special examination is necessary; usually some urinary obstruction is present which requires relief.

VAGINITIS

Inflammation of the vagina or of the vulva and vagina as it occurs in infancy and childhood is chiefly of two varieties. The most frequent of these is due to lack of cleanliness. In general mothers seem very hesitant about the detailed cleansing of the external genitalia of their children, and later about teaching the children to cleanse themselves. Secretions accumulate, decompose, and not only give rise to an unpleasant odor, but actually set up inflammatory processes. Usually these are of mild degree, but they can be severe enough to cause an active discharge. This variety of vaginitis can be prevented and usually cured by ordinary cleansing measures.

Less frequently is encountered vaginitis due to a specific bacterium, the gonococcus. Among adults this variety of infection is looked upon as a social disease. Among girls, however, it is contagious, and it is nearly always innocently contracted. It is distinguished from other varieties of vaginitis chiefly and definitely by identification of the specific bacterium in the discharges. Bacteriological examination of the discharge is usually the first measure undertaken by the physician. This variety of vaginitis responds promptly to penicillin or other antibiotic treatment.

CONVULSIONS

The common type of convulsion is a condition in which the child loses consciousness, becomes rigid and then has spasmodic jerking movements of the face and extremities. They may be very brief, may last several minutes, or occasionally a longer time. They may be repeated, the child having a series of short convulsions.

A convulsion is merely a symptom and the possible disease causes are many. Infants have convulsions more easily than do adults. Sometimes convulsions usher in some acute infection such as pneumonia. In fact, the onset of some acute infection with rapid rise in body temperature is perhaps the most frequent cause of convulsions. A convulsion is very alarming to the parents, but in itself it is not serious except as the underlying cause may be serious. Sometimes the underlying cause is not readily found. In the case of pneumonia, for example, several days may elapse before the diagnosis can be made with certainty. Whether or not the diagnosis can be made at once, the indication is to bring the convulsions under control and take measures to prevent their recurrence. The most effective remedies are sedative drugs, and these must be administered or prescribed by the physician according to the individual indications. A hot bath is often used in an endeavor to control a convulsion. Wrapping the baby in blankets and applying a hot-water bottle or electric pad to the feet is equally effective and considerably less disturbing.

The foregoing discussion concerns chiefly those convulsions associated with fever. Those occurring in infancy without fever are most frequently a symptom of tetany, a condition caused by changes in the calcium and phosphorus content of the blood. The relief of convulsions of this type is most readily and advantageously brought about by the use of certain mineral salts. These and the method of their administration would be chosen according to the preferences of the physician.

Convulsions which occur without fever and which recur from time to time and for which no definite cause can be found are usually classified under the term epilepsy. These require prolonged treatment with drugs under the management of a physician.

FEEDING IN ACUTE ILLNESS

It has been mentioned previously that any acute illness lowers the digestive capacity of the infant and consequently may be a cause of vomiting, or diarrhea, especially when the usual type of feeding is continued. It has been mentioned also that the underlying infection may be obscure, and the difficulty erroneously attributed entirely to the gastro-intestinal tract. Because the continuance of the usual diet is so likely to lead to disturbance in the presence of acute illness, it is desirable to make certain alterations.

It is often beneficial to remove some or most of the fat from the milk and to discontinue the more solid and less easily digestible foods. If the illness is prolonged it will be found necessary to continue to give fair amounts of food, even though a certain amount of digestive disturbance is present, for otherwise the general nutrition will suffer greatly. The baby must be given enough food to keep up his resistance in order that he may be aided in overcoming the disease.

VOMITING

Vomiting may occur in infancy from many causes. The most frequent cause in the otherwise normal baby is some factor which produces distention of the stomach. This may be produced by too large a feeding or by feeding at such short intervals that the stomach is only partially empty when the next feeding is given. The stomach may be distended by the presence of a large amount of swallowed air in addition to the usual feedings. The effects of distention are obtained with tight clothing or abdominal bands. Occasionally the infant has a small stomach capacity, and the feeding of the usual volume of food causes distention. The remedy for all of these distention-producing factors is obvious, once the cause is determined.

The next most frequent cause of vomiting is illness. Almost any acute infection in the infant will produce this event. Vomiting in the acute infections is largely the direct result of irritation of the stomach by the fermentation of food which lies in the stomach unusually long because of the impaired emptying power of the stomach. An excess of fat in the diet may act in this same manner, by delaying the emptying of the stomach. Other less common causes of vomiting depend upon stomach irritation or the ingestion of spoiled foods or inappropriate foods.

A few babies vomit merely because of an apparent desire on their part to do so. This is spoken of as "rumination" in certain instances in which the food is voluntarily brought up for no good reason. In occasional cases babies seem to vomit as a defense reaction against certain foods or against forced feeding. In cases of voluntary vomiting a change in the method of management is indicated. A temporary complete change in environment including caretaker often is all that is necessary.

Any obstruction in the intestinal tract leads to vomiting. The varieties of obstruction are numerous, and all are serious. Some of these seem to have a gradual beginning, as in the obstruction at the lower end (pylorus) of the stomach, which is noticed in the first six weeks after birth; and some may have a sudden onset associated subsequently with evidence of great prostration, as in cases in which one part of the bowel becomes looped into the part immediately next to it.

This is not a complete enumeration of the causes of vomiting, but the discussion includes the most important causes from the standpoint of frequency.

Thus, vomiting may be produced by such simple and easily remedied conditions as overfilling of the stomach, or it may be a symptom of some very serious condition which demands immediate medical attention.

COLIC

In practically all instances intestinal colic in infancy is associated with the presence of gas in the intestines. This gas may have either one of two sources. It may be air which has been swallowed and which has passed beyond the stomach, or the gas may be the result of fermentation of sugar within the intestinal tract. For permanent relief of colic the cause must be abolished. Swallowed air should be made to pass upward after each feeding. Since underfed babies are more likely to swallow air, one should make certain that the food supply is ample. Fermentation may be the result of overfeeding or of the presence of a large quantity of sugar. The correction of overfeeding at the breast has been discussed. When colic occurs in the breast-fed baby in the absence of overfeeding, often the giving of an ounce of boiled skimmed cow's milk before each breast feeding will bring relief. In the artificially fed baby the sugar may be reduced in quantity or altered as to variety. It should be made certain that the baby is receiving sufficient food.

Effective simple measures for temporary relief are enemas or hot applications to the abdomen. In cases of severe colic sometimes an opiate (paregoric) or other drug is required temporarily to give relief.

CONSTIPATION

With the rare exception of certain congenital defects, the causes of constipation in infancy can be classified chiefly into two groups. One group includes those instances in which the residue of food left for excretion is too small to constitute sufficient stimulus to intestinal movement. A small residue is usually the result of underfeeding, though it may also be due to the giving of a type of food which is absorbed to an unusually high degree. The other group includes those instances in which the fecal mass becomes so firm or putty-like that it is moved along with difficulty. This type of constipation is not seen in the naturally fed infant. In the artificially fed infant it is dependent chiefly upon the relative proportion of milk to sugar. A high-milk, low-sugar diet tends to produce the dry type of stool, and thus this kind of constipation; whereas a low-milk, high-sugar formula is laxative.

In the treatment of constipation in infancy drugs ordinarily should not be used except as a temporary measure, pending dietary adjustment. When a drug cathartic is considered necessary, milk of magnesia is usually satisfactory in doses of one to two teaspoonfuls. Instead of drugs it may be preferable to use enemas or suppositories also as temporary measures. In practically every case it will be found that constipation can be relieved by appropriate alteration in the diet, and an earnest attempt to establish a regular habit.

In cases in which the food residue is small it is desirable first to make certain that the food intake is adequate. Additional measures are the feeding of fruits and vegetables somewhat earlier than the customary age, or if these are already being given, to increase the amount. Strained orange juice is not laxative, but prune juice is.

In cases in which it is desirable to alter the nature of the fecal mass a favorable result often may be achieved by increasing the amount of sugar in the formula. If moderate and reasonable increase in the sugar does not give relief, a change in the type of sugar is advisable. Certain sugars are more laxative than others. Milk sugar is more laxative than some of the malt sugars, although the syrupy malt sugars (malt soup extract) are the most laxative of all the sugars. Although constipation may be relieved by decreasing the amount of milk, this should not be done unless the quantity taken is well above the requirements which have been stated previously.

DIARRHEA

In general it may be considered that diarrhea is the result of irritation or abnormal stimulation of the intestinal tract. Because of the unusual stimulus the intestinal movements are increased in intensity, and food material is passed along at a rapid rate. Because of this rapid rate of passage some of the food and much of the water are not absorbed, and as a consequence the stools are fluid and often contain a fair proportion of undigested food.

The increased stimulus may be caused by infection and inflammation of the intestinal tract. In this group belong bacillary and amebic dysentery and typhoid and paratyphoid (salmonella) infections. With better hygiene and improved care of milk and other food these infections are much less common than formerly. In each of these infections the stools show evidence of the disease. In the dysenteries pus and often blood are present. In all the infections the cause can be determined by bacteriologic examination. Prompt determination of the cause is important in order that appropriate treatment may be given. Bacillary dysentery responds promptly to sulfonamides and antibiotics. Typhoid infection responds to chloromycetin. We have very useful remedies for amebic dysentery.

A type of diarrhea difficult to manage is one that occurs epidemically among newborn babies. Many of these diarrheas, if not all, are the result of a virus infection for which we do not yet have a specific remedy. Most of the babies recover if expert medical and nursing care is given.

Diarrhea, often accompanied by vomiting, may occur as a complication of infection elsewhere than in the intestinal tract, such as an inflammation in the ears. In these instances the diarrhea responds to treatment of the infection and to appropriate changes in the diet.

Diarrhea may occur as a result of taking improper food or food that has been contaminated by bacteria which produce toxic products in their growth.

Even perfectly proper foods may be a cause of diarrhea if they are given in excess of the infant's ability to digest and absorb them. For example, almost any infant can be made to have diarrhea by increasing sufficiently the amount of sugar in the diet.

In many instances the cause of diarrhea can not be determined. In such cases response may be expected to appropriate dietary changes.

Some food loss occurs in diarrhea, but the most serious effect is water loss. In the usual mild diarrhea the baby is not particularly ill and the water loss seldom becomes important. However, when diarrhea is severe and prolonged, severe and even fatal dehydration occurs unless measures are taken to keep the body supplied with fluid.

Even though the diarrhea may not be primarily dependent on the diet, certain alterations in the diet are desirable when the diarrhea has occurred. First, it is desirable to allow the intestinal tract to empty. It is customary for some physicians to give a cathartic to hasten the emptying, but this is not necessary. During a brief period, when the tract is emptying, water but no food should be given. The fasting period need not be more than a few hours, in cases of mild diarrhea, although its duration depends upon the severity of the diarrhea and the general condition of the infant. In a few cases of severe diarrhea fasting may have to continue for several days. The first food after the fast may advantageously be one which is high in protein and low in sugar and fat. Boiled skimmed milk is a customary means for fulfilling these requirements. As the diarrhea improves, sugar and fat are gradually replaced in the diet.

MALNUTRITION

Malnutrition may be due to a low food intake, or to failure of absorption. A common cause of malnutrition is failure to offer the infant sufficient food. The body continues to burn food materials whether or not sufficient food is given. If the ingestion and absorption of food are inadequate, the body burns its own tissues. It is thus possible for extreme malnutrition to occur even to the extent of causing death. Malnourished infants are more susceptible to infection than are the better nourished. These infections only add to the difficulties in improving the nutrition.

Another common cause of severe malnutrition is loss of food by chronic or frequently recurring diarrhea together with the underfeeding so often employed in the treatment of diarrhea. Chronic infection anywhere in the body tends to decrease the appetite and to increase the tendency to diarrhea and increase the food requirement.

When malnutrition is caused solely by underfeeding, the remedy is obvious. When it is caused by diarrhea, which in turn is dependent upon infection, the management is more difficult, but even so, careful treatment will usually bring about recovery.

RICKETS

Rickets is a disease of nutrition in which the chief fault lies either in a deficiency of calcium and phosphorus in the diet, or an inability on the part of the body to make proper use of these materials. If the infant receives sufficient milk, the amount of calcium and phosphorus will be adequate. The proportion of these two substances relative to each other affects their absorption. However, when the intake of vitamin D is adequate or with a sufficient amount of sunshine or ultraviolet energy, calcium and phosphorus are well utilized from a customary diet regardless of their proportion. The greater frequency of rickets in late winter and spring is explained by the small amount of available sunshine.

The most striking effects of rickets are seen in the bones because bones have such a large proportion of calcium and phosphorus in their structure. The mineral deficiency associated with rickets causes them to be softer than normal and more easily bent and deformed. When the minerals are not being laid down in the bones, the softer tissues (cartilage) continue to grow at the ends of the long bones; this enlargement develops at the wrists, ankles, and at the points of growth of the ribs. As a result of rickets the skull is often late in closing, the teeth delayed in eruption.

The effects of rickets are seen also in the muscles, which become more lax and weakened. Infants with rickets are likely to be delayed in such muscular acts as sitting, standing, and walking. Infants with rickets are subject to profuse sweating and often to restlessness.

The symptoms which have been enumerated are chiefly those of the well advanced disease. The milder disease is much more frequent than the severe. The same changes take place in the milder disease, but these changes are more difficult to detect. The accurate diagnosis of rickets in the mild disease is made easier by X-ray examination of the bones.

In a few cases of rickets very marked and alarming symptoms appear which are associated with a decrease in the amount of calcium in the blood. When these symptoms occur, the condition is termed "tetany," or "spasmophilia." Tetany may exhibit itself in the form of convulsions or as a spasm of the larynx which causes obstruction and difficult breathing; or as a peculiar spasmodic state of the hands and feet. All these symptoms subside promptly with suitable medical treatment and their return is made impossible by the effective application of the same measures as bring about the cure of rickets.

Rickets is a disease which is easily prevented and easily cured. Prevention is preferable. Any infant who receives the amount of milk that he should is thereby receiving sufficient calcium and phosphorus. If he receives a teaspoon of cod-liver oil daily or 400 units of vitamin D from some other source, the chances are that no rickets of any significance will develop. The same factors that are effective in prevention are equally effective in bringing about the cure of this disease.

CELIAC DISEASE

In celiac disease the child is unable to digest and utilize fats, starches, and sometimes sugars. Sensitivity to gluten from wheat or rye grains is the cause of this disability. In this condition fats such as butter, cream, and fried foods are excluded from the diet along with wheat and rye. Special milk preparations have been developed for such infants.

CYSTIC FIBROSIS

This is a hereditary disorder which involves the pancreas. Mucus accumulates in the lungs and other tissues. Such cases require continuous care by the physician to overcome the symptoms. The National Cystic Fibrosis Research Foundation, 521 Fifth Avenue, New York 17, can supply much helpful information.

CHAPTER VIII

The Prevention and Treatment of Infectious Disease

MORRIS FISHBEIN, M.D.

ABOUT ONE HUNDRED YEARS have passed since it was first shown that germs actually cause disease. In the intervening period hundreds of germs have been identified definitely as associated with certain diseases that attack human beings. In 1880 the germ associated with typhoid was isolated. Since that time such important diseases as tuberculosis, diphtheria, glanders, pneumonia, cholera, lockjaw, undulant fever, meningitis, dysentery, plague, syphilis, whooping cough, gonorrhea, leprosy, and many other specific infections, have been definitely related to invasion of the human body by specific germs or viruses or other living organisms.

ABOUT GERMS

Few people really know what a germ looks like or how it invades the human body. Germs are so small that it takes three hundred billions of an average germ to weigh a pound. They multiply rapidly under favorable conditions. One germ can produce two new ones in twenty minutes. Anyone who has tried to estimate how much money he would have by beginning with a penny and doubling his fortune every hour can realize how rapidly germs multiply. If a germ divided and made two new ones every hour it would, at the end of a day, have sixteen and a half million descendants.

Doctors identify the germs that cause disease in various ways. First they take some of the material from the infected saliva or from the discharges or from the blood of the person who is infected. They examine this under a microscope. The germs are seen as little round dots, or as rod-shaped organisms, or even as long, slender filaments when they are greatly magnified under the microscope. Like human beings, the germs tend to live preferably in certain forms, sometimes two together, sometimes a group of many, sometimes a chain. Some germs are surrounded by capsules, usually a sort of fatty envelope that enables the germ to resist attacks in the body or in the blood of the animal it invades. Other germs have little tails like fins which enable them to move about.

There are still people foolish enough to talk about the germ theory. Germs are no more a theory than are plants, birds, and other living things that live and reproduce. The power of most germs to cause disease can be tested on animals. When the germs are injected into animals they produce changes in the tissues of the animal which are specific for the germs concerned. A pneumococcus in the lung of a man produces pneumonia; first a consolidation of the lung due to invasion by red blood cells and other material and later a softening of this mass and a clearing up of the lung if the patient lives.

When the typhoid germ gets into the human body it produces ulcers in the intestines, and germs are found in the ulcers. When the meningococcus gets into the linings of the spinal cord and brain it sets up an inflammation of these linings, which are called meninges; then the person has meningitis, an inflammation of the meninges. When the spinal fluid is examined the germs can be found in the fluid.

These tests which were developed by the great Robert Koch, with Louis Pasteur, a founder of modern bacteriology, constitute the acid tests for determining with certainty that any germ is associated with the production of a certain disease. If the germ can be found in the infected tissues, if the germ can be artificially grown outside the human body, if the germ can then be injected into an animal like the monkey and produce in that animal a condition like that in the human being from whom the germ was originally taken, it is the cause of that particular disease. Anyone with a reasoning mind should be willing to grant that the germ actually causes the disease.

INCUBATION PERIODS

The common contagious diseases include measles, scarlet fever, diphtheria, whooping cough, mumps, chicken pox, and German measles. The best way to avoid these diseases is to keep away from people who have them. However, this is not so easily done, since many parents do not feel their responsibilities greatly and do not see to it that their children, when ill, are kept away from other children. Really the chief responsibility rests on the parents of the sick child for the prevention of infectious diseases rather than on the parents of the well child.

Most of the common infectious diseases are caused by organisms which get into the body and then begin their action. A certain amount of time elapses between the period when the germ first gets in and when its visible manifestations appear. This is known as the incubation period, and it varies with different diseases. For instance, in meningitis it is from two to four days, in erysipelas from one half to three days, in measles from ten days to two weeks, in German measles from five days to twenty-one days, in scarlet fever from a few hours to a week, in smallpox from ten days to two weeks, in typhoid fever from six days to twenty-five days, and in chicken pox from four days to sixteen days.

In most of these diseases an eruption occurs in the surface of the body. These eruptions have characteristic distribution on the skin, so the physician asks particularly as to whether the redness first began on the face, the neck, the hands and feet, the abdomen, or the chest. The eruptions also differ greatly in their appearance: from tiny red spots to large red patches, from tiny pimples to crops of blisters.

Practically all of these conditions are likely to begin with a mild cold. In some of them the sore throat is severe; in most of them there is fever, slight headache, dizziness, nausea or vomiting. Obviously it is not safe to disregard any of these symptoms, particularly when they appear in a child.

The excretions which carry disease include the material that is coughed from the throat, that is spread by spitting, by sneezing, or that may pass from the body in the form of discharges of one kind or another. Therefore, mothers should guard particularly against contact of a well child with one that is coughing, sneezing, spitting, or that manifests any of the other signs of infectious disease that have been mentioned.

RESISTANCE TO INFECTIOUS DISEASE

Four factors are chiefly responsible for infection of the human body: First, the presence of a germ with sufficient toxic power to grow in the body; second, a sufficient number of these germs to overcome attacks by the body against the germ; third, some special condition in the body that makes it possible for the germ to live and grow; and fourth, some method of getting the germ into the body.

Were it not for the fact that human beings develop within their bodies conditions which make it difficult for germs to live and grow, the human race would long since have been destroyed by the bacteria. However, the resistance which the human being has is not absolute. The constitution of the human body changes from time to time. Resistance is decreased when the body is greatly undernourished, when a person is exceedingly fatigued, when he has been exposed to sudden severe changes of temperature, or in several other ways.

Therefore, the line of defense varies in its intensity from time to time. When the enemy is sufficiently numerous, or sufficiently strong, it breaks through. For this reason, even in the most severe epidemics, some people escape, although there are conditions in which practically everyone attacked is unable to resist. Such conditions occur, for example, when a population among whom a disease has never previously appeared suddenly comes in contact with it. This occurred in the Faroe Islands when measles was brought by a ship carrying white men; at that time more than half the population of the islands died of that disease.

Sometimes the resistance of the body to one disease is broken down by a mild attack of another previous disease. For instance, a person who has had influenza, diabetes, tuberculosis, or some other chronic disorder, may thereafter develop pneumonia, typhoid fever, rheumatic fever, or tuberculosis much more easily than he would have previously.

CARRIERS OF DISEASE

Frequently people who are healthy carry about in their bodies germs which do not attack them but which have sufficient virulence, toxicity, strength, or poison to invade the body of another person and in that person to cause disease. A person who carries the germs about is called a "carrier." Should the carrier suddenly have his own resistance lowered by any of the factors that have been mentioned he might suddenly be invaded by these germs, although previously they had not been able to set up infection in his body.

There is no doubt that all of us are constantly being invaded by germs in contaminated food and water, in breathing, in touching infected items with our hands, which are then conveyed to the mouth and nose. Germs occur on money, in clothing, and on various other objects. However, the dosage of germs received through such contacts, or the virulence of the germs, may not be sufficient to bring about disease. The exposure of the germ to fresh air and sunlight, and the fact that it is trying to live on a substance not suitable to it as a habitation, may prevent its multiplying and may cause the germ itself to lose its strength.

Under other circumstances, germs multiply in tremendous numbers, so that the human being who comes in contact with them sustains a massive assault. For instance, an infected fruit peddler may use saliva to polish the fruit, and the germs might grow well on the fruit thus polished. Germs may be deposited with sewage in running water and multiply tremendously in the sewage. When the water from the contaminated stream is drunk by a human being he gets in enough germs to cause prompt infection. Sometimes an infected food handler is employed to mix a potato salad, to bake a custard, or to make a pie which is then kept under insanitary conditions before being eaten, so that the germs multiply profusely. When this occurs anybody who eats the infected food may become seriously infected, as occurred recently at a picnic when eight hundred people became sick from eating infected potato salad.

PATHS BY WHICH GERMS INVADE

Germs can get into the body in all sorts of ways: with food and water, by inhaling, through open wounds on the skin, by the bite of an insect, as occurs with mosquitoes in malaria and yellow fever, ticks in Texas fever, fleas in plague, and tsetse flies in African sleeping sickness.

When the means by which the germs get into the body are understood, scientific medicine develops methods for keeping them out. When the means are not fully understood, as occurs, for instance, in infantile paralysis, prevention is difficult.

Often the germs produce disease by developing a poison which is then absorbed by the body. After absorption, the poison acts on the nerves or the muscles or the blood vessels. Sometimes the germs themselves gradually break up, and the products of their disintegration are poisonous. Again clumps of germs float around in the blood and cause death by developing in overwhelming numbers in the blood. On other occasions the germs may attack certain organs of the body and so injure these organs that death ensues.

It has been said that the germs like to pick out certain places in which to live under the conditions which suit them best. This happens, for instance, with a germ called the pneumococcus which settles in the lungs and produces pneumonia, but which also may infect the eye or the spine. It occurs with the germs of meningitis, which practically always settle on the coverings of the spinal cord and of the brain, the typhoid germ which settles in the intestines, the germs of lockjaw and of hydrophobia and of epidemic encephalitis which attack the nervous system. There are some germs, like those of tuberculosis or syphilis, which may affect any tissue in the human body although preferably entering by way of the lungs or mucous membrane. There is tuberculosis of bones, of joints, of the eye, and of the nervous system. The organism that causes syphilis actually attacks every organ and tissue in the human body.

RESPONSE OF THE BODY TO GERM INVASION

When germs get into the body and release their poisons the tissues react usually in definite ways. One of the reactions of the body is fever. This is apparently due to the effects of the poisons of the germs on the nervous mechanism of the body which controls the body temperature. Associated with the fever there is speeding up of the chemical changes that go on in the body, so that there may be perspiration and, as a result of the increased activity, a loss of weight. For this reason it has become customary to feed fevers rather than to starve them.

Associated with the disturbance of the nervous system there may be dizziness and loss of appetite, also vomiting and an increased activity of the motion of the bowels. This helps to cause loss of material from the body. Due to accumulations of fluid or swelling of tissue there may be aches and pains in the joints and in the muscles. The interference with the action of the kidney may cause fluid to be retained in the body. The blood usually responds by an increase in the number of the white blood cells, but there are some conditions in which the number is decreased, notably influenza and typhoid fever.

Because the fever is considered to be one of the mechanisms of the body in defense against the attack of germs, scientific medicine does not always attempt to reduce the fever too suddenly or too rapidly by the use of drugs. A fever that is not exceedingly high or prolonged for any length of time is not especially harmful to the body, particularly if the amount of fluid in the body is watched and enough of the right type of food is put into the body to prevent too great a wastage of the tissues.

A normal temperature is 98.6 degrees F. A great many investigations indicate that temperatures over 100 degrees F. are unfavorable to the growth of bacteria and may inhibit the action of some of the poison developed by the bacteria. As will be shown later in the discussion of many of the infections which attack human beings, it is much better to prevent infections than to endeavor to treat them after they have been established.

STAMPING OUT DISEASE

By scientific methods applied since the nature of the germs and their methods of attack on the body have been discovered, certain diseases are now practically eliminated as of exceeding danger to mankind. Yellow fever occurs now in only a few isolated spots throughout the world. In the United States the number of cases of typhoid fever has been so greatly reduced that many young physicians never see a case even in the hospitals where they take their training. Cholera and plague are limited to the remoter areas of China and India and are seldom if ever seen in the United States.

Mankind has undergone progressive changes from the beginning of time; the diseases of man, particularly such as are caused by living organisms, likewise undergo such changes. True, some diseases have been overcome and eliminated, but new diseases constantly appear and demand consideration. The development of new methods of transportation and conveyance, such as the airplane and the ease of intercommunication between various portions of the earth, have brought into the temperate zone the diseases of the tropics which were formerly limited to such areas.

Many a great civilization has fallen because of the development, endemically or epidemically, of diseases that were previously under control, or because of the introduction of some new disease that had previously been considered a rarity. The great civilizations of Greece and Rome fell because of epidemics of malaria. In the United States today certain forms of infections of the glands, certain forms of infestation by tapeworms, and similar disorders, are seen with comparative frequency, whereas formerly they were practically unknown.

The time will never come when man will be free entirely from the fear of disease. The battle is unending, but more and more mankind can celebrate the fruits of victory. As diseases change and as new diseases appear, scientists observe them in their earliest stages, determine their causes and their modes of transmission, and prevent their development.

PREVENTION OF INFECTION

The prevention of disease must be related to our knowledge of the way in which infectious disease gains entrance into the body. Everything possible must be done to see that the germs in the person who is infected do not get out and thus get into contact with other people. If this could be done in every case, many infectious diseases would probably disappear.

If everything possible is to be done, all of the sheets, pillow cases, clothing, handkerchiefs, and, in fact, everything touched by a person who is infected, will have to be sterilized by boiling or by steam under pressure before being permitted in contact with other people. All of the excretions from the body of the infected person must be disinfected by proper antiseptics or by burning. The person with a discharge from the nose, such as occurs in the common cold, might at all times wear a face mask. To carry out completely these procedures would mean such an obstruction and hampering of the usual routine of existence that it not likely to be generally adopted.

The next step is to do everything possible to prevent infected material from being passed from one person to another. This means complete control of food, drink, and air, also the earliest possible detection of human beings, animals, or insects which carry disease, the control of such carriers and their possible elimination.

A human being who is carrying typhoid cannot be eliminated but must be controlled. Since there are millions of persons who carry disease constantly, it is not likely that this source of infection will ever be brought completely under control. Moreover, there are some diseases of which the cause is not definitely known, and it is unlikely that healthy carriers of such diseases will ever be controlled until the cause of the disease is known.

PERSONAL HYGIENE

The best step that the average person can take to prevent infectious disease is to raise his individual resistance by practising the best possible personal hygiene. This means the eating of a suitable diet, the securing of sufficient exercise and sunlight, and enough rest to give the tissues of the body opportunity to recuperate from fatigue.

Moreover, it is possible to aid resistance to certain infectious diseases by injecting the human being either with blood that has resistance, such as the blood from a person who has recovered from the disease, or by injecting serums from an animal which has been infected with the disease and which has in its serum substances opposed to the disease. A considerable number of such specific preventive serums and vaccines will be discussed under each of the infectious diseases as it is considered.

INCIDENCE OF INFECTIOUS DISEASE

The number of cases of the various infectious diseases varies from time to time. There have been great epidemics of influenza such as the epidemic of 1918, in which tremendous numbers of people were involved, whereas there have been minor epidemics in which relatively few people were concerned. Cases of influenza are difficult to differentiate from the common cold. The reports of the United States Public Health Service indicate about 700,000 cases of influenza in 1929, but if all of the conditions resembling influenza were included, the number would be many millions.

The figures for such conditions as measles (about 366,000), chicken pox (216,000), scarlet fever (182,000), mumps (103,000), and whooping cough (197,000) are relatively accurate, since the large majority of such cases are reported. Everyone knows that the rate of incidence of tuberculosis has dropped greatly. The number of deaths from this disease has dropped from 275 per hundred thousand people in the United States to around 12.5 in 1953.

Notwithstanding that typhoid fever can be completely controlled by proper measures, thousands of cases of typhoid fever still occur annually in the United States. Notwithstanding that we have in vaccination and in isolation certain methods of controlling smallpox, a considerable number of cases and deaths from this disease are still reported.

CLEANLINESS AND INFECTION

If infectious disease is to be prevented and brought under control, people must learn to know the nature of disease, the method of its spread, and the methods of prevention. They must do everything possible to keep themselves in such fit condition that infectious disease will not readily attack them.

Much infectious disease can be prevented by keeping as clean as possible, including frequent bathing with plenty of soap and water. Thorough washing of the hands with plenty of soap, particularly before eating, will destroy millions of germs which may otherwise infect human bodies. Vaccination against smallpox is important for everybody. Children should be protected against diphtheria by the use of diphtheria toxoid or toxin-antitoxin. When there are epidemics of typhoid or of other infectious diseases, physicians should be consulted as to the desirability of using other specific vaccines, serums, or antitoxins. Remember that most infectious diseases are spread by contact with persons who have the disease or who may be recovering.

TREATMENT OF INFECTIOUS DISEASES

In the treatment of most of the common infectious diseases, rest in bed is absolutely necessary. The diet should invariably be mild and bland, depending largely on milk, but supplemented with well-macerated vegetables and occasionally with enough thoroughly macerated liver or lamb's kidney to supply the necessary iron and vitamins that are needed in the diet.

For many of the specific infectious diseases there are now specific methods of treatment. For example, there are serums, vaccines, or antitoxins available in scarlet fever, measles, diphtheria, whooping cough, tetanus, meningitis, erysipelas, and undulant fever. In some of the conditions, moreover, the blood serum taken from a person who is convalescing from the disease has been found to have virtues in certain instances.

Typical of the treatment of most of the infectious diseases is the usual method of handling measles. Every child with this disease should be put to bed and kept there, with light covers, as long as it has any fever and for a few days thereafter. If the eyes are irritated, they may be treated with iced cloths soaked in a cold solution of boric acid. The doctor may prescribe the application of an ointment which will keep the lids from getting sticky. The itching and burning of the skin which frequently occurs in the infectious diseases is often relieved by bathing with a simple solution of bicarbonate of soda or a calamine lotion.

The doctor will treat the cough, if it is distressing, by small doses of sedative drugs. The restlessness, headache, and general discomfort may also be relieved by small doses of aspirin or similar remedies, as the doctor prescribes. When, however, any patient develops serious complications or symptoms, such as dullness, stupor, or convulsions, whenever he breathes rapidly or turns blue, it is well to have the physician in immediate attendance. Under such circumstances, the application of a bath, a pack, or a proper remedy may mean a turning between the tendency toward recovery or the tendency toward a more serious condition leading to death.

The details of the treatment of infectious diseases are discussed much more fully in the chapters dealing with individual diseases. The sulfonamide drugs and the antibiotics have revolutionized the treatment of infectious diseases. Penicillin, aureomycin and terramycin are most widely used with chloramphenical or chloromycetin in typhoid. Thus far specific substances are not available for chickenpox and measles. The forms of sulfonamides most widely used are sulfadiazine and gantrisin. Even when not specifically used sulfa drugs and antibiotics control secondary infections such as those of the throat, sinuses or meninges.

CHAPTER IX

Infectious Diseases of Childhood
MORRIS FISHBEIN, M.D.

DIPHTHERIA

IN A NOVEL, *The Marriage of Simon Harper,* by Neil Bell, appears an account of a diphtheria epidemic in a small town in England in the period just preceding the discovery of diphtheria antitoxin. The author depicts graphically the child who is severely infected by this disease. Tchekhov also depicts the horror of this deadly disease in an earlier day. Its conquest has been as dramatic as any struggle known to man.

The condition begins with a sore throat and with repeated attempts to expel, by spitting, the membrane that forms in the throat. If the disease continues, severe paralyses prevent swallowing and injure the heart. There comes a period when breathing becomes impossible, and finally, death. No one who has read such a description or who has actually seen a child with this condition, and who has then seen the marvelous effects of a suitable dose of antitoxin given early in the disease, can fail to appreciate what a great blessing this conquest has been for mankind.

In an earlier day, the physician would frequently be called in the middle of the night to the bedside of a gasping child. Then he would either suck the membrane from the throat by mouth-to-mouth suction or through a tube, if one was available. In severe cases he sometimes opened the windpipe with a knife to permit the child to breathe through the throat beneath the membrane.

Then came the great discovery by the German, Von Behring, and by Roux, a pupil of Pasteur, that an antitoxin could be prepared which would overcome the poisons of this disease. Since that time, there have been developed preparations called toxin-antitoxin and toxoid which can be injected into children early in life and which will give them immunity, or protection, against being infected with diphtheria.

In 1883, shortly after Pasteur had announced his discovery of the germ causation of disease, Klebs and Löffler isolated the germs that cause diphtheria. These germs are known as diphtheria bacilli. They are found in the membrane which appears in the throat of a person infected with diphtheria.

In order to determine whether or not infection is present the physician takes a smear from the throat and sends it to the health department, which then studies the germs to see if they are the germs of diphtheria. By taking a smear one means merely the introduction into the throat of some cotton on the end of a stick, which collects a small portion of the infected material. This is deposited on a preparation which permits the germs to remain alive until they can be studied.

There are various ways in which diphtheria may be spread from an infected person to a well one. The germs have been found on the bedclothing, on handkerchiefs, candy, shoes, hair, pencils, and drinking cups used by infected children. They are, of course, found in any discharges coming from the noses or throats of children who have the disease or who are recovering from it. There are, moreover, healthful carriers of diphtheria who, although they have recovered from the disease, still carry the germs about and distribute them to people who have not had the disease.

It is not safe for anyone to gamble on the possibility that a child infected with this disease does not really have diphtheria but simply some mild throat infection. Most of the serious results can be avoided if the child is seen early in the course of the disease and if proper treatment is given immediately.

If a child complains of sickness, and particularly of sore throat of the type mentioned, a physician should examine it promptly. A physician should be summoned immediately if the child complains of swelling of the neck or of any croupy condition with hoarseness. Early attention is particularly important in small children, because 85 per cent of the deaths from this disease usually occur in the first five years of life. Children are much more likely to catch diphtheria than are grown people. Moreover, the disease is likely to get a better start in a child, before it is properly diagnosed and treated, than in the case of a grown-up person.

The child should not be released to play with other children until it has been pronounced free from the germs. Cases are known in which germs capable of causing diphtheria have been carried in the throats of children who have recovered from the disease for as long as ten months. In more than 10 per cent of all cases a few of the germs can be found in the throat two weeks after all signs of the disease seem to have disappeared from the throat, and in 1 per cent of the cases the germs are still found in the throat four weeks after the child is apparently well.

It is the duty of the physician in charge of the patient to pronounce it well, and he will not wish to do this as long as the germs are still in the throat. Sometimes, when the germs persist for longer than three or four weeks, it is necessary to use active antiseptics in the throat; in a few instances the germs have persisted until the tonsils of the child have been removed.

Whenever a child appears to be ill with a high fever, when it complains of pains in the throat, when it is dull and apathetic, and when white spots are seen in the throat or on the tonsils, a physician capable of making a diagnosis should see the throat and should have immediate charge of the child's care. The more the throat is involved, the greater the spread of the membrane in which the germs are found. The longer the time that the poisons developed by the germs are permitted to get into the system, the more danger there is of death or of serious complications. Hence it is urged that such cases be diagnosed as early as possible, and that when diagnosed large amounts of antitoxin, to be determined by the doctor in charge, be given promptly.

It used to be thought that from 3,000 to 5,000 units of antitoxin were sufficient for a first dose, in the vast majority of cases. Most physicians now prefer to give 10,000 units of antitoxin immediately, and in severe cases 20,000 to 30,000 units of antitoxin as a first injection. The danger of death, or of various forms of paralysis, or of serious complications is far more likely from the disease than from any excess amount of antitoxin. Most strains of the diphtheria germ are sensitive to penicillin and this is beginning to be given routinely in treatment. Throat cultures become negative earlier in patients who receive penicillin.

The child will be immediately put to bed and it will have prolonged rest in bed in order to prevent serious complications. The development of such complications demands particularly the constant care of a physician.

Years ago, a physician named O'Dwyer developed a method for permitting persons with diphtheria to breathe when the membrane had developed to such a point that it obstructed the throat. This method includes the use of gold tubes, called intubation tubes, which an expert can pass through the throat and from the throat into the larynx, or breathing tube, thus permitting the child to breathe. The use of such tubes requires expert knowledge; they are a most valuable method in certain types of cases.

As the condition improves under the use of suitable doses of antitoxin, the membrane disappears, and the child usually coughs up the tube and gets rid of it. In other instances the physician easily removes the tube when it is no longer needed.

During the first few days of diphtheria the child should have a liquid diet as nourishing as possible, including plenty of milk and eggnog and cereals. Thereafter its diet may be gradually improved, particularly with substances that will aid the rebuilding of blood which may have been injured by the infection.

In the prevention of diphtheria in recent years chief reliance has been placed on the use of the Schick test, on toxin-antitoxin and on toxoid. The Schick test is simply a method of injecting a very small amount of the toxin of diphtheria into the skin. Those people who have in their blood antitoxin against the diphtheria poison will have a negative test. On the other hand, those who do not have antitoxin or who cannot develop it will have a positive Schick test.

In a positive Schick test the spot at which the toxin was injected becomes red and slightly raised within twenty-four to forty-eight hours. The application of Schick tests in thousands of cases has shown that about 8 per cent of newly born and young infants are susceptible to diphtheria, which means that they are likely to become infected if exposed to the disease. The remainder are not likely to have the disease at this early age because they have from their mothers a certain amount of resistance to the disease. This is gradually lost, however, so that from 30 to 40 per cent of children will be susceptible at one year of age, and about 65 per cent at five years of age. Apparently, through mild infections, this susceptibility then begins to decrease so that approximately 30 per cent are susceptible at ten years, and 18 per cent at fifteen years.

In the presence of an epidemic it is, of course, desirable that Schick tests be performed on all of the children exposed so as to know which ones are to be especially watched and which ones are to be immediately immunized against the disease by the use of toxin-antitoxin or toxoid. Millions of children have been given toxin-antitoxin and toxoid without the slightest harmful reactions, so that it has become customary in most large cities where there are competent health departments to recommend immunization of all children against diphtheria. Your family doctor will inoculate all the children against diphtheria. You should have this done as soon as possible.

Few people understand the difference between toxin, antitoxin, and toxin-antitoxin. When a horse is injected with the poison which diphtheria germs develop, he develops in his blood a substance which opposes the poison of the diphtheria germ. The poison is called toxin.

The material in the blood which opposes the poison of diphtheria is antitoxin. If a child does not have enough of this antitoxin in its blood to overcome diphtheria infection, the physician gives it antitoxin to help it. If a child has been exposed to diphtheria, and it is necessary very promptly to give it something to help it ward off the disease, antitoxin may be injected.

However, this antitoxin does not protect for a long period of time. It must be remembered that it has been elaborated in animals and not in the patient's own body, and that therefore its effects wear off in about three weeks. Of course, if a person has diphtheria, the antitoxin, when injected, helps to overcome the disease, and when the person recovers he has developed in his own body his own antitoxin, which is one reason why no one seems to have this disease twice.

If one is injected with small doses of toxin or poison, he builds up resistance to diphtheria in his own body. If it is desirable to stimulate his resistance-building factor still more, it is necessary to give him larger doses of toxin. However, such a procedure would be unsafe. Therefore, it is customary to add antitoxin to the toxin, which prevents it from working harm but does not prevent the body from responding to the injection of the toxin by building up more resistance. Toxoid is merely toxin detoxified by the addition of formaldehyde.

Few people realize the background of the way in which the body opposes disease. The process is called immunization. The terms vaccination, inoculation, injection, and similar terms refer to the fact that the substance is being put into the body in order that the body build the materials to oppose it.

Quite recently the preparation called toxoid has been developed for use in protecting children against diphtheria. Toxoid does not contain any horse serum, but is merely toxin detoxified by the addition of formaldehyde. It is used in the same way that toxin-antitoxin is used and serves to stimulate the development of immunity, or of resistance to diphtheria.

There are some people who react unfavorably to injections of antitoxin because they are sensitive to horse serum. Hypersensitivity of this kind is the same type of hypersensitivity that produces asthma, or hay fever, or eruptions of blisters, or similar manifestations. When there is a possibility that a child is going to be especially sensitive to antitoxin, the physician can find out by injecting under the skin a small amount—one or two drops—of the antitoxin and then waiting for an hour to see if there is going to be a reaction. Whenever a reaction appears it can be combated by giving suitable preparations of drugs which serve to control the reaction.

TREATMENT OF DIPHTHERIA

In the treatment of diphtheria, the antitoxin, as has already been mentioned, has been of the utmost importance. A delay of two, three, or four days in giving antitoxin may mean damage to vital organs in such manner that they can never recover completely. Moreover, the first dose of antitoxin that is given should be large enough to control the disease. This antitoxin is usually injected by the doctor in the back below the shoulder blade, but sometimes into the thigh or under the breast. In very severe cases the antitoxin is injected directly into a vein; in less severe cases, into the muscles, and in the milder cases, under the skin.

In the vast majority of cases a striking improvement is seen shortly after the antitoxin is injected. The improvement is demonstrated by a fall in the fever and a favorable change in the general condition of the patient. Usually within twenty-four hours after a sufficient dose has been injected, the membrane in the throat stops spreading, becomes softened and loosens up, and the swelling goes down.

There are, of course, patients with diphtheria who come to treatment so late that the antitoxin seems to be of little help, but even in these cases it exercises a tremendously beneficial influence in comparison with the effects when no antitoxin is given. In an occasional case of diphtheria there is sensitivity to the antitoxin, so that the patient may have a severe eruption or a reaction. These are exceedingly rare, developing perhaps in one out of every one thousand people. So far as is known, death from severe reaction to the serum occurs in only one in about seventy thousand people. These reactions occur more often in people who have had severe asthma or who have developed sensitivity to horse serum following a previous injection.

The heart is usually subjected to a severe strain in diphtheria, so that the patient should always be at rest in bed. Moreover, the heart must be watched carefully for several weeks after the patient recovers to make certain that it has not been damaged in any way.

There was a time when it was customary to wash the nose and throat of a patient with diphtheria with all sorts of gargles and sprays, usually of some alkaline solution. Nowadays it is customary to leave the nose and throat alone. In most instances when there is a foul odor in the throat, a mild wash or gargle may be desirable.

Antitoxin is supplemented with penicillin in cases of diphtheria to control secondary infections and because it helps to prevent formation of diphtheria toxin.

In the very severe cases of diphtheria, when the patient seems to be strangling because of lack of air, it may be necessary, as previously mentioned, to pass an O'Dwyer tube into the larynx so as to permit breathing. In the still more severe cases, an emergency operation is sometimes done, the physician opening the tube that leads to the lungs so that the patient is able to breathe. These cases are, however, exceedingly rare, since a powerful diphtheria antitoxin has been introduced, and since the vast majority of doctors give a large dose of antitoxin immediately, as soon as the patient has been examined and the diagnosis has been made.

Most patients stop showing germs of diphtheria in the throat after three or four weeks. Others continue even after several courses of treatment with

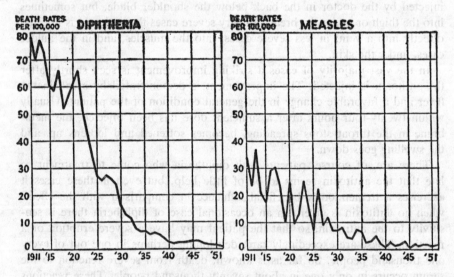

Fig. 9. Principal communicable diseases of childhood. Standardized annual death rates per 100,000 total persons. Ages 1 to 14 years.
(Courtesy of Metropolitan Life Insurance Company)

penicillin. The virulence of the germs should be determined by the state laboratory before the doctor relinquishes control of the patient.

In several communities in this country, notably, Auburn, N. Y., and New Haven, Conn., where almost the entire population of children has been immunized against diphtheria, the disease has been practically eliminated. The prevention of this disease by application of the various methods that have been described represents one of the greatest contributions of modern medical science to the welfare of humanity. Recent tests show that 80 per cent of the children who have been immunized by the use of toxin-antitoxin or of toxoid remain immune for at least ten years after the injections. It is reasonable to believe that we may yet see the time when diphtheria is no longer a menace to any civilized child.

MEASLES

Measles is one of the oldest diseases known to modern medicine. There is some evidence that it may have existed in the early Christian Era. It is even described in the writings of physicians of the seventh and ninth centuries. However, it was for a long time confused with scarlet fever, and it was not until the seventeenth century that it was clearly distinguished from scarlet fever. Moreover, it was occasionally confused with smallpox, and it was not definitely distinguished from smallpox until the eighteenth century.

Two of the greatest names in English medicine are associated with these two observations. Thomas Sydenham distinguished measles from scarlet fever, and William Withering, who introduced the use of digitalis, distinguished measles clearly from smallpox. The English word measles resembles a word in Sanskrit, *masura,* and the German word is *masern.*

For a long time it was generally believed that every child had to have measles. In fact, mothers used to expose their children to the disease with the idea of getting it over. Now it is known that the disease is definitely transmitted from one person to another, and that it is possible, by exercising precautions, to avoid the disease in most instances.

Measles is essentially a disease of childhood. More than half the cases occur in children under five years of age, and more than 90 per cent occur in children under ten years of age. There are occasional epidemics of measles in which considerable numbers of people are affected, even people of advanced years. In such cases it is usually found that the people concerned have come from rural areas and that they have not previously been exposed. For example, there were severe outbreaks of measles among the soldiers in the training camps in 1917 and 1918, because large numbers of recruits came from farms, ranches, and remote districts and had never had measles before.

Measles among a people who do not have anything resembling resistance through heredity may be a most serious and fatal disease. A terrific epidemic of measles occurred in the Faroe Islands in 1846. There were 7,800 people on the Islands and 6,000 of them had the disease in a few months. There was also a great epidemic in the Fiji Islands in 1875. A British ship carrying measles brought the disease to the Islands. Out of a population of 150,000 there were 40,000 deaths in a few months. Part of this was due to the great virulence with which the disease attacked a community without resistance. Much of the fatality is ascribed to the fact that so many people were sick at the same time that there were not enough well people left to take care of the sick. Some people died of starvation, and many died from lack of care.

As with diphtheria, measles is spread mostly through direct contact with those who have the disease. Apparently, the virus or poison that causes the disease is present in the secretions of the nose and throat. Hence it is spread by coughing and sneezing. Fortunately, the virus which carries the disease is injured by exposure to air and sunlight, so that it is seldom likely that measles is carried from one person to another through the medium of a third person or an animal. For this reason it is quite safe for doctors and nurses who see cases of measles to go in the open air to visit other patients.

However, it is well for those who take care of patients with measles to observe all of the precautions that are associated with the care of infectious disease generally. This means thorough washing of the hands after visting a patient, the wearing of a clean gown on entering the room, and removal of the gown on leaving. Moreover, the dishes, bedding, and other materials associated with the child sick with measles must be boiled before they are used again.

Two new methods have been developed for prevention of measles; one involves the injection of serum from a child who has recovered; another includes the use of a protein substance called immune globulin taken from the blood donated for transfusion, which contains anti-substances against infectious diseases. These methods are applied particularly when there is an epidemic.

Before any discovery is accepted as certainly established in relationship to the cause of an infectious disease, as has previously been mentioned, it is necessary to grow the germ outside the body and to reproduce the disease in animals by injecting the germ and to find the germ invariably associated with the disease.

Hektoen gave measles to two volunteers by inoculating them with blood from measles patients. The condition has been similarly produced in a monkey. The virus has been isolated and grown by Plotz and by Rake and Shaffer.

From the time when the child first comes in contact with a case of measles, and thereby develops the likelihood of catching the disease, until the disease appears, is usually twelve to nineteen days. This is known as the incubation period. During this period the patient does not have symptoms. However, he does develop early three definite signs which permit a physician to diagnose the disease in its earliest stages. These signs include fever, running nose and watering of the eyes, and an eruption on the mucous membranes lining the mouth. Measles is particularly infective during the stage before the rash appears when the nose is running and the child is coughing and sneezing.

The inflammation of the eyes differentiates measles from other infectious diseases, in which this symptom is not common. The child avoids the light and, as has been mentioned, the eyes are moist and full of tears. Particularly interesting are the little spots which appear on the sides of the mouth and on the palate and which resemble the rash that is later to appear on the skin. These little bluish white spots, surrounded with an area of red inflammation, were described by a New York physician named Koplik and are commonly called Koplik's spots. A Dutch physician on an isolated island described them earlier, but his report did not circulate; hence Koplik's name goes with the spots.

Three or four days after the running nose and the slight fever appear comes the rash. The child breaks out on the face, the mouth and chin, and then over the trunk, arms, thighs, and legs with red spots which enlarge and join together. The color is purplish red. During this period the child is likely to be sicker than at any other time in the course of the disease. He may have lack of appetite, a coated tongue, even looseness of the bowels; there may be a slight cough and other disturbances related to the lungs.

The child with measles should be placed in a room alone and not permitted to come in contact with other children. Particular attention must be given to the prevention of chilling, because this is especially harmful in measles. The secondary complications affecting the lungs are far more serious than the disease itself. The room should be well ventilated, but care must be taken to avoid drafts by placing screens properly before open windows. This does not mean that the room is to be kept stuffy or hot. It is the draft that should be avoided.

For years it was customary to keep darkened the room used by a child with measles because of the trouble with the eyes. Now it is realized that strong sunlight should be excluded because glare will cause pain in the eyes. The child should not be permitted to read nor should there be a brilliant artificial light. If the child complains particularly of the light, colored glasses may be worn. If the eyelids tend to stick because of the slight inflammation they may be bathed with boric acid solution or with plain warm water, which removes the crusts and prevents pain and irritation.

During the period of restlessness the child will sleep better if it is given a warm sponge bath just before going to sleep. This serves to cool the child and to bring down the fever slightly. It also avoids chilling. After the sponge bath the skin may be powdered with any light, clean talcum. This helps to avoid irritation.

It is not necessary to cover the child with heavy woolen blankets or to use flannel sleeping garments. The child should be kept warm but not made uncomfortable.

The food to be taken by the child with measles should be chiefly light and fluid as long as there is any fever. Just as soon as the fever disappears and the child begins to convalesce, plenty of nutritious food should be supplied, particularly foods containing iron and vitamins, as these will help to build up the depleted blood. Laxatives and cathartics should be given only on the order of a physician. It is much better to keep the bowels regular by the use of proper foods. It is also well in these conditions to give plenty of fluids, including drinks tending toward alkalinity, such as orange juice and lemon juice.

When a person has an infectious disease he builds up in his blood materials for opposing the disease. When he recovers, the material remains. For this reason the person who has measles, scarlet fever, or another infectious disease, usually has the disease only once. For this reason also it has been found helpful, in the presence of severe epidemics of measles, to inject into those who are exposed small amounts of the blood of those who are getting over the disease. This procedure has been found to be safe. It seems to minimize the severity of the disturbance if it does not prevent it. In addition to serum from convalescents, ordinary adult serum and placental preparations have been used.

It is the contagious material from the patient with measles that spreads the disease. This contagious material is found chiefly in the excretions from the nose and throat. Every possible step must be taken to prevent other children from coming in contact with these excretions. Occasionally also there are infections of the ear with discharges. The discharges from the ear may also contain the infectious substances, although quite frequently the ear is infected secondarily with other germs, such as the streptococci, which are always present in the throat.

When the resistance of the body is broken down by any one disease a human being becomes susceptible to infections from others. Measles is particularly important in this regard. It has been noticed that epidemics of measles are frequently followed by invasion of other contagious diseases, such as whooping cough, chicken pox, diphtheria, and scarlet fever. Measles is noted also for lowering resistance to tuberculosis so that children who have quiescent infections from tuberculosis in the glands, the bones, the joints, or the lungs may develop activity in these foci when they become infected with measles.

It is a mistake to consider measles a trivial disease. Perhaps many children do not die of measles, the number approximating in this country seven thousand per year. Diphtheria causes twice as many deaths, scarlet fever half as many, and whooping cough about the same number. However, there are many complications which cause serious conditions that are carried through life. Of all the deaths from measles, 75 per cent occur in children under five years of age. If a child gets measles before it is one year old, the chance of its dying is fifty times greater than in measles in a child between five and fifteen years of age.

In measles, antibiotics and sulfonamide drugs are of immense importance for preventing and controlling secondary complications such as may affect the eyes, nose, sinuses, throat, ears, lungs, heart or kidneys. The streptococcus, pneumococcus, meningococcus and tuberculosis are most frequent secondary invaders.

Whenever a case appears in a school, the parents of other children should be warned that a case has occurred and that they should be on the lookout for symptoms of infection in their own children. Parents should be warned particularly to keep their children who have measles, or who are just recovering, away from other children who may not have had the disease.

New in the prevention of measles is the use of immune globulin, derived from blood. Injections of this substance carry resistance against the disease. The complications are less frequent if the disease occurs and the severity less.

When a child with measles is put to bed promptly and given satisfactory care of the type that has previously been mentioned, it tends to get well. The prevention of the complications in measles is largely due to the kind of attention that is given. Careful management, skillful nursing, and early control of complications by competent medical attention make all the difference between prompt recovery and the possibility of permanent complications or death.

GERMAN MEASLES

German measles brings on one of the reddest eruptions of any disease that affects mankind. Its scientific name is *rubella,* and in German it is called *Rötheln.* Because of its red eruption it is frequently confused with scarlet fever or with measles. Fortunately, it is not nearly so severe a disease, although it is highly contagious.

From fourteen to twenty-three days after a child comes in contact with another who has had German measles it will begin to feel ill and break out with the eruption, which occurs first on the chest and face and then gradually spreads over the body. There is not much fever in most cases. However, the lymph glands, particularly those at the back of the neck, swell up and get hard, a condition that seldom occurs in other infectious diseases. Associated with this swelling and hardness of the glands at the back of the neck there will be tenderness and even stiffness.

It is important to make sure about the cause of such tenderness or such stiffness of the neck because many of the conditions of infection which concern the nervous system, such as meningitis, brain fever, and infantile paralysis, also develop stiffness and pain on motion of the neck. There are conditions in which lymph glands are infected in which the glands later soften and develop pus which has to be released by an opening. In German measles, however, the glands gradually soften and disappear without developing pus or matter.

The doctor tells the difference between German measles and ordinary measles by the absence of the spots in the mouth and by the slightness of the condition, by the nature of the eruption and by the absence in measles, in most cases, of the hard spots at the back of the neck.

Few, if any, people die of German measles. The disease usually proceeds toward prompt recovery. The chief trouble with it is that it causes loss of time from school. Seldom is anything required in its treatment except good care, a mild diet, cleansing of the throat by proper gargles, and the early care of any secondary complications.

Since the chief danger from measles has been the secondary complications, early use of penicillin and sulfonamides has lessened complications and made mortality minimal. At the earliest sign of infection of ears or chest the antibiotics are administered.

German measles and other virus infections are especially serious for pregnant women, since such infections during early months of pregnancy are now definitely related to deformities in the new born child. Gamma globulin from serum of persons recovering from German measles is given to pregnant women not less than eight days after contact or exposure to a case of German measles, as a method of protection.

SCARLET FEVER

No doubt scarlet fever was known to the ancients, but it is only within the last ten years that its nature has actually been thoroughly elucidated. It is an acute infectious disease that comes on suddenly, with a red rash which disappears gradually and is followed by peeling of the skin.

For many years it was known that a germ called the streptococcus was associated with scarlet fever, but it is only recently that the definite relationship of this germ to the cause of the disease has been established. The proof is in the fact that the germ can be found in the throat, the blood, and other tissues of people who have the disease, that the disease can be produced in human beings by putting the germs into their bodies, and that there is a reaction in the skin of a human being who does not have the disease when the toxin or poison taken from the germs is inoculated into the skin.

Scarlet fever usually comes on in epidemics that are worst in the winter or fall. The chief factor necessary is contact, usually of a child, with someone who has the disease. Most of the cases develop in children between five and twelve years of age. There is probably something that the child gets in its blood from the mother which in most cases prevents children below one year of age from catching the disease.

Scarlet fever does not spread nearly as rapidly as measles; apparently only about one in ten people who come in contact with cases of the disease later develop it. It is, of course, possible that people are infected with mild attacks of scarlet fever which are overlooked, and that as a result they are later protected against the disease. Scarlet fever is one of those diseases which happen once in a person's lifetime and then are not likely to happen again. In other words, one attack of the disease protects.

Occasionally scarlet fever is spread through milk or through the excretions or secretions of persons who are infected, but the spread through food is far less frequent than the spread directly from person to person. Most people are interested to know whether or not the scales or the skin that peels off after scarlet fever will transmit the disease. Apparently the scales will not spread scarlet fever unless contaminated with the secretions of the nose and throat.

From two to four days after a person has been in contact with someone who has had scarlet fever he will have a chill and complain of severe sore throat. If the person affected is a child, he is likely to be nauseated and vomit. Promptly the pulse becomes rapid as the fever goes up. The fever may rise as high as 102 to 104 degrees. There is severe headache. Then bright red spots about the size of a pin point appear, usually first on the neck and chest, then rapidly spreading over the rest of the body. The face is flushed because of the fever, but the eruption on the face is seldom severe.

After two or three days the rash or eruption begins to fade, and in about a week the skin appears to be normal in color. Then ten days to two weeks after the disease first appears the skin begins to peel. Great patches of skin may come off the hands and feet, but over the rest of the body the skin comes off in small scales. Occasionally the teeth, the hair, and the fingernails also are affected by the destructive process. An interesting symptom of scarlet fever is the appearance of the tongue. Because of its bright red appearance and because the tissues of the surface of the tongue swell so as to show tiny pits, the tongue of scarlet fever is called a strawberry tongue.

Scarlet fever in many instances is a fairly mild disease. When, however, it is complicated by certain forms of invasion of the kidneys, the ears, the glands or the joints, it may be most serious and destructive.

Until recently there was no certain method of confirming the diagnosis of scarlet fever, no certain method of determining whether or not a person who had not had the disease was likely to be infected on exposure, no method certainly useful in treatment except to put the patient to bed and to protect him against complications, such as is the general method of treatment of all infectious diseases.

Then Drs. George F. and Gladys Henry Dick in Chicago, and Drs. Dochez and Avery in New York, developed information relative to the germ and to the poison that it produces, which led to knowledge of a specific character. They found that a germ of the type called the streptococcus is responsible for scarlet fever; that it produces a poison or toxin which can be found in the material in which the germs grow; that this toxin, when injected into the skin of a person who has not previously had the disease, would produce a severe reaction, whereas in those who were protected against the disease it would not produce a reaction. They found, furthermore, that the injection of a small amount of this toxin or poison in a human being, after it had been made harmless, would cause the person to develop resistance against scarlet fever. Also a horse may be injected with this poison or toxin. The horse will then develop in its blood an antitoxin which is valuable in overcoming scarlet fever.

Since these discoveries were announced, many thousands of persons throughout the world have been tested with the Dick test. Many thousands of persons have been injected or inoculated with the toxin so as to free them relatively from the danger of contracting scarlet fever.

Because scarlet fever is not an extremely widespread disease, it does not appear to be worth while to inject every child with the preventive toxin. However, when a child has been definitely exposed to the disease, or when a girl is going to work as a nurse in a hospital where there are frequently cases of scarlet fever, it is probably advisable to give them the benefit of the preventive inoculations against scarlet fever. There are few, if any, records of severe accidents or injuries following the use of these preventive methods.

Scarlet fever varies in its severity from time to time, from epidemic to epidemic. In the presence of a severe epidemic with numerous serious complications, it is more advisable to inoculate against the disease than under other circumstances.

Because of the danger to other children from a child or an adult who has scarlet fever, the patient should be promptly put to bed and kept separate from other people for about six weeks. If there are discharges from the nose and throat or from the ears the patient should be isolated until all discharges have ceased. These discharges are extremely dangerous in spreading the disease.

Beyond this placing of the patient in a separate room, attention must be given to protecting the kidneys and the heart from the special strains associated with activity at a time when they are exposed to the actions of the poisons that come from the germs. Therefore, every patient with scarlet fever should remain in bed for at least three weeks. It is customary to give a light, soft diet consisting mostly of liquids until the fever has disappeared, and then gradually to add cereals and similar soft foods until the peeling has begun. Then it becomes necessary to build up the tissues and the blood again. This can be done by feeding plenty of milk, fresh vegetables, foods rich in vitamins, mineral salts like calcium and iron, and more protein than is allowed in the active stages of the disease.

It is important to avoid exposure to cold. Therefore, the patient should be bathed with sponges of lukewarm water. Sometimes the skin may be oiled, which aids the peeling and prevents irritation.

In most cases the throat can be let alone because the initial soreness and swelling soon disappear. If, however, there is severe pain from the sore throat, the usual mild gargles may be used. It is well, however, that only persons who have already had the disease should be in contact with the patient and help him with these procedures.

There is no certain method of preventing the complications that affect the kidneys in so many cases of scarlet fever. All that one can do is to make sure that the patient is quiet and that the diet does not throw an undue burden on the kidneys. For this reason it is customary, during at least the first two or three weeks, to eliminate meat and eggs from the diet.

In treating scarlet fever doctors usually prescribe remedies that will prevent headache and pain, giving small doses to avoid irritation of the kidneys. If earache occurs, the ears are closely watched so that the eardrum may be punctured and the infectious material allowed to escape before there is danger to the internal ear from pressure of the poison and danger of mastoiditis. If the infection is virulent, these complications may develop in spite of every precaution.

The discovery of the sulfonamides and of penicillin has revolutionized the treatment of scarlet fever. Penicillin, aureomycin, terramycin or sulfadiazine will suppress streptococci in the pharynx. Penicillin and erythromycin have been proved effective in treating scarlet fever. Most patients recover with few complications when properly treated with these drugs, and the incidence of complications is much less. These drugs are apparently specific against the streptococcus that is associated with scarlet fever. So efficient is penicillin against the scarlet fever streptococcus that routine administration has also been proposed for prevention of infection when there are epidemics. However, antibiotics for the ordinary use are not recommended although they are used prophylactically during epidemics. Serum and antitoxin are given with penicillin in seriously toxic cases. Penicillin also eliminates the streptococcus from carriers.

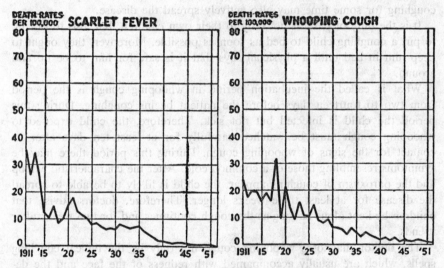

Fig. 10. Principal communicable diseases of childhood. Standardized annual death rates per 100,000 total persons. Ages 1 to 14 years.
(Courtesy of Metropolitan Life Insurance Company)

WHOOPING COUGH

At least four hundred years ago diseases were described which resemble what is called whooping cough today. It was known in Scotland as the "Kink" which meant a fit or paroxysm. This condition is one of the most difficult with which health officials and physicians have to deal. A few cases appearing in any group of children spread rapidly to include all who have not had the disease previously.

Whooping cough causes more deaths than do most of the other infectious diseases of childhood. It is fatal chiefly to the very young, and the immediate cause of death is nearly always some secondary infection. In older children whooping cough is quite frequently followed by pneumonia or tuberculosis and is especially menacing from the point of view of these complications.

A germ was found in connection with the disease in 1906, by two Belgian investigators, Bordet and Gengou.

The chief epidemics of this disease occur in winter. Whooping cough is transmitted, of course, by the material coughed out from the lungs. It has been shown that the explosive cough which occurs in this condition can throw droplets of infected saliva six feet or farther. Far too frequently parents permit children to begin playing with other children just as soon as they are without fever. Yet these children, if they continue to cough, may be active in spreading the disease to children who have not had it. Moreover, there is evidence that whooping cough is infectious in its earliest stages, so that children who are not put to bed and kept isolated until after they have been coughing for some time may also actively spread the disease.

It is the duty of parents not only to their own children, but also to others, to put a coughing child to bed as soon as possible. Moreover, they ought to keep him in bed until a physician says that it is safe for him to be up and around.

What is called the incubation period in whooping cough is the period from two to fourteen days before the patient begins coughing. During this period the child is infected but not sick. Therefore, the child exposed to whooping cough must be watched carefully for at least ten days after its contact for the signs of whooping cough. During this period there may be symptoms resembling those of a common cold. After the characteristic whoop and the paroxysm of coughing appear, the child is likely to be able to spread the disease for at least three weeks longer. Therefore, doctors advise that children be kept alone as long as the cough continues and for two weeks after it ends.

The doctor diagnoses whooping cough not only by the typical coughing spells, which are usually accompanied with redness of the face and the development of a thick, sticky mucus in the mouth, but also by changes which occur in the blood in this disease. Not only do the white blood cells increase in number, but a particular form of the white blood cells, known as the lymphocytes, mononuclear or single nucleus cells, increases even more than do the others.

As has been said, the chief danger from whooping cough is not from the disease itself, but from the secondary pneumonia and changes which may affect the heart and lungs.

The total period of quarantine may be as long as six weeks. In attempting to control whooping cough all sorts of methods of prevention have been tried, including inoculation of the blood from people who are recovering from the disease, the injection of germs that have been killed, with the idea that these injections will stimulate the body to form anti-substances against the germs of the disease, and many similar measures. The use of the vaccines, which means a mixture of killed germs, is established as valuable in preventing whooping cough in children who are exposed, and also in diminishing the severity of the symptoms. Several specific vaccines have been developed and the use of such preparations for prevention is now generally recommended. Preventive inoculations begin as early as six months of age. Booster doses of vaccine are given at four year intervals.

As soon as the child who has had whooping cough is free from fever and any other serious symptoms, it is customary to permit him to be about, particularly where there are sunlight, warmth, and fresh air, but the child should not be exposed to air that is too cold.

Because the coughing spells are frequently accompanied by vomiting, such children sometimes lose weight and may suffer from a lack of water in the body. Hence, the parents must aid the physician in seeing to it that the child has sufficient water and also that it eats between meals, if necessary, or in fact whenever it can retain food, so as to keep up its nutrition.

Because coughing may bring undue pressure into the abdominal cavity and thereby cause rupture or hernia by pushing the abdominal contents through the wall, it is advisable in some cases to put an abdominal binder on the child, which helps to support the abdominal wall and, at the same time, gives the child comfort during severe coughing.

Although the use of various drugs does not cure whooping cough, sedatives which a physician can prescribe lessen the severity of the coughing. Streptomycin, chlortetracycline and polymyxin are new antibiotics successful in whooping cough. Other antibiotics to be tried include chloramphenicol and oxytetracycline. The whooping cough vaccines now available are more efficient in preventing the disease and lessening its severity.

One of the simplest methods of relieving a cough is to inhale warm steam perhaps medicated with a little tincture of benzoin. Fill a cup with boiling water, drop in a teaspoonful of the tincture of benzoin, and inhale the hot steam for five or ten minutes. Such medication is more useful for an ordinary cough than for whooping cough, however. In this condition, frequently, the only way to get relief is by taking sedative remedies that are so strong they can be taken only with a doctor's prescription.

As in other types of infectious disease, all drops from the nose and throat should be disinfected, and all articles contaminated by such discharges, if they are without value, should be disinfected or burned.

In keeping up the nutrition of the child, it is well to rely primarily on milk and the use of vegetables containing plenty of vitamins and mineral salts.

In preventing the spread of whooping cough everyone must coöperate. If parents know of other children in the neighborhood who have whooping cough and who are being permitted to play outdoors with children who have not had the disease, the health department should be notified. In most communities the parents who have children with whooping cough are permitted themselves to go to work and to go outdoors, although the children are kept under isolation. However, a sign on the door to the effect that whooping cough is present in the household will inform other parents of the fact and will enable them to take suitable precaution so that their children may not undergo any unusual likelihood of catching the disease.

CHICKEN POX

All sorts of names have been applied to chicken pox, not only by the public, but also by physicians. In some parts of the country it is known as water pock, glass pock, sheep pock, and crystal pock. These names obviously are related either to some resemblance of the blisters to similar conditions occurring in animals, or, in fact, to the resemblance of the blisters to water or crystal. Scientifically, the condition is called *varicella,* but it was also called *variola spuria,* or spurious smallpox, because it was so frequently mistaken for smallpox.

The cause of chicken pox is a virus. The viruses of chicken pox and herpes zoster or shingles resemble each other. Chicken pox in children may induce shingles in adults. Shingles, whether in children or adults, may be followed by epidemics of chicken pox. The condition occurs most often in children and, because it is so highly contagious, spreads rapidly. Usually a person who has had the disease once does not develop it again. The infectious agent is present in the blisters. The blisters appear early and break almost as soon as they appear. Probably the disease may be spread before the eruption is visible in the form of blisters. About two weeks after a child has been in contact with children who have chicken pox, it will probably come down with this disease.

The blisters on the skin appear in groups, usually first on the back, the chest, and the face, but most profusely on those parts of the skin that are covered by clothing.

As has been mentioned, the condition may be spread not only from contact with infectious material that is in the blisters, but far more frequently through some infection that may be inhaled.

A physician's daughter, sixteen years old, developed a slight sore throat and was immediately isolated in a room in the upper story of her home. On the following day she was found to have the eruption of chicken pox. An eight-year-old brother who was with her on the previous day was kept in a distant part of the house, but sixteen days later he also came down with chicken pox. His only possible contact with the disease was through his sister.

Nobody knows how long a person who has chicken pox remains infectious for others, but it is safe to keep the person who is recovering away from other people until the skin is entirely free of the original crusts.

Chicken pox is not a particularly serious disease, since it is seldom associated with high fever or with much depression. Usually the fever disappears in from one to three days, although it may last four or five days. With the exception of German measles, chicken pox is probably the mildest of all the infectious diseases that attack children.

Usually all that is necessary in such cases is to make certain that the child does not scratch the spots with the likelihood of secondary infection. The finger nails of children should be closely trimmed to prevent such scratching. If it cannot be stopped in any other way, the hands may be enclosed in mittens of cloth or celluloid, or tubes may be put about the elbows which will prevent bending the elbow and scratching.

Ordinarily, the blisters, if let alone, will last a few hours, break, dry up, and form a crust. This crust disappears in from two to four days.

The diet is mild and soft. Mild, warm baths are used, and it may be desirable for the physician to prescribe powder to prevent itching, or ointments and antiseptic solutions to prevent secondary infection.

Chicken pox seldom concerns older people. Most children have had it by the time they grow up. If, however, they have not had it, they may get the disease later. Chicken pox can be exceedingly inconvenient for a grown-up person, but the most important step for a grown-up person is to make certain that he really has chicken pox and not smallpox.

After a patient recovers, it is merely necessary to wash the bedding thoroughly with hot water and soap and to clean and air the room in which the patient has been while sick.

It is also well for everyone who is in contact with the child to wash the hands thoroughly after leaving the room and preferably to wear a gown or covering while in the room.

The giving of sulfonamides or penicillin and the application of tyrothricin to the blisters prevent secondary infections. The lesions of shingles may require sedative ointments. Reports indicate the possibility that ultraviolet irradiation of air or glycol vaporization may help to prevent spread of chicken pox in schools.

MUMPS

Of all the annoying diseases that afflict the child, and which also occasionally attack the adult, mumps is the one most likely to arouse the risibilities of those in the vicinity. Swelling at the sides of the face gives the person who is infected a distinctly comical appearance. There is a current superstition that the person with the disease cannot eat pickles and that anything sour will pucker up his face like the phenomena that follow the eating of a green persimmon.

There is no doubt that the condition is infectious, because it spreads rapidly wherever it gets a start among a group of young people. Cases have been described as long ago as one hundred fifty years, and there is reason to believe that something resembling mumps was described by the famous father of scientific medicine, Hippocrates, 500 years before the Christian Era.

In 1934 the cause of mumps was definitely established to be a filterable virus.

Most often mumps appear in a child from five to fifteen years of age from 14 to 21 days after exposure to infection. Because the glands most commonly concerned are the parotid glands, just in front of the ear, the disease is called scientifically parotitis. The Germans fondly call it *Ziegenpeter,* which perhaps has some reference to a goat.

In most cases, mumps is a mild condition. It occurs usually during the cold season of the year. Out of 150 epidemics, only 21 occurred in the warm months. The mouth becomes dry and there is pain on chewing or swallowing.

Mumps is primarily a disease of adolescence, but cases have been observed in a woman eighty-four years of age, and in a man ninety-nine years of age— no doubt, both in their second childhood.

Mumps is probably spread from one person to another by the saliva. Occasionally a third person may become contaminated with this infectious saliva and, although himself not infected by the disease, carry it from a sick person to a healthy one. Study of the disease shows that it is most contagious during the early days, and that once convalescence begins it is not nearly so dangerous. For this reason it is not customary to quarantine or isolate cases with mumps for more than two weeks.

Beyond the stiffness of the jaw and the pain on opening the mouth, which are associated with the swelling of the glands, the person with mumps usually has little trouble. There are, however, cases in which the mumps seem to spread particularly to the glands of sex. When this occurs, it is a serious complication. There are instances in which the ability to have children has been irreparably damaged by this secondary complication. Incidentally, the complication is more likely to occur in grown people than in children. With the complication of this character there may be fever that is fairly high.

There is not much that can be done about mumps, except to make certain that the person is absolutely quiet and that there is no secondary complication in the form of pus infection. When this occurs either in the glands in front of the ear or in the sex glands, a competent physician can be of much service. Gamma globulin from cases of convalescent mumps is used in treatment. Cortisone or ACTH has been reported helpful in controlling the inflammation. In the majority of cases the condition gets well without any complications. Usually it is mild. Aureomycin has been helpful in the secondary complications of mumps.

The usual treatment of infectious diseases, already described, is ordinarily applied by good physicians in cases of mumps. The attention of the physician is necessary so that he may detect possible complications at the earliest moment. Since aureomycin and chloromycetin are effective against viruses they are now being used in severe cases of mumps.

People who have had mumps should be kept under observation for at least three weeks, to make sure that the condition is fully healed and that no further complications are likely.

INFANTILE PARALYSIS

Of all the diseases that strike dread to mankind, none is more feared by mothers than acute poliomyelitis, or, as it is more commonly known, infantile paralysis. This is an acute infection in which the inflammation attacks the tissues in the front part of the spinal cord. Possibly it has occurred throughout the centuries, but it was first widely recognized as an epidemic disorder around 1887, since Medin described the epidemic of that year in Stockholm in a paper published in 1891. No doubt, previous to that time, cases of this disease were confused with meningitis and paralysis due to other disorders.

The majority of cases of this condition occur in young children, afflicting boys and girls in about equal proportions. There are, however, numerous cases in which the condition attacks older persons, among the most conspicuous examples being Franklin D. Roosevelt, who was infected late in life.

A virus, or infectious agent too small to be seen with the microscope, is recognized as the cause of this disease. The virus can be cultivated outside the body on living tissue. Several different types of poliomyelitis virus have been isolated. Its infectious character is certainly established through transmission from one animal to another. There seems to be reason to believe that the disease is spread through contamination, possibly by direct contact with those having the disease, and possibly also by healthy carriers of the infection. The virus is found regularly in material excreted by the bowel and this may also be a source of infection. Virus can also be recovered from contaminated flies. The appearance of the paralysis usually follows three or four days of fever and disturbances of digestion. In some cases the preliminary symptoms are so slight that the paralysis is the first symptom noted. In other cases, the paralysis may be so slight that the condition is unrecognized except for the fact that the child happens to be sick at a time when infantile paralysis is prevalent in the community. The disease usually appears 7 to 14 days after exposure and the incubation period may be from 5 to 35 days.

Infantile paralysis usually begins to appear in many sections of the United States in April, increases during July and August, diminishes in October, and disappears by November. In the northern part of the United States it reaches its highest point in August and September. However in the Southern States, the high point is reached somewhere between December and May. While the condition occurs usually in warm weather, it is not especially a disease of tropical countries. It is most frequent in the temperate zone. By far the vast majority of the cases have occurred in northern Europe and in the northern part of the United States.

The disease attacks rich and poor alike and appears equally in good and bad sanitary situations. Whereas 95 per cent of those attacked are children, the condition seldom occurs during the first year of life. This may be due to the fact that the infant, during this period, is separated from the community generally. It is also due, however, in some part, to the fact that the mother transmits to the infant at birth a certain amount of resistance against this as well as other infectious diseases, and that perhaps a year is required for the immunity of this character to wear off.

In any event, when infantile paralysis is present in a community, any child with the slightest symptoms of a cold or a fever should be given most careful study by a physician.

Those who have been exposed to infantile paralysis should have temperatures taken regularly for a period of at least three weeks so as to detect the onset of fever and symptoms at the earliest possible moment. During times when there are epidemics in the community, children should not be allowed to mingle with crowds, and travel should be discouraged. The occurrence of fever, headache with vomiting, drowsiness, and irritability when disturbed, flushing, congestion of the throat, and notable sweating during a period when infantile paralysis is prevalent in a community should be looked on with suspicion. Any evidence on the part of the child of stiffness of the back and resistance to movement of the neck is to be considered as a suspicious symptom, demanding the most careful medical investigation.

Careful epidemiologic studies indicate that a community has 200 abortive or non-paralytic cases for every one paralytic case of poliomyelitis.

Since 1952 inoculation against infantile paralysis has been practiced, at first using gamma globulin, and more recently by the vaccine which was developed by Salk. Enders grew the virus types in pure culture outside the body on monkey kidney tissue. Salk combined the three chief viruses in a vaccine. Doses are given two weeks apart; then after a lapse of seven to ten months a booster dose is given. By fall of 1955, in a nation-wide mass inoculation program, more than twenty million doses had been given to ten million children under 14 years of age.

The secretions and excretions from the patient with infantile paralysis should be handled exactly like we handle the material from the patient with typhoid. Particularly dangerous is hand-to-mouth infection. Everyone associated in the care of a patient with infantile paralysis in its early stages should make certain to wash his hands with soap and water each time he is near the patient.

EARLY DIAGNOSIS OF INFANTILE PARALYSIS

As soon as infantile paralysis is well established it becomes important to have a careful examination of the muscles in order to find out which are permanently involved so that plans may be outlined for treatment leading to recovery of the power of motion.

Among the remedies used in the treatment of infantile paralysis it is necessary to mention first absolute rest in bed. This is important in avoiding any unnecessary irritation to the affected tissues. Research has shown the significance of fatigue and exhaustion in extending and making paralysis more severe.

Among the most important factors in giving relief from serious pain and depression in this condition, good nursing is especially to be emphasized. Good nursing in infantile paralysis must be exceedingly gentle. It must minimize as much as possible any movement of the patient and avoid any unnecessary output of energy. The physician can prescribe various drugs which tend to keep such patients quiet. The nurse may aid in giving warm baths which help in bringing about relief.

One of the recent discoveries which gives comfort is the artificial respirator. Machines have been developed into which the child's whole body may be put and its breathing motions kept up automatically. The National Foundation for Infantile Paralysis, Inc., 120 Broadway, New York, has central depots for respirators and makes them available for communities which have a high incidence of bulbar poliomyelitis. Twelve respirator centers provide complete care.

In acute cases the Sister Kenny treatment is used. It includes routine use of hot packs to prevent spasm of muscles and early education and reëducation of affected muscles.

Once the active disease has passed, it is necessary to make a complete examination of all the muscles to find out which have become weakened and which have lost their functions entirely; then the weakened muscles may be benefited. In cases in which some functions have been lost entirely, reëducation of the muscles may be used to enable children to walk and to carry on other activities. Throughout all treatments it is necessary to guard against too much fatigue. Children should not be encouraged to walk too soon. They should never be allowed to stand in a deformed position. If the legs are too weak, splints may be applied, and corsets, jackets, and braces may be worn in order to aid in supporting the weakened tissues.

Exercise in water has developed a great vogue, particularly through endorsement of the Georgia Warm Springs Foundation by former President Roosevelt. The chief advantages of the use of the swimming-pool method are the aid derived from supporting the limbs by the buoyancy of the water. Even under the best of conditions, however, the swimming pool itself is not a cure for paralyzed muscles. It is the training given in the swimming pool by competent teachers that brings about restoration.

The number of deaths from infantile paralysis varies greatly in different epidemics. In the great epidemic which occurred in New York in 1916, 27 per cent of those attacked died.

Of the greatest importance in the care of such patients is the proper handling of all their normal functions. They should be moved sufficiently often to prevent the occurrence of bed sores. There is danger of pneumonia. The patient should not be allowed to lie continually on the back. If he cannot swallow the mucus and saliva which develop in the mouth, he must be turned so that these will be drained out. More decently the development of mechanical devices to aid normal breathing during the period when the lungs are paralyzed has saved many lives.

The majority of children who have had infantile paralysis still retain the ability to perform certain movements but lack the power to make other movements. For this reason general exercises which are good for normal people are not suited to the unequal movements of these patients. Here are some suggestions for the mother who is to aid with daily treatment:

1. The patient must know what movement he is to do and must try to do it, after which he relaxes and lets the mother put the arm or leg back in the starting position ready for him to try again.

2. The mother should understand that it does not strengthen the muscles if she moves the leg back and forth. The patient must try and should not be helped until he has done as much of the movement as his strength allows; then the rest of the movement should be finished for him while he still tries.

3. The mother may make any of these exercises harder by resisting the movement with her hand. This resistance should not be given until the movement can be performed strongly and correctly, without help, ten times. When resistance is given, it should be smoothly graduated to the movement throughout, being great enough to make the muscle work hard to perform the movement, but never great enough to stop it or make it jerky.

4. The patient should never be allowed to turn or twist his body in order to get the part to the desired position, since this will entail the use of muscles other than the ones it is desired to strengthen. If he is unable to do the movement correctly, the mother must guide the limb with her hands, being careful not to help unless it is necessary.

5. The exercises must be done every day to obtain benefit—in the morning, before the muscles become tired, is the best time. Each exercise should be done about five to ten times, with a stop to rest whenever the movement is done less well than the time before. Fatigue should be strenuously avoided and is to be judged better by the relative success in the performance of consecutive movements than by the expressed feelings of the patient. Weakened muscles may be tired by overactivity so that they cannot work as well, without the patient's being conscious of fatigue.

6. As a general rule, it is better not to give as exercises the movements which the child can do pretty well, for fear of producing a deformity from the pull of the stronger muscles, but instead to have him try to do the movement which he finds difficult. For instance, if a parent says that the child can pull the leg

up but can't put it down, or can turn the foot out but can't turn it in, that child should have exercises of pushing the leg down and of turning the foot in, the mother being very careful not to allow him to do the stronger movements.

A physician selects exercises which are graded according to the amount of the deficiency of the muscle, and gradually increases the scope of the exercise to be performed as the weakened muscles straighten. No exercises of any kind are recommended for use during periods of active inflammation in this disease.

As an example of how a handicapped person can overcome his disability of this type, it is well to recall the story of Sir Walter Scott, who lived one hundred years ago. He was one of twelve children, the first six of whom all died in infancy. In the period in which he lived deaths among babies were frequent. Indeed, the infant mortality rate was in many places as high as four hundred per thousand, which means that two out of every five infants that were born died before they were one year of age. Today the rates vary from fifty to one hundred per thousand.

In fact, Scott himself almost succumbed because his parents employed for him a nurse who was tuberculous and who concealed this fact. Fortunately the famous professor of chemistry, Dr. Black, discovered it and notified the parents, who then dismissed the nurse. Even at that time the risk to the child of being nursed by a tuberculous woman was understood.

When Sir Walter Scott was eighteen months old his first serious illness overtook him. Apparently he suffered with the cutting of teeth and a fever. On the fourth day thereafter he was found to have lost the power of his right leg. His parents consulted every possible type of medical practitioner, both scientific and unscientific, and, all of this being without success, he was finally sent to the country to recuperate. This was, of course, an attack of infantile paralysis, not sufficient to cause death but sufficient to produce permanent crippling, for Sir Walter Scott was thereafter lame for the rest of his life. It was probably excellent advice to send the young boy to the country to recuperate.

As Scott himself said, "The impatience of a child soon inclined me to struggle with my infirmity, and I began by degrees to stand, to walk, and to run. Although the limb affected was much shrunk and contracted, my general health, which was of more importance, was much strengthened by being frequently in the open air, and, in a word, I who in a city had probably been condemned to hopeless and helpless decrepitude, was now a healthy, high-spirited, and my lameness apart, a sturdy child."

CHAPTER X

Transmissible Diseases

MORRIS FISHBEIN, M.D.

TYPHOID FEVER

I F THE CASE RATES and death rates for typhoid fever that existed in 1890 prevailed now, the city of Chicago would have in 1955, 60,000 cases of typhoid fever and approximately 6,000 deaths. Instead, the city of Chicago has had in recent years regularly less than 20 cases and seldom as many as 5 deaths. In Chicago from April 1, 1890, to April 1, 1892, there were 2,372 deaths from typhoid fever representing approximately 24,000 cases. Compare that figure with the population of that day to the great population of Chicago at present and the low incidence of typhoid. What a tremendous benefit modern scientific preventive medicine has been for all of mankind.

In an earlier day, the family doctor claimed that he could smell typhoid fever. His guess was likely to be accurate, since one out of five seriously sick people whom he saw was likely to have typhoid fever. There was a time when any doctor could definitely count on the financial returns from typhoid fever, and they were usually sufficient in amount to permit him to send all his children to college.

Typhoid fever is an acute infection caused by a germ which used to be known as the typhoid bacillus and which is now called *Salmonella typhosa*. The germ can be found in the blood of a person seriously sick with the disease, and in 80 per cent of the cases is found in the stools or excretions of the sick. The germ is spread from the sick person to those who are well by means of the excretions, by soiled food and clothing, particularly by contaminated water and milk, and to a large extent by people who carry the disease; that is to say, they themselves have been sick and have recovered, but they still have in their bodies germs which reside frequently in the intestinal tract and also in the gall bladder, and which may get out of those places and infect other people.

There was a time when cases of typhoid fever occurred from the use of ice made from water in polluted streams. Today the vast majority of ice used in this country is made artificially from clean water, and there is no danger of typhoid. Milk used to be a common source of typhoid germs; and milk products such as ice cream, butter, buttermilk, and cheese were also known on occasion to carry the germs. Once the eating of infected oysters was a prominent cause, because the oysters were developed in contaminated water. In fact, the best fattening grounds for oysters were known to be in and around sewers. Now the control of oyster breeding in uncontaminated water, and suitable methods of storage and transmission for oysters, have largely eliminated the shellfish as a source of contagion. Cases have been reported due to the eating of raw vegetables which had been fertilized with contaminated materials or watered with contaminated water.

It was thought for a while that flies were more responsible for spreading typhoid fever than any other cause, but today it is not believed that transmission by flies is important, however, the fly does feed filthily and may transmit any condition associated with the filth on which it feeds.

FLIES CARRY FILTH

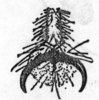

BECAUSE
BRED IN
FILTH

Hairy foot of a fly   *Bacteria colony in fly's footprint*

A FLY OFTEN CARRIES 6,600,000 BACTERIA ON ITS HAIRY BODY

FROM		TO
Manure pile		*Milk*
Garbage can		*Baby's lips*
Privy vault		*Baby's bottle*
Spittoon		*Food*
Sick room		*You*

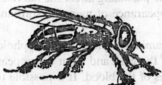

Fig. 11. A fly is the most dangerous animal known.
(Courtesy of International Harvester Company)

Typhoid fever used to follow a long and serious course once a person became infected with it. After a person gets the germs in his body, from three to twenty-one days elapse, known as the incubation period, during which the germs develop and liberate their poisons. The average length of time is ten and a half days. The condition begins with the usual symptoms of infection, such as headache, pains in the body generally, a feeling of exhaustion and loss of appetite. Sometimes there are chills. Quite frequently there is nosebleed, and almost invariably there is disturbance of the action of the bowels in the form of constipation or diarrhea. With the coming of modern methods of treatment using chloromycetin the duration of the disease has been shortened and its severity diminished. The fever is brought under control in a few days.

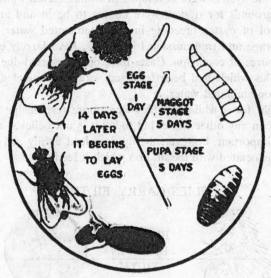

EGG STAGE
1 DAY
MAGGOT STAGE
5 DAYS
PUPA STAGE
5 DAYS
14 DAYS LATER IT BEGINS TO LAY EGGS

Fig. 12. Life cycle of a fly.

In addition to the loss of appetite, there is a tendency to the formation of gas with bloating of the body; and sometimes, because of the ulcers in the bowels and the bloating, sudden severe hemorrhages from the bowel. Sometimes the infection and the poisoning affect the nervous system so that there is delirium and even the appearance of mental disturbance during the course of the disease.

The physician who examines a patient with typhoid fever makes his diagnosis from the history of the case and from the appearance of the symptoms, and also by careful studies of the blood. It is possible to examine specimens of the blood and to determine by the use of a test, called the Widal test, after the Frenchman who discovered it, whether or not the condition is quite certainly typhoid fever. Any serious complications such as hemorrhage, perforation of the bowel, and changes in the heart action and in the nervous system, demand prompt and careful attention by a competent physician.

A person who has typhoid fever must be kept alone and preferably cared for by an experienced nurse. The room should be screened if the condition occurs during the summer, when flies are a common pest. Because the person with typhoid may remain long in bed in severe cases he should have a bed with a firm mattress, and arrangements must be made to change the bed linen any time it is soiled. The patient must be bathed at least once a day and the back

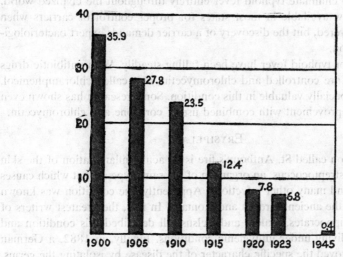

Fig. 13. Typhoid is in retreat in the registration area of the
United States.

and buttocks kept clean in order to prevent secondary infections. It is also important to see that the mouth is kept clean and rinsed each time after food is taken.

There was a time when it was thought advisable to starve patients with typhoid fever. The condition interferes with the nutrition of the patient, so that present methods involve the giving of a diet of from 3,000 to 3,500 calories. Then the patient will not lose weight during the course of the illness.

A vaccine made of the killed germs of typhoid fever is of value in preventing the disease. This was quite certainly proved during World War II. Anyone who is likely to be exposed to the taking of contaminated food or water ought to be vaccinated against typhoid fever. In the entire American army during World War II there were only slightly over one thousand cases of typhoid fever among something like five million enrolled troops. If the rate for typhoid which prevailed during the Spanish-American War had existed, there would have been approximately a million cases.

It is customary to give three injections of the vaccine against typhoid fever at ten-day intervals, although the intervals between injections may be shortened in time of necessity. Obviously, the giving of such vaccines is the work of a physician or of a trained nurse, since the average person cannot inject himself and does not understand the technic of preparation. Only rarely indeed are there reactions of a serious character following the injection of ordinary doses of antityphoid vaccine.

Persistent attention to water supplies and disposal of sewage, pasteurization of milk, education of the public in hygiene, and the control of typhoid carriers will eventually eliminate typhoid fever entirely throughout the civilized world. Means are now available in most states for proper control of carriers when they are discovered, but the discovery of a carrier demands expert bacteriological investigation.

The rates for typhoid fever have been falling steadily. With antibiotic drugs complications are controlled and chloromycetin, also called chloramphenicol, has proved especially valuable in this condition. Some research has shown even more rapid improvement with combined use of cortisone and chloromycetin.

ERYSIPELAS

The condition called St. Anthony's fire is an acute inflammation of the skin caused by the streptococcus, an organism of the same type as that which causes scarlet fever and many other infections. Apparently, the condition was known in the time of the ancient Greeks and Romans. In fact, the greatest writers of those days, Hippocrates, Galen, and Celsus, all described this condition and credited it to living under unhygienic conditions. Finally, in 1882, a German investigator proved the specific character of the disease by isolating the germs.

Erysipelas occurs most often during the months from October to March, and in fact reaches its highest frequency in March. The disease is not so common in children as in persons between the ages of twenty to sixty. Men apparently have erysipelas more often than do women, perhaps because men are more frequently exposed to physical injuries and bad weather conditions during the winter months.

Erysipelas starts most often in a wound, abrasion, or rubbed place on the skin, and particularly in those places where the mucous membranes, such as those which line the nose and the mouth, join the outer skin. In hospitals, in the past, there were frequently epidemics of erysipelas because the infection was carried from one patient to another by attendants. Nowadays the great danger of erysipelas in a surgical ward has been recognized, and a person with erysipelas is promptly put in a room by himself and attended by a nurse who is not attending other people. In cases which occur in homes under ordinary conditions it is necessary to make certain that the other people in the family do not come in too close contact with the patient. The spread of this disease is almost always by the hands of the person who is taking care of the patient.

Erysipelas usually begins with a severe fever and a chill and associated with this all of the usual symptoms of an acute poisoning of the body such as headache, loss of appetite, vomiting, and, in the case of a high fever, perhaps some delirium.

The disease usually lasts from five to ten days, the average being eight days. When the erysipelas affects large areas of the body it may continue for as long as fifteen days.

Usually erysipelas begins on the face and extends from day to day, so that it eventually covers the entire side of the face, including the eyelids, which become enormously swollen and filled with fluid. Sometimes the swelling is sufficient to close the eye completely. Then the disease spreads onto the ear, which thickens tremendously, and finally reaches the line of the hair, where it stops abruptly. In other cases it may spread down the back. In many instances the condition begins on the bridge of the nose and spreads rapidly to each side so that it forms what is called a "butterfly" pattern.

Often any natural boundary such as the hair line, the nape of the neck, and places where the skin is tight over the cheek bones, will stop the spread of the disease.

When the inflammation of the skin stops, the fever begins to drop. Sometimes the skin peels where it has been greatly swollen. If the disease occurs again and again, almost a permanent thickening may develop, which is, of course, exceedingly unsightly.

The doctor is able to diagnose erysipelas certainly by studying its general character and also by examining the blood in which the white cells are found to have been increased tremendously.

The most serious complication in erysipelas is a secondary infection. Under such circumstances the swelling changes to abscess. In the vast majority of cases erysipelas is not a fatal disease. In young infants and in old and sickly people it may be exceedingly serious, but in general it causes a death rate per year of about three people for each hundred thousand in the community.

Numerous remedies have been developed for the treatment of erysipelas, including the use of ultraviolet and X rays, antiseptics, antitoxins, and all sorts of chemicals, especially the newer derivatives of sulfanilamide. Doctors used to attempt to control the disease by painting on iodine, silver nitrate, and similar preparations, but modern authorities feel that these accomplish little, and besides may so hide the spread of the disease as to interfere with its control. Sulfanilamide, sulfapyridine and sulfathiazole prevent the growth in the blood of the germs that cause erysipelas. These should be prescribed by the doctor. If the eyelids are involved, it is customary to drop some mild antiseptic solution, which the doctor will supply, directly into the eyes. The new drugs like penicillin control the disease in most cases.

Dr. Konrad Birkhaug recommends the use of compresses soaked in an ice-cold solution of magnesium sulphate (or Epsom salts). If these cloths are kept cold and applied repeatedly, they offer great relief by lessening the tightness of the skin and diminishing the burning pain and swelling. This will not, however, stop the spread of the erysipelas.

Since erysipelas is caused by a streptococcus, the condition is now controllable by the use of the antibiotics, particularly penicillin, aureomycin and terramycin and by the use of sulfadiazine. These new remedies have made unnecessary the use of biologic preparations like antitoxins. The manifestations on the skin are treated with direct application of specific remedies. Since erysipelas arises in most instances from a small beginning, early and prompt treatment of scratches and minor infections has greatly reduced the total number of cases of erysipelas. Cold compresses are often soothing and some physicians recommend moistening the compresses in a mild solution of aluminum acetate (Burow's solution, 1:1000).

Because erysipelas, like other infectious diseases, tends to break down the blood and weaken the patients generally, it is well to give people who are sick with erysipelas plenty of fluids, actually forcing them to drink not less than ten and as many as sixteen glasses of water daily. It is also well to have the food easy to digest and nourishing, in fact, what is ordinarily called a nutritious soft diet. There is danger in using too much cathartic because of irritation of the bowels during the presence of a serious infection.

A person who has once had erysipelas is likely to have it again. Such people should be exceedingly careful about picking the nose or scratching the ear. If these parts of the skin are irritated, they should be kept covered with mild ointments or cold cream.

TETANUS OR LOCKJAW

The ancient Greeks knew about lockjaw. Indeed, the father of modern medicine, Hippocrates, described it and made some statements about the likelihood of recovery which are still good. It was not, however, until 1865 that it was thought to be infectious. The germ was not described until 1886. Today it is possible to isolate the germ, to grow it artificially, and to produce lockjaw in animals by injecting the germs into their bodies. The germ is called *Clostridium tetani*.

The poison produced by these germs is one of the most powerful poisons known. Most people used to think that tetanus, or lockjaw, was always caused by scratching the skin with a rusty nail. Today it is known that the rusty nail produces the disease because it is contaminated with material containing the germ of tetanus.

When this germ gets into the body by any means whatever, it sets up inflammation of nerve tissue. Because these germs have a special predilection for certain nerves, the condition called lockjaw is produced.

Certain types of wounds are more likely to cause tetanus than others. Most important are wounds which are deep, penetrating, lacerating, or crushing and which, because of that fact, permit particles of foreign matter containing the germs of tetanus to go deeply into the tissues and to remain there. This germ lives much better in the absence of oxygen. When it is pushed deep into a wound it is without oxygen and therefore is under the best possible conditions for its growth. The effects are produced more by the poisons produced by the germs than by the germs themselves. Indeed, it is believed that the poison, or toxin, is transported by the lymphatics and that in this way it reaches the nerve tissues.

The germs of tetanus seem to live preferably in the intestinal tracts of cattle, horses, and man. Because the germs are fairly widespread it is remarkable that the disease is not more common. Apparently, however, it is necessary for the germs to get deep into the tissue through a wound in order to multiply and produce the disease.

In the United States somewhere around one thousand to thirteen hundred deaths occur each year from tetanus. The number is less now than formerly because of the disappearance of horses and manure from city streets, because of the diminution of Fourth of July accidents associated with explosives, and because of the use of new methods of prevention which were not formerly generally available.

Tetanus usually begins about seven days after the wound which permits the germs to get into the tissues. It may, however, come on somewhat later or, rather rarely, earlier. The first signs are a sense of drawing pain in a wound with the twitching of muscles near by; also the usual signs of infection such as irritability, headache, chilliness, and fever. Then comes the stiffness of the muscles of the jaw and neck which gives the disease its name.

It becomes more and more difficult to open the mouth, and finally the jaws may be clamped shut and the neck rigid. Attempts to open the mouth intensify the spasm. Due to the fact that the muscles of the face are contracted, the corners of the mouth are drawn back and the eyebrows raised. This gives the person a typical grinning appearance which is described by the scientists as *risus sardonicus*—in other words, a sardonic expression.

Eventually, of course, other muscles and nerves are involved so that there are serious spasms and convulsions. In fact, there may be from three to forty spasms in an hour. The whole body may be involved, including even the muscles of the bowels and of the bladder. Of course, when the heart and the breathing muscles are involved, the condition is fatal.

Even under the best of treatment, patients with lockjaw may die because of the potency of this poison. Much depends on the time at which the antitoxin is given and on the amount. Of greatest importance is the prevention of lockjaw through the proper treatment of people who have been wounded, at the earliest possible moment. It should be taken for granted that a wound acquired in localities where the soil is likely to be contaminated, such as wounds acquired in fields, stables, and farmyards, or such as gunshot and powder wounds, are infected.

A physician who treats such a case will probably open the wound widely, removing any clothing, soil, or other visible contamination that may be present, and then treat the wound with proper antiseptics such as tincture of iodine or hydrogen peroxide to destroy the germs that can be reached. The opening of the wound is especially important, because this germ multiplies in the absence of air. Opening of the wound permits air to be present. It also permits removal of contamination, and it allows the antiseptics to reach the infectious material.

It is also important at this time to inject under the skin the specific antitoxin against tetanus, and perhaps to give another injection one week later.

If the disease develops in spite of preventive treatment, the patient should be placed in a quiet room, preferably in a hospital. The room must be kept darkened, and all noises or vibrations prevented, because they may serve to stimulate spasms. It may be necessary even to use an anesthetic to prevent these spasms. In order to feed the patient it is sometimes necessary to pass a narrow tube through the nose and down into the stomach, because the jaws may be so tightly clamped as to make it impossible to get food into the body otherwise. Someone must be constantly with the patient to prevent injury from convulsions and to guard against sudden death from paralysis of the breathing.

Several reports have appeared on beneficial effects of combined treatment using antibiotics such as penicillin or terramycin with antitoxin.

In no condition is the constant and immediate attention of a competent physician, and at the same time good nursing, so important. This makes the difference frequently between life and death. The antitoxin which opposes the poison must be given early in the disease and in large doses. Because of the great irritability of the patient it is sometimes necessary to put him to sleep in order that the antitoxin may be given. Under the best of treatment it is possible to save the lives of from one half to two thirds of the people who are infected.

RABIES OR HYDROPHOBIA

The word *"rabies"* is Latin for madness or rage. "Hydrophobia" means fear of water and thus defines what seemed to be the most significant symptom of the disease. It is one of the oldest of the diseases definitely classified by man. Around 100 A. D., Celsus recommended cauterization of wounds produced by mad dogs. As early as 1804, long before the nature of the disease was discovered by Pasteur, it was known that the saliva of a person or of a dog that had the disease would transmit it. Since, however, no means was known for preventing its spread, sufferers at that time were sometimes put to death by strangulation or smothering because people so greatly feared the disease. Until the time when Pasteur made the great discovery which freed mankind from fear of hydrophobia it was customary, as a means of treatment, to burn with a redhot iron the flesh of a person who had been bitten by any mad animal.

Some strange superstitions about hydrophobia still remain. One is that it commonly occurs in the "dog days." It has been believed that the danger from mad dogs was greater at that time than at any other. There is no evidence to support this view, because the bites of mad dogs occur at any time. They are likely to be more frequent from April to September than from October to March because dogs run loose more often and more generally in the spring and summer than they do in winter.

When a mad dog bites another animal or a human being the disease is transmitted by the saliva, which contains the poisonous virus. It is called a virus because it is so small that it will pass through the pores of a clay filter. The time when the disease attacks is from fourteen days on. There are wide variations in the period of incubation, in fact from ten days to twelve months, but in the vast majority of cases the onset follows the bite in from twenty to ninety days. It is rarely less than 15 days or more than 5 months.

During this period of incubation the person may show only signs of restlessness and apprehension, sometimes of irritation or tingling and pain at the site of the bite. However, when the disease begins, the horrible symptoms which give it its name reach their peak. A slight huskiness of the voice and a sense of choking are followed by severe spasms of the muscles of swallowing and breathing. There is shortness of breath. So severe are the symptoms following any attempt to swallow that the affected person will refuse to take water. This, of course, gave rise to the name hydrophobia, or fear of water. Eventually the convulsions and spasms may affect almost the whole body, and the nervous system is so sensitive that the slamming of a door or a sudden draft of wind will bring on an attack. Finally, the spine may stiffen and bend and death result from paralysis of the apparatus of breathing.

Because the affected person or animal is unable to swallow, thick saliva accumulates and drips from the mouth. Because of the paralysis of the muscles of breathing the breath comes in harsh gasps. The person who is infected does not necessarily foam at the mouth or bark like a dog, but the nature of the symptoms is such as to give people this impression.

Because of the great danger associated with this disease, everything possible should be done to prevent its spread. At times when hydrophobia, or rabies, is prevalent in any community the lives of both dogs and children may be freed from menace by protecting them from exposure to the bite of a mad animal. Homeless animals should be picked up and disposed of by the usual methods. A failure to enforce the laws regulating the control of homeless animals represents nothing in the way of friendship for the animal and exposes innumerable human beings to the danger of one of the most serious of diseases.

The dog that is kept in a good home is usually watched carefully, kept from contact with savage dogs, and is not so likely to be involved as the one that runs free. However, any dog may suddenly bite a human being, under provocation or sometimes without provocation. Because of the terrible possibilities of rabies, there is only one course to follow after a dog bite. The animal should be penned up or kept secured for at least ten days, during which time it will either die or develop the symptoms of hydrophobia, if it has that disease.

Far too often, when police are called to kill a dog suspected of hydrophobia, the dog is shot in the head or the head crushed with a club. This should not be done, because it is difficult for a laboratory to examine the brain of the dog when it is too severely injured.

The diagnosis of hydrophobia is made by examination of the brain of the animal under the microscope. When this disease is present the brain contains certain substances known as Negri bodies, which can be seen by the investigator. If there is the slightest suspicion that the dog which has bitten a person was mad, the Pasteur treatment for the prevention of hydrophobia should be begun immediately. If there are bites on the face or even on the hands it is wise to commence immediate treatment because of the short time which usually elapses when bites occur in these places. Otherwise it may be safe to delay for a few days to make sure that the animal was rabid or mad.

The wounds should be immediately cauterized with carbolic or fuming nitric acid. The Pasteur treatment is administered by any private or state laboratory. Moreover, it is available to physicians in any village or town through material that can be supplied by pharmaceutical houses. In the Pasteur treatment a special vaccine is used which is prepared from the brains of rabbits that have been injected with the disease. In these tissues the virus has been attenuated by passage through many animals and by other treatment, such as drying. There are no contra-indications to the use of this treatment.

The success of the Pasteur treatment for preventing hydrophobia is almost certain. Failures occur in less than one half of one per cent of the cases in which it is used. Notwithstanding the fact that information concerning this disease has been widespread for many years, there are still more than one hundred deaths annually from the disease in the United States. These are preventable deaths. Once the disease has developed, the physician can do much to relieve suffering and should be in constant attendance for this purpose.

Control of rabies includes measures which prevent dogs from biting, licensing of dogs, seizure and destruction of stray dogs, quarantine or muzzling of dogs during outbreaks of rabies and subjection of all imported dogs to six months quarantine. These measures eliminated rabies from England and Canada. Vaccination of dogs against rabies is recommended where quarantine cannot be enforced or where the disease prevails among wild animals.

VINCENT'S ANGINA

In 1898 a French physician named Vincent described an infection of the mouth and throat due to a peculiar spiral organism called *Treponema vincentii* and *Borrelia vincentii*. Apparently the disease occurred only in man, was accompanied by slight general disturbances with but a small increase in temperature, but there was pain on swallowing, enlargement of the glands, and a yellowish gray membrane in the mouth and throat. Because of this membrane, the disease was often mistaken for diphtheria until the differences were clearly established.

Sometimes the germs responsible for Vincent's angina were found in mouths that were not infected, but which were in bad condition. Occasionally also the disease appeared to be especially favored by fatigue, chill, exposure, improper food, or the excessive use of alcohol or tobacco. During World War I the disease spread widely among the soldiers and was given the common name of trench mouth, a name which has persisted.

In this common infection penicillin has already been established as especially curative. With good dental care and suitable application of such remedies the condition is controllable. Penicillin is taken by injection, as an application to the infected areas and in troches dissolved on the tongue. Bacitracin troches have also been used successfully.

When the disease is once established, it may be treated by the repeated use of solutions of hydrogen peroxide or by the application of a paste of sodium perborate, as the physician or dentist may advise. In severe cases treatment includes injections with sulfanilamide or neoarsphenamine and also local application of drugs. For prevention it is also advisable to have the teeth clean and smooth and to discontinue tobacco as long as any evidence of the disease remains.

UNDULANT FEVER OR BRUCELLOSIS

Years ago, British soldiers quartered on the island of Malta developed a disease in epidemic form which was called Malta fever. Later, as the disease spread about the world it became known as Mediterranean fever. Finally, it was called undulant fever because of its intermittent character; that is, the fever went up and down in waves. Three types of organisms are now known as causative including *Brucella melitensis, Brucella abortus* and *Brucella suis*. The condition is related to contagious abortion of cattle.

The menace of undulant fever is not the menace of epidemics of yellow fever or even of influenza. The disease insidiously creeps into a population and gradually affects increasing numbers of people. Fortunately, it is likely to spread slowly, if at all, in American communities, because milk is the most important medium in transmitting the disease. Since 1900, milk supplies in the United States have been controlled through suitable public health laws and measures. Milk is made safe for human consumption by pasteurization, in which the milk is heated for a sufficient length of time to destroy dangerous germs.

Before 1927, undulant fever was regarded as a curiosity when it occurred in a human being in the United States. Since that time cases have appeared in practically every state of the union. In the great majority of cases the taking of raw milk containing the germ, which is identified also as the one which causes contagious abortion of cattle, was demonstrated to be the source of the infection. Apparently the condition is more likely to be spread by goat's milk than by that from cattle, particularly since the goat's milk is not usually as well controlled in its assembling and distribution as is the milk of cows. Moreover, the infection is more generalized among goats than among cattle.

From ten to thirty days after the person becomes infected with this disease he has the usual symptoms associated with an infectious disorder—weakness, tiredness, chilliness, loss of appetite, general aching, chills and fever. The condition develops slowly, so that frequently weeks may pass before the person who is infected considers himself sick enough to call a physician. He is inclined to believe that he has something like a persistent cold or rheumatic condition and that it is hard to break up.

Eventually, the symptoms of a person who has contracted undulant fever develop with sufficient fullness and persistence to make him realize that he is subject to a serious complaint. The physician who examines the blood of a patient with this disease finds that changes have taken place in the blood, and it is possible for a laboratory to make the kind of test that is made on the blood in typhoid fever and to determine with certainty that the patient is infected with undulant fever.

The disease resembles many other infectious diseases, such as typhoid, tuberculosis, malaria, or almost any other infectious disorder. In a few instances, perhaps two out of every one hundred cases, death may occur as a result of the seriousness of the infection or from secondary complications.

Of course, the way to avoid undulant fever is to avoid milk that has not been properly pasteurized. Men who work in packing houses where they come constantly in contact with infected animals should, of course, take the necessary precautions in their work. Men with wounds or abrasions on their hands should be certain to wear gloves and perhaps to clean their hands thoroughly at frequent intervals.

The real control of this disease will rest on the ability of government bureaus and of the veterinary industry to eliminate the condition from domestic animals.

The patient who has undulant fever must be handled in much the same way as one who has had typhoid. He must be put into a separate room; the health authorities must be notified; all of the excretions and secretions must be sterilized before they are disposed of in any way. This means either burning, boiling, or the use of proper antiseptic solutions. The patient, of course, must remain in bed and be properly fed to overcome the loss of weight, the anemia, and the weakness that are due to constant chills and fever. The wearing effects of such conditions on the body are extremely serious in producing changes in the nature of degeneration of important organs.

A treatment with sulfadiazine and streptomycin or with aureomycin or chloromycetin or terramycin has been found most effective in treating undulant fever. The drugs are administered by the doctor. There is also a vaccine which is occasionally helpful. Artificial fever treatment is now recommended alone and combined with drug treatment.

Amebiasis and Dysentery

Since the outbreak of amebic dysentery, from a source in two Chicago hotels during 1933, the world has become increasingly aware of the menace of this disorder, which was formerly considered a tropical disease. Instead of being caused by an ordinary germ, this condition is caused by a large type of organism known as the *entameba histolytica*. This organism gets into the large bowel, and once there sets up symptoms that are exceedingly serious. Moreover, the organism may spread to the liver particularly, or to other organs of the body, and there set up secondary places of infection which are also a menace to health and life. Although this condition was formerly unheard of in the northern portions of the United States, more recent evidence indicates that from five to ten per cent of all the people of this country are infected.

The organism which causes this disease multiplies in the bowel and gives off daughter cysts. These cysts are passed out of the body with the excretions, and if they reach food or drink in any way are naturally swallowed. They pass through the stomach and small intestines and then get into the upper portions of the large intestines. Here they divide up and multiply organisms which invade the walls of the bowels.

Ordinarily, the entameba histolytica which infects mankind comes in food or drink that has been contaminated in the manner suggested. After a person has had the disease and recovered, he may carry the organisms in his bowel for long periods of time, and as a carrier of the disease is constantly able to transmit it to other people. These carriers, who apparently are healthy or who have mild symptoms of the infection, are the ones most concerned in transmitting the disease.

Occasionally, however, the disease is transmitted by impure water supply. It has been shown that the cysts of the entameba histolytica may live for days and several weeks in water, depending on the temperature of the water and the number of bacteria in the water. It was thought in the past that these methods of transmission were of comparatively little importance in this country, except in the rural districts where people deposit their excretions on the soil, and where wells and springs are the chief sources of the water supply.

More recently, it has been found that any severe contamination of the water supply in a large building may result in the spread of amebic dysentery.

In China and Japan human excretions are frequently used as fertilizing material for vegetables. This is a serious menace to health, because it has been shown that the cysts of this parasite will remain alive in the moist excretions for as long as two weeks, and when they contaminate the vegetables, they may in this way transmit the disease.

It has also been shown that it is possible for the fly, which feeds on excretions, to carry the organism and deposit it on food. The most common method of transmission of this disease, however, is through the contamination of food and drink by food handlers who happen to be carriers of the entameba histolytica. The food handlers concerned may be waiters, cooks, dish washers, or any other kitchen personnel in a family or in a large hotel.

Inasmuch as the organism may live in the intestines for months or years without producing serious symptoms, it is not possible to say just how long a time is required for infection to develop. However, there is some good evidence that the swallowing of the cysts of entameba histolytica is followed in from ten to ninety-five days, with an average period of 64.8 days, by the beginning of the symptoms which are characteristic in this disease. Usually the disease comes on suddenly, but often it begins with mild diarrhea which gradually becomes worse. When the disease begins suddenly, there is severe abdominal pain with nausea and vomiting and a chilly sensation. The irritation of the bowel becomes acute, and the patient tries to evacuate the bowels repeatedly. This irritation may be so constant that the number of actions of the bowels will vary from six to eight in twenty-four hours to as many as thirty to forty actions of the bowels in twenty-four hours in severe cases.

As a result, the patient becomes exhausted, complains of aching in the back and great weakness in the legs, and is likely to be mentally depressed. There may be little or no fever; even in severe cases the temperature reaches at most from 100 to 102 degrees, but in very severe cases may go higher.

As a result of the extensive action of the bowels, such patients have tenderness in the abdomen, the skin appears sallow and jaundiced, and the patient loses weight rapidly. The doctor will want to examine the blood to find out how much the red cells of the blood have been injured and also whether or not there is any significant rise in the number of white blood cells. Frequently the distinction between this condition, appendicitis, and peritonitis will depend on a careful examination of the blood.

In times when amebic dysentery is prevalent and physicians are naturally on the lookout for it, they are likely to check up the cases. However, in the past physicians have not been particularly aware of this disease; certainly not in the northern parts of the United States. Since the diagnosis is made with certainty only after the excretions have been examined under the microscope in order to determine whether or not entameba histolytica is present, it is not safe to make a diagnosis until such a microscopic study has been made. At the same time, the man who makes the laboratory study must make certain that the ameba is the real entameba histolytica and not a form of the other amebas that live in the bowels without causing symptoms. He must also distinguish between the dysentery that is caused by the ameba and the dysentery which follows infection with some bacteria.

There are certain ways in which the community may protect itself against amebiasis. Much depends on having a properly guarded water supply, on the proper disposal of sewage, the protection of food from flies, and on suitable examinations and treatment of waiters, cooks, dish washers, and other food handlers in public eating places.

Chlorination of water will sterilize it so far as bacteria are concerned, but it takes one hundred times as much chlorine to kill the cysts of the entameba histolytica as it does to kill bacteria in water. In fact, the addition of this amount of chlorine to water would make the water unfit for drinking. Therefore, whenever water is heavily contaminated with entameba histolytica, the only way to make it safe is to boil it: obviously a difficult matter for any city water supply.

In controlling food handlers, it is necessary that they be examined at fairly frequent intervals, and that their excretions be examined in the laboratory to rule out the presence of the organism.

Fortunately, there are now available several methods of treatment which have been established as useful in controlling amebic dysentery. All of the remedies concerned are potent. Since they are powerful remedies, they are dangerous if taken in excessive dosage and should never be taken except under the advice and control of a physician. Among the remedies most commonly used today, and proved to be valuable, are chiniofon, carbarsone, and vioform, also milibis and various combinations. The drug called emetin, which is much used in this condition, is especially valuable in controlling the symptoms of the disease and is usually given early in order to bring about prompt recovery of the patient.

Aureomycin, chloramphenicol and terramycin have all been used successfully. Amebiasis is difficult to cure and relapses are frequent.

TULAREMIA

For the last thirty years market men have known about a condition called "rabbit fever." About 1911 cases were described under the name of deer fly fever. Finally, in 1912, investigators of the United States Public Health Service found a plague-like disease among the squirrels in one of the counties of California and discovered that this disease was caused by a germ which they named in honor of Tulare County, Calif., the *bacterium tularense* now called *Pasteurella tularensis*. Then, Francis, another investigator from the United States Public Health Service, found in 1919 that this germ which caused both the plague-like disease of rodents and deer fly fever could infect human beings with a condition which was named tularemia. Francis later examined the livers of a thousand rabbits offered for sale in the markets of Washington, D. C., and found at least one hundred seventy of these rabbits infected with the same germ.

While the disease caused by the bacterium tularense is not an especially serious disease, seventeen out of four hundred twenty people who had it died. The human being who becomes infected with this germ usually does so in the handling or dressing of rabbits sick with the disease. The rabbit sick with tularemia is not likely to be active. Health authorities warn particularly against eating rabbits that can be knocked over with a stick. If the rabbit gives a good chase and has to be shot with a gun it is probably not a sick rabbit.

The person who has tularemia develops swellings of the skin with the formation of abscesses, swelling of the lymph glands and nodules, and small spots of infection in the internal organs. The typical history of such a case is that the man in question or the woman in question dressed wild rabbits, that he or she had at the time a sore on the finger, and that shortly thereafter the sore developed into an ulcer; then the glands became involved, and finally other organs of the body.

Rabbit meat, even from rabbits infected with this condition, is harmless as a food if it is thoroughly cooked, since a temperature of 133 degrees F. will kill the germ. It is safer, however, for everyone who is dressing rabbits for use as food to wear rubber gloves during the process.

This condition can be transmitted from one animal to another, including the human being, by means of deer flies, wood ticks, rabbit ticks, and lice; and such creatures as the sheep, the coyote, the cat, the quail, and the grouse may be infected, as well as rabbits and squirrels. However, as far as is known, the horse, cattle, dogs, and chickens have not been infected with this disease. In the Eastern states it is most likely to occur during November, December, and January.

Most people who become infected with tularemia have to go to bed from ten days to three weeks, and sometimes recovery is slow. There is no specific serum. The discovery of streptomycin provided a new specific treatment for tularemia that is quite effective. Aureomycin, chloramphenicol and terramycin are also effective.

Sometimes it is necessary to put hot packs on the spots of infection and then to open the abscesses in order to relieve the pressure of the broken-down material. In this infectious condition, as in every other, it is wise to convalesce slowly, since any disease with considerable fever and infection throws a strain on the heart and the circulation.

MALARIA

Authorities in medicine have attributed the fall of the Roman and Greek civilizations to the development of malaria among the population. Certainly, malaria can devitalize any person.

Any community that is willing to spend sufficient money to stamp out the disease can do so. Malaria is becoming less prevalent in the United States each year. Nevertheless, a million people in the United States constantly suffer from malaria. Possibly one-third of the people in the world are infected. Malaria has been called the greatest single destroyer of the human race.

The physician diagnoses malaria by the characteristic symptoms, which include regularly recurring attacks of chills and fever, the presence of an enlarged spleen, and the presence of the malarial parasite in the blood of the sick person. He must not only diagnose malaria but also the special form that is present.

The plasmodium, as the organism which causes malaria is called, was discovered by the famous scientist Laveran, who received the Nobel Prize for this discovery. Ross and Grassi, a British and an Italian investigator, proved that the organism of malaria is transmitted from one human being to another through the bite of the anopheles mosquito.

Although malaria has practically disappeared as one of the great medical problems in large cities, the disease is still to be found in many rural communities, particularly in the southern portions of the United States.

In river valleys and creek bottoms malaria has been found to be highly endemic, averaging fifteen cases for every one hundred persons. The worst infection is always found in the immediate vicinity of some lake, pond, or marsh which could be the natural habitat of the malaria mosquito. The dis-

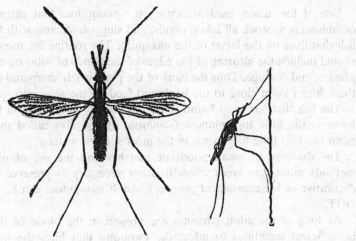

Fig. 14. Female malarial mosquito (enlarged).

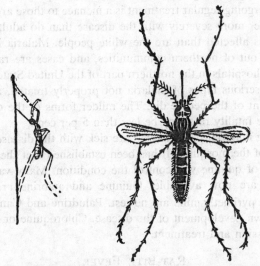

Fig. 15. Female yellow fever mosquito (enlarged).

trict extends about a mile in every direction from the pond, which marks the range of flight of the mosquitoes.

Country club ponds must be watched particularly, as these artificial pools have been found frequently to be excellent breeding places for the mosquito.

The malaria mosquito bites most frequently at dusk. If it has fed on a sick person and then bites a well one, the latter is likely to be supplied with some malarial infection. In summer resorts where the population is mixed, including people coming from all sorts of localities, the chance of infection is greater.

One of the means used to destroy the mosquitoes that carry the malaria organisms is to stock all lakes, ponds, and sluggish streams with the variety of fish that lives on the larvæ of the mosquito. The routine for mosquito control should include the clearing of the edges of the ponds of willows, cattails, water grasses, and floatage. Thus the bank of the pond is left sharp and clean, so that the fish can swim close to the bank and feed on the mosquito wiggletails.

The fish that has been found to be most active in feeding on the mosquito larvæ is the little top minnow *Gambusia affinis,* also called the pot-bellied minnow. This little fish swims in the most shallow waters.

The drainage of small ponds or marshes and the use of oil sprays are methods suitable to areas where it is not necessary to preserve the pond for decorative or for amusement purposes. Adult mosquitoes can be destroyed by DDT.

As long as the adult parasites are present in the blood of the individual in sufficient quantities to infect the mosquito that bites the individual, the person is a possible conveyor of malaria. Since the parasites remain in the blood for months, providing that the individual is not properly treated, anyone who is not undergoing regular treatment is a menace to those around him.

Children suffer more severely with the disease than do adults. Negroes apparently are less affected than are the white people. Malaria has been practically stamped out of northern communities, and cases are rarely seen even in large charity hospitals in the northern part of the United States.

In the more serious types of malaria not properly treated, anywhere from 10 to 30 per cent of the people die. The milder forms of the disease become chronic, and the fatality rate may be less than 5 per cent.

In controlling malaria, patients who are sick with the disease are protected from the bites of the mosquito. It has been established that the regular use of sufficient doses of quinine will control the condition. Many varieties of antimalarial drugs are now available. Quinine and atabrine are best known. Primaquine and pyrimethamine are newest. Paludrine and Camoquin can arrest the full blown development of the disease. Chloroquine or Aralen is used both for suppression and treatment.

RAT-BITE FEVER

When human beings are bitten by animals of the rodent type, including incidentally not only the rat but the weasel and the pig and occasionally, as will be seen later, even the cat, they are sometimes infected with a peculiar organism called a *Spirillum* which produces a disease of the whole body. This disease is characterized by short attacks of fever alternating with periods without the fever, and also an eruption on the skin. Such cases have been known in the United States for a century, and medical journals have reported approximately one hundred.

The usual course of such a case is as follows: After the person has been bitten, the wound heals promptly unless a secondary infection occurs. From one to three weeks after the date on which the patient was bitten, the spot of the bite becomes red and swollen, and the person who is infected develops the usual symptoms of infections in general: namely, headache, general pains and fever, sometimes a chill and a general feeling of sickness. Finally an eruption appears, at first most prominent in the region of the wound, but later spreading over the body.

From this time on, attacks of fever will occur every five or six days, sometimes less frequently. Gradually the person loses weight and may become exceedingly sick due to the loss of nutrition and general health. Somewhere between 6 and 7 per cent of the people who are infected eventually die of the disorder, but the tendency is for the majority to recover.

There have been instances reported in medical periodicals of children who have been bitten by rats when left alone by their parents, particularly when they live in basement homes or poverty-stricken tenements. Of course, a cat may become contaminated through its hunting of the rats.

The doctor makes his diagnosis of this condition not only by the symptoms that have been mentioned, but also by finding the germ which causes the disease in the wound, and sometimes in material taken directly from lymph glands near the wound. There are also cases in which people have been bitten by rats and become infected, not with this organism but with the usual germs that cause infection, such as the staphylococcus and streptococcus.

Formerly this condition was treated like syphilis, with salvarsan or arsphenamine or, as it was more popularly known, "606." Now penicillin seems to be fully effective in rat-bite fever, as in syphilis.

ROCKY MOUNTAIN SPOTTED FEVER

As was shown years ago in investigations made by Dr. Theobald Smith, many diseases of man are transmitted by the bite of a tick. Among the most serious of these is the condition called Rocky Mountain spotted fever, an infectious disease seen frequently in eastern Idaho and the Bitter Root Valley of Montana, but also occurring in most western states and occasionally in eastern portions of the United States. This condition occurs most commonly in men because of their occupations as surveyors, foresters, hunters, fishermen, sheep herders, or cowboys. These occupations expose them to the bite of the tick. If bitten, women and children are just as likely to become affected.

The tick is found on the rodents in the areas mentioned, and from these rodents picks up the organisms which it then transfers to man when it bites. From four to seven days after he is bitten, the man comes down with the disease. At first there are loss of appetite, general aches and pains, and slight fever. Then suddenly there is a chill followed by a high fever. This may reach 104 or 105 degrees. At first there are severe headache and backache with pains in the muscles. Even the skin may be tender. Eventually the nervous system may be involved, with restlessness and lack of sleep and even disturbance of the action of the bowels.

About the third to the seventh day, the infected person breaks out with tiny pinkish spots which generally appear first on the wrists and ankles, and which give the disease its name—spotted fever. In serious cases the spots run together. Since they are due to blood, they gradually turn purple. The fever remains high for a week to ten days and, if recovery occurs, falls gradually. In the fatal cases death occurs from the seventh to the tenth day, with high fever.

The physician is able to make his diagnosis certain by examining the blood, in which he finds not only changes in the blood cells but also specific reactions which are certain evidence of the presence of the disease. This condition resembles the old typhus fever, or jail fever, as it was called when jails were almost universally unsanitary, which is transmitted by the bite of a louse.

The use of paraminobenzoic acid has been recommended and also aureomycin, terramycin and chloromycetin. The diet should be nutritious and high in carbohydrate. Plentiful liquids are given. Most serious complication is pneumonia.

The obvious method of preventing this disease is to avoid the bite of the tick which causes it. This has been attempted in some places through eliminating rodents and through dipping cattle. As a method of prevention this has not, however, been extremely successful.

Investigators of the United States Public Health Service have developed a vaccine made of the ground-up bodies of the ticks. This is found to be a protection against infection with this disorder and can minimize severity.

GLANDERS

Most farmers think of glanders as a disease affecting horses and mules, but occasionally it attacks human beings. It has been reported also in cats, rabbits, sheep, mice, and various wild animals of the cat tribe.

Because the disease is commonly transmitted by horses and affects horses more frequently than any other animal, it is now rarely seen in large cities, from which horses have practically disappeared.

In the first twenty years of the present century there were seven cases of glanders in the wards of the Bellevue Hospital, New York City, but since then, not a single case has been seen.

Glanders is caused by a germ known as the bacillus of glanders. From three to five days after the germ gets into the body, the symptoms first appear. There are the usual symptoms of infection, such as nausea, headache, vomiting, chills, and some fever. Quite soon, however, nodules appear on the skin, associated with inflammation of the lymphatic ducts and glands near the places where the abscesses are located. Sometimes a hard nodule develops which ulcerates and breaks down, discharging a profuse, sticky substance. If the disease attacks the lungs it gives symptoms like those of pneumonia.

Nowadays, a diagnosis of glanders is hardly likely to be made unless the condition described happens to occur in someone who is constantly working around horses. The acute infection is very serious in the human being, and most of the patients die.

In the control of a disease like glanders, everything depends on stamping out the source of the infection in the animal which transmits it. Hence, it is recommended that practically every animal with glanders should be promptly destroyed and the stables thoroughly disinfected, including all harness and watering buckets. All animals that have been exposed should be examined for the infection and kept under observation until well past the time when there is any likelihood that the infection may develop in them.

A doctor who takes charge of such cases treats them usually by the surgical method of opening the abscesses and draining away the infectious material.

PSITTACOSIS OR PARROT DISEASE

In 1904, three cases of psittacosis or "parrot disease" were reported in Boston. In the fall of 1929 an outbreak of this disease was reported in Buenos Aires, and more outbreaks have since been reported in the United States. In Hamburg, Germany, twenty-eight cases, with five deaths, occurred in the fall of 1929. In the epidemic of psittacosis which occurred in Paris in 1892 there were forty-nine cases and sixteen deaths, and it was reported that the infection had been caused by parrots brought from South America.

When psittacosis occurs it begins with a chill and fever, with a good deal of weakness and depression, and usually some inflammation of the lungs.

"Parrot disease" is essentially a medical curiosity and need occasion little alarm among the people of the United States. The symptoms resemble those of other infectious diseases, and one should be certain that the disease is actually psittacosis and not pneumonia or other infection of the lungs.

Obviously, the first step is to get the suspected parrot and to find out whether or not it contains the germs which are responsible. In addition to parrots many other bird pets occasionally become infected, including love birds, cockatoos and parakeets.

The occurrence of this condition is another demonstration of the fact that we are likely to contract diseases from all sorts of contacts and that it is not safe to demonstrate too much fondness for our animal neighbors.

Psittacosis has been known for a long time as a disease of parrots, but the first cases of pneumonic infection traced directly from parrots to man were described in 1879 in Germany.

The proof of the fact that human infection has come from the parrot depends on isolation of the germ from both the parrot and the affected human being.

In parrots, psittacosis is highly fatal, killing from 50 to 95 per cent of the infected birds. The disease can be transmitted from one parrot to another by infected feathers, food, water, dishes, or the soiled hands of attendants. Mice or insects may carry the infection from one cage to another. When a parrot becomes infected it gets weak, loses its appetite, has diarrhea, and is likely to die in a few days. Then the germs will be found in practically all of its organs.

As might be expected, a disease that can pass from parrot to man may also infect chickens, rabbits, mice, and guinea-pigs. It is interesting that this disease which chiefly infects the intestinal tracts of birds strikes the lungs in man. In many instances the infection is due to the fact that the parrot is fed by the mouth-to-mouth method. Not infrequently, however, it occurs merely from handling the sick birds, and not infrequently the person in a family who becomes sick passes the disease on with infected hands to other members of the family.

Fortunately, this disease is rare in civilized communities, probably because parrots are not nearly so frequent as pets as are other animals and birds, and probably also because the disease kills the parrots so rapidly that the likelihood of infection is lessened.

The occurrence of cases of psittacosis in the United States is new evidence of the fact that methods of transportation, exchange of products among various nations, and the complete abolishing of boundary lines between peoples make it impossible any longer for a nation to be isolated. The disease of one people will sooner or later appear among others.

The sulfonamide drugs help to stop the growth of the virus. Aureomycin and terramycin are also effective in checking the disease.

EPIDEMIC ENCEPHALITIS

No one knows when the first epidemic of lethargy associated with fever and destruction of brain tissue first afflicted mankind, but several observers have pointed out that Hippocrates, the famous father of modern scientific medicine, himself described an epidemic of this character which appeared in the spring and continued on into the autumn, at which time it was more fatal. It was suggested that there were similar epidemics in the sixteenth century in various parts of Europe. At the end of 1890, such an epidemic occurred in southern Europe and was described under the name of *nona*.

The modern condition called epidemic encephalitis was described in Vienna in 1917, during the World War, and was given the name *encephalitis lethargica* because it is an inflammation of the brain associated with drowsiness and somnolence. The disease spread to England and to the United States and Canada; it seems possible, however, that there were individual cases in the United States before 1915.

Encephalitis means inflammation of the brain. Now many different causes of such inflammations are recognized. Transmitted by insects are St. Louis encephalitis, Japanese B, Australian X, Western equine, Venezuelan equine and Russian tick borne encephalitis. These are distinct from the condition called *nona* or epidemic lethargic encephalitis.

Epidemic encephalitis occurs most frequently in February and March but may occur at any time of the year. The condition is caused by a virus and at least seven different types of virus more or less closely related to each other have been distinguished. Principal varieties include the so-called eastern type and western or St. Louis type. The disease seems to have been more common in the United States and in Europe than on other continents. It is quite mildly contagious, but outbreaks have been reported in schools, asylums, and barracks in which large numbers of people are housed.

There has been much research in an attempt to find a preventive serum based on the discovery of virus. The virus may be transmitted to humans from lower animals like birds, rats, horses or domestic pets. Such conditions as the louping ill of sheep, X disease of Australia, "B" virus disease in monkeys, and other virus diseases are believed to be related in a group.

In most cases of encephalitis the disease occurs in three stages: first, the beginning, which is sudden; second, a milder condition following the first acute condition; and, finally, a sort of chronic condition in those who recover. In the acute stage there are the usual symptoms of infection, such as fever, weakness, headache, and running of the nose, but in addition in these cases there are quite frequently double vision and emotional disturbances indicating that the brain has been affected. Most of the patients become lethargic or sleepy at the beginning of the disease and remain in this condition until the recovery from the acute stage has taken place. There are, however, other cases which actually have insomnia, and there are some who are lethargic in the daytime and awake at night.

While these patients seem to be completely unconscious, there are recorded instances in which the patient who apparently slept was aware of everything that went on in the room. The brain was affected in such a manner that the patient could not speak or let other people know that he heard what was being said. In association with the somnolence or lethargy in many of these cases there is a delirium in which the patient may have emotional outbursts, delusions, or periods of depression. An exceedingly interesting phenomenon is the development of what is called occupational delirium, in which the person who is affected dwells constantly on the occupation; the orator continually makes speeches, the teacher lectures, the accountant adds figures.

In association with the primary symptoms that have been mentioned are many other symptoms indicating that the nervous system has been involved, such as paralyses, convulsions, tremors, and similar disorders.

After the patient has recovered from the first stage, which may have been slight—in fact, so slight as hardly to have had medical attention—comes the second stage of this disease, in which the patients are weak and say that they have been sick since an attack of influenza. They remember that they were drowsy, but they never feel well, and they are likely to be called neurasthenic or hysterical or simply plain lazy by their families. However, the condition is likely to go on to the time when anyone can realize that these patients are seriously sick, since they begin to develop symptoms like those of Parkinson's disease, or the shaking palsy. In this condition the face is mask-like, the arms and legs are held rigid, the movements are slow, the speech monotonous, and the thumb and forefinger move rather constantly in a pill-rolling movement.

In association with this there may be an apparent oversupply of saliva with some drooling from the mouth because of the changes in the muscles of the face.

There develop frequently in the later stages difficulties of behavior in children who tend to become moral imbeciles. These children are cruel, disobedient, destructive, abusive, rather filthy in their habits, and may actually become a menace from the point of view of their lack of sanity. Without a recognition of the disease which is involved such children are frequently brought before the courts and treated as criminals rather than as invalids. In the same way adults occasionally develop strange mental conditions following encephalitis and constitute a problem for those responsible for their care.

None of these patients are actually sleeping over months or years, but the mentality is seriously disturbed, and the rhythm of sleep may be changed.

Unfortunately, scientific medicine has not yet developed any specific method of treatment that will prevent this disease or arrest its progress. It does, however, attempt to aid these patients by what is called symptomatic treatment, treating each of the symptoms as it develops by well established methods. A number of serums and vaccines have been tried. These patients have been injected with non-specific proteins in the form of typhoid vaccine; malaria germs have been injected to produce shock and artificial fever; and artificial heat has been tried, but thus far the results are quite inconclusive, and no one can say definitely that any of these methods of treatment actually stops the progress of this disorder.

During 1938 outbreaks of a form of brain inflammation or unconsciousness called encephalitis broke out in North Dakota, Minnesota, Vermont and Massachusetts. In the same area at the same time there were numerous cases of a form of inflammation of the brain among horses called equine encephalomyelitis. The investigators proved that both conditions were caused by a virus of a certain type and that this virus is also to be found in a disease that affects the field mouse and other rodents, as well as partridges and pigeons. With an understanding of the nature of the disease which has thus been made available it only remains to find the chain of communication from the animals to man. Then it will be possible to prevent the further appearance of the disease among human beings.

These conditions are diagnosed by doctors through laboratory studies which demonstrate neutralizing or complement fixing antibodies in a patient's serum two weeks or more after infection. Both types of antibody persist for two years at least. After death the conditions found in the brain are not specific, but a diagnosis can be made by the demonstration of virus through intracerebral inoculation of mice with brain tissue. The virus is virulent for mice, monkeys, rabbits, guinea pigs, rats and sheep.

CHAPTER XI

The Respiratory Diseases
MORRIS FISHBEIN, M.D.

THE COMMON COLD

WHEN WILLIAM OSLER wrote his *Principles and Practice of Medicine,* the most popular textbook of medicine ever published, he began with typhoid fever, probably because typhoid was one of the most serious and incapacitating diseases affecting a vast number of people. Students learned to study diseases according to the way in which William Osler systematized knowledge of typhoid. Today typhoid is definitely under control and really disturbs but few people.

Now one of the most widely used textbooks of medicine begins with the common cold—and rightly. Infections of the nose, throat, and sinuses are responsible for more than one half the time lost by wage earners due to sickness. Everybody knows how to cure a cold, and, even if he does not, will tell *you.* You can put your feet in a mustard bath, drink several glasses of hot lemonade, carry a buckeye in your right rear pocket, wear an iron ring, indulge freely in many of the widely advertised remedies, and even take some of the beverages that once required a doctor's prescription and about which the government expressed considerable doubt as to curative value— and at the end of three days you will probably begin to get well almost regardless of the treatment.

The common cold is essentially a self-limited disease. Unfortunately, however, it does not, like an attack of measles or scarlet fever, induce in the person who has it a resistance or immunity which will prevent him from having a cold soon again. People who have colds seem to have them often. Those who are easily susceptible constitute about 23 per cent; they have colds four or more times a year. Sixty per cent of people have colds two or three times a year and 17 per cent once a year or not at all.

There is a great difference between the common cold and epidemic influenza of the type that devastated the world in 1918. That was a definite infectious disease, highly contagious, affecting vast numbers of people and causing a terrific number of deaths. The history of medicine shows that at least eight great pandemics of influenza had previously swept the world, beginning with one in 1580, the seventh occurring in 1889–1892. The common cold is something quite different.

CAUSES OF COLDS

Changes in the weather have been incriminated as a cause of colds from the time of Hippocrates. Geologists, geographists, physiographers, and biometricians have tried to find certain relationships between changes in the weather and the occurrence of colds; as a result, some definite knowledge is now available. Most colds occur in October; then comes a slight drop in the incidence, with a new peak in January and in February, working up to a rather high point in March; then another gradual drop with a low rate in summer, the rate rising gradually to the October maximum. From October to April, whenever the maximum temperature, the average temperature, or the dry bulb temperature falls below the ordinary figures, there is a slight tendency of the incidence of colds to rise. It has not been found, however, that there is any relationship between the maximum temperature, humidity, rainfall, wind velocity, sunshine, or atmospheric pressure. In the warm period, from April to October, whenever the maximum temperature, the average temperature range, the dry bulb temperature, the vapor pressure, or the pecentage of sunshine falls below the ordinary level, there is likely to be a rise in the number of colds. Apparently there is a great deal in the general effect of atmosphere on the human being, but it is rather difficult to determine just how these effects are brought about.

Some time ago investigators in a large clinic proved that the ability of a person with rheumatism to predict a change in the weather is an actual ability, and that it is based on changes that take place in the body before the change in weather occurs. The opinion of at least twenty centuries that there is a definite relationship between sudden changes in the weather and catching cold tends to be borne out by modern scientific investigations but is not absolutely established. A professor of hygiene in the University of Amsterdam found a definite relationship between changes in temperature and the occurrence of the common cold in seven thousand people who kept a careful record of their colds while he kept a record of the weather. If it can be shown that difficulties with the heat regulation of the human body are fundamental to catching cold, the obvious way to prevent colds will be to develop methods for keeping the heat of the body constant.

The noted British physiologist, A. V. Hill, believes that cold weather brings about a large number of colds because people shut themselves up in warm, stuffy rooms and perspire; then submit themselves to the outdoor air without proper protection. The statistician for our largest insurance company found that a sudden drop of 10 degrees in the temperature brought an increase of eighteen colds per week among 6,700 employees in his office.

Moreover, Prof. E. O. Jordan of the University of Chicago discovered that 90 per cent of colds occur at a time when there is less ventilation in both public and private dwellings. Here certainly is well established evidence that changes in the weather are associated with colds.

Everybody has experienced the development of a cold following a night in a sleeping car, a swim in the pool, or a shower bath immediately after being overheated by exercise. Investigators are convinced that the overheated and dehydrated air in the homes and in offices in the United States lowers the resistance of the membranes of the nose; then germs, which are almost constantly present among human beings, begin their work of infection.

There are several ways of emphasizing this fact. Extreme cold does not cause colds. Eskimos seldom have colds. A group of explorers found on visiting one Eskimo settlement that there was not one cold among the Eskimos from the tiniest infant to the most ancient patriarch of the tribe. Seventy-two hours after the expedition, which included several people who had colds, arrived in the settlement, practically every one of the Eskimos developed the characteristic symptoms. That ought to be sufficient proof that there is some transmissible agent which produces the infection. It correlates with the fact that germs do well on new soil.

Obviously, therefore, some search must be made for a specific virus as a cause of the common cold. When the cause is isolated, specific measures of prevention may follow. It is conceivable, indeed, that not one but several different organisms may produce the symptoms.

Granted that the cold is caused by an infectious organism, there must apparently be other factors or all of us would have colds all the time. These factors constitute what are called predisposing causes. Tobacco, dust, gas, the amount of sleep, sitting in a draft, constipation, perspiration, and footwear have all been suggested as possible predisposing elements. A research made by investigators at Cornell University failed to incriminate definitely any one of them. Changes in the weight and quality of underwear that is worn have been suggested. Enough evidence is available to indicate that the wearing of woolen underwear is not a panacea; besides, it itches!

Experts in diseases of the nose and throat feel that obstruction in the nose and enlarged tonsils are important in relationship to the number of colds. Numerous studies recently made failed to prove that either one of them is a certain factor. Obstructions in the nose ought to be taken care of because they interfere with breathing and perhaps bring about congestion. Enlarged and infected tonsils are a menace to health and should be removed. But the person concerned may have just as many colds, if not more, after these factors are attended to than he had previously.

Our modern methods of living may be largely responsible for the increased incidence of colds. We are crowded together in offices, in motion-picture houses, at football and basketball games. We are packed into elevators and subway cars. We breathe constantly, cough frequently, and sneeze unexpectedly in one another's faces. Moreover, our hands are constantly in contact with door knobs, pencils, dishes, and other utensils, also handled by other people. We carry our hands to our mouths and to our noses and thus transmit by what is called hand-to-mouth infection.

SYMPTOMS OF COLDS

Because of its symptoms and its rather poorly understood character in relationship to other diseases, the common cold is variously called by a number of high-sounding scientific titles, in most instances related to the part of the body particularly affected. What is known as a head cold is called coryza. Because of the increase in the temperature and the outpouring of fluid from the nose, the cold has been called acute catarrhal fever. Because the running is principally from the nose, it has been called acute catarrhal rhinitis. If the throat is hoarse, the portion affected may give the title to the disease so that it becomes acute pharyngitis, acute laryngitis, or acute tracheitis.

These anatomical designations nevertheless hardly convey the stuffiness, the chills, the irritability, the loss of appetite, and the other symptoms that are commonly associated with this disorder. The chief changes in the tissues involved are those which affect the mucous membranes of the nose and throat. The lining of the nose is red and swollen, and from it pours continuously the fluid that causes much sniffling and blowing. With the sniffling and blowing comes irritation of the skin around the nose and mouth, and, if the trouble extends down far enough, there is coughing without much discharge from the throat. The mouth is held open during sleep so that the tongue becomes thick and coated.

PREVENTION OF COLDS

What everyone wants to know is how to prevent a cold, how to stop a cold, and how to cure one. In every infection of the human body three factors are concerned: First, contact with the infecting substance; second, sufficient virulence in the infecting germ to overcome the resistance of the body, and third, sufficient resistance in the body to overcome the infecting germ.

The human family, particularly in large cities, is so crowded that it is practically impossible to avoid contact with those who have respiratory infections. Our modern apartment dwellings are simply great barracks into which families are packed, and individual dwellings are like cans into which the individual members of the family are crowded closely together.

If a single organism is responsible for the common cold, it may, of course, vary in virulence from time to time exactly as diphtheria, scarlet fever, and similar infections vary in their potency. However, what is called a variation in virulence may really be the reflection of lessening of resistance or the development of a new generation that has not the resistance of a previous generation. One conception of epidemic influenza emphasizes the fact that it occurs in cycles of some thirty years which permit the development of new generations of human beings not capable of resisting the infection. Since the germs are living organisms, it is conceivable that they may vary in their power from one occasion to another exactly as human beings vary.

Germs may be affected exactly as human beings are affected by the atmosphere in which they live, the soil on which they rest, the diet on which they thrive. The organism of the common cold may die readily on the surface of the skin but grow happily on a mucous membrane. It may die readily on a normal mucous membrane, but multiply exceedingly on a mucous membrane that has been vitiated by the continuous residence of its possessor in a hot, dry, stuffy, dusty room. Here then comes the question of proper ventilation as a factor in the onset and in the prevention of the common cold. Investigators from the United States Public Health Service studied various ventilation systems in their relationship to catching cold by children in seven schools in Connecticut. In three schools ventilation was controlled by windows, in three by fans, and in one by a special ventilating system. About thirty-six hundred pupils attended the schools. Records were kept of their absences, the daily temperature of the rooms, and the occurrence of coughs and colds among the children. The total number of absences on account of coughs and colds among the children in rooms with artificial ventilation was much larger than that among those in rooms ventilated by the open-window method—indeed, almost twice as much. Of course, the children were in school only eight hours of the day. This need not be taken, therefore, as a general condemnation of all mechanical systems of air conditioning. Assembly rooms, theaters, motion-picture houses, and places seating great crowds of people simply cannot be properly ventilated by the open-window method. In general, however, authorities on ventilation are agreed that window ventilation provides the best system for changing the air and keeping it healthful.

The most serious problem is the question of proper heating and the provision of sufficient moisture in the air. Private homes should be heated to 68 or 70 degrees, and large halls to 60 or 65 degrees F. The large halls require less heat because human beings will provide from their own bodies enough extra heat to make up the deficiency. Equally important with heat is moisture. A sufficient amount of humidity prevents chilling. Moisture can be obtained either by special devices built into furnaces which are now widely advertised and which have been proved to be efficient, or by special electric devices which have been developed for moistening the air.

The common impression that chilling, dampness, and fatigue are predisposing factors in catching cold is, as has been shown, supported by much good scientific evidence. The theory is that chilling and dampness induce a cold through disturbing the heat-regulating mechanism of the body by sudden evaporation of moisture from the surface of the body. For example, one who is quite well may sit in front of an electric fan and get up after fifteen minutes with the nose congested and with all of the beginning symptoms of a cold. The draft from the electric fan brings about chilling of the surface of the body and disturbs the circulation of the blood in the mucous membranes of the nose.

Conditioning against colds has behind it the acceptance of many hygienic authorities. The technic of conditioning involves the building of resistance through proper hygiene and a few special measures directed specifically against the predisposing causes. One of these technics is the cold-bath technic. A cold shower is all right for anyone who wants it, provided he rubs himself thoroughly thereafter with towels so as to restore a brisk circulation to the congealed surface. The majority of people probably do better with a lukewarm bath taken primarily for purposes of cleanliness and only secondarily with the idea of benefiting resistance to disease.

There is also the conception that children may have their resistance increased by wrapping their throats and chests with towels wrung out of cold water. There is no good evidence in favor of this notion. Then there are the mothers who believe that they help the health of the child by baring to the wintry blasts the portion of the leg from the calf to the upper third of the thigh. It remains to be shown that any child had its resistance to colds increased by this exposure.

Certainly the biometricians have not credited such statistics as are available in favor of conditioning to cold by subjecting one's self unnecessarily to it. The reasoning in favor of the procedure is only symbolical, like the suggestion that the proper treatment of smallpox is to put the patient in a room with red velours hangings.

Germs in general succumb to sunlight. For human beings it is a pleasant measure. Hence the argument early advanced that exposure to the rays of the sun or to the rays of ultraviolet from the artificial sun lamp, using either the carbon arc or the quartz mercury vapor burner, would aid in building resistance to colds. The Council on Physical Therapy of the American Medical Association, after examining all of the evidence that could be offered in support of such measures, has withdrawn its approval from sources of ultraviolet that are advertised as beneficial in the prevention of colds. Perhaps the ultraviolet does enhance the power of the body in some generally beneficial way, but certainly it has not been proved that its effects are specific against respiratory diseases. Indeed, the exact words of the council are, "As far as normal persons are concerned, the claim that exposure to ultraviolet rays increases or improves the tone of the tissues or of the body as a whole, stimulates metabolism, or tends to prevent colds, has not been conclusively substantiated."

Vaccines Against Colds

Another measure of which much is heard in these advanced times, when people are beginning to understand medical progress and medical methods, is ˌhe use of the vaccine for the prevention of colds. The hoi-polloi refer to the use of vaccines or of any other substances administered by injection as "shɔts." Physicians build resistance against typhoid fever by injecting the patient with vaccine made of killed typhoid and paratyphoid germs. The injection of these killed germs stirs up the tissues of the body to resistance against the constituents of the typhoid organism. Some physicians inject mixtures of the killed bodies of germs frequently found in the noses and throats of people with colds, with the idea of building resistance to infection by these germs. There are two reasons, however, why many scientists do not approve the use of the "shots" in the cases of people with frequent colds. First, it has not been shown that any of these germs are specifically the cause of or definitely related to the colds; second, it has not been shown that the injection of these germs will stimulate resistance. Two viruses known as influenza A and B are associated with symptoms like those of a cold and vaccines against these are available. Another cold or influenza virus is called virus X. Most colds are mixed infections.

TREATMENT OF COLDS

First, everybody who knows advises rest in bed until the temperature is normal, with head of the bed elevated in order to make breathing easier. Actually, only hygienists or people who are quite serious in medical affairs go to bed when they have a cold.

The skin is usually so uncomfortable that a sponge bath with water of a temperature about 98 degrees F. is desirable, and the skin may be fairly well rubbed with a rough towel after the bath. If the bowels are inactive, it is advisable to clear them of their digested and undigested contents. The clearing may be accomplished either by washing out from below or by the usual laxatives administered above.

Fever burns tissue. Hence the diet during a cold should consist of nourishing food. Since appetite is lost in most instances anyway, food should be appetizing and enjoyable. A child should not be forced to eat what is repulsive, particularly in the presence of disturbed appetite. Let the child have what it wants. Many physicians administer sugar and fruit juices with a view to providing calories and to preventing the acid reaction which is believed to be favorable to the persistence of the cold.

The common home remedies, such as bathing the feet in mustard baths, perspiring freely under hot blankets, drinking quantities of hot lemonade and orange juice, are time-tried helps to comfort. Of a similar character are the home remedies employed to lower fever and to diminish pain. Of this type is aspirin, a widely used home remedy. Any good aspirin will do, and fifteen or twenty different pharmaceutical houses now make it available. Aspirin, like every other remedy, is a two-edged sword, capable of damage when employed improperly as well as of good when given in proper dosage at the right time. A new remedy is a mixture of codeine and papaverine that must be prescribed by a doctor.

Diets for Colds

Then there is the specific diet. Rats which have had in their food an insufficient amount of vitamin A begin to develop a breakdown of the mucous membranes of the nose and throat. Rats that are fed sufficient amounts of vitamin A do not develop such changes. From this it has been argued that human beings who eat proper amounts of vitamin A or even excess amounts should be able to preserve the integrity of their mucous membranes and thereby avoid colds. Such experiments as have been done over short periods of time not only on chimpanzees but also on human beings do not support the idea strongly. These experiments, of course, cover but a few months, whereas the entire life of the rat is but ninety days, and a week in its life may be approximately equivalent to seven years of human existence. Whether or not excess vitamin A taken over a period of seven years eventually produces an immunity to colds remains to be studied and probably will not be. Human beings do not lend themselves readily to seven-year experiments. Even presidents get only four-year terms and eight seems to be the limit. Russia seems to be satisfied with a five-year plan.

Nose Sprays for Colds

A man with an eruption wants something to put on it. A man or woman with a running nose wants something to put in it. Hence the development of innumerable antiseptics, sprays, ointments, and lotions for administration in the common cold. There are drugs which dry up the secretions, but apparently that is not the road to cure. There are other drugs which increase the secretions, but the duration of the cold still seems to average three or four days. The experts in diseases of the nose and throat feel that the discomfort when too great should be relieved by one of the sprays which diminish secretions, and which include either the old adrenalin or the modern ephedrine. For years camphor-menthol solutions and preparations of oil, camphor, menthol, and eucalyptus have been used to give relief in nasal irritation. The actual worth of such preparations in curing the cold is doubtful. Their value in securing comfort is considerable.

Most recent in the control of colds are the antihistaminic drugs, used alone or combined with aspirin or phenacetin or sprayed in the nose with camphor or menthol or privine. Such preparations are useful in colds which begin as a running nose due to allergy and these constitute a large percentage of all colds.

General Treatment

When the chest seems tight, a mustard poultice is sometimes helpful. This may be bought ready made in the drug store. If it is to be made at home, a paste is made by mixing ordinary household mustard and flour stirred together with warm water as described in the package; it is then spread between two layers of thin muslin. This plaster is put over the upper chest of the patient until the skin becomes quite red. It usually requires from fifteen to thirty minutes.

When the cough is relieved, the discomfort in the chest usually becomes less. Many remedies are used to loosen the cough, most of them being what are called expectorant remedies, containing ammonium chloride. The dose of ammonium chloride usually prescribed is eight grains to each teaspoonful. This is given every two hours. The ammonium chloride is put up with some pleasant syrup. Sometimes sodium citrate, taken in ten-grain tablets mixed with lemonade or warm water, will help to loosen the cough.

Most important in this condition is taking plenty of water. A person with a cold should take a half tumblerful every hour while awake. The water can be as is, or as lemonade or orangeade. If a more alkaline drink is desired, a little baking soda or sodium bicarbonate—usually about 10 grains—may be added to the lemonade.

There are lots of people who think they want a cathartic every time they have a cold, to clean out the system. Really the cathartic, when the cold begins, does not seem to make a great deal of difference. Somtimes it is so irritating as to induce a condition much more discomforting and worse than the cold itself.

SUMMER COLDS

Beyond the common cold there comes with the beginning of spring another type—the allergic cold, rose cold, summer cold, or hay-fever. The spring or rose cold is due to sensitivity to various protein substances derived in the spring primarily from the dandelion, the daisy, maple, and poplar, and also from various other pollens of weeds and grasses. The season and the nature of the sensitizing agent depend on the location in which the person lives and the kinds of grasses and flowers in his vicinity. The symptoms of onset are much the same as those of the common cold, but with most of the emphasis on the redness of the eyes and on the sneezing. That type of cold is a special condition prevented and treated by proper diagnosis and attempts at desensitization.

If you must blow your nose, be careful not to blow it in such a manner as to force the infected secretions from the nose through the eustachian tube into the ears. Always keep one nostril open as a safety valve. Be careful to protect yourself so as not to develop the secondary complications of bronchitis and pneumonia. The cold itself is not a fatal disorder. The complications of colds in the form of infected ears, bronchitis, pneumonia, cause long maladies and many fatalities. Try going to bed for a day, give yourself a fair chance, and get well soon!

PNEUMONIA

At those seasons, with increasing cold and exposure, and when epidemics of influenza strike in various parts of the country, the number of cases of pneumonia increases rapidly and also the number of deaths. The number of deaths varies from year to year, apparently related to the severity of the climatic conditions and also perhaps to changes in the nature of the germ that causes the disease.

This germ is known as the pneumococcus, a round germ which passes with the discharges from the mouth and nose of the infected person to others, and which may occasionally be carried by a healthful person who is not himself infected, and thus is distributed to others. It has been found that the germs causing pneumonia may be divided into many types. There seems to be reason to believe that the overcrowding and the innumerable human contacts associated with modern life aid in the dissemination particularly of diseases of the mouth, nose, throat, and lungs.

Since normal persons may have the germs in their breathing tracts without having the disease, there may be factors related to the person himself which are concerned with the question of whether or not he will develop the disease. Any factor which will break down the resistance of an individual will tend to cause him to become more easily infected.

A direct injury to the tissue of the lung, such as might occur from inhaling a poison gas, or such as might occur from inhaling some foreign body which would cause an irritation, will open the way for infection by the germ of pneumonia.

The disease occurs in people of all ages but is rather rare during the first year of life. It is much more serious during the earlier and later years of life than it is during the middle period. The rate of incidence and death is high during infancy, decreasing up to the age of ten, and then gradually increasing up to the age of forty, when it again begins to become exceedingly high.

For some reason pneumonia is much more serious in the colored race than in the white. It also follows frequently after such conditions as measles, smallpox, scarlet fever, and even after typhoid. There seems to be good evidence that exposure to severe fatigue, bad weather and to malnutrition give the germs of pneumonia greater opportunity to attack. For some years it has been believed that hard drinkers were more likely to suffer with pneumonia than others, but this has also been related to the fact that hard drinkers occasionally lie out in the open and are exposed to rain and freezing temperatures for long periods of time.

Modern evidence points to the fact that crowding is an important factor in the occurrence of pneumonia. The disease is more frequently found in the city than in the country and is probably more fatal in the city than in the country. The chance for infection from one person to another is much greater where people are crowded together. In trains, street cars, theaters, motion-picture houses, in tenements and under similar conditions, human beings come into contacts that are intimate for fairly long periods of time. Under such conditions germs pass directly from the mouth, nose, and throat of one to another.

When the germs of pneumonia attack the lung it becomes filled with blood, so that quite soon the person begins coughing and spitting material which contains the red streaks showing the presence of blood in the lung. This lung is, however, rather solid because of the presence of the material in it. The physician, therefore, fails to hear the air passing because of the obstruction in the air spaces. Moreover, when he thumps the chest over the lungs it gives forth the dull sound of a solid object rather than the resonant reverberation of one which is full of air.

After a time, depending on the severity of the condition, the lung begins to clear up, the breathing takes place with less difficulty. At the same time the fever goes down.

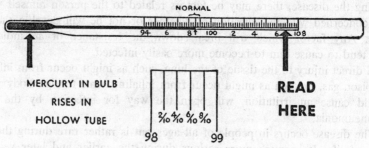

Fig. 16. To read, look along the sharper edge between the numbers and the lines. (Reproduced by permission of the National Tuberculosis Association.)

Pneumonia sometimes begins suddenly with a chill, pain in the chest, vomiting and coughing and difficulty in breathing. In other cases there may be fainting and weakness. In the serious stages of pneumonia the fever may vary from 104 to 106 degrees. Because of the difficulty in getting the blood through the lung there is great stress on the heart. Furthermore, the obstruction to the circulation causes the patient to develop a blue color which indicates that the blood passing through the lung is not receiving enough oxygen. Especially valuable is the use of X-ray to make certain of the diagnosis in pneumonia and to differentiate between lobar and virus pneumonia.

Most people know that the usual case of uncomplicated pneumonia used to last from a week to ten days and that then it cleared up by what is called a crisis; or more slowly by what physicians call lysis, or a gradual dissolving of the disease. In those cases that clear up by crisis the patient suddenly begins to get better and within a few hours is without high fever. He feels much bet-

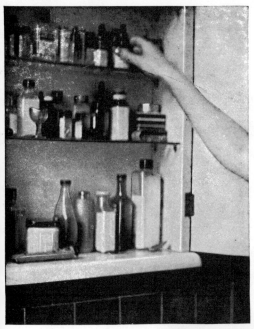

Typical medicine chest.
(Courtesy of H. Armstrong Roberts)

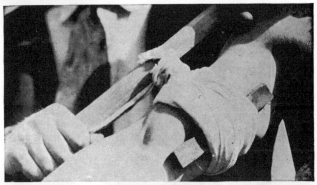

Application of tourniquet.

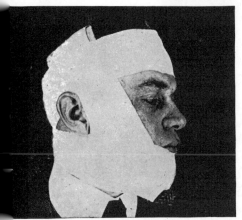

Modified Barton bandage. It may be
used with or without plaster.

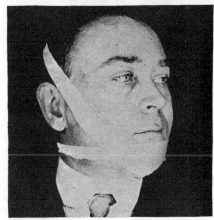

Four-tailed bandage in place. This is a
good emergency bandage.

(Courtesy of R. C. J. Lyons, University of Michigan)

PLATE I

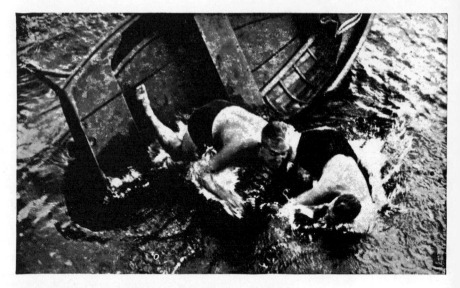

Wrong way of saving a drowning person.

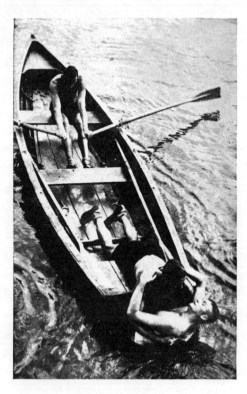

Right way of saving a drowning person
(Courtesy of Acme Newspictures, Inc.

PLATE II

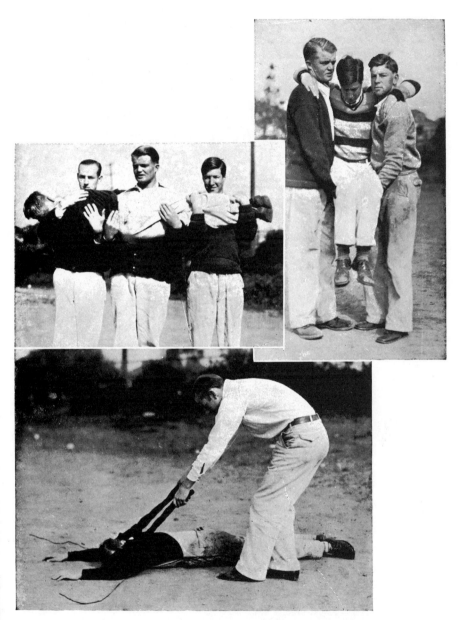

Above left: Method of carrying person with serious injury. *Above right:* Basket method of carrying injured person. *Below:* Method of removing injured person from contact with live wire.

PLATE III

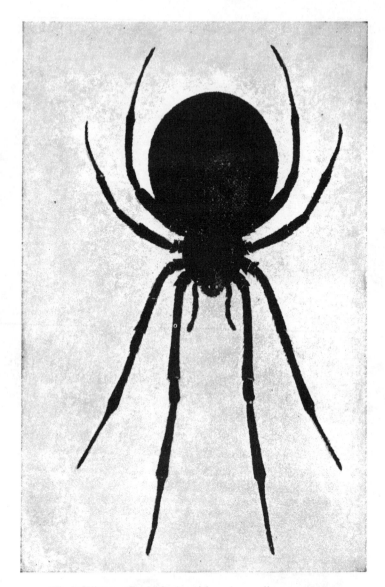

Black Widow. Coal black, with red or yellow spot on the abdomen, identified as *Lathrodectus mactans;* otherwise familiarly known as the "Black Widow." She is really our bad spider.

PLATE IV

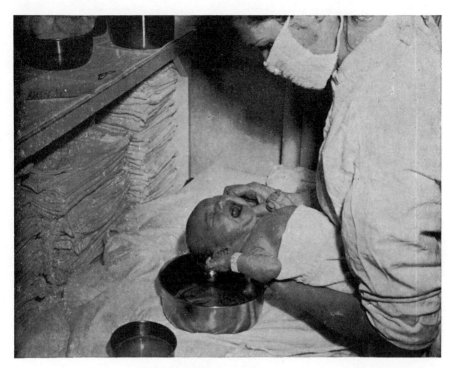

Bathing the baby.

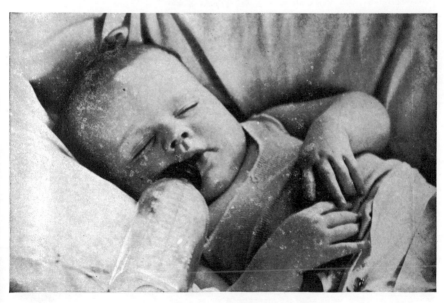

Permitting child to sleep with nursing bottle in mouth may deform face.
(Courtesy of Ruth Alexander Nichols)

PLATE V

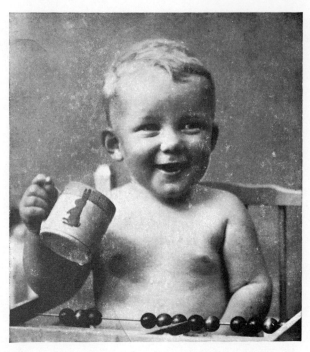

As soon as possible, the child should be taught to drink
from a cup. This is an aid to weaning.
(Courtesy of H. Armstrong Roberts)

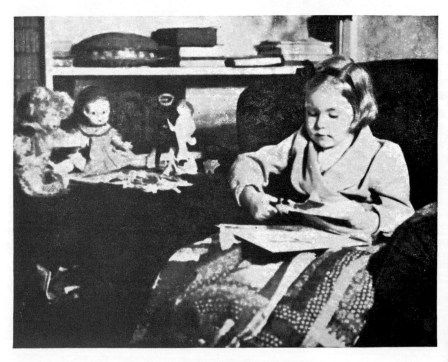

Amusement for bed-ridden child patient.

PLATE VI

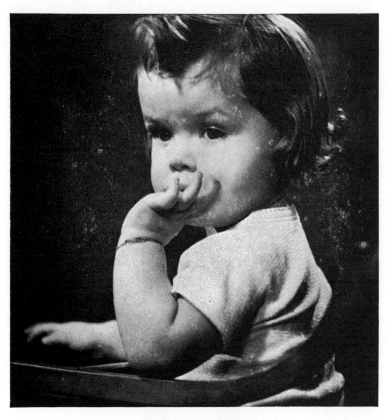

Thumb sucking.
(Photo by Black Box Studios)

Thumbs deformed by sucking.

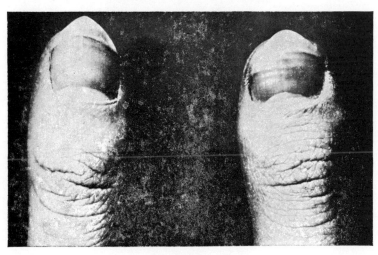

PLATE VII

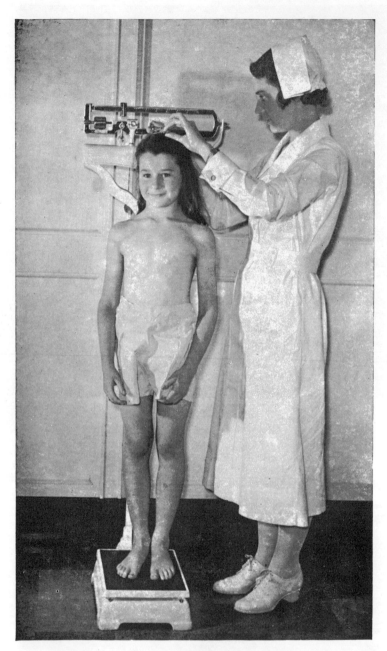

A weekly weighing of the child indicates state of nutrition.
(Courtesy of U. S. Public Health Service)

PLATE VIII

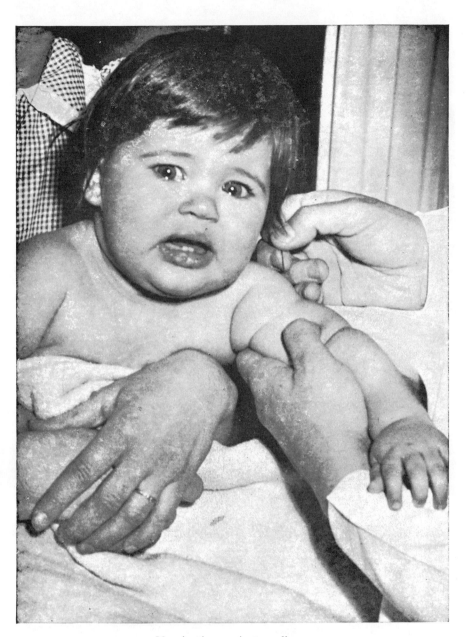

Vaccination against smallpox.

PLATE IX

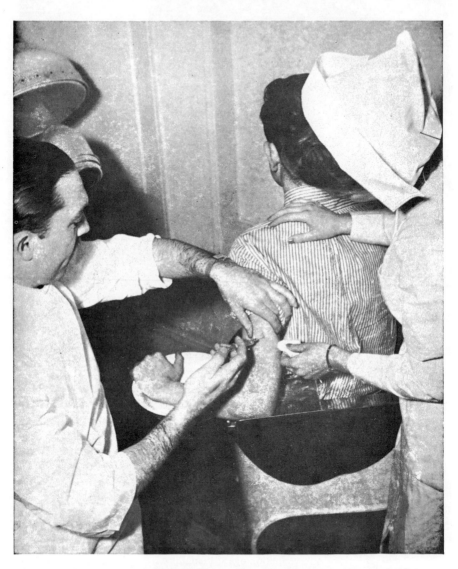

Inoculation against typhoid.
(Courtesy of Keystone View Co., Inc.)

PLATE X

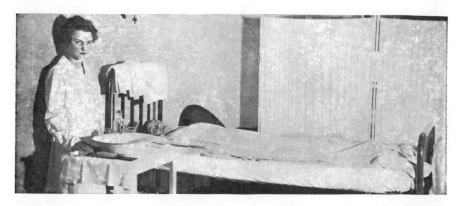

Patient ready for bed bath.

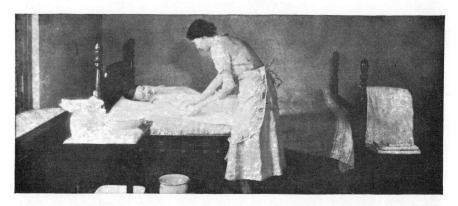

Bathing the patient. Place a towel lengthwise beneath the patient's arm, and bathe gently with the wash cloth wrapped around your right hand. Notice the orderly arrangement of bathing necessities on the stand and the linen on the chair. The bed is raised up on blocks in order to prevent back strain.

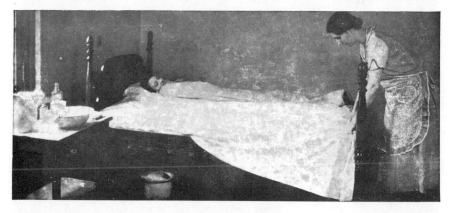

Making the patient's bed. The bed linen is changed after the bath. Have the patient roll to the side opposite you. Loosen the soiled bottom sheet and roll it up against the patient's back. Spread the clean sheet over the vacated area.

PLATE XI

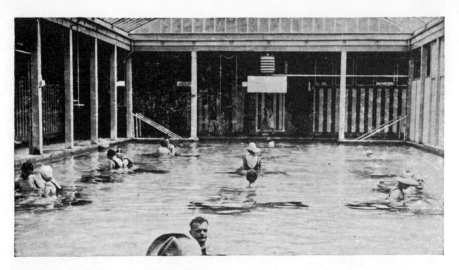

Pool at Warm Springs Foundation for treatment of infantile paralysis.

Class outdoors for incapacitated children.
(Courtesy of Holmes I. Mettee)

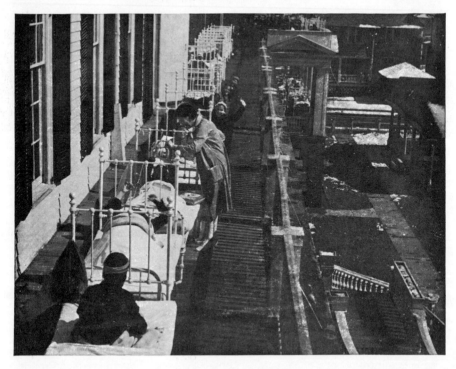

PLATE XII

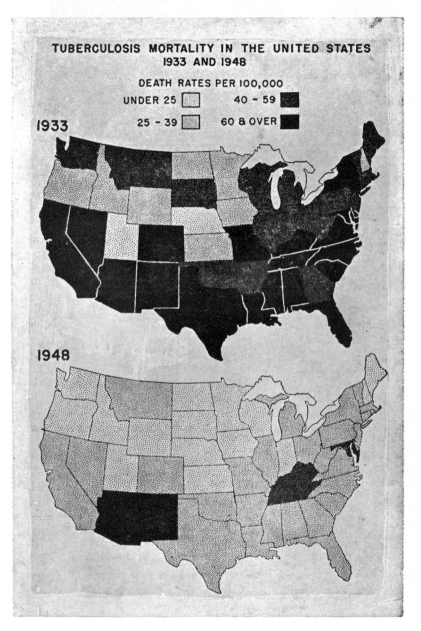

Tuberculosis mortality in the United States 1933 to 1948. Provisional data by place of occurrence, collected by the National Tuberculosis Association.
(Courtesy of Metropolitan Life Insurance Company)

PLATE XIII

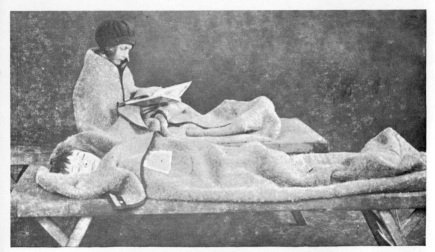

Children suitably dressed for outdoor study and sleep.
(Courtesy of International News Photos, Inc.)

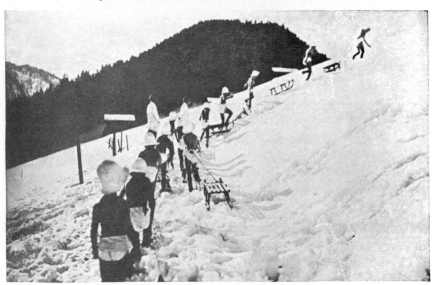

Outdoor sun bath. (Courtesy of Keystone View Co., Inc.)

Indoor sun bath.

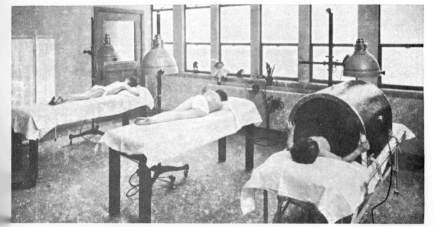

PLATE X

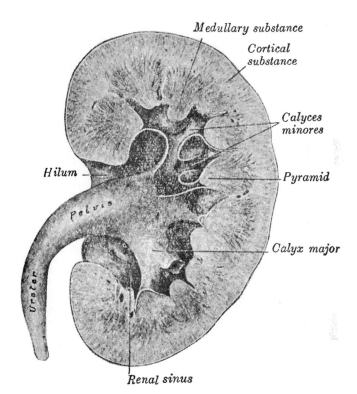

Medullary substance

Cortical substance

Calyces minores

Hilum

Pelvis

Pyramid

Ureter

Calyx major

Renal sinus

Vertical section through a kidney, showing the pelvis, calyces, and the cortical and medullary substance.
(Reproduced by permission of Longmans, Green & Company, Inc., London, from *Gray's Anatomy, Descriptive and Applied*)

PLATE XV

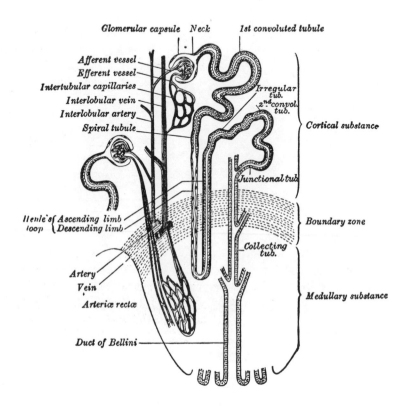

Glomerular capsule Neck 1st convoluted tubule

Afferent vessel
Efferent vessel
Intertubular capillaries
Interlobular vein
Interlobular artery
Spiral tubule

Irregular tub.
2nd convol. tub.

Cortical substance

Junctional tub

Henle's { Ascending limb
loop { Descending limb

Boundary zone

Collecting tub.

Artery
Vein
Arteriæ rectæ

Medullary substance

Duct of Bellini

Diagram of a functional unit (nephron) of the kidney
and its blood supply.
(Reproduced by permission of Longman's, Green &
Company, Inc., London, from *Gray's Anatomy, Descriptive and Applied*)

PLATE XVI

ter, his pulse is better, his breathing is slower, and in every way he is improved. In most instances the recovery is gradual. Recovery is due to the fact that the blood of the patient has developed the power to overcome the germ of the disease.

In preventing pneumonia bear in mind that contact with those who are infected is the chief source of its spread. Certainly, a baby should not be taken into a room in which someone is suffering from pneumonia. Mothers must do everything possible to prevent their children from coming in contact with other children who have running noses, coughs, colds, and sore throats. It is especially important to protect children against sharp falls in temperatures which, through centuries of experience, have been associated with the onset of fall and winter colds.

In some cities people with pneumonia are isolated, as with other serious infectious diseases. This has not yet been done on sufficiently large a scale to permit accurate estimation of the worth of the procedure, but there is reason to believe that its effect may be definitely for good.

The person attending a patient with pneumonia should wear a clean gown which is changed before contact with other people. The hands should be thoroughly cleaned with soap and water after attending the patient. The room of the patient should be kept as clean as possible and thoroughly aired, washed, and sunned after the patient's recovery.

When a person is isolated for an infectious disease the utensils, bedclothing, personal clothing, handkerchiefs, and other material in close contact with him should be sterilized. They should be kept separate from similar materials used by other members of the family.

Most important in the care of the patient with pneumonia is to keep him as quiet as possible, both mentally and physically, and to give him the best possible nursing care. The difference between good and bad nursing may mean the difference between life and death.

Because of the importance of proper care and nursing in such a case, most physicians feel that a patient with pneumonia is better off in a hospital than at home. Moreover, it is better to get the patient under good care early and not to wait until he has reached a critical stage before transferring him to a hospital.

The patient with pneumonia should have a large, well-ventilated room with plenty of access to good fresh air. This does not mean that a patient with pneumonia is to be exposed to storm and stress. In inclement weather it is much better to prevent such additional exposure. The patient himself is frequently the best judge as to when he is breathing with most ease and least distress.

The number of visitors must be kept to a minimum. The patient should not have to worry about troubles in the family or business affairs and must be kept flat on his back for at least a week after recovery has begun. Only gradually is he allowed to assume a sitting posture.

The diet in this condition, as in any serious infection, must be chiefly liquids such as soups, gruels, milk, and soft-boiled eggs. Occasionally it is well to add milk sugar to keep up the energy. Rest and quiet are more important even than nourishment in the serious stages of pneumonia. When recovery has begun, feeding is gradually extended so as to aid the improvement of the blood and the broken-down tissues.

It is well for patients with pneumonia to have plenty of water. This does not mean, however, much more than two to three quarts a day. The patient will not drink unless the water is given to him when he is quite sick. Under such circumstances it is perhaps best to give water with a teaspoon, giving small amounts frequently, or to have the patient suck small pieces of ice.

Of greatest importance in the treatment of pneumonia is the care of a competent physician. He himself must direct the nursing and determine its value. He himself must administer proper remedies at the proper time in order to support the extra work of the heart, in order to relieve stress from the circulation, in order to permit the patient to sleep, and in order to control the actions of the bowels, the skin, and of all the other organs. There is no substitute of any kind for the type of care that a well-trained physician can give in this disease.

The use of oxygen in the treatment of pneumonia has been elaborated of late and is found to be exceedingly valuable. Tents have been developed which may be placed over the patients as they lie in bed, and many large hospitals have oxygen rooms into which the entire bed may be moved and in which the nurse may remain and attend the patient. Oxygen is not to be considered an emergency measure to be applied when the patient is at the point of death, but instead one which is to be used promptly when the physician feels that it is required.

While any of the sulfonamide drugs are useful in the treatment of pneumonia, most frequently used nowadays is sulfadiazine, which is less toxic. Penicillin, chlortetracycline and oxytetracycline as well as newer antibiotics are valuable in the attack on the pneumonia germ. Large amounts of penicillin can be given by injection into the muscles and a sufficiently high level of penicillin maintained in the blood to bring about prompt control of the infection.

The former fatality rate of 25 to 30 percent in pneumonia has now dropped to 5 percent.

ATYPICAL VIRUS PNEUMONIA

The pneumonia that is caused by the pneumococcus is now recognized as quite distinctive from the atypical virus pneumonia, which is milder. Fortunately virus pneumonia is not as serious a disease as lobar pneumonia. Deaths from virus pneumonia are exceedingly rare.

Aureomycin and terramycin are most recommended in this condition. The drug is best given in a half glass of milk.

TUBERCULOSIS

The protection of mankind against tuberculosis is based on two principles which were formulated by the famous Pasteur and Robert Koch. The first is to preserve the child against infection with the germ of tuberculosis by removing it from contaminated surroundings; the second is the isolation of the sick and the education of the well in the prevention of the disease.

Tuberculosis is a social disease in the sense that it affects groups of mankind as well as individuals. Second, it is involved with the economic status of those who are infected. For example, in Vienna in 1913 deaths from tuberculosis were five times higher in the poorer quarters than in the better class quarters.

Tuberculosis attacks all races, all ages of mankind, and indeed all classes of human society, but it is largely a disease of poverty and malnutrition. All of the available evidence indicates that the number of deaths from tuberculosis per hundred thousand of population is steadily decreasing throughout the world. There seems to be some question as to just why this trend has taken place. The decline in the death rate from tuberculosis began long before the era of bacteriologic discoveries and of modern hygiene based on such discoveries. The reason may be not only a change that has taken place in the germ of tuberculosis, but probably also a change has taken place in the nature of man.

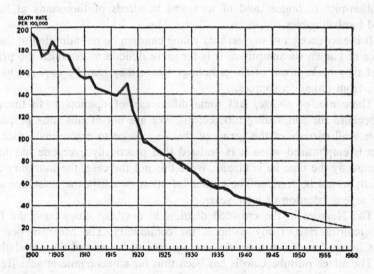

Fig. 17. Decline in tuberculosis mortality in the United States expanding death registration states since 1900.

(Courtesy of Metropolitan Life Insurance Company)

The death rate drops among people who have had tuberculosis for many decades. The death rate rises when tuberculosis comes into a country area or into a district in which the population has previously been relatively free from tuberculosis. There seems to be evidence that the coming of the industrial era with crowding and long hours of labor produced a higher death rate for this disease. Then came the protection of labor, particularly of child labor, social hygiene, improved nutrition and improved housing, with a lowering of the rates for tuberculosis.

With the truly extensive knowledge of tuberculosis which we have, its complete prevention ultimately should be a possibility. However, perfect success in a problem of this kind is not likely in a day, a month, or even a generation.

The path to prevention seems to be clear. Young children must not be exposed to infection, or, in any event, the possibility of infection in young children must be reduced to a minimum.

Let us consider what this means in our modern civilization. Human contacts have been multiplied enormously. Today the home has largely disappeared in our great cities; instead, we have the apartment house, housing from three to fifty families. Obviously under such circumstances children are exposed not only to their own parents and relatives, but to vast numbers of other children and other families.

The child of an earlier day played in its own backyard at least until the age of six. Today it goes early to nursery school and thereafter to kindergarten. Moreover, human beings now assemble in crowds of thousands in motion-picture houses and of tens and hundreds of thousands at baseball and football games.

It is easy enough to suggest that young children be not admitted to the presence of known consumptives. It is far more difficult to establish the principle that they be kept out of all gatherings where they may be exposed to infection from unknown sources.

There are, of course, still some differences of opinion as to the proper procedure for eliminating tuberculosis. We are not at this time prepared to isolate all carriers of the germs of this disease or to exterminate them. The fact is emphasized when it is realized that practically everyone has had the disease by the time he is fifteen. Were this not the case, the mortality among adults would be terrific. The earlier infection establishes a resistance against the severe infection of later years.

The Negroes in the crowded districts in northern cities have the highest tuberculosis rate of any group in the community. The Mexican population of Chicago has eleven times the average rate of the rest of the population.

The attack on tuberculosis has been thus far an economic attack. Realizing that it is primarily a disease associated with bad hygiene, great importance has been placed on physical well being.

The treatment consisted largely of good diet, sufficient rest and fresh air.

Special attention was paid to housing and types of employment, to the prices of food and wages, since it has been shown that a drop in wages is usually related to an increase in tuberculosis.

In the United States the number of beds available for patients with this disease increased from 10,000 in 1904 to more than 100,000 in recent years. Moreover, there has been a tremendous growth in open-air schools, preventoriums, clinics, and dispensaries.

With the development of new methods of diagnosis and treatment of tuberculosis the demand for sanitarium beds is decreasing. In 1954 and 1955 many sanitariums for tuberculosis were closed, including the famous Trudeau Sanitarium at Saranac Lake, N. Y. More and more patients are being treated while ambulatory with the newer drugs including streptomycin, paraminosalicylic acid (PAS), isoniazid and cycloserine.

In tuberculosis, we know the cause of the disease: namely, the germ of bacillus of tuberculosis. We know the method of transmission, which is from the patient with the disease to the person who does not have it, particularly the child, and occasionally through infected milk and food.

We know that the disease could be prevented by complete isolation or extermination of those who have it, but we cannot apply such procedures on a suitable scale, simply because social conditions do not permit the application of such stringent procedures.

Tuberculosis is a social disease because it spreads where there is poverty, malnutrition, overcrowding, bad housing, exposure to the elements and similar social disabilities. Since the disease is spread chiefly from a person who has it to those who do not, the condition could be controlled by isolating all persons who have the germs in their sputum and who spread them about. Since this is not possible, we endeavor to increase resistance to the disease by inoculating great numbers of people with BCG vaccination. We try to detect the disease in its earliest stages by the use of the X-ray and the tuberculin test. If patients are treated in such early stages, they tend to recover promptly and do not become active spreaders of the disease.

The condition requires rest in a sanatorium under controlled conditions with plenty of good food, fresh air and sunshine, and good hygiene. The ailing lung can be put at rest by artificial pneumothorax, by the operation called thoracoplasty, by suitable posture and by cutting the phrenic nerve.

Doctors know that the X-ray alone is not the only method of detecting tuberculosis. Before a final decision is made the doctor wants to obtain specimens of the sputum so that he can look for the presence of the germ of tuberculosis. He may wish to study the specimens by use of the microscope. He may wish to inject a guinea pig with the material to see if the guinea pig will become infected. Sometimes when the examination of the sputum is negative, material from the stomach (which is secured by washing the stomach with a tube) is then examined for the presence of the germ of tuberculosis. The doctor will also wish to obtain a careful record of the person's life and of his symptoms.

He will wish to check the observations by studies of the chest, by percussion or thumping or by listening with the stethoscope.

The following hints for good hygiene in tuberculosis come from the National Tuberculosis Association:

"Babies and little children must stay out of your room. You must insist on this, because they are very likely to catch your germs. The best plan is to send them somewhere else to live while you are sick.

"Do not allow pets in your room.

"Never allow anyone or any animal to eat the food or drink that has been in your room. Left-over food should be burned; if liquid, poured into the toilet.

"Do not let visitors come close to you, shake hands with you, handle your things, or put their coats, hats, gloves, etc., on your bed.

"Never kiss or allow anyone to kiss you! This is a hard rule to obey—probably the hardest for most families. You will have to be the one to insist on it, since if you forbid kissing and remind the family of the danger, they will be less likely to think you want to be kissed, or are feeling hurt at their neglect. Kissing is a very easy way to spread your germs. Show your real affection for your family by refusing to kiss or be kissed.

"Your doctor or nurse will teach your family what to do with your dishes, linen, and other soiled articles, but the most essential thing for you to remember is this: *Protect others from your sputum!*

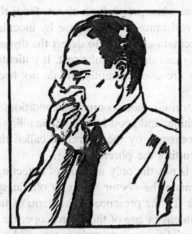 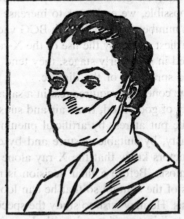

Fig. 18. How to cover mouth and nose. *Left:* Use of paper tissue. Nose and mouth both covered. *Right:* Mask made of folds of gauze (at least four thicknesses). (Reproduced by permission of the National Tuberculosis Association)

"Your sputum (spit or phlegm) is dangerous because there are tuberculosis germs in it. Everything your sputum soils is dangerous to others. Therefore you must catch your sputum when it comes as spit or spray from your mouth and nose in sneezing, coughing or spitting. You do this by covering your nose and mouth with paper tissues or soft old rags and burning them after use. Your supply of tissues should be placed beside your pillow or on the bedside table where you can reach them without stretching. Then do as follows:

"1. Take one or two and hold them in your cupped hand, protecting your hand and fingers. You may need two thicknesses of material.

"2. Cover both your nose and mouth.

"3. After use, drop the tissue into a paper bag (grocery bag, or one made of newspaper) pinned to the side of your bed or bedside table, where you can reach it without stretching and without missing.

"When the bag of soiled tissues is about three-quarters full, it should be taken out by your family helper and burned. Do not fill the bag so full that anyone has to touch the soiled tissues in unpinning and holding the bag.

"Never cough, sneeze or spit without using the paper tissue or rags in this way. Always turn your head away from anyone when you cough or sneeze. Later, when you are up, the doctor may let you use a sputum cup (a metal container with a paper filler), but tissues are safer.

"Try to remember that everything soiled or sprayed by the moisture from your nose and mouth is dangerous to others. Be careful! Have your set of toilet articles, toothbrush, towels, shaving kit, and, if allowed, smoking supplies. You can save your family helper many steps and much trouble by being careful about this rule of separate belongings. Your linen and dishes must be boiled before being used by other members of the family."

DIET IN TUBERCULOSIS

The diet is important in the treatment of tuberculosis. Some people simply do not get enough food. Many people are badly fed because they do not know how to select the right foods and to make the best use of what food they have. There seems to be not the slightest question but that malnutrition has an extremely unfavorable effect on the death rate from tuberculosis.

The charts of deaths from tuberculosis show a high peak in earliest infancy, then a definite drop in the rate during later infancy and school age, and a rise at the beginning of adolescence. This points definitely to the periods when children must be most closely watched for the development of symptoms and when everything possible must be done to keep up their nutrition and to see to it that they have plenty of rest and good hygiene.

CONTROL OF TUBERCULOUS CATTLE

Of special importance in the prevention of tuberculosis is the control of tuberculous cattle. The germ of tuberculosis of the type which lives in cattle is rather rare as a cause of tuberculosis of the abdomen, the glands, the bones, and the joints. There are certain methods for controlling tuberculosis in cattle which are now subject to legislation in this country.

In the first place, milk for children, unless coming from cattle free from tuberculosis, must invariably be pasteurized, and in fact it is probably better to pasteurize all milk for children—at least there is more certainty of safety. Second, it is desirable to stamp out tuberculosis among cattle. This is commonly done by testing cattle for the presence of the disease and then destroying all that are infected, at the same time compensating the owners for the loss of the animals.

CLIMATE IN PREVENTION AND TREATMENT OF TUBERCULOSIS

While it is possible for a person to recover from tuberculosis in almost any climate, climatic factors nevertheless play a considerable part in the speed of the recovery.

In considering climate one is concerned not only with temperature and humidity, but also with wind, dust, and storms, with rain, the character of the soil, the sunshine, and many other factors.

Heat or cold in great excess are dangerous to health and may be fatal to life. The effects of temperature on the body are dependent to a great degree on humidity.

Warm moist climates are generally believed to have a depressing effect. Cold, dry air is stimulating, but demands a capacity for response from the individual.

If the body is not able to respond properly to cold, dry air, as is the case with persons who have been greatly weakened by long continued illness or by old age, the effects of cold, dry air may be harmful.

Excessive moisture has a relaxing effect which may predispose to infection. The movement of the air materially influences the temperature and the humidity.

If the air is hot and moist, movement of the air will aid in elimination of heat. If the air is very cold, there will be an increased demand for heat produced from the body. If the air is both moist and cold, conditions are extremely uncomfortable and may be harmful.

There is no one best climate for tuberculosis. In other words, proper treatment under scientific conditions is more important than climate alone.

Some types of patients never should be moved in search of climate. This includes patients who are severely ill in the early stages of the disease or in the late stage of the disease. In such cases, complete rest in bed either at home or in an institution in the home city is the first step in treatment and should be continued until the patient is able to travel without risk.

The cost of invalid care almost anywhere is from $50 to $100 per week. Therefore, at least $2,500 to $5,000 per year must be available for the care of the invalid if he is to go to any health resort.

When the burden of providing for one's self in a strange land is added to those of the disease itself, the invalid has a handicap to overcome which may result in the difference between life and death. Good food and lodging are just as necessary as plenty of sunlight and fresh air.

The satisfaction of the patient's mind is of the utmost importance. A mother will not get well if she is constantly worried about the condition of the children that she has left at home.

A business man will not recover as well in a strange climate as at home if he is constantly worried about his business. It is for this reason that many institutions have grown up near all of the large cities in our country.

The routine of treatment in such instances is of greater advantage than any possible advantages to be derived from climate. The biggest advantage of an institution is the fact that the patient can be educated in the proper routine of life leading to recovery.

The second reason for treating a patient in an institution rather than at home is the advantage of a change. Wealthy people, when tired, experience a tremendous improvement in their general physical and mental tone by a complete change of environment.

This is all the more true of those with tuberculosis. People who live in apartments or tenement houses frequently do better merely by transfer to a day camp near the seashore or in the country.

The advantages of open-air life and open-air sleeping are now recognized by common experience. These increase the general tone of the body, quiet the nervous system, and favor relaxation and sleep.

Perpetual sunshine will not prevent tuberculosis, and excessive sunshine is exceedingly irksome to many people.

Dr. James Alexander Miller has drawn certain conclusions which should be borne in mind by every person with tuberculosis who may contemplate a change of climate.

Here they are:

1. The regimen of regulated rest and exercise, proper food and open-air life, is the fundamental essential in the treatment of tuberculosis. Suitable climatic environment makes this open-air life more easy, enjoyable, and beneficial.

2. When these essentials are assured, a change of climate is of definite value in a considerable number, probably the majority, of cases, but with the proper regimen many cases will do well in any climate.

3. Any change of climate involving the fatigue of travel is contraindicated in acute cases with fever or hemorrhage, or in very far advanced and markedly debilitated cases. Absolute bed rest is the one essential here.

4. No patient should be sent away in search of climate who cannot afford to stay the reasonably to be expected time and to have the necessary food, lodging and care.

5. Competent medical advice and supervision are essential.

6. One of the most valuable assets of change is the education of the patient. This may, of course, be obtained in a suitable environment without reference to climate, as in a sanatorium near home.

7. Selection of a suitable locality is an individual problem for every patient, depending upon his temperament, tastes, and individual reaction to environment, as well as the character of his disease. The advising physician should have an appreciation of these as well as a knowledge of the particular environment to which the patient is being sent. Contentment and reasonable comfort are essential.

8. There is no universally ideal climate. For each patient there may well be a most favorable environment, if we are wise enough to find it.

9. There is a reasonable amount of evidence that certain medical types of cases are more favorably influenced by certain conditions of climate, everything else being equal. For example, reasonably cold, dry, variable climate, such as is found in the mountains, for young or vigorous constitutions which will react well. Dry, sunny climates for laryngeal cases and those with marked catarrhal secretions. Equable mild climates at low altitudes for the elderly and those of nervous temperaments, as well as for those with arteriosclerosis, weak hearts, or marked tendency to dyspnœa.

10. Successful selection of climate and environment for cases of tuberculosis requires wide knowledge of human nature, of places, and of the disease. This can only be acquired by patience, skill, and experience.

SKIN TESTS FOR TUBERCULOSIS

Many years ago it was proved that almost every human being has tuberculosis before he dies.

Indeed, the vast majority of people become infected with the disease in childhood and recover. However, a considerable number do not recover, and these represent the constant mortality from this disease. The death rate from tuberculosis has been cut tremendously through the advancement of modern medical science and modern hygiene.

In order to detect cases as early as possible and to apply as soon as possible suitable methods leading toward recovery, several systems have been established. The first is to examine all school children physically and by means of the X-ray and to give all of them the tuberculin test. The tuberculin test is a simple skin test, less painful than a pin scratch and much less dangerous.

One of the advantages of such a procedure is the fact that during the physical examination for tuberculosis, it is also possible to detect any other disease which may happen to be attacking the child.

Another method is to select from among school children those who seem particularly likely to have tuberculosis and to limit the examination to them. When a child is found to be positive to the tuberculin test, a thorough study is made of its physical conditions, then the X-ray examination is made. The X-ray reveals even small changes which may have taken place in the lungs.

If a child is found to be susceptible to tuberculosis or in a very early stage it can be put under a course of hygiene which will aid its prompt recovery in the vast majority of cases.

One of the modern developments in the care of tuberculosis is the establishment of the preventorium to which children are taken who have very mild degrees of tuberculosis or who come of families in which tuberculosis is prevalent. There they have opportunity to recover under the best conditions.

REST IN TUBERCULOSIS

Since rest is the most important single measure in aiding recovery from minimal tuberculosis in its early stages, the provision of adequate facilities in a sanatorium is fundamental to the control of tuberculosis in any community. Some states already have more beds than they need because of lowered number of cases.

In any ordinary year there are some fifty thousand deaths from tuberculosis in the United States. On the basis of five active cases for each death there would be about a quarter-million active cases of the disease always among us. The vast majority of people with this disease cannot be taken care of in institutions and the chief purpose of the institution may be to instruct a considerable number of people how to take care of themselves.

Rest, fresh air, and food, it has been repeatedly emphasized, are the important trilogy by which the person with tuberculosis must regulate his life. The sanatorium teaches the person how to follow this trilogy automatically and as an everyday procedure.

The person with active symptoms must have absolute rest. As symptoms quiet down the competent physician is able to tell the patient how much exercise is to be taken along with the rest to secure the best results. To most people fresh air means a lusty breeze pouring through a window or below-zero weather on an outdoor sleeping porch. It is important to realize that fresh air does not demand physical discomfort. Windows may be kept open, but the temperature should be equable, and drafts are unnecessary.

One of the chief values of the sanatorium is to teach the patient the routine facts regarding such matters as rest, exercise, diet, and fresh air. It will teach him also how to prevent the contamination of clothing, dishes, and other human beings with the organisms that are in his body. It will teach him his limitations in work and help to find work that he can do.

Thus will it have fulfilled a most useful function and when he is improved sufficiently to be on his way, the place he occupied will be filled by another pupil, and he will go out to help educate the public.

TREATMENT OF TUBERCULOSIS

For many years all sorts of specific remedies have been tried on the tuberculous, and millions of dollars have been mulcted from the people for patent medicines.

The first drug proved to be specific against the germ of tuberculosis is streptomycin. It seems to have established value in tuberculous meningitis, in miliary tuberculosis (which spreads rapidly throughout the lung) and in very severe cases of tuberculosis when there is secondary infection with pus in the chest cavity. The drug is also of value in tuberculosis of the kidney, the peritoneum and of the intestines. At present physicians do not believe that streptomycin should be used in the mild, early cases of tuberculosis because these cases are best cured by older technics which establish suitable resistance in the patient. The use of streptomycin in tuberculosis, combined with para-amino salicylic acid (PAS), and the combination of streptomycin with drugs like promin or diasone or tibione, which are sulfonamide derivatives, may bring about even more satisfactory improvement. The drugs are not a cure for tuberculosis; they supplement bed rest and specific methods of resting the lung.

Newest among drugs in tuberculosis are preparations of hydrazides of isonicotinic acid called isoniazid including remiofon, marsalid and pyrazidin. They bring about improvement, aid appetite and give a feeling of well-being. Another new drug proved efficient is cycloserine.

People with tuberculosis suffer frequently with fever and sweating at night. When these symptoms become oppressive, the doctor can prescribe drugs which will control them. An alcohol rub at bedtime or a sponge bath with luke-warm water containing about one gram of alum to the ounce is also helpful.

One of the most severe symptoms that may occur in a patient with tuberculosis is bleeding from the lungs. The appearance of this symptom is a danger signal which should cause the patient to lie down immediately and to get medical attention at once.

In the sanatorium in which the patients are treated for tuberculosis, one o the most useful remedies thus far developed is artificial pneumothorax. Thi involves the injection of air into the chest cavity, which serves to put the lung at rest. The same effect is also brought about by cutting the nerve which leads to the diaphragm, or by performing surgical operation on the ribs.

Tuberculosis could probably be completely controlled if every case with germs in the sputum could be isolated until freed of germs.

MENTAL ASPECTS IN TUBERCULOSIS

One of the most important factors in the care of the tuberculous is the co-operation of the patient in the handling of his disease.

In a thesis prepared in the University of Minnesota, Blanche Peterson insists that the most important single factor in the cure of tuberculosis is an intelligent attitude of the patient.

Doctors, nurses, and social workers endeavor, therefore, in every possible way to influence the patient to assume an intelligent and constructive outlook.

A questionnaire sent to a score of leading physicians who have specialized in this subject resulted in the almost universal response that reasonable and courageous attitudes are highly constructive. The worst states are those of fear, anxiety, and depression.

The patient with tuberculosis who becomes discouraged, hopeless, pessimistic, or rebellious is difficult to treat and aids in his downfall.

When a person first learns that he has this disease, he is likely to be upset and depressed. Knowing nothing of modern care, he is likely to feel that the disease will be promptly fatal.

If, however, the physician who makes the diagnosis will tell the patient that help is possible, that the disease is curable if treated sufficiently early and sufficiently long; that dozens of persons have achieved world-wide fame even though suffering from this disease, he is likely to have a different attitude and to coöperate fully in treatment.

Courage and reasonableness can come only with complete understanding of the situation. For this reason the health education of the tuberculous has come to be one of the most important factors in the control of this condition, and a vast literature has been developed for the purpose.

Practically every tuberculosis sanatorium and tuberculosis society now publishes books and pamphlets which are helpful in informing the tuberculous of the important facts relative to their condition.

The National Tuberculosis Association, 1790 Broadway, New York City, publishes much material that is useful. Such books as the guides and calendars for the tuberculous, edited by Lawrason Brown, are exceedingly helpful.[1]

Above all, the persons living with and surrounding the tuberculous must realize that it is their duty to keep the patient in a hopeful frame of mind and not treat him as a helpless invalid from the moment the diagnosis is made.

HEALTH HINTS FOR THE TUBERCULOUS

Here are some hints for people with tuberculosis. Many of these hints constitute excellent advice regarding hygiene for everyone who is slightly run down, whether tuberculous or not.

1. Never exercise to the point of fatigue. If you find yourself tired, you have done yourself harm.

2. Rest comes before exercise. By resting a surplus of strength and energy is built up and stored in the body.

3. Aim to spend as much of each day outdoors or in absolutely fresh air as possible. The air, to be fresh, need not necessarily be cold.

4. Ideal food should be appetizing, nutritious, and not too bulky. If appetizing and not nutritious, it will not nourish you; if nutritious and not appetizing, you will not eat it; if too bulky, however appetizing, it upsets your stomach.

5. Eat up to the limit of your digestion. It is the food which is digested and absorbed, and not what is put into your mouth, which will do you good. A glass of milk with each meal is advisable. Raw eggs are not as digestible as cooked eggs.

6. If your digestion is poor, tell your doctor.

[1] *Laws for Recovery from Pulmonary Tuberculosis.* Lawrason Brown, Saranac Lake, N. Y.

7. Eat your meals at regular hours. Do not take reading matter to the table.

8. Approach and leave each meal in a rested condition. Never eat when tired. Never exercise immediately after eating.

9. In winter, wear warm, light, or medium wool underwear; in summer, ordinary summer cotton underwear.

10. Never wear heavy underclothing or chest protectors.

11. Let your shoes be stout and warm in winter and wear warm woolen socks, by all means. Woolen socks at night are often a great comfort. In winter, a flannel shirt is much more comfortable than anything else. When sitting out in winter, have an extra wrap near by.

12. If you get overheated and perspire, change your clothing and rub dry.

13. A healthy condition of the skin is most important. A warm bath once or twice a week if ordered by your physician is advisable, and a cool sponge bath or a tub bath in the morning if your doctor permits it. The water should be cool but not ice cold. If you do not have a proper reaction after your bath, if you feel chilly or are blue, the water is too cold. Ask your doctor about it. See that your room or bathroom or wherever you take your bath is warm.

ULTRAVIOLET RAY IN TUBERCULOSIS OF THE LARYNX

Tuberculosis of the larynx has been considered, until recent years, one of the most dangerous forms of the disease, leading usually to fatality.

The drugs such as streptomycin and isoniazid are used. Tuberculosis in any part of the body demands careful treatment with the methods that are used for tuberculosis of the lungs and special methods designed for kidneys, skin, larynx or other part that may be involved.

With the discovery of the apparatus which yielded ultraviolet rays, in the form of the carbon arc and the quartz mercury vapor lamps, it became possible to apply concentrated sun's rays directly to the larynx. In order to get the rays directly to the laryngeal cords, various systems of mirrors have been devised, and also quartz stems along which the ultraviolet rays pass.

It has been found that people who are very frail, those with advanced tuberculosis of the lung, and those who have very severe lesions in the throat are treated better by means of the mirror reflection than by other methods.

A steel mirror will reflect about 44 per cent of the valuable rays into the larynx whereas ordinary glass mirrors absorb these rays and reflect only about 9 per cent. It has been found that practically all of the patients treated by direct sunlight to the cords tend to heal.

CONCLUSIONS

Particularly of importance in controlling the spread of tuberculosis is the use of dispensaries in which the disease can be diagnosed in its earliest stages and properly controlled. Experimentation with the method of vaccination against tuberculosis by Calmette has not yet gone sufficiently far to warrant its general adoption in this country.

The most powerful social factors in controlling the disease are housing, nutrition, and education. In educating people it is desirable to educate them not only in general hygiene but also especially as regards the prevention of tuberculosis. The regular examination of school children and teachers, studies of the nutrition of the school child, and education of those who are infected in methods of preventing the spread of the disease are significant factors.

The preventive institutions against tuberculosis today include holiday camps, open-air schools, preventoriums for children who are perhaps not certainly infected with tuberculosis but in such poor state of nutrition and general health that they offer easy prey to the disease, and certainly removal of children as soon as possible from contact with adults who are infected.

CHAPTER XII

Stress and Disease
HAROLD G. WOLFF, M.D.

O UR LANGUAGE BEARS WITNESS that men have been long aware that feelings and bodily changes are related. A few indicative phrases are:

> He got red in the face; he was pale with rage; it took one's breath away; he got into a cold sweat; it makes me sick; it turns my stomach; he had a lump in his throat; he got a weight off his chest; he trembled with fear; he shook with rage; he had cold feet.

Industry has not been blind to these facts. A thousand people sweat approximately 100 pounds of moisture in one hour under ordinary conditions, but under the emotionally charged conditions of a thrilling motion picture the moisture output rises to 150 pounds per thousand persons.

Bartlett's *Familiar Quotations* has in its index nine columns of phrases including the word "heart." Roget's *Thesaurus* has "heart" in the index more often than any other word. Indeed, "heart" has become a symbol of the human spirit, thus, "hard-hearted," "warm-hearted," "cold-hearted," "steel-hearted." We continually use words that indicate our knowledge that the body participates in reactions to experience. How pertinent these bodily changes are to health, and how these changes begin to disturb a man's effectiveness and jeopardize his life, will be seen in the following pages.

SKIN

The skin offers dramatic demonstrations of change during stress. For example, the minute vessels of a man's skin were tested as regards their ability to retain blood within them, called, for convenience, capillary tone. The left arm was forcefully struck, and immediately a red area appeared which began to swell, and the deterioration of the capillary tone was charted. The skin of the right arm behaved in the same way even though it was not struck. The left arm gradually returned to its former state; the right arm reached that state a little sooner. The experiment was repeated, but, instead of bringing the ferrule down onto the forearm, it was brought just short of the arm. Even though no injury was inflicted by this sham blow, the skin of the left arm behaved just as it had before. That of the right arm did not respond. Gradually the left returned to its former state. In other words, this person, through his skin, reacted not only to an actual blow but also to the symbol of a blow by putting into his tissues a certain amount of fluid, perhaps representing not only a reaction to tissue injury, but also a means to protect him from injury. The whole procedure was repeated, except that this time the subject was told what was going to happen; after the expected sham blow, no bodily change took place.

Another man with a complaint of hives was studied. A record was made of the ability of his capillaries to hold their contents. Instead of striking him with a ferrule, we discussed a situation involving his family which made him feel as though he were being hit. At the same time, his skin behaved as though he were actually struck, and he developed "hives." In a little while they disappeared. In this instance a bodily pattern serving to protect from injury was used in a way in which it was of no specific value.

A man's skin was tested for ability to react to stroking, and to the chemical poisons, histamine and pilocarpine. His skin was insensitive to all of these. He was then exposed to a discussion about his family troubles which made him feel as though he were "taking a beating." At the height of his reaction the very same mechanical and chemical stimuli that failed before to produce an effect produced a great effect, seen as hives. In other words, he became at this time vulnerable to a great many assaults, not only to the effects which came from the discussion of his family troubles, but also to other noxious influences. He was, at that moment, in a weakened or vulnerable state. With reassurance he soon returned to his original condition.

Stenographic records of remarks during such bodily changes were made. During a conversation in which a man was developing hives, we heard: "They did a lot of things to me and I couldn't do anything about it." "I was getting pushed around." "I had to sit and take it." "I was taking a beating." "They were cracking a whip over me." "My mother is constantly hammering on me." "He walked all over me." In other words, while his body is acting as though it were "taking a beating," he feels as though he were being exposed to such an assault. The organism deals with an assault in a given way and uses that pattern again and again, sometimes in reaction to noxious interpersonal relations where it can serve no useful or appropriate end.

STOMACH

A man was offered food which interested him, and immediately the measured blood flow in the lining of his stomach increased. (Fig. 19.) A record of the mechanical action of the stomach showed that it was churning and contracting. Also the digestive secretions had increased in amount, i.e., the stomach was preparing for the act of digestion even though the man was only look-

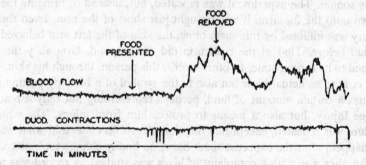

Fig. 19. Changes in blood flow and motility associated with the sight and smell of appetizing food.

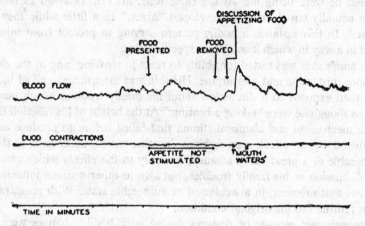

Fig. 20. Changes in blood flow and motility associated with the discussion of appetizing food. (Note the absence of changes with the sight and smell of unappetizing food.)

(Reproduced by permission of the *Journal of Clinical Investigation,* from "The Measurement and Recording of Gastroduodenal Blood Flow in Man by Means of a Thermal Gradientometer," by Richards, Wolf and Wolff)

ing at food. When the food was removed, the blood flow and contractions gradually returned to their initial level. Other food was offered which did not appeal to him; his "appetite" was not stimulated and consequently there was no change noted in the function of his stomach. (Fig. 20.)

Next, the food was removed from view, and instead of introducing something he could see or smell, food that he liked was discussed. (Fig. 20.) Immediately his stomach prepared for digestive activity. Words symbolic of food rather than food itself were the stimuli. A topic which was extremely poisonous to this patient was then presented. During an absence due to illness, his business partner had carried on some shady business deals which had brought him disrepute. As he discussed his partner's behavior he became exceedingly angry, and his stomach and upper gastro-intestinal tract acted as though they were preparing to digest. (Fig. 21.)

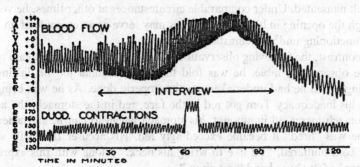

Fig. 21. Gastroduodenal blood flow in man. Increase in duodenal blood flow accompanying anxiety, tension, and resentment. (The pressure is calibrated in mm. of water.) The rise in the upper recording indicates an increase of blood flow in the walls of the duodenal portion of the intestine, during an interview which aroused feelings of anxiety, tension, and resentment.

(Reproduced by permission of the *Journal of Clinical Investigation*, from "The Measurement and Recording of Gastroduodenal Blood Flow in Man by Means of a Thermal Gradientometer," by Richards, Wolf and Wolff)

One of our subjects, "Tom," now about age sixty-five, experienced a serious accident when he was nine. He came home from school one day, thirsty and warm, and mistakenly drank scalding hot clam chowder. He thus blocked his gullet and could not swallow. In order to keep him alive surgeons created a hole in his abdomen leading to his stomach, and through this opening he has since fed himself twice a day for more than half a century. He is a good citizen, father, and worker. He is shy, taciturn, with strong feelings about "respectability" and his capacity to take his place in the community. He is now employed as a helper in the New York Hospital. He comes into the laboratory every day, and the blood flow in his stomach lining is measured—the more blood flow, the redder the lining; the less blood flow, the paler the lining. The secretion of gastric juices and the churning activity of his stomach are also ascertained. At the same time a note is made of his current fears, hopes, wishes, frustrations, and satisfactions.

On one occasion while "Tom" was in the laboratory a physician entered saying that a certain important protocol, the safekeeping of which was Tom's responsibility, was missing. Gradually he grew pale in face and stomach as his terror increased. The troubled doctor opened and closed drawers, muttering imprecations. He finally found the protocol and left. Tom said, "I was scared that I had lost my job." This statement has to be seen in symbolic terms. The man was in terror that he had lost his position not only as our fellow worker, but also that he had "lost face" as one who had been entrusted with responsibility. His stomach was pale, hypoactive, non-functioning. It was "out of condition," distended, and digestion was slowed. He complained of flatulence, food remained in the stomach a long time, he experienced gaseous eructations, and felt nauseated. Under comparable circumstances at other times, he vomited through the opening in his abdomen. This may serve as an example of an organ hypofunctioning under circumstances of stress.

In contrast, the following observation was made on Tom when, again resting on the observation table, he was told that an additional job of dusting and cleaning which he had undertaken was improperly done. As he was being told about his inadequacy Tom got red in the face, red in the stomach, the acid in his stomach increased in amount, his stomach began to churn, and when told that he was "fired" it became exceedingly red. His accuser then left, whereupon Tom muttered, "I'd like to wring his neck." Along with this expression of anger he felt abused and "put upon."

Such changes in the stomach may last for weeks. The acid secretion and the color of the stomach before, during, and after a period of crisis are exemplified in the following situation: Receiving a small salary, Tom was obliged to accept the contributions of a benefactor who meddled in his personal affairs. This threatened his independence and he repeatedly made efforts to throw off his benefactor. Finally, during a two-week period the meddling was particularly irksome, and his stomach exhibited a high acid secretion and a deep red color. A slight raise in salary enabled him to be rid of his benefactor, and his stomach returned to its former state.

Also studied was another man who had a similar abdominal aperture through which his stomach could be viewed. The lining of the stomach had a pink color when he was tranquil. But when a certain doctor was mentioned whom he hated because he believed he had failed to diagnose his illness, which he feared was to cost him his life, he became exceedingly angry. He sputtered and became profane, and his stomach mucosa became dark red. Thus as part of his reactions to the poisonous topic involving his hates and fears, impulses went down the vagus nerve which converted the mucous membrane of the stomach from a resting state to one of readiness for eating, and one, which if sustained, could lead to ulcer formation. It became necessary to cut this major nerve to the stomach, i.e., the vagus. After surgery, discussion of this same doctor was associated with every outward show of anger, but there was no change within his stomach.

ATTITUDES

Feelings are part of our reaction to events. They should not be spoken of as causing bodily changes. What one feels is not truly causative, but only another manifestation of one's reaction to experience. In other words, when something happens to you, you develop an attitude which has two components. First, what meaning has this experience for me? Secondly, what do I do about it?

This attitude is, for the most part, unconscious. When a person rids himself of something by vomiting because it is disgusting or unattractive, he expresses a characteristic attitude. Recorded statements included: "I wish it hadn't happened." "I didn't want this." "Why did it have to happen?" "I wish things were the way they were before." "I wish I hadn't gotten into this." "I wish I hadn't listened to him."

Much has been said concerning the conscious versus the unconscious, but an appraisal of the *meaning of a situation for the individual person* is far more relevant. If it be conscious, it has a chance of being dealt with; if it be unconscious, it is less accessible and the person may suffer its effects for indefinitely long periods. Often matters are so dreadful and so overwhelming that they are dismissed from consciousness. But to repeat: important for consideration is, "What is the *meaning* of an experience or a stimulus or a threat or a statement?" and then, "What do I do about it?"

BOWEL

Four people with abdominal apertures allowing views of the large bowel gave us much information about the connection between the bowel and life experiences. One man had a thumbscrew arrangement put on top of his head. He willingly volunteered, although he knew that he was going to be hurt. Painfully squeezing his head with the thumbscrews caused his bowel to get red and to contract. He felt angry and anxious, but placidly accepted the assault. The second man, despite the fact that he wished to participate and knew what was going to happen, became angry and showed it. Indeed, he would not permit the experiment to continue. Also, this second man had, in reaction to exactly the same stimulus under the same circumstances, precisely the opposite bodily reaction as did the first man. His bowel got pale, and contractile activity stopped. A general principle is thus exemplified: Here were two people exposed to the same assault, yet, because its meaning was different, they experienced opposite reactions. The assault engendered a distinctly individual attitude in each of the men, leading to different ways of meeting the threat and danger.

In a similar study it was observed that a person's bowel when he was in a state of relative tranquillity was pink in color. During a period featured by dejection or sadness, it became pale and relaxed. During a period with anger it contracted and became dark red, and a balloon inserted within the bowel showed it to be hypermotile. Also, about twenty minutes after eating, it became red and hypermotile even during a period of tranquillity. This is the so-called gastrocolic reflex and it is the basis of the urge to empty the bowel shortly after meals. It serves a good purpose, but it is not good for this condition to be maintained by anger. The same man was observed on another day after lunch, under ostensibly the same circumstances, but reacting to the lunch not at all as regards to change in color and blood supply of his mucosa, or the contractile state of his bowel. He was dejected because of an unfortunate and humiliating incident involving a neighbor which occurred just a few hours before. The subject under these circumstances would have no urge to evacuate the bowel and indeed might consider himself "constipated."

THE SIGNIFICANCE OF THE TOPIC

When a topic is introduced that sets off a given reaction during an interview, it does not mean that the subject matter is the key to the person's life difficulties and that if this particular problem be solved, all of his troubles would end. The topic under discussion is merely representative of many which are looked upon as threats and reacted to in a similar way. For example, we discussed with a sensitive man something about his sister-in-law. This man's bowel trouble, known as ulcerative colitis, began shortly after the death of his mother upon whom he was overdependent. He was devastated by her death. He duly assumed the position of head of the family with vigor, but without conviction or effectiveness. His younger brother married and brought into the home a woman who, by her attitude and behavior, threatened the patient's position as head of the family. Merely discussing this woman caused his bowel to contract and become dark red. His sister-in-law had become a threatening symbol. He reacted to many other threats in the same manner. The bowel acted as though it were trying to get rid of an irritant.

A sailor, with similarly exposed colon, believed that because of his religious affiliations he was not given a "good berth" on ship. Discussion of the problem caused his feelings to be roused, anger expressed, and his bowel to contract, become overactive, and dark red. He was easily diverted, however, and within a few minutes the bowel became paler and relaxed. Again, within a few minutes he felt much threatened and challenged by questions which he took to indicate that his integrity was in doubt, and again the bowel became dark red and contracted vigorously.

The overcontracted, hypermotile gastro-intestinal tract with a dark red mucous membrane becomes very fragile. When a person is relaxed and tranquil, a negative pressure of up to 200 mm. of mercury applied to the bowel surface may be withstood for six minutes without damage or bleeding. But when a person subject to ulcerative colitis becomes insecure and angry and the bowel is in an overactive, congested state, it takes very little—say 60 mm. of mercury pressure for 1½ minutes, or even the gut's own contractions—to cause the tissue to tear and bleed. Under these circumstances when bleeding so readily occurs, many small erosions and ulcers may appear. In other words, this exposed portion of mucous membrane goes to pieces under circumstances that can have little to do with the nature of the colonic content or the feces. These damaged areas may become the sites of serious hemorrhage which occasionally cause death.

Thus a stressful life circumstance or a symbol thereof evokes protective reactions—in this particular instance, the desire to get rid of something by pushing it out of the gut, by vomiting, or diarrhea. The person feels angry, resentful, hostile, as well as anxious and apprehensive, although his outward behavior may be passive at the same time. Concurrently manifesting itself, although not causally related, is altered function of the colon with increased contractility, increased blood flow, engorgement, alteration of secretion with bleeding, tearing of the gut, erosions, ulcerations, hemorrhages, and perhaps secondary infection. (Fig. 22.)

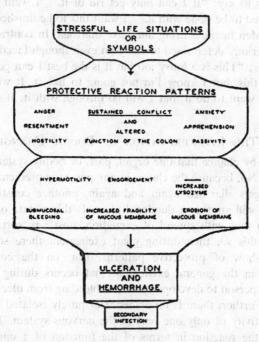

Fig. 22. A schema suggesting the relationship of life situations, emotional reactions and bodily defects which lead to ulceration of the colon. (Reproduced by permission of the Association for Research in Nervous and Mental Disorders, from "Life Situations," by Dr. William J. Grace)

On the other hand, when a patient bleeding profusely from the bowels, with fever and weight loss, makes contact with another human being who helps alter his attitudes, re-establish his self-esteem, re-establish his faith and trust in himself and others, his body may also restore itself. In so doing, his temperature becomes normal, he gains in weight, and the body diarrhea, which is the inappropriate expression of the drive to get rid of something, stops.

Constipation and diarrhea are opposites in their functional significance. Diarrhea serves to rid the organism of some noxious agent it has inadvertently admitted by mouth or otherwise and is associated with increased redness, contraction, and heightened motility of the bowel, so that as quickly as possible the noxious agent may be emitted. Constipation is associated with a large, relaxed, pale bowel showing ineffective contractions of the terminal portions, with retention of ingested substances for longer than the usual periods. Contraction of the muscles around the outlet further impedes the ejection of the bowel contents.

What does such a person feel? What attitudes does he express at the time that these patterns are being enacted? The person with diarrhea or ulcerative colitis is likely to say: "If I can only get rid of it." "I want to get this over with." "I wanted to be done with it." "I want this to be finished." "I want it to be all over." Men facing a firing line have diarrhea. In contrast, the one with constipation, grimly determined to carry on even though faced with little hope of change, says: "This is a lousy job but it is the best I can get. I will have to keep on with this, but I know I'm not going to like it. It will never be any better. I don't want to do it, but I will go through with it. It's no good, but I won't quit."

THE INTERPRETATION OF BODILY CHANGES

Is it purely by chance that one organ, part, or bodily system is used rather than another? No, because the choice in any person is predictable. One person under stress gets diarrhea again and again, another constipation, another vomiting, and still another a duodenal ulcer. Is this a state of general excitement only, so that with spread of excitation most any sort of change may occur? Were this so, then during great excitement there should be an indiscriminate show of protective patterns. But, on the contrary, there is evidence that in the general excitement that occurs during battle it is uncommon for a person to develop asthma, or bleeding from ulceration, colitis, or peptic ulcer. Further, there is no evidence of purely isolated responses representing the activity of only one part of the nervous system. Thus it does not help to view the reaction in terms of the function of a unique part of the nervous system or of any particular endocrine gland.

The person at times of stress is using protective or adaptive patterns which have in their literal application a highly useful purpose, i.e., to improve ventilation, to maintain nutrition, circulation, or to get rid of a poison. When dealing with a poison it is useful to vomit or have diarrhea. When dealing with one's sister-in-law it is of no use. In the latter instance it is inappropriate, and therefore may become an excessively prolonged pattern of action; appropriately used, it serves a good end, but when used awkwardly and, because of that, excessively, the person may be damaged.

That does not mean that these patterns in action do not serve a useful purpose. A good display of tears with frustration, for example, will often make one feel better. A pattern in action—running, jumping, crying out, weeping, vomiting—brings with it a degree of tranquillity even though no resolution has occurred. But the price is often high, and if the pattern continues in operation excessively or too long, tissues may be damaged. The person who shows such an uneconomic and inappropriate use of equipment is punished accordingly.

AIRWAYS

A man was examined as regards the color of his nasal mucous membranes by simply looking into his nostrils. Day after day the color of his mucous membranes went along in a steady way, as contrasted with that of another man. The latter's nasal mucous membranes were red one day and pale the next, red on one side and pale on the other. When a person is exposed to smelling salts, he suddenly gasps, and the mucous membrane of the nose gets dark red and swollen; water pours out, and he hardly can get any air through; he may not be able to speak; his chest seems held in a vise. It would appear that he is attempting to neutralize, wash away, and shut out a very unattractive feature of the environment. When exposed to rose pollen, a sensitive man developed symptoms of "hay fever," and his nose reacted as it did when exposed to smelling salts. He attempted, seemingly, to shut out, wash away, and neutralize the noxious agent to which he had been exposed. He exhibited a proper use of the nose.

But consider a woman with a long history of nose troubles, resulting in several operations. She couldn't get air freely, and her nose seemed to be stopped up much of the time, particularly at night and especially when her husband was in the room smoking. It was suggested by her physician in an interview that perhaps her troubles were related to her attitudes and her husband. She violently rejected the suggestion and burst into tears. The mucous membrane on the inside of her nose became dark red and there was much secretion and swelling. A little while later it appeared pale, boggy, and solidly occluded. This woman acted as though she were shutting out, neutralizing, and washing away some noxious agent. Figure 23 shows what took place in her airways during the discussion. The membranes of this woman's upper airways became redder, more swollen, wetter, and the air passage was completely closed.

These changes may last minutes, or days, as exhibited by an ambitious young physician who was much concerned with his career and was obliged to work intimately with a professional partner in his hospital some years his senior, but junior in experience and wisdom. He resented working with this colleague and feared that his future was jeopardized by the inadequate performance of his associate. Their relationship deteriorated rapidly. During a two-week period, while his conflicts with this colleague were most severe, he exhibited red and swollen mucous membranes, with quantities of fluid pouring out and scarcely any space for the passage of air. He developed headache, which he called "sinus headache," and had red eyes, tender swollen flushed cheeks, and tender forehead. His nasal mucous membranes were exceedingly sensitive to touch. During an interview the mucous membranes swelled further, additional secretion poured out, and increased quantities of pus cells appeared in the secretion. It was possible to separate these men, and soon thereafter the patient became

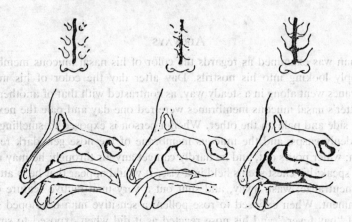

Fig. 23. Diagrammatic representation of the turbinate bones and their mucous membrane coverings and their appearance in various stages of swelling. Obstruction to air passage is indicated schematically by arrows. Note that minor deviations in the septum (see vertical line in upper pictures) may become important when the turbinates are swollen. (Reproduced by permission of Charles C. Thomas, Publishers, from *The Nose* by Holmes, Goodell, Wolf and Wolff)

symptom free and his nasal mucous membranes became paler and much less swollen, with little secretion and no obstruction.

Summative effects are evident when one kind of noxious stimulus is added to another. A patient was brought into a room containing a constant amount of circulating pollen in the air. She had "hay fever" in the pollen season and was sensitive to this pollen, and as she sat in this room her mucous membranes began to redden and swell slightly. Then, in addition to the irritating pollen, a topic concerning her troubles and her quarrels with her father was introduced. Immediately her symptoms were greatly augmented and her airways became obstructed. She was then reassured by the words of her physician, and, despite the fact that she remained in the room laden with pollen, the membranes were restored even to their initial state, akin to that noted before she entered the pollen-laden room. In this instance, then, the more important noxious agent of the two seemed to be her relation to her father, rather than to the pollen, although both were operating.

An anatomical defect in the nose, present since birth, can under certain circumstances take on importance in middle life or later. For example, a deviated septum which has been present for a lifetime may become important when one's relations to others become of such a nature as to call forth the protective reaction of shutting out, washing away, and neutralizing. A man may then need to have his septum removed to allow more air to get through his nose.

The asthmatic person is closely akin in his pattern of reaction to the one who has trouble with his nose. Indeed, an asthmatic reaction seldom occurs without nasal involvement. It becomes evident by direct inspection that threatening topics cause the mucous membranes of the bronchi to become redder, wetter, and the lumen to become smaller. During a series of observations, topics calling forth feelings of bitterness, regret, and failure also precipitated asthmatic attacks.

Sensations of "air hunger," tightness in the chest, and "butterflies in the stomach" are sometimes experienced under stressful circumstances. Tight, unpleasant feelings of pressure in the middle of the chest may be mistaken for pains originating in the heart. These may result from a cramp of the diaphragm, a sheet of muscle separating the lungs and heart from the contents of the abdomen. When an X-ray picture of the diaphragm of a person in a relaxed and tranquil state is compared with that of his diaphragm when he is anxious, the latter shows a contracted state which would make it difficult to take in more air. There may be a fluttering sensation and sometimes cramps just underneath the heart.

SPECIFICITY OF REACTIONS TO STRESS

When presenting a protective or adaptive reaction, people do not necessarily exhibit the whole of the reaction pattern; fragmentation of the pattern is characteristic. If one wished to shut out an unattractive experience, one could close off the entire airway system, but, actually, the reaction involves a small part of the pattern—that involving the nose. If one did not want to take something into the stomach, one could close the mouth, shut off the gullet, and vomit, but, actually, only a piece of the pattern, such as the closure of the gullet, may be exhibited.

Also, there is specificity as regards reactions during stress. Any kind or amount of stress doesn't evoke just any or all kinds of reactions. Observations were made by a distinguished physician in Holland who, during the bad years of Holland's occupation by the Germans, was able to examine a number of patients with ulcers of the stomach. He attended their medical needs before the Germans came and attended them also after they were put in concentration camps because of their religion. Before the war they were wealthy, comfortable, and successful merchants. They suffered a good deal with their stomachs. In the concentration camps their plight was horrible; they never knew in the morning whether they would survive that day. Life was filled with much stress, yet these people lost all manifestations of their peptic ulceration. The ironic aspect of it is that many of them regained their peptic ulcers and symptoms when they returned to "Main Street." The specific type of stress which had engendered the ulcer in their stomach lining was absent during the terror of their stay in the concentration camp.

A group of people with intense and frequent headaches were missionaries in Japan. During the heyday of their missionary activity they suffered considerably, even though esteemed and presumably effective. When these people were put into Japanese concentration camps, with all the deprivations entailed, they lost their headaches. When they were freed at the end of the war, the headaches returned. These instances indicate that danger has to have a specific meaning to a person in order to produce specific changes.

People may exhibit one and sometimes two of these protective or adaptive patterns. You may at one time have vascular headaches and at another time peptic ulcers; sometimes you may have them both together. Certain combinations, such as ulcers of the large bowel occurring with ulcers of the stomach, are uncommon.

Thus tissue derangement may be considered a part of an adjustment which was meant to protect the individual, including swelling, edema, reduction of blood supply to tissue, tenderness, inflammation, erosion, hemorrhage, ulceration, pus formation, changes in secretion, and lowering of the pain threshold.

Over-all Mobilization Patterns

So far, considerations have included patterns involving portals of entry— the mouth and airways—and portals of exit—the rectum and anus. Under certain circumstances the organism may exhibit general mobilization for action. If a man runs upstairs or exercises vigorously, he increases the output of blood from his heart with each beat: his heart rate is increased, his blood pressure goes up, and the amount of resistance offered to the flow of blood by the minute vessels in the tissues of the body is decreased. Such reactions, by insuring a good supply of blood to muscles, serve to make his actions more effective.

Similarly, in an interview in which some important relationship to another person is discussed which causes you to be frankly anxious and frightened, you act just as though you were running upstairs, or preparing for battle. A patient came to us in a tense, anxious state, complaining of pounding heart and breathlessness. Climbing a certain number of steps caused his already augmented stroke volume (the amount of blood ejected by the heart per beat) to be further increased. The heart rate also was increased. As the patient's general life adjustment improved, his circulation gradually improved, so that ten months later the same effort produced a minimal but effective response. At this time his state was relatively tranquil and relaxed.

A man ostensibly loved but actually hated his mother, although he never admitted this even to himself. He presented a bland exterior during an interview, but his blood pressure rose and the resistance offered to the passage of blood by blood vessels of many of his organs mounted. His blood became much stickier and coagulated more readily. During the interview concerning his relations with his mother, his blood pressure went up sharply and, as a part of his generally increased resistance to the flow of blood, the amount of blood that went through the kidneys was much decreased. With the increased stickiness and clotting proclivity of the blood, he might have damaged organs further.

This clotting device serves presumably to help the animal stop bleeding during mortal combat, but when it is used every time a person comes in contact with his mother, it follows that he might appreciably damage his kidneys and perhaps his brain. Again, a device that serves to protect and prolong life is called into action so inappropriately as to threaten a man's very existence. On the other hand, a patient with elevated blood pressure did, by a restoration of self-esteem and by changing attitudes toward his environment, gradually, over a period of a year and a half, bring down the level of the blood pressure to the average.

Another feature of the mobilization reaction to threats results in backache. The amount of an individual's muscle contraction is indicated by the firmness of the muscle when it is felt. It can be shown also by a record of the electrical disturbance in the muscle, which roughly parallels in amount the magnitude of contractions. While a man was exposed to a discussion aimed to bring into focus feelings of hostility and anxiety, contraction of the big muscles of his back and legs increased, presumably in readiness for action, for fight, or flight. Being thus contracted for long periods, but not actually associated with movement which brings also relaxation, they began to hurt. When topics that interested him and brought him esteem and satisfaction were discussed, the muscle activity was reduced, but with a reconsideration of the threatening matters, the muscle contraction was again increased and again he had backache.

Similar painful contraction occurs in the muscles of the head and neck. Headaches can persist for days, weeks, or months, due to the sustained contraction of the sheet of muscle at the top of the head and neck when an individual is exposed to an environment which calls forth the need to be on the alert against assaults that may never come but always threaten. Electrical records of these muscles were recorded during such a headache and showed much contraction. A few weeks later, after the patient had had an opportunity to express something of his anxieties and fears and had adopted another attitude, the sheet of muscle was no longer contracted and the headache ended.

Blood vessel headaches, such as migraine, constitute a most important bloc of man's discomfort. A person with migraine headache may exhibit large, swollen blood vessels on the side of his head. A woman suffering with many headaches of high intensity came to the doctor on the first of September. She had had bad relations with her child and, frightened by the intensity of her anger, feared she might injure her child. She had no headache for nine days after telling this story to an understanding physician. However, the matter was rediscussed with her on the tenth day, and inadvertently her feelings of guilt and hostility were roused again (Fig. 24.), and a headache was precipitated. The headache was ended by the introduction of an agent which causes swollen blood vessels to come back to their original shape.

A similar headache was induced in a woman by an interview involving her husband, concerning whom her hostile feelings were barely suppressed. During

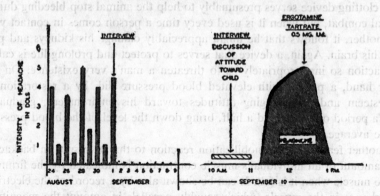

Fig. 24. Precipitation of a migraine headache in a woman following a
stressful interview concerning her feelings of guilt and resentment
toward her child, which evoked anger.
(Reproduced by permission of *Psychomatic Medicine*, from "A Form
of the Dynamics of the Migraine Headache," by Wolff and Marchissen)

discussion of this topic a headache developed as the large arteries of her head
began to swell and painfully to pulsate. Instead of using an agent causing the
blood vessels to constrict, this woman's faith in her doctor was utilized. When
an intravenous injection of neutral salt water solution was then given, the
vessels constricted and her headache stopped. In other words, normal salt was
capable of terminating this woman's headache just as would an active, con-
strictor agent.

Stock Factor and Organ Inferiority

Why don't we all have the same bodily reactions during stress? Why do
some of us get high blood pressure, others peptic ulcer, still others ulcerative
colitis, others asthma, and others headache? We might as well ask: "Why are
we different? Why do we look at the same assault or threat differently?" And in
this rests the answer. In looking at it differently, we are prepared to meet it
differently. These reactions represent our individual ways of meeting a threat.
Do we run toward it? Do we run away from it? Do we try to avoid it? Do
we try to act as though it didn't exist? Do we wish to fight but dare not? All
these and more are possible ways of dealing with a threat. Now why is it that
individuals of some families have headache, hypertension, or stomach trouble?
Again, we might as well ask: "Why do dogs of certain breeds easily learn to
retrieve birds, or fight fiercely, or follow scents? Why do beavers construct
dams? Why do squirrels hoard nuts?"

The implication is that there are proclivities handed down; its easier for a
bird dog to learn to be a bird dog. It doesn't follow that the proclivity leads to
disease, it only means that it's easier for an individual to meet his problems
in some ways rather than in others.

Thus he has inherited a proclivity which makes it easier for him to use a particular pattern. In addition, a way of dealing with life is shown every day by parents, and the child gradually takes it on as his way. For example, the individual whose parents have headaches would be likely to have a headache when the going is tough. But it doesn't mean that his life needs to be given over to headaches if he understands his nature, his way of looking at things, and how much of the latter he has learned from his parents, and that he can learn other ways, too.

Moreover, the repeated or prolonged participation of a given organ in a protective pattern cannot be construed as evidence of the weakness or inferiority of that organ, even though, because of such participation, it fails to maintain its structural integrity. The individual may be said to be in a weak or vulnerable state, but the organ can hardly be said to be weak and, indeed, may be especially well developed and strong for long periods before it finally fails.

CULTURE AND STRESS

It is doubtful if man has ever considered himself under more stress than he does today. A most conspicuous feature of our time is rapidity of change in values and customs. Cultures with opposite emphases, as, for example, Japanese and American, concerning parents, property, and relations with children exhibit the same disorders; thus the cultural values alone cannot be the prime factor. But in any rapidly changing culture a man's faith in his customs, habits, intuitions, his leaders, teachers, and parents is shaken.

With a cultural emphasis upon the desirability and need to face a "changing world," a man is mistakenly led to believe that long-term values and basic human relationships are also changing. Undoubtedly rapid and relatively superficial changes in mores bewilder those who cannot separate the wheat from the chaff. To be sure, there have been rapid changes in attitudes toward property and possessions; women's place politically and economically, and in manners. Also subject to rapid change have been the amount of social mobility, the precise symbols of power and prestige, the desirability or amount of "outdoing" one's neighbor. But there is no change in such basic elements in human societies as belief in man and in the desirability of his survival; recognition of his tribal nature and his responsibility to the group; certain aspects of a man's relationship to his mate; acceptance of adult and parental responsibility and the giving of effective support during childhood.

Two persons out of three exhibiting stress manifestations can be significantly relieved. The thoughtful doctor can do much to indicate that first things come first and to give support while the individual reorients himself. A responsible person of authority who helps the sufferer regain his self-esteem and change his attitudes can help him restore his body to more appropriate patterns of functioning. Certainly we can get courage from the knowledge that when we pursue a goal, we pay a price. If we know what the price is, we may then decide whether the goal is worth the cost. There are aims more important than comfort, and occasionally even more important than health. But when you know what price you are paying for your goals, you may decide that your values are poor and, by changing your attitudes, restore yourself.

EPITOME

The stresses to which man is exposed include assaults by many living forms that aim to invade as parasites or to destroy; by meteorologic and climatic crises; by mechanical, electrical, and thermal forces that operate upon man merely in terms of his mass and volume, and by elements of the earth's crust that man manipulates for his comfort and delight or to satisfy a passion for destruction.

Man is further vulnerable because he is so constituted that he reacts not only to the actual existence of danger, but to threats and symbols of danger experienced in his past which call forth reactions little different from those to the assault itself. Since his adaptive and protective capabilities are limited, the response to many sorts of damaging agents and threats in any given man may be similar, the form of the reaction to any one agent depending more on the individual's nature and past experience than upon the particular injurious agent evoking it. Finally, because of its magnitude and duration, the adaptive-protective reaction may be far more damaging to the individual than the effects of the noxious agent *per se*.

Also—most important—man is a tribal or group creature with a long period of dependence and development. He is dependent for his very existence upon the aid, support, and encouragement of other men. He lives his life so much in contact with men and in such concern about their expectations of him that he is jeopardized as well as supported by his fellows; indeed, he may feel more threatened by cultural and individual human pressures than by other environmental forces. He must be part of the tribe and yet he is driven to fulfil his own proclivities. These pressures and the conflicts they engender are ubiquitous and create a large portion of man's stress.

In other words, in times of stress bodily changes and feeling states are evoked, representing a reaction to something that threatens us. What is its meaning? What do we do about it? Do we run? Do we try to get rid of it by vomiting? Do we grimly hold on? Do we try to act as though it never was? Do we try to deal with it by non-participation? All of these action patterns are associated with bodily changes and concurrent feelings, and bring with them a degree of tranquillity. But when used too long, they damage tissue and threaten the life that they might have prolonged.

CHAPTER XIII

Arthritis, Rheumatism, and Gout

HOWARD F. POLLEY, M.D.

ARTHRITIS, RHEUMATISM, and gout are among the oldest diseases known to affect human beings. Hippocrates, a Greek physician called the "Father of Medicine," described these conditions graphically many centuries ago. Evidence of the occurrence of these diseases even before his time has been found in mummies and excavations from other ancient civilizations. The widespread occurrence of these diseases in the United States at present is indicated by the presence of some form of rheumatic disease in more than 11,000,000 people in this country.

The terms "arthritis" and "rheumatism" have been used synonymously at times, but as a result of advances in our medical knowledge, physicians can now recognize almost a hundred different kinds of arthritis and almost another hundred kinds of rheumatism. Arthritic diseases are those that affect singly or in various combinations the tissues of the joint: (1) the *cartilage*, (2) the adjacent *bone*, and (3) the *synovial (lining) membrane*. Rheumatism, by contrast, affects tissues *outside* the joint, sometimes spoken of as "the soft tissues." These tissues include the fibrous tissue or capsule immediately surrounding the joint and also lining or enveloping bundles of muscles and sheaths of nerves, ligaments, tendons, and bursae. Terms such as "fibrositis," "tendinitis," "bursitis," "myositis," or "myalgia," depending on which structure is affected, or the term "periarthritis," meaning around but not in the joint itself, may be used in describing the location of the rheumatism. Rheumatism may affect a person who also has arthritis, but rheumatism can and often does occur without arthritis.

There are both acute and chronic types of rheumatism and arthritis. Persons of any age and either sex may have practically any of the various types of arthritis and rheumatism. The most common type of arthritis is known as *osteoarthritis,* which can be found to some extent in almost all persons past middle age. Hence this type of arthritis is often attributed to the results of "wear and tear" of use of joints of the body over a long time. Fortunately, though most persons may acquire some evidence of osteoarthritis, symptoms from the presence of the osteoarthritis occur only infrequently. Hence the presence of osteoarthritis is not necessarily evidence that a person's "rheumatic" or "arthritic" symptoms are the result of this type of arthritis.

Another type of arthritis of particular significance is *rheumatoid arthritis*. Physicians find that about one out of three patients who have symptoms of arthritis have this type of arthritis. It can affect persons of any age but tends to occur more commonly in the young adult years. Women are affected by rheumatoid arthritis two or three times as frequently as are men.

The most common types of rheumatism include *bursitis, fibrositis, tendinitis* or *periarthritis* in the various parts of the body in which these tissues are particularly subject to rheumatic involvement. Another kind of rheumatism that is common is that which results from muscular and nervous tension and emotional fatigue. This is sometimes called *"psychosomatic rheumatism."*

Gout is a special type of metabolic disorder of the bodily functions which may be manifested by the occurrence at various times of either arthritis or rheumatism. Gouty arthritis (or bursitis or rheumatism) is related to the body's inability to dispose properly of chemicals, known as purines, eaten in certain foods or accumulating (as urates or uric acid) as a result of certain metabolic processes within the body itself. Gout almost always affects men past middle age, although occasionally it occurs earlier than this. Gout affects women only infrequently (about one case in fifty), and then usually late in life. Gouty involvement occurs in the region of the "bunion joint" of the great toe, other joints of the feet, the ankles, and occasionally the knees, hands, wrists, or elbows. Usually only one joint or tendon or bursa is affected at a time. Attacks of gouty arthritis develop rapidly, and the affected area becomes red, warm, and painful. The acute episode may last for a few days or perhaps weeks before it completely subsides. Even after the acute attack is gone, however, the basic derangement of bodily metabolism continues to exist and may require treatment. If the disease continues uncontrolled, multiple joints or articular areas may be affected and there may be gouty deposits in the bone and joints or bursae or ligaments which may be affected. This ultimately can result in a change from an acute to a chronic gouty arthritis. Similar gouty deposits are sometimes found on the ears and also can occur in the kidneys. Treatment for gout may include a special diet and drugs. This is discussed under the heading "Treatment of Arthritis, Rheumatism, and Gout."

CAUSES OF ARTHRITIS AND RHEUMATISM

Arthritis and rheumatism, like diseases of other organs of the body, can result from a number of causes, some known and others as yet unknown. These include (1) injury, (2) heredity, (3) infections, (4) allergies, (5) tumors, (6) metabolic disorders, and (7) other factors.

INJURY

Injury to joints or related soft tissues may be either acute such as might be encountered in a fall, an automobile accident, or in the course of strenuous sports, or chronic injury such as that which might result from less severe but repeated daily injuries, such as those resulting from certain occupations or from other disadvantageous use over and over again of a certain joint or related tissues.

HEREDITY

Arthritis and rheumatism can be produced by hereditary influences. The occurrence of a peculiar but common type of osteoarthritis in end joints of the fingers called "Heberden's nodes," is an example of hereditary or familial development of osteoarthritis. The arthritis of the hemophiliac or "bleeder" is another example. This is more serious but fortunately is not common.

INFECTIONS

Arthritis and rheumatism can result from a number of different types of infections, including streptococcal and staphylococcal infections, pneumonia, meningitis, tuberculosis, venereal diseases, typhoid fever, undulant fever, and many others. Because of the infections which occur predominantly in children, certain types of infectious arthritis and rheumatism occur more frequently in younger than in older persons. Despite intensive investigations and long search, no germ or virus has been found to be the cause of osteoarthritis or rheumatoid arthritis.

ALLERGIES

Allergic reactions, or perhaps more properly reactions of hypersensitivity, may affect tissues involved by rheumatism or arthritis. Unusual sensitivity to drugs or proteins "foreign" to the human body, for example, may result in arthritis or rheumatism. When this type of arthritis or rheumatism occurs, it can be described as an inflammation without an infection.

TUMORS

Like other organs of the body, the joints may be affected by new growths or tumors, but fortunately these are rarely encountered in persons who have arthritic and rheumatic diseases.

METABOLIC DISORDERS

Changes in metabolism or the way in which the body performs its work may affect the joints and related skeletal tissues, thus resulting in arthritis or rheumatism. A deficiency of vitamin C, for example, may result in a disease called "scurvy" in which there may be rheumatic complications. A disorder in the body's ability to handle the purine substances in certain foods results in the condition known as gout, which has been described. Similarly, a disturbance or upset of the balance between the various hormones of the body may affect the condition of joints or result in certain types of rheumatism.

OTHER FACTORS CAUSING ARTHRITIS AND RHEUMATISM

Some physicians have suspected from time to time that arthritis and rheumatism may result from disturbances of circulation or disturbances of function of the nervous system. Lowered physical resistance, emotional upset, stress, shock, fatigue, and the like are other factors which might be of considerable importance to the development of certain types of arthritis and rheumatism.

In general, climate is neither a cause of nor a cure of arthritis or rheumatism. A few specific types of arthritis and rheumatism may be related to certain climates or geographical areas, but people in all parts of the world can and do have many of the common types of arthritis and rheumatism.

SYMPTOMS OF ARTHRITIS AND RHEUMATISM

Persons with arthritis and rheumatism often have a background of acute or chronic stress or strain. This may be of either a physical or mental nature or both and may be an important indication which will permit early recognition of the symptoms of articular or rheumatic diseases. Sometimes the first symptom is not directly related to the joints, but is more in the form of tiredness or exhaustion or generalized aching and stiffness. There may be loss of weight, appetite, and strength. The sensation of swelling of joints or muscles may be recognized by the person affected even though it may not be detected by careful examination of the affected areas. As would be readily recognized, these symptoms of a more or less general nature are not always indicative of arthritis or rheumatism. A person with such symptoms should rely on the advice and judgment of his physician in evaluation of these symptoms.

SYMPTOMS OF ARTHRITIS

The main symptoms of arthritis or rheumatism are pain, stiffness, limitation of motion, and swelling of affected areas. Pain from arthritis and rheumatism varies from dull to sharp in severity, or may be described as "like a toothache" or "knifelike." In some types of rheumatism burning sensations and feelings of "pins and needles" and numbness may occur in affected areas. The pain may be fleeting or constant and may vary from one location to another or may occur only in an isolated area. The affected area may be warm or hot to touch, and there may or may not be some degree of redness or discoloration of the overlying skin. Pain of arthritis and rheumatism is often characterized by its "ups and downs," but may disappear without returning or may progress either slowly or fairly rapidly.

Patients with rheumatism and arthritis often complain of "stiffness." When rheumatic stiffness is aggravated by rest, it is often relieved by mild exercise and easy movements of the affected areas. When the stiffness is more directly related to fatigue, it may be relieved by rest and inactivity.

Limitation of motion of an affected area may result from pain on motion and consequent avoidance of that painful motion or may be related to muscular weakness or imbalance in muscular function. Sometimes limited motion also is attributed to fatigue. In other instances roughening of the smooth, shiny, cartilaginous surfaces of the joint may be the basis for limitation of motion. Creaking noises or crepitation on motion may also result from such changes in the joint surfaces, but the creaking sounds may be produced just as readily by friction in tissues outside the joint. Hence such sounds do not necessarily indicate that a joint is damaged or even diseased.

Swelling may occur either outside the joint or inside the joint. Swelling outside the joint often can be attributed to generalized fatigue or disturbances in the balance of function in small blood vessels which become "sluggish" in their capacity to remove or circulate the body fluids. Swelling of this type may produce the sensation of rings becoming temporarily tight on fingers or shoes tight on the feet. This type of swelling may occur either after periods of rest and inactivity or in parts of the body that are dependent or hang down during much of the time that a person is not resting.

Swelling that occurs inside the joint results from the collection of fluid in the joint in an amount in excess of that normally produced by the lining (synovial) membrane for lubrication of the joint. This may occur with certain types of inflammation, infection, injury, or other disorders. Local heat or warmth outside the joint often accompanies the collection of excess fluid, although when excess fluid has been present for some time there may not be apparent local heat, warmth, or redness of the covering tissues.

TREATMENT OF ARTHRITIS, RHEUMATISM, AND GOUT

As is to be expected, the treatment of arthritis or rheumatism depends on the type of involvement present. To determine this a careful medical examination is usually needed. When a cause of arthritis or rheumatism such as infection, allergy, tumors, or metabolic deficiencies is found and can be corrected, the arthritis or rheumatism subsides.

When a removable cause of the arthritis or rheumatism cannot be found, treatment is generally directed toward helping the patient (1) improve the ability of his natural bodily functions to cope with the arthritis or rheumatism, and (2) (when needed) maintain as nearly normal joint function as is possible. Thus in the treatment of arthritis and rheumatism both the daily activities and the periods of rest need to be considered carefully; neither should be minimized or slighted. Adequate rest and sound sleep, a mind free of worry and daily activities free of anxiety and tension go a long way toward improving the body's ability to cope with the presence of extra inflammation, infection, or other factors requiring special effort by the bodily functions. *How* well this is accomplished is generally more important than *where* it is done. The position of joints during resting hours should be favorable to use of the joints when rest is not needed. This is discussed in the following section on "Physical Therapy." An occupation that protects affected joints and muscles, minimizes fatigue and loss of bodily energy and resistance may be another means of improving the natural bodily resistance against arthritis or rheumatism.

It is sometimes advisable for persons who have arthritis or rheumatism to sleep in a warm room, wear warm socks, mittens, or a head covering, in addition to the bedclothes, or use an electric blanket. Whether any exposure to the sun is desirable is determined by the type of arthritis or rheumatism present. Such persons must rely on the advice of their physician regarding this matter as well as for advice concerning the amount of exposure to sun that is desired.

Extra care to protect against exposure to infections is usually desirable, especially when resistance is low or when fatigue is present. Attention to dental and other bodily hygiene also constitutes an important aspect of the general bodily care of the arthritic or rheumatic patient.

A well-balanced diet, including meat, vegetables, fruit, and dairy products, is usually advisable. The details of a normal diet have been presented in another chapter in this book. The physician can decide when dietary supplements (such as vitamins and iron) are indicated. Many dietary fads have appeared from time to time, but, in general, the arthritic or rheumatic person does best to eat the type of food which would be best for him if he were not troubled by arthritis or rheumatism. It is generally advisable for rheumatic and arthritic patients to avoid being overweight in order to provide additional protection to weight-bearing joints.

The diet for patients with gout and gouty arthritis usually requires restricted use or entire elimination of foods containing significant amounts of purine substances. Wild game and fowl, meats derived from animal organs, such as liver, kidneys, sweetbreads, brains, and so on, contain large amounts of purine and are especially to be avoided. Certain other meats and meat extracts used in soups and gravies may be allowed in the diet, but amounts are generally restricted. Alcoholic beverages are generally excluded from the diet, but coffee, tea, cocoa, milk, and fruit juices can be permitted. A person with gout can best determine his particular dietary requirements by detailed consideration of his individual needs with his physician or a dietitian instructed by the physician.

PHYSICAL THERAPY

Since efforts to improve a person's general physical condition may involve spending extra time in bed each day, special attention may need to be given to the maintenance of joint function that will be as useful as possible when the patient does not require rest. Pillows under knees or hands, and arms folded over the chest, for example, are positions usually to be avoided during resting hours. Judicious use of splints, sandbags, lightweight plaster casts, a board under the mattress of the bed, and other supportive measures, however, can be helpful in maintaining a desirable position. During the waking hours and when a person is up and about, strains or pressure on affected joints and soft tissues should be avoided. The additional support of various types of corsets, braces, properly supporting shoes, and other similar devices also can give some assistance. Even when joints have already been affected and *normal* function is not to be anticipated, it still may be possible to obtain some degree of *useful* function. This can be the difference between the person's being self-dependent, that is, in his being able to earn a living or care for a family, and not being able to do these things. Various types of physical therapy are available and can be used to help an arthritic or rheumatic person improve his condition as much as possible.

Heat and Massage

Heat in almost all forms is one of the best measures of physical therapy which arthritic and rheumatic patients can use to good advantage. Occasionally, however, heat will not be indicated or will need to be used limitedly. Applications of heat increase the circulation and induce rest and relaxation in a painful muscle, joint, or other skeletal tissues. Many devices are available for the application of heat in the patient's home, including ordinary electric light bulbs, heat lamps and pads, warm tub baths, applications of warm or hot towels, woolen or flannel materials. Applications of paraffin or use of hot and cold contrast baths, when properly carried out, are other effective methods of utilizing heat. Care must be taken to avoid burns and overheating. It is advisable to consult a physician regarding the details of such treatment.

The application of heat is sometimes followed by massage performed under the direction of a physician or by either a trained physical therapist or a member of the patient's family who has been properly instructed in such treatment. The use of mechanical devices for massage may be hazardous and hence is not advised. The duration and type of massage vary with the type of rheumatism or arthritis, and specific instructions are also required for proper use.

Heat and massage, besides being of value in relieving symptoms of arthritis or rheumatism, also serve as a good preliminary to therapeutic exercise.

Therapeutic Exercise

The use of exercise as well as the type of such treatment which may be advisable is determined by the type of arthritis or rheumatism which may be present. "Therapeutic exercise" is designed to maintain or obtain as nearly normal strength, endurance, and range of motion in affected joints and muscles as it is possible to obtain. A person's ordinary daily activities rarely serve as a suitable substitute for therapeutic exercise, but when properly undertaken, therapeutic exercise, including postural and deep-breathing exercises, can and should be performed daily. The conscientious application of the appropriate therapeutic exercises for whatever period of time they are needed constitutes one of the best approaches to the problem of how useful articular function may be regained or maintained in many types of arthritis and rheumatism. Therapeutic exercise should be undertaken only on the advice of a physician and when specific instructions regarding such treatment are made available. A physician may use a pamphlet such as that prepared by the Arthritis and Rheumatism Foundation of New York City or other supplements to supply additional information for effectively carrying out a program of home physical therapy.

TREATMENT WITH DRUGS AND OTHER MEASURES

Simple analgesics such as aspirin (acetylsalicylic acid) or closely related chemicals of the salicylate family are often of aid in giving relief from the pain of arthritis, rheumatism, or gout. Many highly advertised and ofttimes expensive patent remedies have utilized this beneficial effect by having the inexpensive salicylates as their principal effective ingredient. When a physician advises the use of aspirin or other salicylates, there should be no hesitancy on the part of the patient to use such treatment to best advantage. Of course, these drugs like many others are not to be used indiscriminately, but a popular opinion that such drugs are "bad for the heart," stomach, kidneys, or other organs is erroneous. Aspirin and other salicylate drugs can relieve painful spasm and are not dope or habit-forming drugs. However, for nearly all types of arthritis and rheumatism, narcotic drugs which can be habit-forming should be avoided. This is especially true when treatment for arthritis or rheumatism is likely to be prolonged.

For the special type of arthritis which patients with gout have periodically, a drug known as colchicine is of particular value. This time-tested remedy has been used successfully for more than a hundred years for acute gouty arthritis, but it usually is not of benefit to other types of arthritis or rheumatism.

Injections of gold salts are sometimes helpful for persons with rheumatoid arthritis. Treatment with X-rays is used only for certain types of rheumatism, such as acute bursitis, occasionally for osteoarthritis, rheumatoid arthritis of the spine, and a few other types of arthritis. Use of vaccines or tonics has now been largely replaced by other types of treatment which are more likely to be of benefit. Occasionally blood transfusions give relief of rheumatism or arthritis, but the use of particular sources of blood such as from pregnant women, the placenta, or afterbirth, for example, has been of very uncertain value. Operations to repair or reconstruct affected joints may reduce disability from certain types of arthritis. With new or better technics, the results of such operations are continually being improved. The limitations of such treatment, however, add a further impetus to efforts to prevent whenever possible the development of disability which might require such operative treatment.

TREATMENT WITH HORMONES

Nearly all the hormones of the body which have been isolated have been tested for their value in the treatment of various types of arthritis and rheumatism. Until recently results of such trials were generally disappointing. However, relatively recently available hormones from the adrenal cortex and pituitary glands have given physicians and their rheumatic and arthritic patients much encouragement that certain hormones may be effectively used in the treatment of rheumatoid arthritis and certain other related types of arthritis and rheumatism. The hormones of the adrenal gland are known as cortisone and hydrocortisone. The hormone of the pituitary gland which currently offers the most promise is that which stimulates the cortex of the adrenal gland to produce the adrenal hormones. This pituitary hormone is called "corticotrophin" and is also known by the letters ACTH. Recently products have been developed called prednisone and prednisolone which have five times the activity of cortisone and which do not affect the use of salt and water by the body.

These hormones are capable of relieving symptoms and signs of the *active inflammation* of rheumatoid arthritis and related types of arthritis, but they have little or no effect when symptoms are the result of damage already developed. When these hormones are used, they usually supplement other treatment such as has already been discussed. When treatment without hormones will suffice for control of the rheumatism or arthritis, treatment with the hormones may not be needed. Thus the use of cortisone for a person with rheumatoid arthritis might be compared in a general way to the use of insulin for a person with diabetes mellitus. If the altered bodily metabolism of diabetes can be controlled without administration of insulin, then the hormone is generally not given; likewise, if the active rheumatoid arthritis can be controlled without cortisone (or hydrocortisone or corticotrophin), the addition of hormonal treatment will not be needed. When additional treatment of rheumatoid arthritis with hormones such as cortisone (or corticotrophin) is needed, it may have to be undertaken for a more or less indefinite period if the anti-rheumatic effects are to be sustained. To obtain the optimal and sustained advantages of hormonal treatment of rheumatoid arthritis, dosage needs to be highly individualized. This requires careful medical supervision of such treatment. However, when use of these hormones is advised by a physician familiar with their use, a person may proceed with the use of the hormones with the same confidence and consideration he would have in accepting an operation if the disease was one that required such treatment.

Cortisone and corticotrophin are used in the treatment of certain kinds of arthritis and rheumatism other than rheumatoid arthritis, but to date there is little basis to encourage their use in the treatment of osteoarthritis, the arthritis of injuries, the rheumatism from fatigue or nervous and emotional upsets, or the arthritis and rheumatism resulting from specific types of infections by germs. Arthritic and rheumatic persons may reasonably anticipate that the further efforts of medical and chemical scientists will improve the physician's ability to affect the course of the various types of arthritis and rheumatism and gout.

RESULTS OF TREATMENT

Use of currently available methods of determining the type of arthritis or rheumatism and adequate application of currently available treatment will provide most patients with considerable comfort and useful joints. Success in treatment is a co-operative venture on the part of the patient and physician. Rarely can the physician facilitate the accomplishment of the objectives of treatment without the expenditure of much time and effort by the person affected.

Most arthritic or rheumatic patients can anticipate a long and useful life, especially when the desire and effort for this are sustained. Improvement sometimes comes when least expected. Though at times the ailment seems to run its course despite effort to control it, in most instances and especially when appropriate precautions are taken to protect affected muscles and joints, some degree of useful function can result. The course of many types of arthritis and rheumatism, fortunately, is generally favorable. A recent large survey of arthritic and rheumatic patients revealed that 88 per cent were able to earn their own living. Ten per cent were able to do limited amounts of work, and only 2 per cent had such limited articular and muscular function that they were not self-dependent. The arthritic or rheumatic person who with the help of his physician utilizes to the fullest every advantage indicated to improve his condition can be well repaid for his efforts.

CHAPTER XIV

Diseases of the Heart and Circulation
NEWELL C. GILBERT, M.D.
Revised by M. F.

INTRODUCTION

THE HEART OF A CHILD *at birth weighs less than an ounce; that of an adult, a half pound. The energy which causes the heart to contract develops in some nervous tissue called the pace-maker of the heart. Apparently its energy is the equivalent of a thousandth of a volt. The heart beats one hundred times a minute in a small child, and on an average of seventy-two times a minute in an adult.*

This pump, because the heart is a pump which circulates the blood throughout the body, moves five hundred gallons of blood a day. During a lifetime the heart beats two and a half billion times and pumps a total of nearly thirteen million gallons. The heart begins working before a child is born and is never quiet until death. The only rest it gets is when its beat is slowed a little or decreased somewhat in its force. The heart never gets a complete rest. This vital organ must therefore be protected in every possible way against damage.

The one disease of the heart which has baffled medical science is known as rheumatic fever. This disease is responsible for a vast amount of crippling and handicapping of young children. Because of its great importance, it is given more than usual consideration in the pages that follow.

About two hundred and twenty-five thousand people die in the United States each year from heart disease. The condition is more expensive in cost of human lives than cancer, but somewhat less expensive than tuberculosis. On those who live, however, the burden of heart disease falls heavily.

Because of the greater realization of the importance of heart disease in relation to the cause of death, and since today it leads all other causes, and since it is estimated that there are at any time at least two million people in the United States suffering from heart disease, this section of any modern home medical book is important.

From the earliest times the heart has aroused the curiosity and interest of man to an extent not equaled by any other organ in the human body except the brain. Most people who get sick are inclined to refer unusual symptoms to the heart. This organ has often been associated with the idea of courage, as in the phrase "faint heart," and the average man is likely to speak of the other person as either "weak-hearted" or "strong-hearted." It was once believed that the heart was the seat of the soul. It is still referred to as the seat of one of life's most interesting emotions.

The heart is one of the involuntary muscles of the body. There are but few instances recorded in medicine in which people were able voluntarily to control the heartbeats. Nevertheless, there is plenty of evidence to indicate that the speed of modern life and the stress of modern emotions modify greatly the work of the heart. There is also evidence that a suitable hygiene in relationship to this organ will lead to longer life.

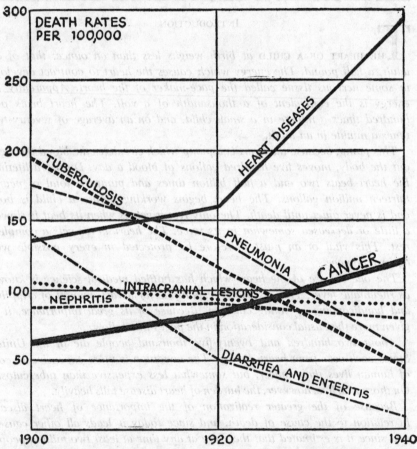

Fig. 25. Changing causes of death in the United States.
(Courtesy of the Graphic Association for Public Affairs Committee, Inc.)

The circulatory system is in reality the transportation system for the body. It carries to the cells, of which every organ and tissue of the body is built, essential materials for construction, reconstruction, and replacement of the tissues broken down by wear and tear. The blood carries fuel, and oxygen to burn the fuel, so that the necessary energy for repair and rebuilding may be obtained; each cell is thus enabled to perform its special function. Many other products, for instance, the secretions of certain glands, must be carried to the cells. The waste products from the cells must be carried away and taken to organs whose duty it is to excrete the waste or the waste may be utilized elsewhere, and made over for certain needs of the body. This circulation system acts perfectly under normal conditions and takes care of the changing needs of each part of the body. When an organ or tissue is doing active work, that part receives an increased flow of blood, while parts at rest receive a reduced amount.

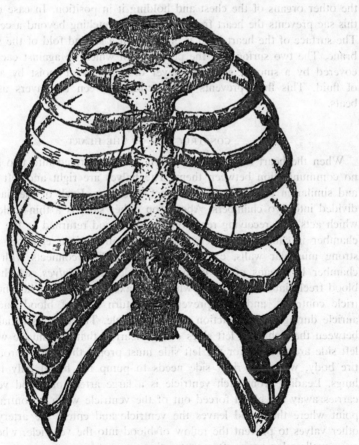

Fig. 26. Position of the heart in the chest cavity.

THE ANATOMY OF THE HEART

The heart is the great central pump which moves the fluid carrying the necessary supplies through the blood vessels to every part of the body. It is a hollow organ with strong muscular walls. Its size is about that of the clenched right fist of its owner. The heart lies just below and to the left of the lower two thirds of the breastbone. Its shape is similar to that of a large pear with the broadened end upward and under the breast bone, and the pointed end downward and to the left, where one may feel the impulse as the heart beats.

THE PERICARDIUM

The heart lies inside a fibrous sac, called the *pericardium,* which is a resistant membrane and which forms a chamber, separating the heart from the other organs of the chest and holding it in position. In case of necessity this sac prevents the heart from dilating or stretching beyond a certain point. The surface of the heart itself is enclosed in a second fold of the same membrane. The two surfaces of the pericardium which lie against each other are covered by a smooth glistening layer of tissue, kept moist by a thin layer of fluid. This fluid prevents any friction between the layers as the heart beats.

CONSTRUCTION OF THE HEART

When the heart is opened it is seen to be separated into two halves with no communication between them. The halves are right and left in position and similar in arrangement. They act in unison. Each of the halves is also divided into two chambers. Above, on either side, is a thin-walled chamber which acts as a receiving reservoir for the blood returned to the heart. This chamber is called the *auricle.* Below the auricle is a chamber with thick, strong muscular walls, called the *ventricle.* This connects with the upper chamber by means of an opening provided with *valves,* which admit the blood freely into the ventricle when it relaxes, but close tight when the ventricle contracts, and thus prevent the return flow of blood back into the auricle during the contraction of the ventricle. The only essential difference between the right and left sides of the heart is that the muscle walls on the left side are thicker; for the left side must propel the blood through the entire body, while the right side needs to pump the blood only through the lungs. Leading from each ventricle is a large artery or blood vessel which carries away the blood forced out of the ventricle when it contracts. At the point where the blood leaves the ventricle and enters the artery there are other valves to prevent the reflow of blood into the ventricle, when its muscular walls relax again after contraction.

THE HEART MUSCLE: THE MYOCARDIUM

The muscle wall of the heart is referred to as the *myocardium*. The entire hollow interior of the heart is lined with a thin smooth membrane called the *endocardium*. This is continuous with a similar membrane lining the arteries. From these terms come the names of diseases in which these tissues are inflamed, such as myocarditis and endocarditis.

The heart muscle itself is supplied with a system of arteries and veins for its own fuel and repair requirements. This is called the *coronary system*. The coronary arteries open from the interior of the *aorta* (the large artery leading off from the left side of the heart). They begin just below the valves which separate the aorta from the ventricle. The flow through these arteries, then, will be greater or less as the blood pressure in the aorta is greater or less.

THE FUNCTION OF THE HEART

The blood returning from every part of the body is brought back to the right auricle by two large veins, one coming from the upper, the other from the lower, part of the body, called respectively the superior and inferior *vena cava*. From the right auricle, the blood enters the right ventricle, which forces the blood through the lungs. There it gives up its carbon-dioxide, carried from all parts of the body, and takes on a fresh supply of oxygen. The blood returning from the circuit through the lungs is returned to the left auricle by the pulmonary vein. The auricles act as receiving reservoirs for the blood. Between the beats of the heart, their muscle walls relax and the chambers become distended with the returned blood. The period between each contraction or beat is referred to as the *diastole,* and is a period of rest and recuperation for the heart.

When the walls of the ventricles relax in their turn, after each contraction, the blood from the distended auricles flows into the ventricles during the relaxation or diastole of the ventricle. Just before the end of the ventricular diastole or period of relaxation of the walls of the ventricle, the muscle walls of the auricle contract, further emptying the auricle and more completely filling the ventricle. A fraction of a second later, the ventricle begins to contract. As the walls of the chamber contract and draw together, the pressure of the contained blood increases; the valves leading back into the auricle are closed and held firmly shut by the blood in the ventricle pushing against them. When the pressure in the contracting ventricle becomes greater than the pressure in the artery, the valves leading into the artery are opened and the contents of the ventricle forced into the artery. At the end of the ventricular contraction or *systole,* the ventricle in its turn relaxes. As it does so the valves leading back into the ventricle from the aorta are closed by the pressure of the blood, thus preventing a reflow of blood back into the ventricle. During the period of ventricular systole the relaxed auricle has again been filling

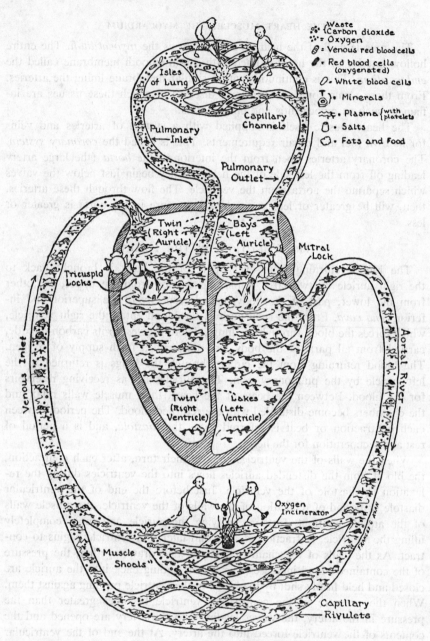

Fig. 27. Circulation of the blood.

The blood, composed mainly of red blood cells, white blood cells, platelets and plasma, enters the heart by way of the superior and inferior vena cava (Venous Inlet). From the right auricle it passes through the tricuspid valves into with blood, whereupon the now relaxed ventricle is again filled. This cycle is repeated, many times a minute, hour after hour, and year after year during life. The heart works constantly, but the amount and speed of its work may be varied.

The heart and the blood and lymph vessels which make up the circulatory system of the body constitute a mechanism equipped to meet every need of the body under normal conditions. This mechanism automatically adjusts itself to changing and varying needs in every part of the body. Provision has been made for almost every contingency that may arise. In addition, nature has given this mechanism a wide margin of safety so that it may still continue to do its work, even after a considerable amount of damage to the heart has been sustained.

Nothing that is said in this chapter should ever lead the reader to form his own opinion without the consultation of a well-trained physician. The purpose of the chapter is only to help the reader to understand the mechanism of the heart, and to understand the disorders to which it may be subject, so as to better understand the physician and his counsel and his advice.

Except in the rare instances in which the structure of the heart is defective from birth, it continues to do its work day after day and year after year without its possessor being conscious of its activity.

Frequently our attention is called to the heart by symptoms which we interpret as symptoms of heart disease, but which are not due to any disease of the heart or to disease of any organ. Sometimes such symptoms may be troublesome. Usually they are due to an instability of the nervous mechanism which regulates the rate at which the heart beats, or to disturbances of the digestive tract, or other organs. Such simple conditions as over-fatigue, worry, or emotional excitement tend to produce such effects. Rest and care usually provide a cure, or at least substantial improvement. Whether the heart is really damaged or not is a question for your physician to decide. He will be guided by an evaluation of the symptoms, by a physical examination and by laboratory methods. If a murmur is present, it does not necessarily have any significance. Murmurs may come and go in a heart that is quite normal. A heart that is normal in size and contour may almost always be assumed to be a normal heart.

---

the right ventricle and flows into the pulmonary artery which carries it to the lung capillaries. It is replenished with oxygen and started back to the heart through the pulmonary veins. When the blood reaches the left auricle it passes by way of the mitral valve into the left ventricle, where it is distributed by the aorta to all the arteries of the body (except the pulmonary artery). In this way the blood furnishes the tissues of the body ("Muscle Shoals") with oxygen and food, and carries away carbon dioxide and waste by means of the veins to the vena cava and hence to the heart, where the whole process is repeated.

CHANGES IN THE HEART

Structural changes in the heart are largely permanent. They may be compensated for in many ways by the body, and there is such a wide margin of safety that the heart may continue to do its work for a normal lifetime in the presence of extensive damage. But such changes are never to be ignored. They are usually due to one of two causes: Infection or disease or the degenerative changes which follow the disease, and which may appear in any of us as we grow older. But a third less frequent cause must be considered, and that is a contusion of the heart due usually to a sudden, sharp blow. The most frequent of such contusions are "steering-wheel accidents," or other incidents in which the chest has received a severe blow. A heart muscle which is forced to work with a blood supply which does not bring it sufficient material for repairs, or sufficient fuel, or sufficient oxygen to burn the fuel, is bound to suffer some damage. Changes in the blood flow to the heart muscle are due in large part to structural changes in the vessel walls, which narrow the vessels. Such changes may result from infection, especially rheumatic fever, or they may occur with advancing years because of reasons which we do not fully understand. There are a very few people who are born with deficiencies in the arterial blood supply to the heart muscle. In many cases the blood supply to the heart muscle is inadequate, not so much because of changes in the arteries, but because the territory which the arteries supply has been greatly increased by an overgrowth of the muscle. This overgrowth has been made necessary by demands for increased work. This increased work may be the result of damage to the valves. It may also be the result of the necessity of pumping blood through narrowed vessels over the entire body, as is the case in high blood pressure.

Temporary, and often only momentary narrowing of the vessels may result from nerve impulses. They may be due to reflex nerve impulses from other organs, as the stomach, gall bladder, or other sources. They may be due to working under extreme nervous tension with insufficient rest and relaxation. Emotional stress may be a factor. Such temporary narrowing of the vessels, oft repeated, may bring on permanent changes.

Overexertion does not injure a normal heart. Uncomfortable symptoms, or if these are not heeded, unconsciousness, stop the overexertion long before the heart is damaged. But overexertion can cause great and perhaps irreparable damage in a heart in which an active infection is present or in a heart previously damaged by infection.

Except, then, for the small group of hearts which are defective at birth, permanent changes in the structure of the heart which interfere with its function as a pump, and which are crippling, are due for the most part to infection, or to the inevitable changes which appear with age, or, very much more rarely, to trauma. If a heart is not able to perform its functions, either structural defects present at birth or structural changes acquired as the result of disease or as a result of a blood supply to the heart muscle insufficient for its needs may be responsible.

CONGENITALLY DEFECTIVE HEARTS

A small number of children are born with hearts which are structurally defective. This defect may occur as a narrowing of the two large vessels which leave the heart, or as defects in the valves of these vessels. There may be defects in the structure of the heart itself which interferes with its work. A rather frequent cause is the persistence after birth of an arterial connection which diverted the blood from the lungs before birth. Such congenital defects may be so serious that the child dies at birth or soon after. In other cases, where the defect is less serious or where its presence is compensated for by some other abnormal condition, the child may survive for varying periods, with some disability, or may even lead a normal life, with the heart doing its work in spite of its handicap.

In some of the children in whom the only evidence of a congenital defect is perhaps only a loud murmur over the heart area and who are normal in growth and development, it is probably safe to disregard the condition if there are no symptoms on exertion. These children should be allowed to live the life of normal children with the usual attention to health and hygeia, but under careful observation. They do not require any medicine for the heart.

However, it is quite a different thing if the child does have symptoms. Such symptoms are shortness of breath on exertion, or occasional fainting spells, or a lack of growth and development for the age. The skin may have a bluish cast, and the fingers may be "clubbed," that is, the ends may be broader and flatter than normal. Formerly such children did not survive, or were invalids or semi-invalids. Now surgical procedures can do a very great deal to restore such children to normal. The risk of doing such an operation is small compared with the risk to future health and life if it is not done. The decision is a matter for the careful judgment of your physician, as is also the choice of a surgeon with special training who is skilled in such work. One point of especial importance should always be kept in mind, that is, the increased likelihood of infection. Particularly to be guarded against is the predisposition to tuberculosis and to those infections which cause additional heart damage, as infective endocarditis. The child must be carefully guarded against exposure to infection, or to conditions which predispose to infection; and the general health must be kept at the highest possible level. Such children should receive the same care as those whose hearts have been previously damaged by rheumatic fever, and the same precautions should be taken. They should be examined at frequent and regular intervals, and any possible question of doubt should be referred at once to the physician for advice.

HEARTS DEFECTIVE BECAUSE OF DISEASE

The illness responsible for more heart disease than any other, and for almost all the heart disease of childhood and early life, is known variously as rheumatic fever, acute rheumatic fever, or inflammatory rheumatism. Chorea, or St. Vitus's dance, is only a manifestation of rheumatic fever.

The name "rheumatic fever" is not apt! The name "rheumatism" calls to mind symptoms of disease of the bones and joints, and rheumatic fever may exist and cause severe damage to the heart without any such symptoms or with symptoms so slight that they do not attract attention.

Fever, while it is doubtless present in some degrees at times during the disease, may be a minor symptom or may remain undiscovered. However, the name "rheumatic fever" has been in general use for so long that it would be confusing to attempt to change it.

MANIFESTATIONS OF RHEUMATIC FEVER IN CHILDHOOD

While we think of rheumatic fever as a disease of the joints and of the heart, it is really a very generalized disease. Its effects are not evenly distributed and it may affect some organs greatly, such as the joints and the heart, while other organs may be only slightly affected, or not at all. The joints may escape damage and the heart may be involved, without any joint symptoms. But the characteristic changes in the smaller arteries may appear anywhere, from the brain down. It is essentially a chronic disease and its course in one form or another may cover a period of months or even years. One does not acquire an immunity as the result of one attack, but the whole process may recur following some slight "cold" or other infection. The disease should never be regarded as cured no matter how complete the apparent recovery after an acute attack, nor how long the apparent recovery may have lasted.

There may never be any acute symptoms. It is, however, usually characterized by intervals of varying duration which come on more or less suddenly and sharply, and by much longer intervals of apparent quiescence, when but slight symptoms or none at all are apparent.

Most of the damage done to the heart occurs during the acute stages, but damage may also be going on slowly, though none the less certainly, during the periods when the disease is apparently inactive.

Rheumatic fever may exist and cause structural damage to the heart without any recognizable symptoms. Frequently unquestionable evidence of heart damage due to rheumatic disease is found in patients whose record, after the closest questioning, furnishes no clue to the time when the damage might have occurred.

The earlier and milder manifestations of rheumatic fever, unless accompanied by some more definite sign, such as rheumatic nodules, or the so-called growing pains, are difficult to differentiate from symptoms occurring in other conditions.

The child may only appear to be below what would be considered the normal health level. Colds and sore throats may appear with more than usual frequency. The weight may be below the normal average, or a loss of weight may occur rather conspicuously and suddenly. Fatigue is present out of all proportion to the play or exertion which brought it on. There may be loss of appetite, symptoms of stomach or intestinal disturbance, headache, nervous instability, or many other symptoms which are not characteristic of rheumatic fever particularly, but which are indicative of mild illness. There may be pallor, and a blood examination may reveal mild anemia, although sometimes the pallor is out of proportion to the anemia actually present. Blood examination may also show an increase in the number of white cells, indicating the presence of an infection, even during these mild and doubtful stages. The pulse may be more rapid than normal. Careful and repeated trials may indicate the presence of fever. A reliable temperature record, especially when only a slight rise is present, requires that even the best thermometer be held under the tongue for fully five minutes. Rectal temperatures are more reliable in children.

In some of these doubtful cases, repeated examination of the urine may show evidence of a mild inflammation of the kidney. This may be related to a silent rheumatic fever, or to one of several mild and more or less silent infections. It should never be neglected, and should be cared for especially by rest and by medication in addition, if the physician thinks it advisable. If such mild cases are cared for thoroughly the occurrence of chronic kidney disease would be reduced to a point where it is very rare indeed, if not ruled out altogether.

There is nothing characteristic of any one disease in the symptoms described. These cases do, however, demand careful examination and reëxamination by the family doctor. It is significant that there is a period of a few months up to three to five years of such indefinite symptoms, which have been called "toxic debility," in the majority of cases, before there is definite evidence of rheumatic fever. It is also significant that in many of these cases of "toxic debility" some evidence of rheumatic fever may occasionally be found on examination. It is during these silent and doubtful stages that some of the unexplained permanent changes may occur. Also, mild infections precede and predispose to rheumatic fever.

"Growing pains" are usually an important symptom and may occur during the doubtful stages. Many such indefinite pains are not significant, but there should always be careful questioning to determine their true nature. If there is any doubt, careful and repeated physical examination by the physician is of the greatest importance. About three fourths of all cases of rheumatic fever have had such pains. They are rather indefinite nagging muscle or joint pains, occurring anywhere, but most often in the legs, in front of the thighs, or behind the knees, or in the so-called "hamstring muscles." Sometimes the child complains of neck pains. Similar pains may occur from many natural causes. But no matter how mild they may be, they constitute an early danger signal. The watchful mother should listen to the child's story in order that the true nature of the pains may be determined.

Another minor manifestation which occurs with variable frequency is the "rheumatic nodule." It is a small round nodule, visible under the skin and movable. It is not tender. The size varies with the location, but on the average is about the size of a small pea. These nodules are most easily found where the tendons join the muscles with the bones, as close to the elbows or wrists, the knees, or the nape of the neck, or over the shoulder or hips, and less frequently over the shoulder blade or the collar bone. The presence of these nodules may be presumed to indicate rheumatic fever, although they have been observed in apparently healthy children, in cases in which rheumatic fever could not be definitely proved.

More frequently the actual onset of rheumatic fever occurs abruptly. It begins with the immediate appearance of joint symptoms or sometimes heart symptoms. There may be a short premonitory stage of fever. Some infection of the upper respiratory passages, such as a cold or sore throat, usually precedes the attack, and there may have been exposure to cold or dampness. In more than half the cases, the attacks begin with an inflammation of one or more joints. There is pain in the joint, which is swollen, tender, reddened, and feels hot to the touch. The symptoms may be severe or mild. The joints may be tender with little or no swelling, or slightly swollen with little or no tenderness. Characteristically the symptoms migrate from joint to joint, with a duration of one to eight days or more for each joint. At a given time, one or several joints may be involved. Fever is present from the start during these stages, and its height varies with each case. Its severity or lack of severity must never be taken as an index of the involvement of the heart.

Pleurisy or inflammation of the membrane lining the chest cavity may be the first symptom of the onset of rheumatic fever. Severe pain on breathing may occur suddenly, without any previous warning, or may follow after a few days of what is apparently only a "cold." The symptom of pain may disappear, and the pleura, or lining membrane of the chest, escape further trouble. Sometimes the pain may be followed by a collection of fluid in the chest cavity. Occasionally the fluid may appear silently without any preceding pain. A form of pneumonia, peculiar to rheumatic fever, may appear at the onset, but is more likely to occur later in the disease.

CHOREA

Chorea, or St. Vitus's dance, is another manifestation of rheumatic fever, occurring rather more frequently in girls, and is limited usually to the early school age. Most cases occur between the ages of five and ten, and most frequently independently of the joint symptoms. The child who has had choreic twitchings will probably have chorea when rheumatic fever recurs, just as the one with symptoms affecting the joints most frequently has joint symptoms when there is a recurrence. In a part of the cases chorea and joint symptoms are present at the same time, or the child may show chorea at one time and joint symptoms at another.

Heart disease ensues in the children with choreic manifestations as frequently as it follows with other signs and symptoms. It does not always follow so promptly, however. Children with the joint symptoms usually develop the heart disease while they are still under observation because of the acute attack, or shortly after, although the appearance of heart disease is often delayed in them also. In chorea the heart disease frequently appears later, after the symptoms of chorea have subsided, or even after a period of years. Chorea is less disabling and is often mild, and does not always attract the attention it should. Occasionally it occurs without being noticed. Sometimes there are only minor symptoms, such as fidgeting, restlessness, or lack of attention and concentration. The lack of concentration may be noticed only at school, or the nervousness may show in the handwriting. There may be loss of appetite, headache, and general nervous instability. The child may be forgetful, irritable, emotional, and may have crying spells. In the less mild cases the nervousness is more evident. There are spasmodic involuntary movements of the face and hands. The child may drop things that he is carrying and be unable to sit still. The more severe cases cannot escape attention. The spasmodic movements are more extreme and pronounced; the face is distorted, and there are uncontrollable grimaces. The tongue may be involuntarily thrust out; the speech may be interfered with.

Choreic manifestations are always worse during excitement or when attention is attracted to them. The choreic movements disappear during sleep. A child with chorea requires rest and quiet surroundings and should never be sent to school. Chorea should be considered as active rheumatic fever and treated as such.

RHEUMATIC INFLAMMATION OF THE HEART (CARDITIS)

Inflammation of the heart and its consequences are as much a manifestation of rheumatic fever as are the joint symptoms or the nodules. It is not to be regarded as a complication or as an aftermath of rheumatic fever, but as an essential part. Rheumatic fever is a generalized chronic infection, doing similar damage to similar tissue in many parts of the body. The damage may be much greater in one part of the body than in another, or it may be more evident, because it may interfere with functions, as in the heart, or cause pain, as in the joints; or it may occur where it produces no symptoms and be silent. The heart may escape, or apparently escape, or the joints may escape, or both may escape and the infection manifest itself in some other way.

The infection may seem to expend all of its energy on the heart, and the effects of rheumatic fever on the heart may appear without evidence of rheumatic fever elsewhere. Occasionally when a child is examined because of an acute attack of rheumatic fever with joint symptoms, or other manifestations, the heart is found to have been already involved at some previous time. In such cases there is always the probability that minor manifestations of rheumatic fever had occurred and were unobserved.

Such cases are not the common rule; more frequently involvement of the heart is associated with or follows one or more of the other manifestations of rheumatic fever. Unless there are symptoms of pericarditis or inflammation of the heart sac, the inflammation of the heart may not be noticed at the onset and for a long period give no indication of its presence.

Pericarditis is an inflammation of the walls of the sac in which the heart in enclosed. As these inflamed walls rub past each other with each beat of the heart, they may cause intense pain. In some cases the pain is absent. Frequently fluid appears between the two walls of the pericardium, separating them, and sometimes causing great distention of the pericardial sac, even to the point of interfering with the work of the heart. This is referred to as *pericarditis with effusion.*

Pericarditis may be the first manifestation of rheumatic fever and may come on suddenly. It more frequently occurs in the course of the disease and in the presence of other manifestations. It always means that an inflammation of the heart is present. Rheumatic inflammation of the heart is to be considered as an inflammation involving all of the tissues of the heart. While one tissue, as the pericardium or the endocardium, may give more evidence of involvement than the other tissues, or may be more extensively involved than the other tissues, the other tissues do not escape.

Except when pericarditis makes an inflammation of the heart evident, signs of heart involvement, or changes in the heart which interfere with its function, may not appear for a long period after the onset of rheumatic fever or even after actual involvement of the heart. Indeed, such changes may not appear until long after all the other symptoms of rheumatic fever have subsided and the patient is apparently well.

Usually in such cases there is evidence that an inflammatory process is still active somewhere. A slight fever is found on careful examination, the pulse is more rapid than normal, and an increase in the number of white cells in the blood may be found on examination. Such a child should be kept in bed under the supervision of a doctor until all possible chance of an active infection of the heart has been ruled out.

The absence of signs of damage to the heart does not mean that an active inflammation of the heart is not present. Such signs of damage are the results of the inflammation, and not signs of the inflammation itself. No child in whom rheumatic fever is even suspected should be allowed out of bed while there remains any elevation of temperature or until after the temperature has been normal for at least two weeks or more and until the sedimentation rate is normal.

Heart damage may be found three or four years or more after an attack of rheumatic fever, without any of the manifestations of the disease having been observed during this period. The patient may appear in good health during the intervening period. In many of these cases, a mild infection may have occurred which escaped observation. In some of these patients, the late appearance of the heart symptoms may be that the vessels which nourish the heart muscle have been narrowed by the previous rheumatic infection. Because of this slow, but progressive damage has been done to the heart muscle. This would be especially true if the earlier attacks had caused changes which resulted in an overgrowth of the heart muscle. New vessels do not come with the overgrowth of heart muscle, and the heart must do its work with the same vessels it started out with at birth.

Because of this possibility of progressive damage occurring after an attack of rheumatic fever, the child should be carefully watched by the parents, and frequently re-examined by the physician.

Rheumatic fever causes what is essentially an inflammation of the whole heart, the enveloping membrane or the pericardium, the heart muscle or the myocardium, and its lining membrane or the endocardium. Because of the inflammation of the endocardium, deformities of the valves develop so that they cannot close properly. This may affect any of the valves, but most frequently the mitral valve between the left auricle and ventricle, and the aortic valve are involved. Less frequently the tricuspid valve, between the right auricle and ventricle, and rarely the pulmonic valve are concerned. The mitral valves may have a deformity which is specially characteristic of rheumatic fever, a narrowing of the valve due to scar contraction following the inflammation, referred to as *mitral stenosis.* Such a deformity also prevents the valve from closing properly when the ventricle contracts. This makes an *"insufficiency"* of the valve (*valvular insufficiency*), so that the blood flows back into the auricle during contraction of the ventricle. This insufficiency of the mitral valve also occurs without the narrowing. It is what people refer to when they say they have a "leaky valve" or a "heart leak."

The heart muscle is invariably involved in the inflammation to some degree, perhaps slightly, or perhaps to a degree which interferes with its efficiency.

Permanent changes may also persist in the pericardium, increasing the work of the heart. The two layers, the one covering the heart and the one forming the sac in which the heart is suspended, may adhere together, so that at each beat the heart not only has to pull against the normal attachments of the pericardium, but frequently against new and abnormal attachments due to inflammation of the outer sac and its attachment to surrounding tissue.

In order to compensate for damage done to the heart, nature causes the heart to enlarge and the muscular walls to become stronger and thicker. In this way it can pump more blood at each stroke and make up for reflow of blood through the damaged valves, or it can pull against the adhesions of the pericardium to adjacent structures. A heart that has been damaged is almost always enlarged and in rheumatic fever may become greatly enlarged. When the heart enlarges in order to compensate for the additional work which it must do, the muscle fibres become longer or thicker, or both. The bulk of the muscle is increased. But as the heart muscle increases in size, it cannot grow any new blood vessels, so that the enlarged muscle must be nourished by the same number of blood vessels that supplied it before it became enlarged. The blood vessels per unit of size are fewer in number, in spite of the increased needs. The body may compensate for this in part by increasing the blood flow through the vessels which are present. But a decreased blood flow, with increased blood needs, may eventually cause serious changes in the heart muscle and the person with an enlarged heart should not leave the entire burden of care to nature, however kindly nature may be, but he should help by not throwing any greater burden upon an already burdened heart muscle. A heart muscle forced to work without sufficient material for repair and without sufficient fuel and oxygen to burn the fuel may suffer further permanent damage.

The Attack on Rheumatic Fever

Most acute infections are produced by a specific variety of germ, which always causes the disease characteristic of that germ when it enters the body under conditions favorable for its growth. In such cases the actual causative organism can be demonstrated in the infected part or in the blood.

In rheumatic fever we have very good reason for thinking that the disease is caused by the hemolytic streptococcus, and usually, if not always, by a group known as Type A, but we can not show the responsible organism in the blood or in the tissues affected. There is a lag between the onset of infection and the symptoms of rheumatic fever. Also, this infection does not cause an immunity, as it usually does in other streptococcus infections. This has led many to assume that rheumatic fever is an allergic response to the infecting organism. Similar responses of sensitization to bacteria or to foreign blood proteins, or even to chemical agents, are seen in other of the so-called "collagen diseases," of which rheumatic fever is one. Perhaps in some cases different streptococci may cause a similar response.

We have reason to think also that very often some mild or not so mild upper respiratory infection, or "cold," may prepare the ground for the advent of the streptococcus infection with its resulting symptoms of sensitization. Usually we do see such a preceding infection.

Rheumatic fever is probably the resultant of many factors in addition to the invading organism. The effects of many different environments on the growth of the germ and of different responses by different bodies to the growth of the organism must be considered. Some of these differences in environment or response may be determined by hereditary predisposition, by the effect of fatigue or exercise, by the effect of previous infections or ill health, or by many factors not accurately known.

There are several general conditions which seem to influence the incidence of rheumatic fever. In the first place it is much more frequent in the Caucasian or white race, although it does occur among all races. While it occurs all over the world, it is much more frequent in the temperate zones. When it does occur in the tropics, it is likely to run a milder course.

Damp climates have been considered an important factor; but apparently a damp climate does not necessarily predispose to rheumatic fever, nor does a dry or warm high climate prevent its occurrence. Rheumatic fever is not especially common in Holland, and is much less frequent there than in England or the northern United States. It is more common on the Mexican plateau than on the Mexican seaboard. In the West Indies it is infrequent. In Puerto Rico, in spite of poor living conditions, it is uncommon among the native population. It does occur in Egypt, but is unknown in the Malay peninsula. Much remains to be learned in regard to the influence of climate as a single factor in the incidence of rheumatic fever. This much can be said, however: that it is less frequent in warm climates and less common where there are no abrupt or sudden changes in temperature. It has been supposed to be less common where there were no abrupt or sudden changes in climate. But in the Malay peninsula it is just as uncommon in the highlands, where such changes occur, as on the coast, where the changes are minimal. The decreased occurrence in warm climates is probably due in large part to a life lived more out of doors.

Bad housing, cold, damp surroundings, or proximity to water courses have been considered important causative factors. There is much to indicate that such conditions may be a determining influence in the occurrence of rheumatic fever, but again there is the low incidence in Holland, and there was a low incidence in the late war among the troops in the trenches.

Rheumatic fever is less common among the well-to-do. While it is probable that social status is a factor, it is probably not as important a factor as would appear at first glance. Perhaps among the well-to-do predisposing ill health and minor infections are better cared for than among the poor. When rheumatic fever does occur it is recognized earlier and managed more adequately, so that there is less probability of serious consequence. Among the well-to-do classes there is less crowding and less frequenting of crowded places of amusement and crowded conveyances. There is much greater chance of transmitting minor infections of the nose and throat from one to another in crowded surroundings.

Probably there is a family predisposition to rheumatic fever. It is also difficult to be sure just how to evaluate the importance of contagion. Rheumatic fever is not contagious in the sense that it is transmissible from one developed case to another. Local epidemics have been reported and ward epidemics have occurred in hospitals. Epidemics of recurrences have been reported in convalescent homes for rheumatic fever patients. These may be explained as epidemics of "colds," or of sore throats, referred to as "upper respiratory infections," which have paved the way for the ever ready strepto-coccus, and which have resulted in rheumatic fever. It must be remembered that those who have already had rheumatic fever are not immune, but are very prone to have a recurrence with any infection.

Rheumatic fever, as such, is not contagious, but the causative strepto-coccus infection is contagious.

Rheumatic fever does show annual variation, in which there are years of increased incidence and years of lower incidence. This would suggest some epidemic influence, although it may be that these variations are due to cli-matic or other causes.

There are seasonal changes also. In the United States rheumatic fever is more frequent in late winter and early spring. In England it is more fre-quent in the fall months.

Rheumatic fever is much more common in childhood; indeed, it is largely a disease of childhood. There are a few cases from three to five years of age, but after five the frequency steadily increases until the twelfth year. After twelve the frequency of the initial attacks decreases, and they are much less frequent after twenty, but do occur with constantly diminishing frequency through old age.

Rheumatic fever, generally considered, is somewhat more frequent in girls, and the choreic manifestations are much more frequent in girls.

The weak and undernourished child seems to have the pre-rheumatic state. This may be a definite constitutional state, due to inherited tendencies, or to repeated minor infections, or deficiencies in diet and general care; or perhaps it is actually a stage of the disease itself. The truth probably includes both views: that it is a definite predisposing constitutional state, and that among the group are many who already show the minor manifestations of rheumatic fever. Such conditions either predispose to rheumatic fever or actually may be a part of it.

Some children are under the standard of weight for their age, are prone to listlessness, and tire more easily than a normal child. Such children have poor appetites, constipation, and other minor and indefinite symptoms. These children are especially liable to recurrent upper respiratory infections, or colds. By the upper respiratory tract is meant the upper air passages, the mem-brane of the nose and pharynx and the lymphoid tissue of the tonsils, ade-noids, and walls of the pharynx. It is a question as to whether these recurring infections are a cause or a result of the subnormal condition of the health. The same question applies to the gastro-intestinal symptoms.

However indefinite may be the effect of these factors on the incidence of rheumatic fever, there can be no doubt of the importance of infections of the upper respiratory tract as a whole. Such infections are almost always asso-ciated with the occurrence and recurrence of the different manifestations of rheumatic fever, with the single exception that there is a less close relationship with the occurrence of chorea.

This of course brings up the question of the relation of the tonsils to rheumatic fever. The tonsils are frequently the portion of the upper respiratory tract most obviously infected, although similar infection may be and usually is present in other portions. The tonsils are only a part of the tissue which may be involved in such infections. Their normal function is to act as a barrier to infection.

The fact that the tonsils are only a part of the tissues which may serve as a point of entrance for the infection must be borne in mind in considering the prevention of rheumatic fever. Normal tonsils serve as a barrier to infection and should not be removed under any circumstances, even if they are larger than normal. The same applies to tonsils which have recurring attacks of infection but are normal between the attacks. The inflammation at such times is due to the fact that the tonsils are acting as a barrier to infection and are bearing the brunt of the attack. Not infrequently, when tonsils of this type are removed, the attacks still recur, in the tissues similar to the tonsils which are part of the throat membrane and which also serve as a barrier.

If the tonsils, however, have constant, chronic infection, they should be removed. Such chronically infected tonsils need not be large. Small tonsils which show signs of chronic infection, associated with enlargement of the glands of the neck and large, ragged chronically infected tonsils, should be removed. Adenoids which are infected or are an obstruction to breathing should of course always be removed. Such a procedure will at least aid in conserving the health of the child and will tend to make attacks or recurrences less likely.

PREVENTION

The prevention of rheumatic fever is largely a matter of attention to the many details which go to insure the best possible general health. Absolute rules for this care cannot be set forth in detail, for just what are the best conditions vary with the individual child. In general they may be summarized in the words "good maternal care." This will mean first of all a quiet, restful home life, free from the disturbing influences which make a "nervous child," with the attendant disturbance of digestion and sleep. It will mean well-ordered and adequate rest periods and supervised recreation. Overfatigue interferes with digestion and rest and predisposes to infection. A rest period of a half hour before and after meals will aid in digestion and nutrition.

The clothing should be warm and adequate. Damp, wet clothing should be changed at once. Fresh air in the home and sleeping quarters is essential. Fresh air need not be damp, irritating air and warm air can be fresh air. Certainly infections of the nose and throat have been made worse by overenthusiasm in the matter of fresh air. Here again individual judgment must be applied to each child.

The diet should be a sensible, easily digested, nutritious diet. Vitamins are sometimes deficient, even in good American homes. That is a matter for your physician to advise you upon.

It is always to be borne in mind that in rheumatic fever in actual practice and in experimental animals, "colds" and upper respiratory infections and the so-called virus infections are found to predispose to streptococcus A infection.

It is also important to remember that rheumatic fever is usually preceded by some minor "cold" or so-called virus infection.

Colds and sore throats are more apt to be contracted from the "droplet infection" of crowds, or crowded places of amusement or public conveyances. Minor colds and sore throats should be watched and treated carefully, and the child should be kept in the house for a period after all temperature has subsided.

Children with chronic throat, nose, and sinus infections should receive especially watchful care at home and be under the observation of a physician. When possible they should be given the benefit of a warm, equable climate, if only for a time, where such infections are at least less frequent.

Antibiotics, and especially penicillin, have been shown to be of value in the prevention of rheumatic fever in two ways. One method is their prompt use in any hemolytic streptococcic infection, in adequate dosage, combined with bed rest and an adequate period for convalescence. This applies to any "cold" of any origin, any one of which may precede an attack of rheumatic fever.

Another method of prevention is the daily use of the antibiotics over a long period of time in cases where there are recurring attacks of "colds" and a history of previous rheumatic fever.

The possibility of sensitization to the drug must of course always be considered. Such sensitization may cause joint pains or hives. There is a possibility, too, that a race of organisms may develop which will not yield to penicillin, or whatever antibiotic is used. Neither of these deterrents is very important, as the drug can be taken by mouth.

On the other hand, sulfa drugs used to prevent rheumatic fever may result in a sensitization which has very serious possibilities. Such a sensitization is rare, but it is too serious to chance. Other drugs are much safer and just as effective, or more so. The treatment of rheumatic fever when it has once occurred is a matter for the best judgment of a good physician. Pressure should not be exercised upon the physician to use some new drug just because it has received a great deal of newspaper or magazine publicity.

ACTH AND CORTISONE IN RHEUMATIC FEVER

One of the most remarkable discoveries of modern times is the value of Cortisone and ACTH in many conditions. They are two of the most active agents which we possess in medicine, but like all extremely active agents, they have great powers for harm as well as for good, and they are to be used only in specific circumstances, according to the judgment of your physician.

Rest and quiet and time, and some of the old, long-tried remedies are often just as effective in the long run, and do not possess dangerous side effects.

ENDOCARDITIS

While rheumatic fever is the one largest single factor in the production of heart disease, other illnesses arise later in life which are also causatives. Just at the time when rheumatic fever is becoming less frequent, endocarditis, or inflammation of the interior of the heart, begins to appear. It may occur in childhood but is uncommon until after puberty, when its frequency increases until some time in the early twenties, at which time it gradually decreases, although it may persist through all ages.

Endocarditis occurs much more frequently in those who have previously had rheumatic fever, and this is especially true of the less acute forms.

There is an acute, sudden, sharp form which may occur at any age, and usually occurs in the course of some severe illness such as pneumonia, childbirth fever, multiple abscesses with pyemia, severe gonorrheal infection, influenza, severe tonsillitis, or recurrences of rheumatic fever. The causative germ is in each case the causative germ of the original infection. This acute severe endocarditis does not bear the same intimate relation to previous heart involvement as does the more mild and more frequent form to be described later and which is known as subacute bacterial endocarditis.

The symptoms of the acute endocarditis are those of a severe acute infection with high fever, chills, and prostration. It is important only as a complication of a very severe infection of some sort quite apart from the heart, but a complication which involves the heart. Recovery is very rare indeed.

The milder, subacute form is of more concern because some cases of this form do actually recover, and others might recover if recognized more promptly. This form is much more closely related to rheumatic fever, and at least 80 to 90 per cent of cases follow rheumatic fever infection. The connection is so close that in many cases there is some doubt as to the separate identity. In the acute form only a little over half are due to the streptococcus, while in the subacute form about 95 per cent are due not only to the streptococcus, but to one type of streptococcus, the *S. viridans,* and the remaining 5 per cent are divided between other forms of streptococci, the influenza bacillus, the gonococcus, and other organisms.

As in the acute form, the infection is practically confined to the endocardium, especially to the valves, where it results in a productive inflammation, causing vegetation upon the valves, with underlying ulceration of the tissue.

The symptoms may be mild indeed at the onset, so mild as to attract little or no attention for a long time. The condition is frequently similar to mild, incipient tuberculosis. There may be only fatigue on slight effort, weakness, feeling of malaise, or slight digestive disturbance, or loss of weight and strength. There may be some pallor, and an actual anemia is often present.

Fever is invariably present, although there may be periods of days when it is absent. It varies from a rise of only a fraction of a degree in the milder cases to higher temperatures in the more sharp types. In the cases associated with the higher temperatures, chills may occur. The pulse rate is usually faster than normal.

The fingers may show clubbing, the spleen is usually enlarged, and the symptoms of the preëxisting heart disease may be accentuated. At some time during the disease what are known as petechiæ, or spots, always occur. They should be watched for constantly, as they occur in crops with sometimes long intervals between them, and last only for a day or two or longer. They are small round red dots, not appreciably raised, and differing in size, rarely larger than a pinhead in diameter, and do not disappear on pressure. They occur most frequently above and below the collar bone and over the chest, but may extend over the abdomen, down the arms, or to the back. They are frequently seen in the white of the eye, where they cannot be confused with minor blemishes of the skin.

Still another sign of the disease is the occurrence of emboli in various parts of the body. These are small fragments which have become detached from the growths on the valves of the heart, and are carried by the blood stream through the arteries to lodge in some distant part. The symptoms and signs will vary with the site of the artery which is occluded by the embolus. Occasionally the lodgment of such an embolus in the brain, with consequent paralysis, or in the spleen, with intense pain, or in the kidney with pain and the appearance of blood in the urine, or in one of the arteries of the extremity, is the first symptom which brings the disease to the attention of the patient and his physician.

Subacute bacterial endocarditis may start with a mild, almost unnoticeable infection, very much like a beginning tuberculosis, or it may start with severe and definite symptoms and a fever which is high from the first. It seems to have lost much of its former significance. We can not be too sure of this, however, as waves of this infection have come and gone. Just at present it does not seem to appear as frequently as it did, due to better general care of rheumatic fever, and better care of other acute infections. The sooner this infection is recognized, the better. The outlook, with penicillin and the other antibiotics, is immeasurably brighter than formerly. In these days most cases recover, instead of just a few, but it is still an extremely serious disease.

SYPHILIS OF THE HEART

Syphilis of the heart and aorta may occur in the twenties but is more common in middle and in later middle life; it is the causative factor in much heart disease first appearing at this time, and especially among certain elements of the population.

Syphilis of the heart may exist silently until extensive or irreparable damage has been done. For this reason repeated blood examinations, like Wassermann or Kahn tests, should be made on those in whom there is any reason to suspect the disease to have occurred, no matter how well it has been treated. Too much confidence should never be placed upon any supposed cure by any method.

The heart should be carefully watched, and the observations checked by X-ray examination, for the infection does not always show in the blood examination.

When syphilitic disease of the heart is known to be present, treatment should be directed primarily at the heart condition, and the underlying syphilis may be treated secondarily and with great caution.

HEART CHANGES IN TOXIC THYROID

In the cases known as toxic thyroid, or exophthalmic goiter, or more popularly known by the misleading name "inward goiter," there is an oversecretion of thyroid material or a secretion which is in some way abnormal.

In these cases there is almost invariably one symptom referable to the heart: the rapid pulse rate. Occasionally there may be an abnormal rhythm, or some shortness of breath, or even pain. The presence of a definite increase in the metabolic rate will confirm the diagnosis.

Such symptoms subside when the abnormal condition of the gland is remedied, by operation or use of new drugs like propylthiouracil or similar agents which control excessive action of the thyroid. Iodine is useful now, as it has always been. In some cases there is some degree of permanent damage, but this is rarely serious and can usually be readily cared for. An abnormal rhythm, such as auricular fibrillation, may be present in cases which have remained untreated for some time. If the rate is too rapid, it can be readily controlled by digitalis, under the advice and direction of a physician.

ANGINA PECTORIS AND CORONARY OCCLUSION

The heart muscle is supplied with the blood necessary for its activity by means of blood vessels which run through the heart itself, dividing and subdividing finally in small capillaries in close contact with each muscle fibre. They bring to the heart muscle material for repair, fuel to furnish energy and oxygen to burn the fuel. They carry away the waste and the results of combustion. They are essential for the life and the activity of the heart muscle.

These arteries have their origin in the aorta, the large vessel leading from the heart, at its beginning, just as it leaves the left ventricle or left chamber of the heart, and just above the valves which separate the aorta from the ventricle. Hence the flow into these arteries will depend upon the pressure in the aorta, at their origin.

The coronary flow is a very perfect mechanism, and an excellent example of the "wisdom of the body." It works constantly all through our lives, supplying the heart muscle according to its needs, with more blood or less, as the occasion demands. Any condition which interferes with the coronary flow, or tends to make it inadequate, may shorten life or result in incapacity.

Some people, very few indeed, are born with a coronary blood supply which is insufficient. They may do very well until the artery walls in middle life change and become narrowed. When this does happen, these patients may have symptoms of coronary insufficiency. On the other hand, these patients may lead a perfectly normal life and die of old age.

In some patients the coronary vessel walls are constricted by the inflammation of the wall which accompanies rheumatic fever, and symptoms of deficient circulation to the heart muscle appear in later life. Other more rare diseases may have a similar effect.

In all of us changes in the coronary vessels occur as we grow older. These may be of very minor importance, or of very great importance. It is interesting, in this connection, to observe how many people live to a ripe old age, with no symptoms at all, even though they may have very hard arteries indeed. Probably "hardened arteries" receive more attention than they deserve. So-called "hardening of the arteries" begins early in life in everyone, and should never alarm us too much.

Nature, too, has provided a safeguard by increasing the connections between the different arteries as we grow older, so that if the flow in one artery in one locality is insufficient, blood may be detoured to it through other highways.

A deficient blood supply to the heart muscle results in definite symptoms, the severity and duration of which depend upon just how seriously the blood supply is interfered with and upon what is interfering with it. When a muscle anywhere in the body is obliged to contract when it does not have a blood supply sufficient for its needs, pain results. The same thing occurs in the heart muscle when it is forced to work with an insufficient blood supply. In addition, it may not be able to do its work adequately, and shortness of breath may result, or even what we refer to as heart failure.

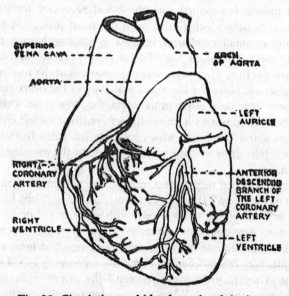

Fig. 28. Circulation and blood supply of the heart.

ANGINA PECTORIS

One of the most frequent and best known episodes resulting from an inadequate blood supply is referred to as angina pectoris. In angina pectoris symptoms are of short duration, because the blood supply is only temporarily diminished, or because it is insufficient for the work of the heart just at that time, as when some extra demand is made on the heart. Such a decrease in the blood supply of the heart might be due to a temporary and transient narrowing of the vessels supplying the heart with blood, due to nervous impulses having their origin elsewhere. Since the flow through these arteries rises and falls with the blood pressure in the aorta, a fall in blood pressure, as occurs during sleep, or as occurs during the day from many causes, might decrease the flow to a point at which it would cause pain. This is particularly the case in a heart whose arteries show the hardening which comes with age, but would probably not cause any symptoms in a more normal heart. Whatever may cause the temporary decrease in the flow of blood in the vessels of the heart itself, it is this decrease and the consequent transient inadequacy of the blood supply to the heart which causes the symptoms.

Pain is the one most important symptom in angina pectoris. The pain is usually under the breast bone, and more frequently under the upper portion of the breast bone, or just to the left of the upper portion. It may remain in that region, or it may radiate to the shoulder, or down the left arm, perhaps only as far as the elbow, or the wrist, or it may extend to the tips of the fingers. Occasionally it may radiate to the right shoulder and down the right arm, or it may radiate to both shoulders, and down both arms. In other persons it may radiate to the left side of the neck or be referred to the lower back teeth. In others it may radiate to the pit of the stomach and be considered as having its origin in the stomach, or it may be felt just below the ribs on the right side. Frequently the pain may never be felt in the chest at all, and be felt only at the points to which it may radiate, as the left shoulder, the elbow, or the little and the ring finger, or the left lower jaw, or the pit of the stomach. The pain is often severe and agonizing, but it is not necessarily so, and may be mild.

Except for these symptoms, associated or appearing singly, there is nothing which characterizes an attack, except that it is of short duration, a matter of seconds or minutes. Attacks lasting hours, or with other symptoms, are not merely angina pectoris.

There are no certain signs which enable the physician to recognize the presence of an attack or to judge of the probability of the future occurrence of such an attack. Nothing characteristic can be found by examination of the heart, or the pulse or blood pressure, or by laboratory methods. The physician must be guided altogether by the story of the attack and such characteristics as the patient tells him.

Attacks are most frequently brought on by exertion. In some persons they are brought on by moderate exertion at any time; in others by moderate exertion only under certain conditions; and in others the attacks may accompany only unusual exertion. Attacks are especially apt to accompany exertion soon after a meal. With an empty stomach a man may be able to walk briskly for a long distance without distress and find himself unable to walk a hundred feet after a meal without symptoms of pain. In some the attacks may follow exertion after any meal, or may follow especially some one meal, as in the evening or in the morning. Attacks are likely to follow a meal which is too hastily eaten, or one which is indigestible, or too full a meal, or one eaten when too tired.

For these reasons, it is best not to eat when tired, nor to eat heavily at any time. It is well to take a rest period before and after each meal and to eat leisurely. The diet should be chosen so as to avoid those foods which are indigestible or which in the patient's experience cause gas.

Anginal pain may occur almost equally easily on an empty stomach. In addition to oxygen the heart muscle also needs sugar to burn with the oxygen. Too low a blood sugar, or exertion with too low a blood sugar, may cause typical anginal pain. This condition may occur with a poorly proportioned diet, or too much insulin, etc. It is a matter of careful consideration by your physician.

A reflex narrowing of the coronary vessels due to impulses arising from various sources may occur. One very frequent such reflex is that resulting from breathing cold air through the nose or walking against a cold wind. This can readily be obviated by holding a muffler over the nose and breathing warm air through the mouth.

Other sources of such reflex effects are gall stones or stomach disorders, duodenal ulcers, diverticula of the duodenum or of the esophagus. A fairly frequent cause is a hiatus hernia, where the stomach pushes up through the opening through which the esophagus descends to the stomach. Just too full a stomach, or an indigestible meal, may be a cause, or an abdomen distended with gas.

Exertion does not necessarily bring on an attack. An attack may come when sitting quietly, especially after a meal. An attack may occur in the early morning hours in the midst of a normal sleep.

Attacks are more frequent in the emotionally and nervously unstable. Any emotion may bring on an attack, but especially anger, grief, or worry. Attacks are more frequent also in the presence of fatigue, and especially of nervous or mental fatigue. While angina pectoris may occur in people in any walk of life, it is much more common in those whose work demands an undue proportion of strain and energy and worry, and who are obliged to do their work under tension, or, what is especially true, those who are so constituted that they do any work under tension, and with an undue amount of nervous energy. This is probably one reason why angina pectoris is more frequent in cities and why it is much less frequent in the more leisurely tropics.

Angina pectoris is by no means the hopeless disease which is often pictured.

It may be serious, but it is possible in many cases for patients to go on for years with recurring attacks, or the attacks may cease to occur and the patient lead a normal life with only moderate restrictions, living within his physicial means. Sources of reflex irritation should be overcome. Patients with angina pectoris usually know about how far they can go without bringing on an attack, and they should conduct their lives accordingly. They should keep in touch with their physician and report at regular intervals. It is possible, also, that the physician may wish occasional electrocardiographic tracings made to confirm his observations. If an attack occurs which is different from those usually experienced, which is more painful, or lasts longer, the patient should get to his home with just as little effort as possible and as soon as possible, and have his family physician called immediately.

CORONARY OCCLUSION

In occlusion of one of the branches of the coronary artery, as well as what is referred to as acute coronary insufficiency, the pain is identical with that of angina pectoris and occurs for the same reason. In angina pectoris there is only a temporary disproportion between the blood supply to the heart muscle and its needs for blood. The pain usually quickly passes away, and no damage to the heart muscle results from the isolated attack. Oft-repeated attacks may eventually cause permanent damage. In coronary occlusion one of the branches of the coronary artery is occluded, just as the term suggests. Whatever the occlusion is due to, the area of muscle supplied by that particular branch is deprived of blood for a length of time sufficient to do serious damage to the muscular wall of the heart, and weeks of time and rest are necessary for the body to make sufficient repairs.

In what is referred to as acute coronary insufficiency an area of the heart muscle is again deprived of its blood supply for a length of time sufficient to do serious damage, although here an actual obstruction of one particular vessel is not seen. The results may not be as serious as when one branch is actually occluded. The differentiation between the two incidents is not defined clearly enough, however, to warrant drawing a conclusion in any one case as regards future outlook or treatment. They should be treated alike.

A patient with coronary occlusion or coronary insufficiency is best cared for in a hospital, where laboratory methods are available to confirm the diagnosis and to check on progress toward recovery. Electrocardiographic tracings are almost always diagnostic, but their absence or lack of characteristic findings should not outweigh the clinical evidence. Oxygen and other emergency agents are always at hand in the hospital, as well as trained observers.

DISORDERED ACTION OF THE HEART

In a large group of cases, especially in early life, there are symptoms regarded often as due to the heart and variously referred to as disordered action of the heart, neurocirculatory asthenia, and, most apt of all, "effort syndrome."

In these cases the heart and the circulatory system are perfectly normal structurally. What is abnormal is the automatic nervous mechanism controlling the heart and controlling all of the activities of the body. This automatic nervous system temporarily responds to smaller stimuli than normal, and when it does respond, overresponds. An exertion which would make the pulse of a normal individual beat only a little more rapidly than normal causes the pulse of such a person to beat exceedingly rapidly. An exertion which would hardly affect the rate of breathing in a normal person would cause rapid breathing in such a person.

During sleep, or when resting quietly or unobserved, the pulse and the respiration are normal. On exertion, and in some cases on slight exertion, the pulse becomes rapid, and there is severe shortness of breath. The hands and feet may appear blue. The hands are cold and wet, even in a warm room. Such patients often complain of what they refer to as dizziness; this is not a real dizziness, when there is a sense of rapid rotation, but is rather a giddiness, a sense of unsteadiness; surrounding objects may appear to sway or turn slowly. Fainting attacks are frequent among such patients and rare in actual cases of heart disease. Some of these patients complain of pain in the heart region.

When they are examined, the heart is always normal in size and normal in every determinable way. If it is not normal, the case does not belong to this group. To add to the difficulties, what is called a heart murmur is often heard. It is the kind of murmur which, although it is heard in heart disease, is also heard in normal hearts, and is not of significance in a heart of normal size. In those belonging to this group, the murmur is rarely constant. It may be heard at one time and a few moments later may have completely disappeared.

Such patients often complain of various other symptoms, which are on a nervous basis. They will in addition show a lack of initiative, an unwillingness to go about their normal duties, and be subject to worry, and fear, and apprehension. Others may lead a normal life, be energetic in their work, but still show the symptoms referable to the heart.

There is always a certain proportion of such people in any population. They are frequently classified as having real heart disease or as having thyroid disease, or early tuberculosis, or as being simply neurotic. Such hearts have been a source of disability in every war, for many decades past.

In the army a period of rest and recreation usually restored the soldier to normal. Of the large number who showed the symptoms on entrance into the army from civil life, or who developed the symptoms in the army, more than half were restored to normal in camps where they were given special care and put on gradually increased exercise.

Care should be taken that there is no underlying minor infection in such cases. An adequate period for convalescence should always be allowed after illness or even a minor operation. When these symptoms are present, rest, recreation, exercise increased gradually and carefully, and attention to the general health should restore the patient to normal.

IRREGULARITIES OF THE PULSE

Some irregularities of the pulse beat are quite normal; others may be significant of conditions which demand the physician's advice. In youth, and again in later life, there is a slowing of the pulse in breathing out, and a quickening in breathing in, which is normal. Sometimes the alternating change in rate may be noticeable. It is never of any significance.

In many people over forty years of age, an irregularity which may frequently attract attention is really an extra beat of the heart coming before the anticipated time, but the long pause following the beat makes it appear as though a beat had been dropped. It is usually described by the patient as a feeling of the "heart flopping over." It is more noticeable with fatigue, or with indigestion, or after too hearty a meal. It often appears with worry or apprehension. The irregularity tends to disappear on exertion and then is more noticeable during the rest which follows exertion. This irregularity is usually of no significance in itself, but is a matter for the physician to decide.

Attacks of rapid heart action coming on instantly, and stopping just as suddenly, occur in some people. They rarely last more than a few seconds or minutes, but they may persist for longer periods. They usually begin in early life. They are inconvenient and troublesome, but not serious. Such paroxysmal attacks occurring later in life may be of real significance, and a physician should be consulted at once.

Another form of irregularity occurs, especially in those who have had a rheumatic infection of the heart, but may accompany other conditions, such as toxic thyroid. In this, the pulse is absolutely irregular in both rate and volume and is more irregular on exertion and more quiet at rest. Because of the usually rapid rate, the ventricle of the heart does not have sufficient time in which to fill at each beat; hence the volume of blood pumped by the heart is less, and is insufficient for the needs of the body. The patient may be short of breath and the limbs may swell.

This condition and the rapid heart rate can always be controlled by digitalis or similar drugs, and may be adequately controlled for an indefinite period of time. This should always be under the guidance of a physician, but the physician should also teach the patient just how to adjust the dosage to meet changing needs. If too little is used, the heart will beat too rapidly, and the volume pumped will be insufficient. If too much is used, there may not be enough beats per minute, and the volume of each beat may be too small, because the drug also tends to make the chamber of the ventricle smaller. The patient cannot have the doctor at his elbow every minute, and the doctor must teach the patient just how to use the drug. Paroxysmal attacks of fibrillation coming on early in life may be of short duration and will go away of themselves, without medication.

Accidental injuries to the heart are often overlooked, because there may be little in the way of symptoms and signs at first, and because the possibility of injury is not considered as often as it should be. Traumatic injury to the heart may result from a variety of chest injuries. By far the most frequent cases occur as the result of motor accidents, and especially steering wheel accidents where the chest is thrown violently against the steering wheel. When ribs are broken or there are bruises and obvious signs of injury, it is not so apt to be overlooked, although even then it may be. However it is possible for the breastbone to be pushed clear back against the spinal column without any fracture of the ribs or breastbone or any bruising of the skin. While this is most apt to occur in youth, it may occur in adult or middle life or later. In such cases the heart can not very well escape damage.

There may be bleeding into the pericardial sac or actual bruising of the heart muscle. There may be hemorrhages beneath the lining membrane or interior of the heart. There may be no evidence of these hemorrhages at first, but they initiate a necrosis of the heart muscle and a rupture of the heart wall days or weeks later.

After such injuries there may be immediate shock with obvious signs of heart damage. In some cases the symptoms may be very slight or none and the injured person protests that he is quite unhurt. Between these two extremes, there is every possible gradation. The symptoms may remain slight, or they may progress to severe symptoms and death. No matter how mild the immediate symptoms may be the heart should be considered one of potential damage, and watched and investigated. In an English hospital seventy-five cases of chest injury had electrocardiographic tracings made, and twenty showed heart damage. Of the twenty, two died, and one suffered some permanent heart damage.

CARDIAC INSUFFICIENCY

When the heart is unable to fulfill its function adequately as a pump, supply sufficient circulation to all of the tissues of the body, such symptoms as shortness of breath, or swelling of the limbs, or swelling of the abdomen may result. Such conditions always, in every case, demand the advice and the care of a physician at once.

SURGERY OF THE HEART

Among the greatest advances in modern medicine are the applications of surgical techniques to correcting deficiencies of the heart, either congenital or acquired. Operations are done to re-route the circulation, to widen large blood vessels like the aorta, to transplant blood vessels from blood vessel banks, to stimulate formation of new blood supply to the heart, and to open constricted valves of the heart. Such procedures are carried out only in hospitals by experienced surgeons with all the special equipment and facilities necessary.

CHAPTER XV

Digestion and Digestive Diseases
SIDNEY A. PORTIS, M.D.
Revised by M. F.

THE TERM "INDIGESTION" *is an unscientific word like dyspepsia, but almost everyone knows what it means. It merely means that the person who suffers with this symptom is having trouble with the digesting of his food or in absorbing it. Some years ago the word "dyspepsia" was one to conjure with. It described the great American disease, now transformed into the possibly more scientific term "nervous indigestion." However, as will be seen in the following pages, there is far more to a consideration of the disturbance of the gastrointestinal tract than merely indigestion or dyspepsia.*

As will be seen from the illustrations accompanying these articles, the gastro-intestinal tract extends from the mouth, through the pharynx, the esophagus, the stomach, the small intestines, including the duodenum, the jejunum, and the ileum. The large intestines include the cecum, the ascending, transverse, and descending colon, the sigmoid and the rectum, to the point of excretion of undigested material and wastage known as the anus. Moreover, this central tube for digesting and absorbing food is in intimate contact with most of the organs of the body which are concerned with aiding the process of digestion and absorption.

The glands empty into the gastro-intestinal tract at various points and provide the secretions that are necessary for digestion. Blood vessels and tubes of various kinds carry away the digested materials and distribute the basic substances for tissue building and repair throughout the body. In the debates that are frequently held as to what are the important tissues of the body, the gastro-intestinal tract will take a very high place.

In the articles which follow, an attempt has been made to discuss the diseases of the gastro-intestinal tract and the organs associated therewith, and at the same time to explain something of the mechanisms involved in the development of these diseases. It might be taken for granted that the control of dietary diseases is practically always dietetic. While diet is important, there are many other factors which are probably even more important in relationship to controlling such diseases. Mechanical, glandular, and infectious causes are probably more frequently responsible for diseases of the stomach and intestines than are merely irregularities of the diet. For this reason the articles which are here included do not provide corrective diets for some of the gastro-intestinal diseases. The subject is, however, discussed in the chapter on diet, and special diets used in some of the gastro-intestinal diseases are there provided.

The mouth is the first organ in which digestion begins. The tongue, with its taste-buds, distinguishes between types and varieties of foods. There is the sense of sweet, sour, salt, and bitter and the feel of the food upon the tongue. The nose with its sense of smell helps to give piquancy to the sense of taste. With the aid of the teeth, the food is chewed; then, emulsified by saliva from the glands on each side of the jaw, it is made easy to swallow. In addition, the saliva begins partial digestion of starches. The more completely the food is chewed, the easier it is to swallow, and later the more readily is it digested.

The esophagus is just a tube that conveys the food from the mouth to the stomach. It is controlled by nerves from the central nervous system in the spine and brain. At its bottom end it is closed by a sphincter (a muscle surrounding the outlet) to prevent too rapid entrance of food or liquid into the stomach. The mucus from the glands of the esophagus is supplied purely for lubrication.

As the food and water enter the stomach, the first really important digestion begins. Here the food is mixed with gastric (stomach) juice. This juice is ordinarily a thin, colorless, or nearly colorless, liquid with strong acid reaction. Belching of sour fluid is a reflection of this acidity. The essential constitutents of the gastric juice are an acid (hydrochloric) and two or possibly three enzymes (digestive ferments) called pepsin, rennin, and lipase. Many patent medicines have been based on these substances. The stomach itself consists of an outer layer, called the peritoneum; a muscle layer, in which the blood vessels and nerves lie; a submucous membrane; and an inner lining called the mucosa. The glands of secretion are in the mucosa, and the absorption of material goes on through its tissues.

The acid of the gastric juice is a mineral acid and is present in considerable strength. It is secreted by acid cells situated in the glands of the mucous lining. The other constituents of gastric juice are secreted normally at the same time as the acid. The pouring out of gastric juice is first started by the sensations of taste and smell; i.e., it is a psychical secretion. Stimuli from the nose and mouth call forth, reflexly, a secretion in the stomach. Secretion in the mouth and stomach may begin by the sight or at thought of food. This is the reason that the mouth waters under such conditions.

Certain foods contain substances designated as secretagogues, which are able to cause a secretion of gastric juice when taken into the stomach. Thus, meat extracts, meat juices, and soups are particularly effective in this respect, while milk and water cause less secretion. In other foods, these ready-formed secretagogues are present in smaller amount or may be lacking.

Of the enzymes or digestive ferments, pepsin is the most important. Peculiarly pepsin acts only in an acid medium. If acid is absent, pepsin remains inactive. The result of digestion in the stomach is to convert the protein of the food into a simpler and more soluble form. Thus proteins are only partially digested in the stomach. Rennin is another enzyme, whose main purpose is to coagulate milk. It is rapid in its action, especially in an acid medium. The fats are not digested in the stomach but are liquefied owing to the body heat. The starches or carbohydrates are acted on not by stomach secretion properly but by an enzyme called ptyalin which is present in saliva and continues to exert its action in the stomach. In this way food is prepared for intestinal digestion.

There is some absorption in the stomach. Little water is absorbed, while alcohol is readily absorbed. Some salts and sugar and the soluble proteins are absorbed slowly, while fats are probably not absorbed at all. The food and the products of the changes in the stomach undergo most complete digestion in the intestinal tract. Here also the final products of digestion are mainly absorbed.

Intestinal digestion begins in the duodenum, the first portion of the small bowel attached to the stomach. It is called duodenum from the Greek words meaning two and ten, because it is twelve fingers long. Digestion is largely completed by the time the food arrives at the end of the small intestine. This is effected through the combined action of three secretions: the pancreatic juice, the secretion from the intestinal glands (*succus entericus*), and the bile. These secretions are mixed with the food beginning in the duodenum, and their action proceeds simultaneously.

The pancreas is a long, narrow gland situated in the back wall of the abdomen. Its secretion into the intestine is composed of three enzymes: trypsin, which splits up proteins; lipase, which splits up fats; and amylase, which digests starch. The direct secretion is distinctly alkaline, in contradistinction to the acid of the stomach. Besides, it has an internal secretion into the blood called insulin, the secretion necessary to prevent diabetes. Thus the food proteins are completely broken down into their finer components—amino-acids— and when absorbed as such, the body constructs its own peculiar type of protein from these split products.

The tissue cells reconstruct from these pieces—or building stones—a form of protein adaptable to their needs and more or less characteristic for the needs of a particular organ. Just as letters of the alphabet may be combined in different ways to make different words, so various amino-acids may be combined to make proteins of different kinds.

Starchy food that escapes digestion in the mouth and stomach is digested in the duodenum, where it is split up into absorbable sugars. The fats are split up into fatty acids, and when the latter are combined with alkaline salts they form soaps. The digestion of fats is materially aided by the presence of bile. The mixture of bile and pancreatic juice digests neutral fats more rapidly. Certain enzymes are secreted by the small intestine. These effect the final stage in preparation of the food for absorption. There is, in addition, a hormone or excitant of gland secretion in the small intestine, called secretin, which stimulates the flow of pancreatic juice.

Absorption takes place readily in the small intestine. Carbohydrates are absorbed for the most part as simple sugars. From the intestines these pass into the liver, where some are stored as glycogen—the material used for muscle action—so that the amount of sugar in the blood is kept quite constant. When a large amount is taken and the liver is not able to take care of it readily, it increases in the blood, and later the excess may appear in the urine, provided the kidneys are normal. Those carbohydrates which escape digestion undergo bacterial fermentation with the formation of acids.

Fats are absorbed with the aid of the bile, especially the bile salts. They, for the most part, do not pass through the liver but get into the general circulation by way of the lymph stream. They are picked up in the lymph directly from the intestine. From the general circulation they are taken to the cells of the body for their use.

Proteins are split up or absorbed in the intestinal wall, and, as explained, pass through the liver for the most part, later to build up the protein of the tissues. Some proteins escape and pass into the large intestine, where they are acted on by bacteria. These bacteria have a most important place in the body economy. For instance, many of the components of the Vitamin B complex are formed in the intestine. Particularly is this true of Vitamin B_{12} which is essential in blood formation and has its specific activity on the liver. The lack of Vitamin B_{12} is seen in patients who have a pernicious anemia. These B_{12} forming organisms are either made inactive or destroyed when people take large amounts of aureomycin and also terramycin which are antibiotics. Folic acid is also manufactured by the bacteria in the intestines and plays an important part in iron deficiency anemias.

The secretion of the large intestine, while it contains much mucus and has an alkaline reaction, does not seem to have any distinctive enzymes. Water is readily absorbed from the colon or large intestine. The alkaline reaction makes the colon a favorable environment for bacteria. Putrefaction is a normal occurrence in the large intestine. The splitting of the protein which escaped small intestinal digestion is completed here. The colon frequently receives incompletely digested food, because the food frequently passes too rapidly through the small intestines before digestion is completed. There are three outstanding conditions in which this rapidity of movement occurs: (1) where the hydrochloric acid is absent from the stomach and the food passes almost undigested into the large bowel, (2) where a deficiency of pancreatic juices exists and there is no digestion so that naturally some undigested food will pass through rapidly and (3) the rapid movements which are interdependent upon increased nervous stimulation. This hypermotility, as it is called, is seen frequently in emotionally disturbed people. All who have increased motility of the small intestines do not necessarily have diarrhea. This may happen in those who have absence of free hydrochloric acid; however, diarrhea is much more common in those who have an absence of pancreatic juice. Finally, in those who have increased movements due to nervous stimulation of the bowel there may or may not be diarrhea. The diarrhea in this last group may be, for the most part, increased movements in the colon. It does not necessarily follow in the physiologic balance of the intestinal tract that just because you may have a rapid movement of the small intestine, you also have a rapid movement of the colon. It can occur but it is not always necessarily associated with it. Many of the products are given off in the stool, while others are absorbed in part and excreted subsequently in the urine. It is well known that excessive bacterial action may lead to intestinal troubles, such as diarrhea, or possibly to more serious interference with general nutrition, owing to the formation of poisonous products.

THE FECES OR "STOOL"

The end products of digestion are excreted, for the most part, by the bowel as the stool; the composition of the excretion from the bowel depends on the character of the food eaten. The color of the stool is usually dark brown or it may be a light yellow to brown where a person has not eaten meats or leafy vegetables as a part of the diet. However, occasionally green stools may be present. Green stools, frequently seen in children, have an acid reaction rather than the usual normal alkaline reaction as described previously. The green reaction in the stool of children where there are acid stools is associated with the changes in the bile. Bile in the presence of acid becomes green and in the presence of alkalinity becomes brown. More recently in the last few years since the introduction of the antibiotic drugs we have seen many patients with large amounts of green stools which are alkaline in reaction. This green stool in these patients is not due to the presence or absence of bile but is due to green pigment producing organisms that can grow when the normal bacteria of the intestine are destroyed by antibiotics. The organism most commonly associated with this green producing alkaline stool is called a pseudomonus. If the diet is composed exclusively of meats, the stool is small in amount and dark in color; with an ordinary mixed diet, the amount is increased, and it is largest with an exclusively vegetable diet, especially vegetables containing cellulose of much crude fiber. When the processes of digestion and absorption are entirely normal, the stool should be well formed and devoid of offensive odor. If it is soft or liquid with a disagreeable odor, there have been indiscretions in diet or some distinctly abnormal causes. In other words, such excretions are an indication of some abnormality in the digestive mechanism. The bad odor is usually due to excessive putrefaction.

When the excretion of the bowel is studied with a microscope the following constituents may be seen or found chemically: (1) Undigested material, such

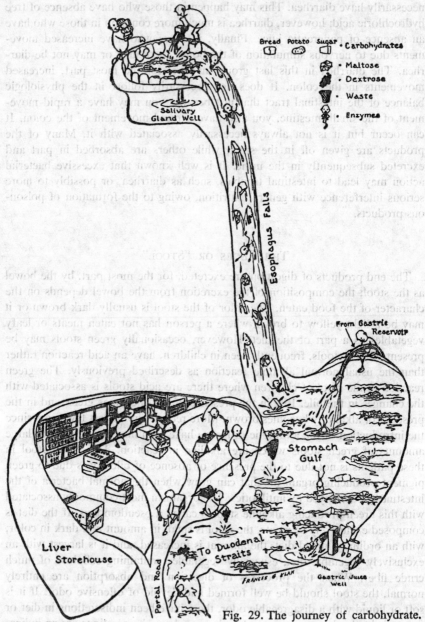

Bread Potato Sugar • Carbohydrates

• Maltose

• Dextrose

• Waste

• Enzymes

Salivary Gland Well

Esophagus Falls

From Gastric Reservoir

Stomach Gulf

Liver Storehouse

Portal Road

To Duodenal Straits

Gastric Juice Well

FRANCES G FLAN

Fig. 29. The journey of carbohydrate.

In the form of sugars and starches, carbohydrate is taken into the mouth where the action of the enzymes in the saliva converts some of the starches to sugar (maltose). The action of the saliva continues down the esophagus to the stomach, where some absorption of the simpler sugar products (dextrose) takes place. Most of the carbohydrate is carried to the duodenum to

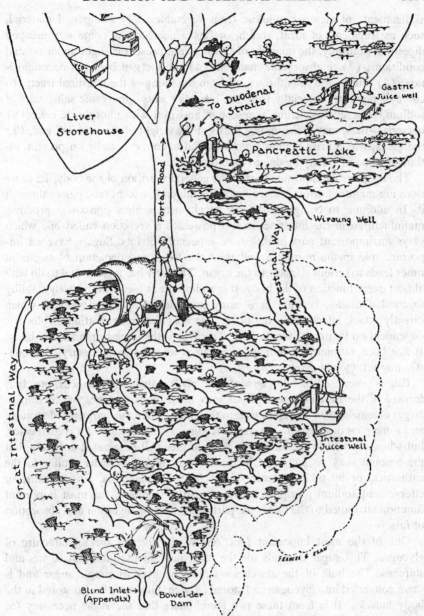

undergo further digestion by the pancreatic juices which enter by way of the duct of Wirsung. Throughout the duodenum and small intestine digestion and absorption continue until all the carbohydrate has been assimilated by the time the ileocecal valve ("Bowel-der Dam") has been reached. The portal vein carries it in the form of dextrose to the liver where the excess of sugar is withdrawn and stored as glycogen for future use by the body tissues.

as ligaments of meat or cellulose from vegetables; (2) undigested material, such as fragments of meat, starch, or fats which have in some way escaped digestion; naturally, the quantity of this material present is slight under normal conditions; (3) unabsorbable material; (4) products of bacterial decomposition; (5) mucus and cells thrown off from the lining of the intestinal tract; (6) color or pigment, especially from the bile; (7) salts—inorganic salts, salts of sodium, potassium, calcium, magnesium and iron with phosphoric acid; (8) bacteria—these may make up two thirds of the weight of the material, and, (9) the gases, which arise mainly from bacterial action, especially on protein, although some of it may be due to swallowed air.

The liver has an important part in the general nutrition of the body. Its functions are manifold. Most of the absorbable material, except fats, passes through it. In addition to being the defense mechanism against poisonous products manufactured in the intestine, it also possesses a secretion called bile which plays an important part in digestion, especially of fats. Sugars have an important rôle in the normal activities of the liver, and depletion of sugars at times leads to serious damage to the organ. The liver has a great deal to do with almost every function of the body. It is an important factor in the body's ability to combat disease because here many immune bodies are developed which directly attack infections in the body. The coagulation or clotting of blood is dependent on its proper functioning. The liver is the largest organ in the body. It has been estimated that it is seven times as large as necessary, this constituting a factor of safety.

Bile is composed of bile pigment, bile acids, salts, water, mucus, etc. It is formed in the liver cells and passes into small ducts or tubes which lead to larger channels; then some passes into the gall bladder, for purposes of storage, and some goes directly into the small intestine. Bile is usually of a golden color, but when exposed to the air it may become green. It is secreted normally, but the amount may be increased by such foods as fats or salts similar to the cathartics, or by taking laxatives like citrate of magnesia, Epsom salts, or effervescent sodium phosphate. As a digestive secretion, the most important function attributed to the bile is the part it takes in the digestion and absorption of fats.

One of the most important functions of the liver is the manufacture of glycogen. This sugar depends for the most part on the intake of sugars and starches. The bulk of the starches reaches the liver as simple sugar and is there converted into glycogen and stored as such. Glycogen is also stored in the body muscles. It is from these two storehouses that the sugar necessary for function of the body is supplied.

METHODS OF STUDYING DIGESTION

With the foregoing knowledge of the physiology and anatomy of the digestive tract, numerous analytical methods and instruments were devised to recognize changes from the normal. The stomach tube has brought to light many facts that were hitherto unknown. When it became feasible to remove a part of the stomach contents and subject it to a laboratory study physicians began to understand, to better advantage, the nature of stomach troubles. The decrease or increase of hydrochloric acid, or its complete absence, and the presence of pepsin are important in the diagnosis of various ailments. For instance, a German physician, Ewald, suggested that the patient first eat a definite standard test breakfast. This consists of a cup of weak tea, without cream or sugar, and a slice of dry toast or an unbuttered roll. This is given on an empty stomach and a part is then removed, in an hour, with a stomach tube and tested.

As was noted in the physiological considerations, acid and pepsin are present in normal stomach juice. If the acid is absent and pepsin is present, the condition is called achlorhydria, which means absence of hydrochloric acid. If both are absent, the condition is called achylia (or absence of chyle or stomach juice). Each of these conditions may be found in different disorders. For instance, in pernicious anemia just the acid is absent early in the disease, but as the disease becomes more severe, both the acid and pepsin are noticeably absent from the stomach juice. As hydrochloric acid and pepsin are secreted according to the needs of the stomach for digestion, there must necessarily be some variation in the amount and character of the stomach juice from time to time. Therefore, during the day the secretion is low or even absent. Because of this, the ordinary test meal as described may not be a true measure of the cycle of secretion of stomach juice. With this in mind, a test called the fractional test was devised. This is carried out by the use of a small soft rubber tube, swallowed, kept in the stomach, and then through this tube small amounts of stomach juice are withdrawn every fifteen minutes for a period of two or three hours. Occasionally even this test does not reveal the presence of acid. Then the doctor gives a weak alcohol solution instead of the ordinary test meal. Sometimes special drugs are used to determine the presence or absence of acid. For instance, a substance called histamine may be given by hypodermic injection to provoke secretion. Finally, certain dyes when given to a person by means of a hypodermic needle may be secreted by the stomach. If acid is able to be formed, the acid cells then secrete the dye.

Likewise, the motor power of the stomach may vary in disease. The stomach may empty too soon, or emptying may be delayed, especially if there is any obstruction at the outlet of the stomach. A full meal is given, and the stomach tube is introduced in seven hours. The stomach should be found empty of food, if its action is normal.

If pus or blood or bile are found in the stomach contents, they are evidences of a diseased condition. Sometimes in cases of obstruction at the stomach outlet, in the absence of hydrochloric acid, lactic acid may be found. This may indicate the beginning of a cancer.

By filling the stomach with a substance that is opaque to the X-ray, the size, shape, and motility of the stomach may be readily demonstrated. Barium sulphate is commonly used; it is added to any palatable liquid, such as buttermilk or malted milk. Lots of times the mere taking of this mixture may cause people to think they are better. By looking with the fluoroscopic X-ray screen, the doctor can detect changes in the peristaltic waves or contractions of the stomach, and any abnormal appearance in the outline of the silhouette or changes in the density of the normal shadows. The fact that the stomach can be manipulated during the X-ray examination under the screen is of greatest importance to detect tender areas, or to fill out parts of the stomach or duodenum under the pressure of the fingers. Thus ulcers and tumors are readily detected. X-ray pictures are made of all abnormal appearances not merely to detect minute changes but to keep a permanent record. This furnishes definite information which is most valuable in the diagnosis.

A large number of people who worry about stomach trouble do not have X-ray evidence of anything wrong with the stomach. This is due to the fact that diseased conditions outside of the stomach often give rise to digestive disorders or to symptoms in the digestive tract.

The gall bladder is X-rayed in the following manner. A patient is given a fat free meal the night before and two hours later is given some tablets containing dye by mouth. This dye has a special affinity for liver and it is passed by the liver cells into the small canals and later into larger canals and finally into the gall bladder. When this dye reaches the gall bladder it is concentrated there and casts a shadow on an X-ray film. This usually takes about 12 hours. It is important that the patient does not eat any food after taking the tablets of dye by mouth. This dye is absorbed from the intestines and by means of the blood stream gets into the liver. Two hours after the first film is taken, or approximately 14 hours after the patient has taken the dye, the night before, another film is taken. This is to determine whether or not the gall bladder can concentrate the dye. The shadow is usually denser than that seen on the 12 hour plate. The patient is then given a fat meal in order to see whether or not the gall bladder will empty properly. The fat acts on the valve that closes the gall bladder and makes it relax. When the ring of muscle tissue, called the ampulla of Vater, relaxes there is usually a contraction in the gall bladder. Therefore the gall bladder should normally empty after a patient is given a fat meal. The size of the shadow on the X-ray film is normally one third to one half the size of the originally filled gall bladder (as seen on the 12 and 14 hour X-ray films). This information permits the doctor to make more accurate diagnoses and also makes treatment, both medical and surgical, more definite.

Formerly gallstones were rarely detected by the X-ray, the chance depending on the amount of calcium (or lime salt) which they contained. Now early cancer of the gall bladder may be recognized in some cases by this method. This gall-bladder dye test was based on a test of the function of the liver.

Occasionally, when the doctor wants special information as to normal and abnormal conditions of the duodenum, which is the first portion of the small intestine just beyond the stomach, he allows a small tube with a metal perforated tip to pass through the stomach until it reaches the duodenum, where it can be retained. This duodenal juice is collected and may be studied for its constituents as outlined under physical considerations. Today, many physicians use this type of drainage to diagnose diseases of the gall bladder. This is accomplished by putting the material under the microscope and looking for crystals of cholesterol, pus cells and cells which line the gall bladder on the inside.

EXAMINATION OF EXCRETED MATERIALS

A routine and systematic examination of the stool (feces or bowel movements) of every patient is of great importance. This enables recognition of diseases of the stomach, liver, pancreas, gall bladder, and intestine. The consistency, shape, size, color, odor of the stools, and gross admixtures of mucus, blood, pus, and worms are all important. Chemical tests are made for blood and bile. The fermentation test determines whether the stool inclines too much to carbohydrates or protein putrefaction. The stools are examined with a microscope for the presence of undigested muscle fiber, fat, starch, pus, blood, or eggs of the parasites. They are also stained with dye to determine bacteria present. Bacterial cultures are made of the stool to determine the type of parasite that may be found in the stained smears. These cultures also reveal whether or not there are any dangerous organisms that should not be present in the stool. If such organisms are present in the stool they are separately cultured and then they are run through a set of broth culture media in which various dilutions of sulfa drugs or the antibiotics have been added. In this way, the physician gets accurate knowledge of the sensitivity of these organisms and will be better able to direct his treatment in a specific manner because of this information which comes out of the bacteriologic laboratory.

ACUTE INDIGESTION

Acute indigestion usually follows the intakes of substances that are obnoxious to the stomach. This condition is rather common today because many of the foods that persons take into their stomachs are either spoiled or infected. There are large epidemics of so-called acute gastrointestinal disturbances, dependent upon the fact that food may not be properly cooked, or that the handlers may contaminate it. It has become a public health problem. People are seized with severe upper abdominal pain followed by profuse nausea and vomiting. This is associated with midabdominal pain which is cramp-like and accompanied by a profuse watery diarrhea. As a rule this is without any fever but the temperature may rise to 100 degrees or slightly higher. The victim becomes acutely dehydrated, is weak, and for a period of anywhere from 6 to 24 hours, cannot hold anything on the stomach. All of the patients recover without any residual symptoms and are no more vulnerable to subsequent attacks than any other person since the initial attacks and the subsequent attacks depend upon the infective organisms. It was thought for a while that this was dependent upon a virus infection comparable to the virus that may cause acute colds.

However, frequently the organism is a staphylococcus which is highly toxic to the body. This may happen in children as well as adults.

Another common cause of acute indigestion is the abuse of alcohol, especially "modern alcohol." The tendency to disturbances of the stomach is increased in people who may have an irritable stomach and may get symptoms with the least provocation. A look into the stomach with a gastroscope will show that the lining of the stomach, called mucous membrane, is red, swollen and covered with mucus and, in some people there may be minute or large hemorrhages. These hemorrhages are beneath the lining of the stomach and do not, as a rule, cause bleeding into the cavity of the stomach. Occasionally the blood may break through and cause a patient to vomit a good deal of blood.

In mild cases, the symptoms are those of slight indigestion such as an uncomfortable feeling in the abdomen, headache, depression, nausea, belching, and vomiting, which usually gives relief. The tongue is heavily coated, and the saliva is increased. In children there are also intestinal symptoms, such as diarrhea, colicky pains, and often fever. The duration is rarely more than twenty-four hours. The severer attacks may begin with a chill, followed by fever which may reach 102 or 103 degrees. The tongue becomes furred; the breath is heavy, and vomiting is frequent. The material vomited first contains food particles and later becomes bile-stained. There may be an associated constipation or diarrhea. The abdomen becomes distended and tender. Herpes (cold sores) may appear on the lips, and these severe attacks may last from one to three days.

Many acute infectious diseases may begin the same way, and great care must be taken to be certain of the diagnosis. In addition, one must ascertain at once if poison such as phosphorus, corrosive sublimate (bichloride of mercury), ammonia, arsenic, lysol, iodine, or similar substances, has been swallowed, so that a proper antidote may be promptly administered. Furthermore, one dare not overlook the fact that appendicitis, peritonitis, or other infections in the abdomen may also begin in this manner. Any delay in making a conclusive and accurate diagnosis of these conditions may be fraught with danger. Finally, many of the deaths reported from so-called "acute indigestion" are actually acute heart attacks, in which the symptoms are more related to the abdomen than the heart. It is rare for anybody to succumb suddenly to a so-called attack of "acute indigestion" which has no other basis than disease of the stomach.

TREATMENT OF INDIGESTION

Some people with indigestion get the idea that there is some one food substance that is responsible for the feeling of fullness, the discomfort, the pain, and the eructation of gas that follow eating. Some of them force themselves to eat with the idea that this will make them well; others eliminate one food substance after another in the hope of finding the offending food substance, almost starving themselves to death.

After the doctor has made a complete examination and finds out that there is nothing organically wrong with the patient that can be reached, and after he assures the patient that he does not have cancer, heart disease, or some equally serious disturbance, he next tries to find what troubles are in the family which cause the patient to lose his appetite and ruin his digestion. Many cases of indigestion are due to the fact that patients have emotional disturbances which produce effects on the stomach. The family physician will be able to talk this out with the patient and thus aid to develop a better family situation and to try to straighten out the emotional difficulties.

Sometimes rest or vacation will have a favorable effect on the person with acute indigestion or dyspepsia, particularly if he goes away from his household and all the people around him. This does not mean a strenuous holiday but an actual rest.

Many persons who seem to be having trouble with their digestions do better with a certain amount of massage and mild exercise. This is particularly the case in stoutly built men who were once athletic and who, following a business career, become flabby and fat. Most important in these cases, however, is the developing of a diet that the patient can take and the teaching of the patient to eat as he should. The smooth diet is the one most frequently prescribed for such patients. In one of the largest clinics in the United States the following smooth diet is regularly advised for persons with chronic digestive trouble:

If you are to give this diet a fair trial, eat no coarse foods with fiber, skins, seeds or gristle. Avoid particularly salads with celery, tomatoes, cucumbers, and pineapple, many of the green vegetables, raisins, berries, jams full of seeds, nuts, and many of the raw fruits. Beans, cabbage, onions, green or red peppers, melons, cucumbers and peanuts are notoriously gassy. If you are living in a boarding house you can stick to this diet by simply avoiding the forbidden foods and eating more of the digestible ones which are put before you.

Avoid sugar in concentrated form and take no candy or other food between meals. Hot cakes and waffles might not be bad if they are properly fried, that is, totally immersed in fat at the right temperature. Avoid eating when in a rush and when mentally upset. Family rows should be held away from the table. Chewing gum may cause distress, as much air is swallowed with the saliva. Digestion is greatly helped by a good chewing surface. If there are any gaps in your teeth have your dentist fill them with bridges. Purgatives often cause flatulence and distress in the abdomen.

The following are suggestions for breakfast: Orange juice, grapefruit (avoid the fiber in the compartments); cantaloupe and melons are inadvisable. Coffee, if desired, is allowed in moderation; it sometimes causes flatulence. If you are sensitive to caffeine try Sanka Coffee or Instant Postum. Chocolate, cocoa or tea, one or two eggs with ham or bacon (avoid the tougher part of the bacon), white bread, toast or Zwieback with butter, any smooth mush such as farina, germea, cream of wheat, cornmeal, or rolled oats (a fine oatmeal can be obtained by calling for Robinson's Scotch Groats); puffed cereals and cornflakes are also allowed. Shredded wheat biscuits and other coarse breakfast foods are not allowed. Bran is particularly harmful. Graham bread is permitted but not the coarser whole-wheat bread.

Suggestions for lunch and dinner: In fruit cocktails avoid the pieces of orange and pineapple. Broths, bouillon, cream soups and chowder are allowed, also meat, fish or chicken, squab or game, excepting duck (avoid the fibrous parts and gristle). Veal may be tried; it is not digested well by many persons. Eat no smoked fish or pork. Crab and lobster had better be left alone. Oysters and sausage may be tried later.

Bread and butter are allowed, and hot biscuits if they are made small so as to consist mainly of crust. Rice, potatoes, mashed, hashed brown, or French fried, are allowed; and later may be added sweet potatoes, hominy, tomatoes stewed, strained and thickened with cracker or bread crumbs, well-cooked cauliflower tops with cream sauce, asparagus tips, Brussels sprouts, squash, beets, turnips, creamed spinach, Italian pastes, noodles, macaroni and spaghetti cooked soft, purées of peas, beans, lentils, lima beans, or artichoke hearts. All skins or fiber should be removed by passing the food through a ricer. Sweet corn may be used if passed through a colander. There are practically no other vegetables that can be puréed to advantage. String beans (large tender string beans which can be used as a vegetable or salad can now be obtained in cans) are allowed if they are young and tender.

No salad should be taken at first. Later you may try a little tender lettuce with apples or bananas, tomato jelly, or boiled eggs. Mayonnaise and French dressing are allowed. Potato salad without much onion may be tried.

Suggestions for dessert are: Simple puddings, custards, ice cream, jello, plain cake and canned or stewed fruits, particularly pears and peaches. Cottage cheese is permissible; other cheeses often cause trouble. Apple, peach, apricot, custard and lemon cream pie may be tried if only the filling is eaten.

In case of constipation, stewed fruit may be taken once or twice a day. In winter the dried pared fruit may be used for stewing. Prunes are probably the most laxative of fruits and if eaten every other morning they will relieve the average case of constipation. They should be cooked slowly until they almost go to pieces. If the skins are still tough they should be discarded. Apple sauce is much more palatable if made from unpared and uncored apples. The sauce is strained later. It may be mixed with a little tapioca or sago. The apples may be baked. Apples, even when cooked, often cause distress. Blackberries and loganberries can be stewed and strained and the sweetened juice thickened with cornstarch. This makes a delicious dish with the full flavor of the berries. Later you may try fully ripe pears and peaches.

Make no effort to drink water. Be guided by your thirst. Avoid excessive use of salt or other seasoning. If you wish to gain in weight eat as much cream, butter, fat and starch as you can. If you wish to lose or stay thin, live largely on vegetables, fruits and salads, with a moderate amount of lean meat.

DIFFICULTY IN SWALLOWING

Many people have difficulty in swallowing. The scientific term is dysphagia. Many nervous people suffer from "lump in the throat." In purely functional or nervous trouble of this kind, there is seldom loss of weight and strength, such as occurs in actual changes of the tissues of the esophagus (the food pipe leading to the stomach). Simple spasmodic contractions of the esophagus may be due either to disease of the wall or to a so-called reflex (referred) spasm from disease elsewhere. The most common type of spasm is at the end of the esophagus (called cardiospasm), where it enters the stomach. Here the esophagus closes down and does not allow the food to enter the stomach. The esophagus becomes larger above the constriction, food is not taken satisfactorily, and the patients lose weight and strength. Sometimes people with this condition become nauseated and may even vomit. In severe cases food may remain in the esophagus for a few days. As a rule these cases recover when the opening is stretched repeatedly at suitable intervals with proper instruments.

In cases of cancer of the esophagus the early signs and symptoms may go unnoticed. However, there ensues gradually increasing difficulty in swallowing, associated with loss of weight and strength. There are numerous other causes of disturbed swallowing because foreign bodies are swallowed and stick. Sometimes patients swallow too much air (called aërophagia). The stomach becomes dilated and swollen, and then it is difficult to force any food down.

The diagnosis of any of these conditions is based on a careful record of the events and, in addition, accurate X-ray observation. Occasionally a long metal (lighted) tube is put down the esophagus and direct observation can be made of the trouble. Sometimes the condition can be treated directly through this tube.

DYSPEPSIA

"Dyspepsia" means difficult or painful digestion. Indigestion, strictly speaking, is perhaps somewhat different from dyspepsia; it denotes failure of digestion rather than difficulty or pain in the process. The two terms are commonly used synonymously and may be understood to include every condition which is associated with an abdominal sensation referable to the stomach after the ingestion of food.

The outstanding symptom of dyspepsia is abdominal discomfort or pain. The healthy person is unconscious of the existence of his stomach; the dyspeptic rarely forgets it. The intensity of the sensation may vary in degree from a slight feeling of heaviness to agonizing pain which is almost beyond endurance. This occurs usually immediately after the intake of food. When the discomfort becomes more evident, it may be a dull, aching pain, or it may be boring, cutting, stabbing, burning, or griping. Occasionally it is so severe that the sufferer is "doubled up" and writhing in pain. It may be aggravated by pressure over the stomach. Vomiting may afford relief, especially when associated with belching, which relieves pressure.

Heartburn is a peculiarly appropriate word. It exactly describes a sensation; a characteristic burning pain felt immediately behind the "chest bone," rising upward and occasionally spreading to the throat. Heartburn is a frequent symptom of stomach disturbance. It is supposed to be due to increased acidity of the stomach and a regurgitation of the contents upwards into the esophagus through a relaxed muscle at its lower end. The acid supposedly irritates the lining of the esophagus. However, some patients without excess acidity in the stomach have heartburn. Heartburn may be due to nervous disturbances of the stomach, particularly those of emotional origin. When the doctor looks into the stomach, he finds no changes at all in the lining of the stomach, there is no redness, no swelling and no evidence of any hemorrhage. On the other hand, when people are sufferers of heartburn of nervous origin, one may find that the folds of the stomach are greatly increased due to increased work of the stomach. The heartburn which occurs at night or in the early hours of the morning is due to increased stimulation of the vagus (wandering) nerve, going to the stomach. This may be related to changes in levels of blood sugar. The pain comes during the early hours of the morning when a sufficient amount of food is not going to the brain. The brain sends these obnoxious stimuli to the stomach which may cause heartburn. This is frequently observed in patients, as will be later shown, who have peptic ulcer. Posture may, at times, seem to favor its development. Occasionally change of position from one side to another, sitting up, rather than lying down, may afford relief. Heartburn tends to occur especially at night and may cause considerable distress by interfering with sleep.

"Water brash," or eructation of sour fluid, may follow a burning sensation in the stomach. It is due to increased flow of saliva, associated with acid eructations and heartburn. Increased salivation is frequently an accompaniment of many forms of dyspepsia. Acid eructations are similar to heartburn, except that the acid is brought up with gas by belching. Many dyspeptics complain of a feeling of distention after meals. This may be associated with flatulence or "gas on the stomach." The latter may be caused by the swallowing of air. A certain amount of air is normally swallowed by everyone with food and saliva, but in some people the quantity is excessive. This is called aërophagia. Flatulence may also be caused by fermentation of the stomach contents.

Vomiting often accompanies indigestion. It may be associated with pain, which is relieved when the stomach is emptied by vomiting. Closing of the upper end of the stomach and the attempt to vomit without bringing up anything is called retching, which is always accompanied by nausea.

In dyspepsia, the appetite is variable. The tongue is often furred, especially when thirst is severe. The breath is offensive, and there is a bad taste in the mouth. However, bad breath may also be due to disease of the nose and throat.

CHRONIC GASTRITIS

Chronic inflammatory conditions of the stomach have again reappeared as a distinct disease, for which the term "chronic gastritis" is applied. The reawakening of this disease has been due to the introduction of an instrument called the gastroscope. This instrument is lighted electrically at the end, and through a series of lenses one is able to see the interior of the stomach. The causes of chronic gastritis are numerous. It occurs frequently in patients who are chronic alcoholics and prolonged and continuous users of tobacco. It may also be due to secondary disease of the teeth and chronic sinus inflammation. Deficiency states, associated with a low vitamin intake, are frequent precursors of the disease. It is seen in such diseases as pernicious anemia and sprue.

In this disease the lining of the stomach may become distinctly flattened out and show evidence of hemorrhages and pigment, which is called the atrophic (wasting) type, or the stomach folds may be distinctly increased, which is called the hypertrophic (overgrowth) type. The symptoms of these conditions are variable. They sometimes resemble that of a peptic ulcer. Patients may complain of a moderate to severe pain in the region of the stomach, and in thin, emaciated people, pressure over the stomach sometimes elicits pain. Acids may or may not be present in normal amounts.

The first step in treatment is to eradicate the possible cause. This is followed by a suitable and easily digestible, non-irritating diet, and in patients with an absence of acids in the stomach dilute hydrochloric acid should be given after meals in suitable amounts to replace the deficiency. Large amounts of vitamins, either by mouth, hypodermically or intravenously, may be indicated in patients with chronic gastritis, particularly the vitamin B complex. Further, the fractions of this complex may be given singly in larger amounts because as a rule the usual "shotgun" vitamin tablets, capsules, or perles, do not contain enough of the specific vitamin to be of definite curative value. Crude liver extract has been injected into the muscles of patients who have definitely shown improvement after this type of treatment. Vitamin B_{12}, which is a fraction of the Vitamin B complex and has to do with blood formation, also has been used in patients with chronic gastritis and anemias which resemble a pernicious type. This is particularly true where a patient has a loss of free hydrochloric acid associated with chronic gastritis.

The relation of chronic gastritis to cancer is not definitely known. However, there are some who feel that a prolonged disturbance of the stomach, associated with a gastritis, may lead to cancer.

GASTROPTOSIS

Many thin, weak people suffer from time to time with vague stomach complaints which, until the advent of the X-ray, were not well understood. The condition called gastroptosis or falling of the stomach is not uncommon. It occurs more often in women than in men. There are many theories as to its cause. Pregnancy, loss of body tone and vigor, and great loss of weight may be factors. Some people are born with the condition.

Most people with gastroptosis are dull and apathetic, have dizziness and headaches and are without appetite. There may be some nausea and even vomiting. Pain, feeling of pressure, weight, fullness or distention of the stomach are common. Small amounts of food satiate them, and they have little desire for food after the first mouthfuls. Sometimes there is a splashing sound in the stomach as water enters it. If the disease is of long standing, patients begin to lose weight and strength. Many remote changes in the body may be referable to the "fallen stomach." It is apparently due to the inability of the food and secretions to get out of the stomach into the small intestine. The duodenum, which is the first part of the small intestine beyond the stomach, may be four to six inches long, or longer. Because of the stagnation and pressure caused by the drag of the stomach the duodenum becomes dilated and larger. When substances are absorbed from the duodenum they are poisonous, and an overwhelming amount, as in the case of this disease, is more than the body can take care of. Therefore, headache, dizziness, nausea, lack of appetite, and consequent loss of weight appear.

The X-ray clearly reveals this difficulty. Furthermore, these patients are more comfortable when they lie down, or even better, if the end of the bed is elevated so that the pressure is relieved from the duodenum. With proper diet and sedatives, these patients begin to gain in weight and vigor. If the treatment is to be accomplished without rest in bed, then a suitable corset and pad to elevate the stomach, to favor more rapid emptying, has been used successfully by some physicians. Some people get immediate relief on getting into the knee-chest position. Either on the floor or on the bed they turn their body upside down with the head much lower than the back. The person who remains in this position for about five minutes will usually experience definite relief. In obstinate and severe cases, operative procedures have been designed to correct the trouble.

ULCER OF THE STOMACH AND DUODENUM

An ulcer is a raw spot in the inner lining of the stomach or duodenum, representing destruction of tissues. The life history of an ulcer is extremely varied. Some heal; others burrow deeper and become chronic; others bleed (hemorrhage); some penetrate through the tissues or perforate. Occasionally this perforation may be sealed by nature. The ulcer may be adjacent to a neighboring organ, such as the pancreas, or it may be sealed by that great protective pad or veil of fat in the abdomen, called the omentum. Sometimes the perforation may remain unsealed and the contents of the stomach or duodenum, or both, get into the free abdominal cavity, called the peritoneal cavity. Then a serious condition of inflammation and infection develops which is called perforation peritonitis. The peritoneum, or membrane lining the abdominal cavity, is involved.

The exact cause of ulcer is unknown. There are, however, many predisposing factors. First, there is a definite tendency in some families to the formation of ulcer. This has been considered to be purely psychological because the patients may inherit emotional tendencies similar to those that existed in their father or mother or both. The condition is more common in the third and fourth decades of life, although it is found in the first decade. Constant abuse of the stomach, eating too highly seasoned foods, or foods too hot or too cold, or not properly masticating foods, may be a factor. The abuse of alcohol and tobacco, especially cigarettes, plays a role in the development of ulcer but is not necessarily its immediate cause. However, hydrochloric acid is practically always present in a benign gastric ulcer or duodenal ulcer. As long as the mucous membrane of the stomach and duodenum are covered by mucus, ulceration cannot take place. What causes the disappearance or the dissolving of mucus at any given point and causes an ulcer to develop, is not known at present. It has been suggested that certain enzymes which will produce a solution of mucus may be secreted in one spot more than another and allow the unprotected gastric mucous membrane to be attacked by the digestive juices. The digestive action of gastric juice is the all important factor in the development of an ulcer of the stomach or duodenum. Observations have been made that certain people have a tendency to develop ulcer in or about the age when hardening of the arteries occurs. This has been debated by many investigators but notwithstanding that a certain incidence of ulcer occurs in elderly people the question of changes in blood supply is significant. Recent studies have indicated that there may be a place for the role of blood sugar in the development of peptic ulcer. When the blood sugar is sufficiently low, more stimulation comes from the brain by way of the vagus nerve to the stomach. When the blood sugar levels are high, such stimulation does not as a rule go over the vagus nerve. This theoretical consideration is made more plausible by the fact that ulcer rarely occurs in diabetics under 40 years of age. Furthermore, if we take all the statistics of patients who have diabetes, we find that the incidence is much lower in diabetics than it is in the population as a whole. Beyond the age of 40, when blood vessels begin to have changes associated with arteriosclerosis, ulcer becomes a more prominent factor. In many laboratories, where statistical evaluation of the ulcer problem has been made, large series of patients who have died with diabetes have failed to show any evidence of peptic ulcer in the stomach or duodenum.

Patients with ulcer have variable symptoms. Most of them complain of a distress which may be a burning sensation (sometimes called heartburn), or a feeling of pressure and weight, or a dull ache, or even a severe pain, sometimes remaining localized to the region of the stomach, occasionally going into the back, or even traveling upward beneath the sternum (chest bone). This distress may come on soon after eating or may be delayed as long as two or three hours. It usually lasts until the next meal, unless it is relieved by taking some medicine. It may awaken the sufferer in the early hours of the morning. It may be seasonal in type, more prone to occur in the spring and fall of the year. As the ulcer becomes chronic, the distress may last throughout the year. But this periodicity of the distress is quite characteristic. Many patients are afraid to eat because eating seems to bring on the pain. Some have found that by eating frequently they are more comfortable. Occasionally, at the height of the pain, vomiting brings relief. This is especially true in those cases in which there is a spasm or constriction at the outlet of the stomach. Patients soon learn to avoid certain foods, especially seasonings, condiments, fried and greasy foods. Tobacco and coffee, as a rule, increase the distress. While pain is an outstanding feature, occasionally the observant patients may notice tenderness in the abdomen high up, just beneath the sternum (chest bone).

As the ulcer grows older, so to speak, certain manifestations may take place. The pain may become more persistent and severe and may only be relieved by natural or forced vomiting. If the scar of the healing ulcer is located at the outlet of the stomach, an obstruction may develop, which will not permit the stomach to empty itself, or the ulcer may have two important complications; notably, hemorrhage or perforation.

Hemorrhage is associated with certain definite symptoms. Even if no vomiting of blood takes place, the person who is bleeding soon finds himself overcome by a sudden weakness with slight nausea. He may break out in a cold perspiration, become dizzy, feel faint and giddy. If the hemorrhage is large he may become unconscious. Sooner or later his stool, or bowel movement, appears black; this is called a "tarry stool." The face becomes blanched; the expression is anxious. The feeling of fear has a tendency at first to increase rather than decrease the hemorrhage. Nature counteracts this by causing a fall in blood pressure and thus lessens the tendency for hemorrhage.

If a person with ulcer vomits blood, which is more common if the ulcer is located in the stomach rather than in the duodenum, he immediately knows the cause of his distress. Anyone who has experienced the sensation of a hemorrhage recognizes the early symptoms promptly on the second or third repetition of the bleeding.

In the case of perforation, the course is much stormier. Agonizing, excruciating pains develop in the upper abdomen. Cold, clammy sweat appears, and the sufferer becomes anxious, nauseated, and may even vomit. The abdomen becomes tense and board-like, and as conditions become more severe, the symptoms become intensified. Unless the ulcer becomes immediately sealed an operation should be performed at the earliest possible time. After 12 hours have elapsed from the beginning of the perforation the life expectancy decreases. However, today with the use of the newer drugs, particularly the sulfa drugs and the antibiotics, fewer patients die of an overwhelming peritonitis than did previously to the discovery of these drugs.

After the ulcer is diagnosed, the choice of treatment depends on the nature of the condition. Some ulcers will never heal with medical treatment alone and should properly undergo surgical operation; others should have medical treatment from the outset. If the patient has ulcer of the stomach and is in or about the cancer age, thirty-five or above, then great care should be exercised as to the choice of treatment. If the ulcer is in a young person, medical treatment can usually be carried out safely. It is important that repeated X-ray examinations at monthly intervals be carried out on all patients who are treated for gastric ulcer, in order to note the progress of the disease. With resistant ulcer, surgery should be used promptly.

If the ulcer is located in the duodenum, medical treatment can usually be carried out unless there is evidence of penetration or obstruction. In the chronic, indolent, and refractory ulcers, surgery probably offers the best end-result. Frequent recurrent hemorrhages may have to have surgical intervention.

Operative procedures for ulcer include removal of portions of the stomach, gastroenterostomy which shunts the food around the area, and vagotomy, which cuts the nerve and stops the acid secretion.

The medical treatment of duodenal ulcer should be primarily directed at decreasing the acidity of the stomach. Efforts should be directed not only to the neutralization but also to preventing or inhibiting the formation of too much acid. This may be accomplished by a definite adjustment in a patient's mental habits, household, and work. Certain drugs which paralyze the vagus nerves which go to the stomach and decrease the secretion of gastric acidity should be given to patients. These drugs form into the atropine group and there are many new synthetic preparations that have been developed. A person with such a nervous system should be put at physiologic rest and this is usually accomplished by the doctor, and the doctor only, prescribing some form of phenobarbital.

It is important that patients undergoing ulcer treatment should be calm, and have few, if any, irritating incidents to disturb their mental equilibrium. Furthermore, the reduction of acid may be accomplished by an easily digestible, non-provoking acid diet. Milk and cream should be important constituents of the diet, and patients should refrain from the use of alcohol, highly seasoned foods, and tobacco, which cause an increased acidity. Fried foods are not well tolerated. Puréed vegetables, puréed or stewed fruit, and fruit juices are distinctly beneficial.

The direct neutralization of the acidity may be accomplished by the use of alkalies (ordinary neutralizing powders), or, more recently, the use of the so-called aluminum salts (aluminum hydroxide and aluminum phosphate, the latter being the drug of choice). Many people cannot stand alkalies and develop a condition called alkalosis (too much alkali). This is particularly true of people beyond fifty years of age. Therefore, one must resort to a neutralization by such salts as those of aluminum which do not cause an alkalosis. It is also important that the diet be sufficiently high in vitamins and that the neutralizing agents not be given immediately after meals, because they have a tendency to destroy certain components of the vitamin B complex.

DISEASE OF THE GALL BLADDER

The most common cause of stomach disorders in the adult is disease of the gall bladder. Such diseases as typhoid, pneumonia, influenza, sore throat, and other acute infectious diseases may leave residual disease in the gall bladder. Gall-bladder disease is particularly likely to occur during and after pregnancy, especially in nursing mothers. Fatty or obese people are also likely to develop this disease. Modern methods of dieting, of omitting meals, of allowing the gall bladder to remain filled too long without its physiological emptying are also important factors. The gall bladder empties when food is taken, especially fatty foods. It is best to eat three times a day to keep the gall bladder functioning well. More recent observations have suggested the role of the nervous system in the development of gallstones. By this I mean the gall bladder does not empty when stimulated by foods which ordinarily would make it empty. This allows the gall bladder to remain filled. The cholesterol which is in the gall bladder may precipitate out. These cholesterol crystals may adhere together to form stones. At first, the stones are purely cholesterol but later calcium salts enter and they may be calcium and cholesterol. These stones also may be pigmented by the bile pigment and they may go into typical gallstones. A person may have a normal gall bladder filled with large numbers of cholesterol stones. However, sooner or later the sharp-edged stones irritate the lining of the gall bladder and the patient develops a real inflammation of the gall bladder called cholecystitis.

The early signs are usually fullness and distention of the abdomen, associated with much belching. The distress comes on, as a rule, immediately after eating, and the patient rises from the table with an "overloaded" sensation. This overloading is due to the sucking in of air, because the muscle at the upper end of the stomach is relaxed and air easily flows into the stomach and distends it. Belching affords relief, but occasionally more air is swallowed in the act of belching, and this leads to greater distention. Fatty, greasy, and highly seasoned foods aggravate the distress. Pain may be present. It may be a dull ache, a sensation of weight, or it may be sharp and severe. It may be constant or intermittent. It may be localized beneath the ribs in front on the right side, or it may go to the back and right shoulder. If it is severe enough to "double one up" and is associated with nausea and vomiting, it is significant of gallstones. Occasionally gall-bladder disease causes a spasm of the outlet of the stomach, which is not only painful but may be accompanied by nausea and vomiting. When the outlet relaxes, the vomitus may be yellow or green.

Headache is a common symptom and is associated with disturbed movements of the first portion of the small intestine. Here absorption may take place. It is not definitely known at the present time whether the absorption of the duodenum is poisonous or whether because of the amount of stasis a definite increase in blood alkalinity may occur. There is some evidence to favor the latter point of view. The sleep is disturbed and fitful. The complexion is often sallow, and patients complain of being "bilious." Constipation is a frequent symptom. If the disease progresses, stones may be formed in the gall bladder, which later become dislodged into the larger tubes carrying the bile and obstruct the flow of bile; then "yellow jaundice" supervenes. Jaundice may be present without stones associated with disease of the liver.

Jaundice first appears in the whites of the eyes. Later, the skin becomes yellow, and still later the urine grows darker and the excretion from the bowels lighter in color. Itching may be a pronounced and aggravating symptom to the extent that severe scratching and abrasions of the skin take place. The jaundiced person becomes dull, apathetic, and lethargic when cholemia (bile poisoning) takes place. People with gallstones are frequently miserable because of irritation and pain, and when a positive diagnosis is made they should have an operation, providing contraindications to operation do not exist. The danger of gallstones should not be under-estimated. Pus may form, which is dangerous, and in a certain group of gall bladders, associated with stones, cancer has been known to develop. Therefore, it is considered good prophylaxis to remove gall bladders with gallstones. There is no medical treatment that will dissolve the gallstones. However, it is to be frankly stated that not all patients with gallstones are considered good surgical risks, and it may be the lesser of two evils to allow a patient to continue medical management without operation.

JAUNDICE

Whenever material from the bile, called bilirubin, gets into the blood there follows a yellowish discoloration of the skin. The skin, the mucous membranes, and even the whites of the eyes become jaundiced. There are, however, several different types of conditions that can cause the passage into the blood of this bile. For instance, an obstruction may occur anywhere in the bile ducts from the smallest channels which develop in the liver to the point at which the bile pours into the intestines. If the obstruction is sufficient, the bile is turned back, and jaundice follows.

The most frequent causes of such jaundice are stones which block the tubes, but occasionally tumors may form and block off the ducts, and in other instances there may be serious infection with inflammation and swelling resulting in obstruction.

Associated with jaundice, itching of the skin is not infrequent. Bile pigments appear in the urine, and therefore it becomes yellow. If the bile does not flow into the intestine, the excretion develops a clay color. Patients may complain of a great deal of nausea, loss of appetite, weakness, and loss of weight, which is due to the impairment of liver function. Frequently hemorrhages occur, due to the lack of absorption of a specific vitamin called vitamin K from the small intestine. It is necessary to have bile present in the small intestine for the absorption of vitamin K.

INFECTIOUS HEPATITIS

One form of jaundice which may occur in children or others has become well identified in medicine today. This type of jaundice is associated with viral disease of the liver. Viral hepatitis had its greatest incidence during World War II when large numbers of our soldiers were exposed to the virus of hepatitis in the foreign lands to which they were sent. They also became carriers of the disease and when they came back to civilian life other people also became infected from transmission of the virus. Apparently this virus gains access to the body by means of the gastrointestinal tract, that is, the foods you swallow. However, there are a large number of patients who have gotten virus hepatitis or serum hepatitis from blood transfusions or blood plasma given in the treatment of the disease. Today a large number of older patients have become seriously ill due to infected blood plasma or whole blood. During World War II large amounts of plasma contained this virus. We did not know at that time that the virus was a factor. Since it became evident that the serum could carry the virus measures have been taken to kill the virus in serum. In many large hospitals and serum centers this method of treating blood plasma is practiced. These patients are given irradiated serum or irradiated plasma. The solution of serum or plasma is exposed to radiation and this radiation kills the virus. Garet Allen found that the virus dies if pooled plasma stands for some weeks at room temperature. Viral hepatitis is a serious disease in older people and not so serious in younger ones. However if it happens in a woman patient beyond the change of life it is an exceedingly dangerous condition and mortality figures as high as 50 per cent have been reported by some hospitals and clinics. The disease, as a rule, starts out with loss of appetite, definite fatigue and even headaches. Sooner or later the patient complains of pain in the right upper quadrant of the abdomen and that is due to a swollen, tender liver. At the same time that this group of symptoms begin to show themselves, jaundice appears in the eyes and the doctor recognizes that the patient has epidemic hepatitis. It usually runs a course of from 8 to 10 weeks and then gradually subsides. During the disease the patient becomes deeply jaundiced, loses his appetite completely, there is a great loss of weight and the patient becomes dull and apathetic. As the liver begins to repair itself, the appetite is first to return and when the appetite returns in a patient who has infectious hepatitis, it is one of the best signs that the patient is beginning to conquer the disease. Keep the patient absolutely at rest in bed, give a high carbohydrate, high protein, low fat diet and additional vitamins. Occasionally the physician may have to inject fluids into the veins. These fluids consist mostly of sugar and sometimes proteins. Frequent laboratory studies are made during the progress of the disease and the doctor knows from the changes in the laboratory studies, whether his patient is getting worse or better. Once the patient begins to get better he usually goes on to complete recovery. However, instances are reported of more chronic changes in the liver known as cirrhosis. If a patient develops cirrhosis following epidemic hepatitis it is of serious import because sooner or later, the patient may have all the signs of an out and out case of cirrhosis of the liver which may be difficult to treat and difficult to get well. Even though you have a badly damaged liver, the liver is able to repair itself in its entirety sometimes and this may even apply to patients who have been afflicted with cirrhosis. No age is spared in this disease; however, since the end of the last War, the condition is seen more commonly in patients who are in their thirties and forties.

Another form of jaundice which closely simulates epidemic jaundice is due to glandular fever. Glandular fever affects the liver in a way similar to infectious hepatitis; however, the prognosis is always much better. As the glandular fever subsides, the liver usually returns to normal. The following diet is suggested for persons who have liver disease and should be followed during the active stage of liver disease.

HEPATIC DIET

FOODS ALLOWED:

Cereals:	One serving daily of any type cooked or prepared cereal, i.e. enriched cream of wheat, farina, oatmeal, cornflakes, rice krispies, etc. Avoid those containing large amounts of bran.
Bread:	Enriched white bread, cracked or honey wheat bread, melba toast, holland rusk, zwieback or white crackers. No rye bread.
Cereal Substitutes:	Rice, noodles, macaroni, spaghetti, vermicelli, or hominy. All to be plainly prepared without the addition of highly seasoned or rich sauces.
Soups:	Lean chicken broth on occasion and vegetable milk soups.
Meat:	Two servings daily of very lean meat, i.e. lamb, veal, beef, liver, chicken or turkey. To be broiled, boiled, or roasted without additional fat. Remove all visible fat and gristle. No gravies or sauces. No pork or pork products, including bacon. Four ounce cooked portion equals minimum serving; may use more.
Fish:	Lean fresh water fish, i.e. perch, pike, trout, bass, or whitefish. All to be broiled, boiled, poached, or baked; none fried.
Cheese:	Three tablespoons cottage or small amounts of cream cheese. No other kinds to be used.
Eggs:	One or two daily. May be either soft boiled, poached, shirred or scrambled over water. None to be fried. May substitute two eggs for one serving meat, fish, or poultry.
Vegetables:	At least three or four servings daily of any type cooked or raw vegetable with the exception of raw onions, radishes, cucumbers, or sauerkraut. All to be prepared without additional fat.
Potatoes:	Mashed, baked or boiled potatoes. None fried.
Fruits:	At least three or four servings daily of any type canned, stewed or fresh fruits with the exception of bananas or avocadoes. One fruit should be citrus, i.e orange or grapefruit or the juice of either.
Desserts:	Fruit as above. Simple puddings, custard, gelatine, sponge cake, and simple wafers.
Beverages:	Three or four glasses of milk daily; may use more. Tea, sanka, kaffee hag, postum, fruit juices and water.
Butter:	Three teaspoons or pats per day.
Condiments:	None to be used except salt.
Sweets:	Sugar, jelly, honey, and hard candy as desired.

FOODS TO AVOID:

Fried foods, oils, salad dressings, nuts, peanut butter, cream. Smoked, spiced or tinned meats or fish. Pork or pork products. Gravies and sauces. Pies, pastries, chocolate and chocolate products. Alcoholic and carbonated beverages. Coffee. Spices and condiments. AVOID TOBACCO.

OTHER CAUSES OF JAUNDICE

Various types of poisons which tend to injure the liver as, for example, poison by arsenic, phosphorus, chloroform, and cinchophen, are frequently associated with jaundice. There are also cases in which certain types of infection actually do spread through a community. Much liver damage is frequent. Unfortunately the sulfanilamide type of drugs may cause jaundice.

One of the most common types of bile in the blood is that which occurs in tiny babies just after birth. This usually tends to clear up in a few days. Patients with jaundice should have a high sugar diet. Further, the protein of the diet should be more than normally needed in order to supply the deficiency due to liver destruction. The sugars can be given by mouth or in concentrated solutions in the vein.

APPENDICITIS

Appendicitis, as the name indicates, means an inflammation of the appendix. This small rudimentary organ, located at the beginning of the colon, a portion of the large bowel in the lower right side, is important in the causation of acute and chronic abdominal complaints.

Acute appendicitis now is recognized as a definite disease. It occurs at all ages, even in infants. The early signs of this condition include mild to severe abdominal pain, which frequently is first felt in the upper portion of the abdomen. After some hours the pain tends to localize in the right lower quarter of the abdomen. The pain usually develops suddenly and is cramplike. It recurs at intervals and at times is most severe. The patient soon has some nausea which may be progressive and associated with vomiting. These early symptoms may increase in severity, and if the inflammation of the appendix progresses there is soon a rise in the temperature of a few degrees. When a blood count is made it shows evidence of infection by an increase in the number of white blood cells. The abdominal muscles on the right side over the region of the appendix are rigid, and to relieve this feeling of tenseness the patient will often bend the right knee.

The examining physician is able to demonstrate the local tenderness over the appendix and perhaps some increased resistance to touch or muscular rigidity in the same region. This is typical of acute appendicitis, and most physicians usually decide on immediate operation in such cases. If after a few hours the pain suddenly diminishes, there may be gangrene or rupture of the appendix, to be followed within a few hours by peritonitis. Hence, although at times in mild catarrhal appendicitis the pain may subside and the patient begin to improve, in the majority of cases this abrupt change should be considered a danger signal for the beginning of peritonitis.

If the sick person does not have medical attention during the first twelve to twenty-four hours, two possibilities may occur. First, the inflammation may subside and thereafter be followed by mild symptoms of a chronic nature. Second, the acute inflammation of the appendix may progress rapidly, giving rise to the so-called pus appendix, gangrene, or rupture with peritonitis. These complications are, of course, extremely serious and may even terminate fatally. When a member of the family develops a sudden pain in the abdomen, like that described, one should never give a laxative, but should call a doctor at once.

Chronic appendicitis is usually the outcome of one or more mild attacks of previous acute appendicitis. The symptoms may be vague and baffling for a long time. Ordinarily there is some abdominal pain, which has a tendency to be colic-like and may not be associated with any nausea or vomiting. In the chronic cases the doctor must make sure that the symptoms are not due to some other cause, such as gall-bladder disease, or stone in the kidney, or ulcer of the stomach, or disease of the colon; then, when the symptoms are clear and the X-ray gives evidence of disease of the appendix, an operation should be done to remove it.

Once the diagnosis of acute appendicitis is made, an operation should be done as soon as possible; this is still the safest course.

No one can predict just what the subsequent changes may be, and no one can foretell whether a rupture of an inflamed appendix with peritonitis may occur. Operation in the uncomplicated cases is comparatively simple and safe.

Ulcer, Gall-Bladder Disease, and Appendicitis

To distinguish between ulcer, gall-bladder disease and appendicitis is difficult. At times the three may be similar. It is not safe for anyone to try to distinguish these for himself. There is severe pain in all of them. The pain in ulcer comes on one-half hour or longer after eating and is relieved by taking some milk or bland food or some alkaline substance. Highly seasoned foods or alcohol make the pain worse. The pain is felt over the pit of the stomach and remains there. The pain in appendicitis, although at first felt in the region of the stomach, later moves to the location of the appendix. The pain has no relation to the taking of food and is not relieved by food or an alkali. The pain in gall-bladder disease is first felt in the upper right side of the abdomen, and it is referred to the right shoulder and back and often to the right shoulder blade region. The pain may be severe, especially in cases that have gallstones, and it may be colicky.

In all three diseases, nausea and vomiting may be present. In ulcer the vomiting brings relief, except in the ulcers that may be in a perforating stage. In the gall-bladder disorders or appendicitis vomiting is persistent, usually without relief.

There is usually fever in acute disease of the gall bladder and appendix, but seldom in ulcer unless the ulcer has perforated the wall of the stomach or duodenum. Likewise, the white cells of the blood increase in number except in the case of ulcer, and they are usually higher in disease of the gall bladder. The physician determines this by a blood count.

If the patient is jaundiced or has a history of a previous attack of jaundice, it is more than likely that the gall bladder contains stones.

At least one half the chronic cases of indigestion are due to disease of the appendix or gall bladder. It is only by careful laboratory work and the use of the X-ray that an exact diagnosis can be made. A host of digestive troubles that are called neuroses are really due to ulcer of the stomach or duodenum or a diseased gall bladder or appendix.

Cancer of the Stomach

Cancer of the stomach is third in frequency among the parts of the body that cancer attacks. It usually appears after forty years of age, but it has occurred in young persons. The cause is unknown. It, as a rule, is very insidious in its onset or it may start out abruptly as a very stormy course. Ulcers of the stomach may change to cancer, but in the duodenum rarely become cancerous. A patient with cancer loses in weight and strength and gets indigestion. If the tumor is at the entrance of the stomach, food cannot enter, and rapid starvation occurs. If the tumor is located at the outlet or pylorus, obstruction occurs, and food will be vomited instead of passing into the bowels. This produces rapid loss in weight. The secretions of the stomach are altered by cancer, and the hydrochloric acid disappears. This interferes with digestion and causes nausea. Sooner or later the tumor ulcerates and bleeding occurs. Due to the fact that the blood remains in the stomach for some time, it becomes dark and altered, and in the vomitus looks much like coffee grounds. Most patients with cancer have pain; the pain may be a dull ache or be boring or severe, depending on the location of the tumor. The pain is usually made worse by food and is not relieved by alkalies, but it may be diminished by vomiting.

Any person in or beyond the middle period of life who develops indigestion, with nausea and pain and loss of weight and strength, should be examined immediately and most thoroughly. More recently stomach contents have been taken from a patient by means of a stomach tube and they are concentrated so that they can be put upon a glass slide and stained. This special staining device originated by Papanicolaou may show cancer cells in the stomach juice so examined.

The only possible treatment in most cases is an operation to remove the growth; if that is not possible, then X-ray or radium treatments may be of benefit. When obstruction occurs, it is necessary to make a new opening between the stomach and bowels, or a gastroenterostomy. This gives relief from symptoms and may prolong life for several months.

Constipation

In constipation there may be retention of the material that should be excreted, for an abnormal time, or merely difficult evacuation of the bowels. Few other subjects in medicine have received more thought and attention. Volumes have been written on it. From the moment of birth until death the question of the daily bowel movement is paramount. The child is asked daily over and over again whether its bowels have moved; naturally this emphasis makes a strong impression which lasts the rest of its life. No other drugs have had greater sales than those that contain laxatives; fortunes have been made by clever advertising of patent medicines, taking advantage of this all-absorbing question of the human animal.

Actually, it is not necessary for the bowels to move every day. It is normal for some people to have an evacuation every other day; in others several days may elapse between actions of the bowels and still complete health be possible.

Until the food eaten reaches the colon, digestive processes are going on in the long small bowel, with absorption of all digestible portions. The material which reaches the colon is in a semi-solid state, and its passage through the large bowel occurs slowly. During this time a good part of the liquid content is absorbed, leaving a more solid residue which finally is expressed as a stool or bowel movement. Naturally, as more food keeps coming along, the bowel contents are finally forced into the terminal portion of the bowels, called the rectum. Normally the rectum does not contain material; when the excrement is forced into it, reflex contractions occur, and the bowels empty themselves of their contents in the terminal portion. This constitutes the act of defecation. Usually this occurs once or twice in twenty-four hours.

There are many different possible causes of constipation. Failure to pay attention to the desire for a bowel movement or to devote sufficient time to it will lead first to a retarded movement and later to constipation. There must be a sufficient amount of residual material or bulk to form a mass of stool to excite activity; hence the food must contain enough vegetables and fruit and salads, if normal evacuations are to continue. Likewise, for normal digestion, the body demands a necessary supply of fluids. If the material in the colon is dehydrated or dried out, the desiccated stool will be difficult to evacuate. For this reason profuse sweating or the loss of fluids due to fever may induce constipation. All diseases which cause body weakness or wasting may be attended by constipation, due to the fact that the muscles necessary for expelling the bowel contents are too weak to act. Any disease causing a narrowing of the caliber of the bowel may be attended by constipation for mechanical reasons. With our newer knowledge of the physiology or function of the intestinal tract and its mechanisms, we have learned more about the problem of constipation. This is particularly true of the influence of the nervous system. For instance, some people may be constipated because they do not move the left half of the colon. The left half of the colon down through the rectum is the expelling portion of the colon and is concerned with the expulsion of the stool. There may be disturbances in this nervous system which lead to the impairment of this function. Drugs have now been developed which stimulate the nerves and overcome constipation. Furthermore, certain drugs which paralyze the bowel in the treatment of other diseases may cause constipation. This poses an important question for the physician for a patient who needs drugs to paralyze the upper intestinal tract and get the lower one to move. I have found that both of these drugs can be given at the same time because they act at different levels in the bowel. A paralysis of one type of nerve and a stimulation of another nerve produces what we call a normalization in the physiology of your intestinal tract.

Finally, the habitual use of purgatives is a frequent cause of constipation. Owing to the irritation of the drugs the colon becomes contracted and tight, or owing to repeated overstimulation it finally becomes exhausted or atonic.

In some cases there may be no symptoms, whereas in others there may be conditions simulating a wasting disease. Early there is, as a rule, a loss of appetite. The patients complain of a foul breath and often notice a coated tongue. Later, mental depression supervenes, and the individual wonders why he has become dull and listless; why his ordinary activities, which formerly caused him no fatigue, now cause undue fatigue; why he is not as alert as formerly; why ordinary problems befuddle him; why it takes him longer to work out things mentally than formerly. He may have headaches, complain of dizziness, and often of ringing in his ears. His friends tell him that he does not look well, that he has a pallor to his skin, and this may be associated with a resulting beginning anemia. Often, in young people, skin eruptions and skin manifestations may be associated with habitual constipation.

Constipation is usually associated with indigestion, so-called dyspepsia; such patients may feel full after a relatively small meal. They frequently belch and complain of undue distention. Often, cramp-like pains are noted, and little relief is obtained from the small, constipated bowel movement. If this condition persists long enough, actual disease of the large bowel may follow. In many cases ulcers of the bowels seem to have their origin in long-standing constipation.

It is important to correct any tendency to delayed bowel movement, especially when this occurs in childhood. Regularity should be insisted on. The bowels should be trained to move the first thing in the morning. An effort should be made to have them move after breakfast each morning.

Exercise and diet are important. The diet should consist of plenty of vegetables, salads, and fruit, in addition to milk, cereals, eggs, and meats. An outdoor, active life is also beneficial for people with sluggishness of the bowels. An occasional enema or mineral oil may be helpful, but the use of laxatives regularly is distinctly harmful.

Along with diet, exercises intended especially to strengthen the abdominal muscles, massage of the bowels, and the drinking of large amounts of water on arising are of distinct help in stubborn cases.

Cathartics are at times necessary for temporary help. Mineral oil and agar are usually tried or some of the substances like cellulose or psyllium seed which act through stimulation by bulk. An enema of olive oil or mineral oil is often necessary when the bowel is in an irritable condition, and plain water may be used for an enema without harm.

Laxative medicines are put up today in tempting forms, such as candy and gum or in chocolate and cookies. Children may take these too often and thus lay the foundation for stubborn constipation in later life. It is best not to take even laxatives, and certainly not cathartics, without the advice of a physician. Vitamin B₁ (thiamin chloride) definitely increases the muscular activity of the bowel and promotes regular bowel habits.

More recently our attention has been turned to what are the natural mechanisms of keeping the bowel more liquid instead of dry. It has been found that if you can increase the bile coming out of the liver, make it thinner and in a larger amount, the stool will remain softer and patients can have a bowel movement. Previously many physicians gave bile salts in order to accomplish this. However, bile acids are far better because they thin down the bile in the liver and therefore allow it to pass out more profusely and in larger amounts. This increased amount of bile is a perfectly normal laxative for the gastrointestinal tract and it should be encouraged to take place in the treatment of constipation.

COLITIS AND DIARRHEA

"Colitis" is a misnomer. More accurately it is an inflammation, either acute or chronic, of the large intestine. The inflammation may be limited to the lining or may involve the other layers of the colon. If the outer coats are involved, adhesions to the intestines may form. The essential cause is bacterial, or it may be a parasitic infection. Constipation is doubtless a predisposing factor of importance, especially in the chronic forms. The large bowel symptoms are often due to faulty digestion higher up in the intestinal tract. When the improperly digested material enters the lower bowel it may give rise to disturbed function. Because the symptoms are referable to the large bowel, the condition is diagnosed as colitis, when in reality inflammation is not present.

Inflammation of the colon frequently accompanies diarrheal diseases. Sometimes such inflammation is a secondary manifestation of certain infectious diseases, such as blood poisoning, pneumonia, smallpox, measles, influenza, and typhoid, and also kidney conditions with anemia. Included under this heading also are the acute diarrheas of infancy, frequently called summer complaint. In the vast majority of cases these are due to infections with germs which are taken into the body as contaminations of foods, principally spoiled milk.

The causes of the acute form of diarrhea include faulty diet or the use of spoiled and contaminated foods. Foods which decompose readily, such as unripe or overripe fruit, ice cream, and sea foods, may cause diarrhea. Sometimes water may carry grave infection. Indeed, infected water is the most common source of such serious diseases as dysentery, cholera, typhoid fever, and paratyphoid fever. In the tropics and even in temperate climates, amebic dysentery is often due to infected water. In the temperate climates bacillary dysentery is the more common.

In certain cases, spoiled meat is the cause. Poisons, such as arsenic, mercury, silver salts, and various cathartic medicines often provoke diarrhea. General toxic conditions, such as blood poisoning, measles, exophthalmic (inward or ingrowing) goiter, pneumonia, cancer, and Bright's disease may cause diarrhea. Certain food deficiences where lack of vitamins plays a rôle, as in pellagra, cause frequent movements. In some cases, absence of the acid of gastric juice may cause diarrhea.

Simple acute diarrhea, ordinarily due to ingestion of infected drinks or food or unripe fruit, is characterized by frequent evacuation of material, which is at first solid or soft but soon becomes chiefly liquid. Colic with pains is common, and straining at stool with a sense of a desire to purge further is evident. There may be thirst, coated tongue, tenderness in the abdomen, and in some cases even fever, especially in younger people. If the attack becomes severe, mucus—slimy material—is noted in the excrement. In severe cases even blood or blood-tinged material may be noted. Chronic diarrheas usually follow acute attacks, and when they persist, further search for the causative factor must be made by the doctor. If allowed to continue without abatement, loss of weight, anemia, profound weakness, loss of appetite, and susceptibility to infections may develop.

CHRONIC DIARRHEA AND DYSENTERY

The two most common forms of chronic diarrhea of the infectious type are bacillary dysentery and amebic dysentery. Bacillary dysentery is due to a specific infection with the germs of dysentery of which there are many types. It is a communicable disease and due, for the most part, to bad sanitation. After one person in a community has the disease, another may come down with it from two to seven days later. The onset is sudden, with griping pains in the abdomen, followed by diarrhea. The bowel movements show much mucus and later pus and blood. There is practically always fever. Along with this, there may be headache, vomiting, malaise, or drowsiness. The abdomen may be tender over the course of the large bowel. Sometimes the onset may be confused with acute appendicitis. If the disease persists, it frequently goes into a chronic form, which may have definite periods of remission, during which time the patient may be comfortably free from symptoms.

Early in the disease, the germs can be isolated from the stool and, in some cases, even from the blood. The most important aid in diagnosis is found in the ability of the serum, or fluid matter of the blood, of the affected patient to "clump" dead dysentery germs together. This scientific test is an almost specific method. On the basis of this fact there is a specific treatment using an anti-serum made from the blood of horses. The disease may for years be unrecognized. Many cases of ulcerative colitis (called non-specific ulcerative colitis) are nothing more than chronic bacillary dysentery with a secondary invading or infective organism. Arthritis is the most common complication of the disease. Sulfadiazine controls many cases of dysentery. Many new forms of the sulfa drugs can adequately control bacillary dysentery. The drugs of choice are those which will remain in the bowel longer and are least absorbable. Noteworthy among this group is sulfaguanidine. Also useful are terramycin and aureomycin which are prescribed by doctors.

AMEBIC DYSENTERY

Amebic dysentery was once considered to be a disease confined to the tropics; now it is known that there are few places in the world where the disease does not occur. About 10 per cent of the population of the United States may be affected. The causative organism is called endameba histolytica. It is a parasite called for short "ameba," and its favorite habitat is the human intestinal tract, especially the large bowel or colon. It frequently penetrates into the blood stream, and thus can travel to any organ in the body. The liver is at times invaded, and an amebic abscess of the liver sometimes results.

In cases with acute dysentery actively moving ameba may be found, while in the chronic cases, even without diarrhea, the ameba may be found in the form of cysts, or collections of fluid. It is in the form of cysts that the disease is usually carried. Individuals who pass these cysts in their stools are called "carriers," though they may themselves never have had the typical acute symptoms.

The infection in the human body can take place only by swallowing the cysts. Food handlers who are carriers have been found occasionally. Some vegetables that are eaten raw may be contaminated when the soil has been contaminated by a carrier. The house fly may carry the cyst from the stool to the food. Hence, one should be careful that vegetables grown in gardens should not be eaten raw, and proper screening should be used to intercept the fly with its burden of filth.

The symptoms of the disease are similar to those of the dysentery caused by the smaller germs. Our recognition of amebic dysentery or amebiasis has been very much improved of late. Parasitologists more readily recognize the presence of the motile amebas in the stool or, by staining preparations, can see them on smears. Furthermore, culture media now are available in which even though the cysts are present they may grow into full size amebas when incubated for 24 hours. This material is then again stained by the same method used in the uncultured stool and full grown amebas are shown to be present. A person may harbor the amebas and have for prolonged periods few, if any, symptoms. The liver is a common site for the amebas to locate outside of the intestinal tract, due to the fact that the blood of the intestinal tract first enters the liver. In the liver, small or large abscesses may result from the action of the invading amebas. The joints are, at times, invaded, producing arthritis, or inflammation of the joints, and the kidneys may be affected, causing bloody urine. It is difficult to eradicate, but prolonged medical treatment usually yields results.

Cancer of the Bowels

Cancer rarely occurs in the small bowel but is fairly common in the large intestine. In the small bowel the cancerous growth usually does not make itself known until obstruction or blocking occurs, due to its filling the inside of the bowel. At other times, the first warning may be bleeding. The symptoms of an obstruction are at first cramp-like pains and later nausea and vomiting.

Cancers may arise in any part of the colon or large bowel but are more common in the lower portions, called the sigmoid and rectum. In the early stages there may be no symptoms. When the tumor grows large enough to obstruct the inside, the typical symptoms of intestinal obstruction or blocking arise. At other times, the surface of the tumor becomes abraded or bruised by the onward movement of the intestinal contents, and infection or ulceration of the eroded surface takes place. Thus, the blood vessels may become exposed and broken, and bleeding follows.

Cancers in the rectum are commonly located just above the opening and are within easy reach of the doctor who examines for them. The person affected may think he has piles, with some bleeding from time to time. The simple examination to make certain should always be made.

Cancer of the bowels may set up secondary growths, commonly in the liver, with jaundice or yellowness of the skin, but the secondary growths may also appear in the lungs or bones.

Early symptoms are frequently absent, and the patient may come to the physician too late for a cure by operation. The symptoms, when they do appear, are constipation, distention and cramps and sometimes diarrhea, alternating with the constipation. If the tumor is in the lower part of the bowels, some mucus and blood may be present with the stool and the patient frequently feels that he has not emptied his bowels.

The X-ray is of greatest value in diagnosing cancer of the bowels. When some opaque material, like barium, is taken by mouth and its course through the bowels is watched by the X-ray, a defect in the shadow can be seen which represents the tumor mass. In order to recognize cancer of the colon the patient is usually given some castor oil the night before. The next morning he is given tap water enemas until the washings of the bowel become clean. He is allowed to eat a light breakfast and then he is sent to the X-ray room. Here an opaque enema made of barium and some mixtures are injected into the colon and these filling defects can be readily seen by the X-ray observer. Occasionally the tumor may be elusive. In these instances the X-ray doctor usually allows the patient to empty the bowel and injects some air into the colon to balloon it out. This is called a pneumocolon. Frequently on films made in this way, the X-ray doctor will determine the presence of a cancer or may even determine the presence of a polyp. Polyps may be benign or they may be malignant. There is still a great debate in the medical profession whether or not all polyps are malignant at their inception or whether most of them are benign. It is difficult at present to give an answer to this problem. Certainly the polyps which occur diffusely after ulcerative colitis are, for the most part, benign and are not malignant. However, 5 per cent of the patients who develop polyposis after ulcerative colitis do develop cancer in one or more places. For that reason polyposis following ulcerative colitis has been considered a precursor of cancerous disease of the colon.

Another technique for diagnosing cancer of the bowels is the use of a long metal tube, electrically lighted, which can be passed into the rectum for a considerable distance, and through it even small growths may be seen; also a small piece of tissue may be removed for microscopic examination.

As soon as the diagnosis can be made, an operation should be carried out to remove the tumor, if possible, and, if that is not feasible, at least a new opening may be made by bringing the bowel just above the tumor to the skin surface. This procedure is called a colostomy. Inoperable cases can sometimes be helped by X-ray or radium treatments.

INTESTINAL OBSTRUCTION

Intestinal obstruction indicates some abnormal abdominal condition which gives rise to an interference with the onward flow of intestinal contents. This may be produced by a large variety of causes. Adhesions resulting from previous operations are the most common cause, as the intestinal loops become entangled in these strands of tissue and become kinked. Hernia, or rupture, may be complicated by obstruction when the bowel falls through the outlet of the rupture and its return to the abdomen is prevented by swelling of all of the structures. Sometimes one portion of the intestine ensheathes or slips into itself; this is called technically intussusception, and is an especially common form of intestinal obstruction in children. Tumors, of which cancer forms the largest group, may narrow the inside of the intestine by progressive growth and prevent normal onward movement of the intestinal contents. The circulation of the bowels may be destroyed by small clots which may lodge or form in the blood vessels, with subsequent loss of vitality and paralysis of the intestine. Intestinal obstruction, or ileus, as this condition is called, may also be associated with numerous conditions, such as peritonitis, kidney stones, and gallstones.

The symptoms depend usually on the suddenness of the onset and the degree of obstruction. When due to adhesions or ruptures, there is usually a sudden attack of severe abdominal pain followed by repeated severe vomiting. These symptoms become more severe with the passing of hours and soon are followed by distention of the abdomen and inability to have bowel movements. Obstruction due to tumors is usually slow in its development and may be preceded by periods of constipation alternating with diarrhea and abdominal pain. Cancers of the rectum and lower colon frequently are associated with bloody excretions and mucus, and the tumor may be felt by the finger or seen by the use of special instruments. With an enema opaque to the X-ray, obstructing growths and gas-distended intestinal loops above the site of interference may be seen by the doctor. However, even in cancer of the rectum, a sudden obstruction may be the first evidence of its existence.

The diagnosis of an intestinal obstruction is usually obvious, but some cases may remain uncertain until operation. The causative lesion must be carefully localized, as this gives a definite plan for surgical relief. The location of the pain and tenderness are valuable aids. The physician may think it wise to see what can be accomplished by the use of enemas for the relief of the obstruction. Obstinate constipation and impaction of stool may produce symptoms which resemble true obstruction, but in them enemas will bring complete relief.

When there is delay in taking care of intestinal obstruction, an artificial opening must be made above the obstruction to permit complete drainage of the obstructed intestine. In the cases in which this is the only remedy, later on a more complete operation can be carried out to join the bowel above and below the obstruction and at the same time to close the artificial opening. It is all-important to recognize, in the cases with the symptoms described, that intestinal obstruction is present and to call a surgeon at once as a life-saving measure.

INTESTINAL PARASITES OR "WORMS"

Several types of animal parasites may inhabit the human intestine. The more common types encountered are the beef, pork, and fish tapeworms; roundworms, pinworms, hookworms, and flukes. They vary in size and shape, some being long and flat, others shorter and round. There are species which are microscopic in size, while others are many feet in length. They usually enter the body by way of the mouth through the intake of food which has been contaminated with the eggs or the adult parasite. After an interval in the intestinal canal the eggs hatch into the adult worms and continue to live, grow, and reproduce. With certain species the embryonic forms are absorbed into the blood stream and migrate through the body, at times lodging in the liver, brain, lungs, and muscle, to return later to the intestine. Along with the contents of the bowels the parasites are excreted in the form of either the adult or the embryo, to be taken up later by animal or man for repetition of the cycle.

The common sources of the worm are infected beef, pork, fish, and contaminated food and water supplies. In hookworm disease the parasite enters the body through the skin.

There are no absolutely typical symptoms produced by worms, and many cases are long free of symptoms. In many instances there is abdominal pain, irregular evacuation of the bowels, itching about the rectum, vomiting, headache, mental depression, lassitude, and loss of appetite. There may be a severe anemia and marked physical and mental underdevelopment. The bowel content will at times contain blood and mucus, and in most instances the parasite or its eggs. Examination of the blood shows an increase in the percentage of certain cells called eosinophiles. In cases of hookworm cr fish tapeworm infestation, the blood may be very watery, owing to a severe grade of anemia induced by the parasite.

The most important feature of the treatment is prophylaxis or prevention. Thousands upon thousands of lives have been spared or made useful through careful attention to sanitation and hygiene. This has been especially true with hookworm. The proper disposal of sewage, careful inspection of cattle and foodstuffs, and proper washing and cooking of vegetables and meats have been responsible for the marked diminution in the number of worm-infested people. The measures used in the treatment of the sick include starvation for a period of twelve to forty-eight hours, purging, and the administration of certain drugs called anthelmintics, which have almost a specific action against the worms. The more common ones in use are male fern, oil of chenopodium, thymol, santonin, and calomel. In cases of fluke infestation, emetine and antimony and potassium tartrate are effective.

CATHARTICS, LAXATIVES, AND ENEMAS

The large bowel is one of the most abused organs in the abdomen. This abuse can be attributed, for the most part, to the drastic cathartics and laxatives which people are in the habit of taking. When one considers that the function of this part of the intestinal tract is purely mechanical and that its labors are mostly concerned with excreting the waste products of digestion and metabolism, it is not at all surprising that many patients develop colon disturbances when they irritate it with drastic cathartics. Nature never intended that severe cathartics be used. It supplied suitable roughage in food to supply mass action in the large bowel. While one may get results from a drastic cathartic or purge, it should also be remembered that there is a concomitant obstipation or "tying up" of the bowels for a few days following this irritation. The patient then often desires another laxative or purge, and there soon develops a so-called cathartic habit. Finally, there is a chronic irritation of the colon due to the persistence of the hard small masses of the stool, and many cases of ulceration of the colon or bowel may thus be due to an apparently innocent cathartic habit.

If laxatives must be taken, one should try to use the natural laxatives, particularly those found in fruits and vegetables. Such foods as meats, bread, eggs, fish, potatoes, and milk give little residue in the large bowel, and these, for the most part, form the bulk of the average American diet. If one finds that fruits and vegetables are not enough to stimulate the bowels, mild laxatives may be used.

Many people resort to various types of enemas to relieve constipation. Just as the colon can be abused from above by drastic cathartics, so can it be abused by irritating enemas injected from below. The prime function of an enema is to produce contractions in the lower section of the large bowel so that this expulsive force may bring about the required movement. This expulsive force is directly proportionate to the overdistention with fluid and not to the kind of irritant used. Such simple enemas as tap water enemas may be used. However, when more drastic enemas are required, they should be used under the direction of a physician.

The colon is an innocent organ bearing the brunt and work of the rest of the digestive tract; its main function is to get rid of the waste products. Do not disturb its function by the habitual use of artificial cathartics, laxatives, or enemas.

CHAPTER XVI

The Kidney: Its Diseases and Disturbances
HOWARD M. ODEL, M.D.

To THE KITCHEN of a great hotel are brought quantities of food, wholesome and pure, catering to each need and taste. In the preparation and consumption of this food, waste accumulates; useless material in which food has been packed, unused and unusable parts of food itself. Avenues are provided for ready elimination of this waste; boxes and wrappings disappear in fire and in chimney fumes; liquids flow into cisterns; garbage is carted off in wagons of the "reduction company." So too in the organization of human bodies, there are veritable reduction companies.

In the human economy, as has been noted in previous chapters, food is the source of all tissue growth and energy. Yet for all modern laws there is no such thing as "pure food"—at least, in the sense that for the human body there exists no food wholly valuable and completely utilizable. Even from that "perfect product," mother's milk, are formed wastes to be discarded. Men foretell, perhaps not too seriously, the day when a hearty meal will consist, alas, of six courses—each a scientifically compounded pill. Even were the prophecy to come true, waste products would develop from the ordinary wear and tear on tissues. The twitch of the tiniest muscle, the lightning wink of an eyelid, the swift flight of a half-formed thought: each is accompanied by, indeed is the result of, the combustion or reduction of some body substance. In the utilization of food and from the growth and repair of body tissues, end products are formed. Carbon dioxide escapes in the flue of the lungs; food residue is discarded by the bowels; water steams out in the breath, escapes in sweat, and is lost in urine. Daily, about 2 quarts of water are eliminated by the lungs, 1 to 1½ pints in the sweat, and about 1½ to 2 quarts in the urine.

ANATOMY AND FUNCTIONS OF THE KIDNEY

The kidneys, forming urine, are one of the chief organs of elimination. Their function is to keep the body free of an excess of substances derived particularly from protein, albuminous or nitrogenous matter—found, for example, in meats, milk, eggs, and body muscle. When such fuel is consumed by the human engine, the ash or residue consists of certain matters that cannot be eliminated readily or in quantity by means other than in urine. Those about which most is known are urea, uric acid, creatinine, sulfate, and phosphate. Since these substances are not only useless, but also potentially toxic, they must be got rid of; otherwise they would accumulate in the body and be injurious to health and life.

So vital is the need for proper elimination that nature has included the kidneys among those organs of which not one but two seem necessary to provide a safe margin of reserve. Man can live, at least for the time being, even after all of one kidney and about half of the other have been removed or destroyed. Yet nature was not unduly profligate in providing this reserve, for the kidneys are unfortunately called on to excrete not only the natural waste of wholesome foods, but from time to time must hastily and efficiently help rid the body of end products of bad food, germs and their harmful toxins, diseased and dead tissue cells, and chemical poisons.

Every such experience provides a hazard for the kidneys, and little by little tends to lower their reserve. Some insults are borne by them silently and uncomplainingly, without signs or symptoms. To some injurious experiences they temporarily succumb, soon to regain apparently full capabilities. From others they may acquire permanent damage. When the burden is temporarily or permanently too great for the kidneys, when the "threshold of their reserve" is exceeded, when their function is appreciably deranged, a train of events occurs, the symptoms and signs of which indicate what is called "nephritis." Considering the great variations in type and degree of such insults met in the course of a lifetime, different types and degrees of nephritis result. Some forms of nephritis may be the expression of an essentially minor and transient difficulty, a condition about which concern need not be felt, readily amenable to treatment and leaving the afflicted person the happy subject of an early cure. Other forms, however, may signify a grave diseased state fraught with great danger, which may destine its victim to an early fatal outcome.

The term "nephritis" means simply inflammation of the kidneys. While modern medicine recognizes many different diseases of the kidney, each essentially a type of nephritis, the term represents to many people one condition and is synonymous with "Bright's disease." Because the first reports of nephritis, made by Richard Bright, an English physician, in 1827, dealt with one of its most serious forms, to some persons nephritis and Bright's disease remain designations with an evil portent, omens of death. Happily this unfortunate point of view is being abandoned, and modern dictionaries define Bright's disease as "a term of very indefinite limitations, meaning, in general, acute or chronic nephritis," or as "any one of a group of kidney diseases attended by albuminuria" (albumin in urine). Fortunately, modern science has provided ways of differentiating among types of kidney disease and of telling whether a given type is serious or not.

ANATOMY OF THE KIDNEY

The average man has eaten beef or lamb kidneys occasionally, but that is about all he knows of kidneys. The kidneys are so placed that they are amply guarded from injury even during such strenuous exercise as the straining and twisting of an athlete at the hurdles or high jump. Situated in the lumbar region, or small of the back, at about the level of the eleventh rib, they are protected by thick spinal muscles behind them and by the peritoneal cavity in front. Thus they are not in the abdomen but behind it. They are further surrounded by a tough fibrous coat or capsule, around which is packed a considerable amount of fat.[1] The right kidney is usually about a half inch lower than the left, probably because the liver is above it, and is a little lower in children and women than in men; it is often easily felt on examination. Such a "palpable kidney," if smooth and not enlarged or tender on pressure, is perfectly normal.

Each adult kidney is about 4½ inches long, from 2 to 2½ inches wide, about 1¼ inches thick, and each weighs on an average ⅓ of a pound. In shape it resembles a large kidney bean, being rounded and curved, with a concave area in the middle of the inner border known as the hilus, where the renal[2] artery, vein, and nerves enter the substance of the kidney, and from which arise the ureters, the tubes that carry urine from the kidneys to the urinary bladder.

On slicing the kidney and laying it open, one can see three main areas. (Plate XV.) The outer zone, the cortex, contains the pinpoint kidney filters, the glomeruli or "little balls." The middle zone, or medulla, is marked by innumerable stripings consisting of microscopic tubules that converge into a number of pyramidal areas. These are connected by many fingerlike projections to a fairly large, smooth-lined, saclike, collecting chamber called the "pelvis." From this pelvis the ureters arise at the hilus. The ureters are hollow tubes about 1/5 of an inch wide, the channel within being only ⅛ of an inch in width. They travel 10 to 12 inches down along the spinal column to the bladder.

Thus each kidney is a tremendously compact area of collecting tubules and of wonderfully small filters, each placed in its minute filter chamber. The filter chambers and tubules are the fundamental anatomic units of the kidney. (Plate XVI.) Each of these units—or nephrons—begins as a little cuplike chamber, 1/200 of an inch in diameter, comprising the filtration chamber, or

---

[1] Placed just above each kidney is the adrenal or suprarenal gland, small organs whose physiologic action is different from that of the kidneys but which sometimes become diseased by extensive inflammations around the kidneys.

[2] "Renal" means "pertaining to the kidney." For its derivation see comment on page 373.

Bowman's glomerular capsule, into which are inserted the filters themselves, which are masses of tiny blood vessels (capillaries), the glomeruli. The walls of the cuplike Bowman's capsule are double, with a narrow space between, since the structure is like a round ball pushed in from one side. These small filter chambers are confined entirely to the cortical substance, and from them arise small tubules, which begin meandering courses to end, many of them together, in large collecting tubules that lead to the kidney pelvis. Just after the tubule leaves the filter chamber, it enters a series of convolutions in the cortex ("proximal or first convoluted tubule") and then dips down into the medullary substance as a thin descending limb 1/1200 of an inch thick, which turns as Henle's loop to ascend again into the cortex where, somewhat thicker (1/600 of an inch), it becomes even more convoluted ("distal or second convoluted tubule") before it finally straightens out to join with myriads of others into the collecting tubules, which empty into the kidney pelvis. Despite all this wandering, the tubule has traversed a distance of only about 1½ inches. The purpose of this extreme migration is to permit it to come in contact, in a minute space, with an extensive meshwork of fine blood vessels. It has been estimated by some that there are about 1,000,000 to 1,500,000 of these tiny units or nephrons in each kidney. In the adult, therefore, the total length of these tubules in each kidney would be from 1,500,000 to 3,000,000 inches, or the equivalent of a channel about 50 to 100 miles long in both kidneys, compressed into a space of only about 20 cubic inches in volume!

STRUCTURE AND CONTENTS OF FILTER CHAMBER

From the great blood vessel of the abdomen, the aorta, a short, thick, renal artery passes to each kidney, entering at the hilus and carrying a large amount of blood under great pressure. At the hilus this artery divides into several branches, which pass to the junction between the cortex and medulla where each again divides, at length forming a small but stout little vessel, the afferent vessel or arteriole, or intake pipe. This enters the capillary tuft in Bowman's capsule. As it plunges into the cuplike depression constituting the filter chamber, it breaks up into two, then four, and finally into about fifty curling, twisting capillary loops, each about 1/2500 of an inch in diameter, which coil and twine in interlacing fashion and then reunite to pass out of the chamber as the outlet pipe or afferent vessel or arteriole. The latter soon breaks up into fine intertubular capillaries that surround the meandering tubules mentioned above, finally reuniting to leave the kidney as the great renal vein.

The tortuous capillary loops within the filter chambers constitute the glomeruli, or filters, and each glomerulus with its little cuplike room forms a marvelous little filtration plant, the basic unit of the kidneys' excretory system. The reason for such an arrangement of glomerular loops can be understood by visualizing the structure of an ordinary room radiator. The steam enters the room through a single pipe, which breaks up in the radiator into a large number of coils before leaving the room again as a single pipe. The many coils increase by so much the radiating surface of the apparatus. Although the glomerular loops are only 1/2500 of an inch wide, their length totals about 1 inch in each glomerulus. If there are about 1,000,000 glomeruli in each kidney, the surface area of its glomerular capillaries is about 0.78 of a square meter for one kidney, or for both kidneys about 1.56 square meters (15 square feet), the approximate area of the top of a dining-room table.

FUNCTIONS OF THE KIDNEY

In simple terms the function of the kidney is to make urine and get rid of it. The first clue to an understanding of its function is obtained by analysis of what substances are found to be continuously present in normal urine, for such substances obviously are not wanted by the body. The urine contains large amounts of water and urea, smaller amounts of sodium chloride (common table salt), potassium, phosphates and sulfates, creatinine and uric acid, and minimal amounts of several other substances. Some are excreted because they are always and entirely useless; others are got rid of because, while they are ordinarily useful, the body already has enough of them to supply its needs. The functions of the normal kidney are further demonstrated by observing what happens when they go wrong, noting what substances accumulate in the blood and tissues and what deficiencies appear in the urine.

As a result of such analyses, the known functions of the kidney can be summarized as follows:

1. It is the avenue of elimination for 40 to 60 per cent of all water liberated from the body. An excess of this vital substance is always present in healthy bodies, derived from food and drink and from cellular activity.

2. It excretes the waste products of protein breakdown: urea, uric acid, and creatinine.

3. It helps to preserve the normal acid-alkaline balance of tissues by excreting excess acids. The system is never "acid," and by "acidosis" is really meant a reduction in the reserve of alkali. All tissues and fluids of the body except the stomach juices and at times the sweat are faintly alkaline. Although large amounts of acids are eaten in food and more is constantly produced by our normal body processes, the reaction (alkalinity) of tissues remains practically constant. The maintenance of an alkaline reserve is of supreme importance, and the extreme delicacy of this balance is appreciated by realizing that death would occur were the reaction of blood to be altered by the minute change equivalent to that caused by adding one drop of even a weak acid to a quart of water. Blood becoming as acid as distilled water or as alkaline as ordinary tap water would be incompatible with life (Marriott).

4. It helps to maintain that normal physiochemical state of body fluids responsible for osmotic pressure by eliminating just the proper amounts of salt and water. When this balance is disturbed one of two things results: water-

logging of tissues (dropsy, hydrops, edema, ascites, anasarca)[3] or the opposite, a condition of body dehydration,[4] desiccation, or water famine.

5. It has been discovered that the kidneys apparently manufacture small amounts of certain substances found in urine: hippuric acid and perhaps ammonia. All other recognized urinary constituents are brought to the kidney already manufactured, and the kidney merely excretes them unchanged. Since the synthesis of hippuric acid and possibly ammonia are but steps in the excretion of unwanted substances, it can still be concluded that the known functions of the kidney are chiefly if not entirely excretory.

PHYSIOLOGY OF THE KIDNEY: HOW IT CARRIES ON ITS FUNCTIONS

The striking anatomic arrangement of glomerulus and tubule led early physicians to regard the kidney units as filters and to believe that urinary components passed through glomeruli into tubules by a sort of suction, or a simple process of filtration (resulting from a higher pressure in the glomerular capillaries). Later, others insisted that the cells, or microscopic units of which living matter is constructed, played more than a passive role in formation of urine and that they had an important part in its manufacture, actually pouring out or "secreting" substances into the tubules. Thus a great dispute arose between the "mechanists" and the "vitalists." While the details of this argument need not be considered, a brief statement of the modern view of kidney physiology will aid in gaining knowledge of some of the different symptoms and signs of kidney disease and the rationale of treatment.

It has been estimated that more than 600 quarts (about 20,000 ounces) of blood (some say 1,000 to 1,500 quarts) flow through the kidneys every day, passing through glomeruli at the greatly reduced speed of about 18 inches per hour (Vimtrup). About 90 per cent of it continues on into the efferent arteries and finally back into the main blood stream, but fluid amounting to about 10 per cent of this volume is taken out in the glomeruli and starts flowing down the tubules. The fluid taken out amounts daily to more than 60 quarts (cited by Harvey); others say 170 to 290 quarts (Rehberg, cited by Wilbur; Richards). Were all of it allowed to continue on down the tubules and be lost in urine, there would be an enormous waste of water causing almost constant urination and producing a tremendous thirst to replenish body fluids. In addition to water, this glomerular filtrate includes not only wastes (urea, uric acid, creatinine, and so forth) but also large amounts of useful substances (sugar, salt, and amino acids), foods that the body cannot afford to lose. The tubules, therefore, prevent this waste by reabsorbing through the cells, of which the walls of the tubules are built, all of the sugar and amino acids and almost all of the water and chlorides, at the same time

---

[3]Dropsy means "hydrops" or "water." Edema means "swelling." Ascites ("bag") means "dropsy of the abdominal cavity." Anasarca ("throughout flesh") signifies "general dropsy."

[4]Dehydrate means "to deprive of or to lose water."

refusing to take back any of the unwanted substances. As a result of this vigorous reabsorption of water (97 per cent or more), the total amount of fluid that finally reaches the bladder to be excreted as urine is only about 1½ quarts a day (instead of 60 or more quarts), in which there is a high concentration of waste products. The latter are not equally concentrated; for example, the amount of urea in a quart of urine is 60 to 100 times that in a quart of blood, but the amount of uric acid is only about 30 times that of blood.

Modern studies indicate, then, that substances pass out of the blood going from glomeruli into tubules in one direction only. Lower down in the tubules some useful materials are restored to the blood by passing through the cells lining the tubules. That the passage of materials through the cells lining the tubules may not be just in one direction, as formerly supposed, is suggested by recent evidence indicating that certain tubular cells may actually take out further waste material from the blood capillaries surrounding the tubules and pour it into the tubules. Thus this waste passes through the walls of the tubules in the opposite direction from the useful substances that are reclaimed by them. By this means, the kidneys are given a second chance to throw off wastes by means of tubular secretion supplementing glomerular filtration.

The co-ordinated activity of the myriad cells in each kidney unit is remindful of a scene in an automobile assembling plant where down along the long runways are placed hundreds of men. Here one is adding a part, there another removing some appliance, until at the end of the runway there rolls off a completed car. As automobiles are thus born at so many an hour, so drops of urine roll out into the bladder at the rate of about four a minute, night and day.

In summary: Both glomerular and tubular cells apparently exhibit definite discrimination in determining just what and how much shall be filtered out of the blood, reabsorbed in the tubules, and eliminated in the urine. By a process of filtration, the glomeruli excrete a filtrate containing substances (except for proteins and cellular elements) in about the same concentration as they exist in the blood, and through the selective reabsorption of useful substances and possibly also some secretion by tubular cells this fluid is further elaborated into the final product, urine.

To demonstrate this graphically, with due apologies for the omission of finer details and at the risk of being taken too literally, I have included a diagram devised in the spirit of modern animated maps by Dr. Philip S. Hench, showing the main essentials of renal physiology. (Fig. 30.)

HISTORY OF KIDNEY DISEASE BEFORE THE TIME OF RICHARD BRIGHT

Almost all information about the kidney and its diseases has been attained in the last century. The term "Bright's disease" is about 125 years old, and previously little indeed was known of the diseases of the kidney. Before that it was not even known that albumin in the urine bore any special relation to nephritis. At the time of the American Revolution, doctors recognized in general only two kinds of kidney disease; namely, stones (*nephritis calculosa*) and

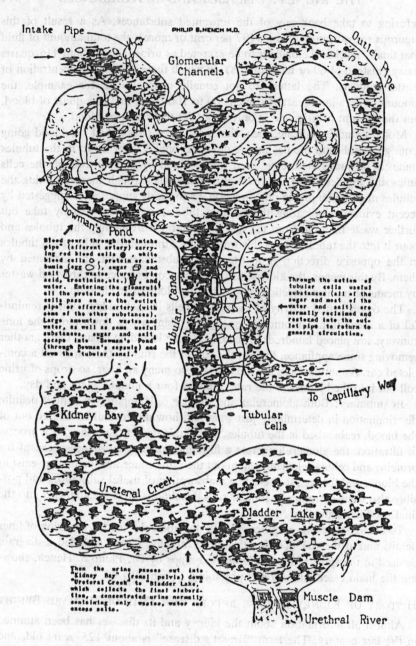

Fig. 30. A little journey through the kidney. The essentials of renal physiology illustrated in the spirit of a modern animated map.

suppurative or purulent nephritis (so-called ulcerated or pus kidney). This much had been known two thousand years before, in the time of Hippocrates, the Father of Medicine, when four diseases of the kidney were described, among them calculus (stone) and abscess.

The development of knowledge of the kidney and its diseases and especially of urine, an analysis of which constitutes modern man's commonest medical experience, is an interesting story. Philologists say that the word "kidney" may have been derived from words meaning womb or egg. Its Latin ancestor *ren* (renal and so forth) is thought to have referred to the midriff, the parts about the heart and liver.[5] Hippocrates (460–370 B.C.) believed the kidneys separated out urine, but Aristotle (384–322 B.C.), who was one of the greatest scientists and philosophers of all time and who carried on extensive anatomic investigations, thought the bladder was the chief site of urinary formation. He believed that the kidneys were not essential to life, but "when they are present exist not of actual necessity but as matter of greater finish and perfection." Galen (A.D. 131–201) had no patience with such "nonsense" and considered that the blood serum percolated through the kidneys. A thousand years after Aristotle, errors still persisted in some quarters, and urine was considered by Protospartharius (A.D. 603–641) as a filtrate of the portal vein of the liver.

Long before this, although the ancients knew little or nothing about the kidneys or the source and purpose of urine, much was written about urine itself. Records indicate that Babylonian physicians at the dawn of earliest civilization (around 4000 B.C.) examined it sufficiently to note changes in color, "worms of urine" (casts) and "knots of thread" (albumin). In old Sanskrit writings twenty different diseases were described, each with its characteristic urine, among them "honey urine." Ten of these diseases were said to be due to deranged phlegm, six to deranged bile, and the remaining four to wind. The diagnoses of diseases, as well as prophecies as to their outcome, were made by those ancient worthies from examination of the skin, eyes, and tongue, but "especially the pulse and urine without which all knowledge of physick is obscure, doubtful and uncertain." From observations made on the urine of patients with fever, Hippocrates wrote: "One may judge what is to take place, for if the urine be thick and more yellowish so much the better, but if it be thinner and blacker so much the worse. . . . When in fever the urine is turbid, there either is or will be headache." And again: "The most deadly of all kinds of urine are the fetid, watery, black and thick. . . . If the urine is passed in

---

[5]The Bible contains many references to "reins" and kidneys, using the terms literally and figuratively. In a literal sense it refers only to the kidneys of animals offered in sacrifice. By law the kidneys and their fatty covering were Jehovah's special share of sacrificial victims. Their peculiar sanctity arose from the belief that, next to the blood, the kidneys were the seat of life and should therefore be returned to the Author of Life. A natural extension of this idea led to their being considered the "seats of passion," the organs of feeling, or man's conscience. It is used in this latter sense in Psalms 26:2— "Examine me, O Lord, try my reins and my heart"—and not as an appeal for a kidney function test as a recent writer implied when he wrote, "Even the Bible mentions as important 'to test a man's heart and kidneys.'"

deficient quantity, with a noise, it indicates either that the man stands in need of purging or that the bladder is diseased."

Urine was held by some to have curative properties, an idea repulsive to others. "It is said that some who have drunk it in the plague have recovered." It was also drunk as a cure for leprosy, putrid ulcers, sprains of the feet, used as antidote for snake bite and deadly poisons and as an application for erysipelas! "The urine of mules suits with arthritic remedies, that of goats and camels is laxative of the belly and hence is given in dropsical complaints."

Through the succeeding centuries, uroscopy, the art of inspection of urine, gradually became the greater part of medical practice. Many recall the numerous drawings in European art galleries[6] that depict the physician of the thirteenth to the sixteenth centuries practicing this art, a subject particularly fascinating to Dutch painters. The urine was always contained in a characteristic flask, of transparent "clere glasse," not flat on the bottom, "but the shape of a very bladder (for the urinall should represent the bladder of a man) and so shall every thyng be sene in his dew place and colore." The container being shaped thus, "the urine should be in natural position as in the bladder." With the spherical base the container could not stand alone, and it was therefore always carried to the physician in a basket of cylindrical shape. The grave-faced physician, dressed in doctor's robe and cap, is always represented as inspecting the urine in a most judicial way, sometimes holding the flask in his hand, at other times examining it while it was held in the hand of a patient or servant, as by some a physician was considered too sacred to hold a bottle of urine himself. Near by, the patient silently awaits the verdict, his attentive expression portraying his pathetic anxiety.

A proper light was most necessary, and the urine was held in such a way that no reflection or refraction from the sun's rays would "make the colour more remisse" and thus interfere with a true observation. As many as twenty different colors were described, each of significance. In addition to the color, the urine was studied as to consistency, transparency, quantity, sediment, odor, froth, scum floating at the top, and substances in the watery part. Grave pronouncements followed such inspection. Cloudy urine at the top of the bottle signified disease of the highest parts of the man's body, alterations in the middle part of the urine related to diseases of the spleen, liver, heart, lungs, bowels, and stomach, and the urinary sediment showed the condition of the lowest parts of the body. Bubbles and frothing indicated evil digestion.

"In an epoch when all clinical methods and investigation were unknown," as Wellcome has aptly put it, "it is natural that the urine should be expected to indicate the disease and its nature, and so as time went on it is not surprising to find that inspection of the urine gradually became more popular in medical diagnosis, as doubtless it appealed, from the spectacular point of view, as strongly to the patient as to the physician." But as imagination increased,

[6] I am informed that there are no such originals in the art museums of the United States.

uroscopy became uromancy and quacks flourished everywhere, traveling the land with their flasks, preying on the gullibility of the people, diagnosing all kinds of diseases and prognosticating all manner of events, from the diagnosis of chastity or pregnancy to the sex of an unborn child.

Naturally a reaction was aroused from time to time against such charlatanism, and frequent tirades were made against the "tricks of the water-doctors" who might go to such limits as did "the physician who saw an oat-grain in a urinal and stated the patient had eaten a horse."

Particularly blameworthy were the attempts of physicians to diagnose the ills of an unseen patient from the analysis of urine sent from a distance. This practice in sixteenth-century England caused the passage of statutes forbidding apothecaries from sending such specimens to physicians, and physicians from pronouncing on any disorder from such an uncertain procedure.

Up to this time, the examination of urine was almost entirely by inspection, not analysis. Discoveries in the seventeenth and eighteenth centuries saved it from ill repute and opened the era beginning with Van Helmont's (1577–1644) studies on the variable weight of urine and ending in the epochal work of Bright (1827), which ushered in the modern period in the study of renal disease. Among these were the demonstration of albumin in urine in the presence of acetic acid (Dekkers, 1694), after boiling (Cotugno, 1764), and in dropsical urine in the presence of nitric acid (Cruickshank, 1798); the determination of its water and solid content (Bellini, 1643–1704), its specific gravity (Booerhaave, 1668–1738), and some of its chemical constituents, such as urea (Booerhaave, 1720; Rouelle, 1771), sugar in diabetic urine (Dobson, 1772), and many others.

THE WORK OF RICHARD BRIGHT

Surpassing all these in importance, as previously stated, was the contribution in 1827 of Richard Bright, distinguished English physician of Guy's Hospital, London, whose name will always be associated with kidney disease. The rare and great honor paid by physicians to colleagues who have made outstanding contributions in certain diseases is to designate that disease by the physician's name. Of the thousands of known diseases, less than five hundred are called in modern medical literature after physicians' names. Of all these conditions the layman, happily unacquainted with disease, is familiar probably with the name of hardly a single one save "Bright's disease." (Saints have fared less well, being honored thus only about twenty-five times.)

In retrospect, Bright's contribution seems a simple one, the demonstration that albumin in urine indicated kidney disease. Its importance rested in making with gratifying precision and clarity the differentiation among several diseased states about which there was great confusion.

In Bright's time, the significance of dropsy and of albuminuria was unknown. Dropsy, an accumulation of fluid in the tissues (extremities, abdomen, or lungs), was thought by some to be a disease in itself; by others, it was considered the result of a variety of diseases, among them disease of the liver, ovaries, lungs or heart, or from certain obstructions to circulatory flow. Albumin had recently been found in the urine in dropsical patients (Cotugno, 1764; Cruickshank, 1798; Wells, 1811; Blackall, 1813), but neither dropsy nor albumin was at that time considered significantly related to kidney disease, which was then thought to consist mostly of stones or the inflammation resulting therefrom. This may seem strange when as early as the sixth century a Roman emperor's physician (Aetius) noted the association of dropsy and hardened kidneys. Four centuries later, Avicenna, the doctor of a Mohammedan caliph, commented on the excessive, thin, watery urine in dropsy, and in 1476, Saliceto, an Italian doctor, wrote on the association of scanty urine, hardened kidneys, and dropsy. But this had apparently been long forgotten. Bright first connected these conditions clearly, albuminuria and dropsy, with kidney disease. He showed indisputably that albuminous urine was present in twenty-four cases of dropsy accompanied by kidney disease, but absent in eleven cases of dropsy associated with liver disease and in four cases of dropsy caused by heart disease. Thus he demonstrated that there were different kinds of dropsy, that albuminuria was a sign of nephritis, and that the dropsy resulting therefrom could be recognized by finding albuminous matter in urine.

Although he mentioned several varieties of nephritis of differing severity, Bright spoke of "this most fatal disease"—fatal enough to bring seventeen of the twenty-four patients to the post-mortem table. While he felt that "where the mischief is less rooted we may undoubtedly do much," he admitted that "some cases defy cure." Thus, by the very strength of his observations, both at the bedside and post-mortem, so important to prove the significance of his discoveries, he unwittingly fostered the notion that this new type of nephritis was a hopeless condition. Then began the era when albuminuria doomed many comparatively healthy persons to fear of an early death. So indiscriminately were dire predictions made on the presence of albumin alone that Bright wrote other papers mainly for the purpose of correcting this misconception. He tried to modify the general pessimistic view by stating that "the disease on which the secretion of albuminous urine depends is in the commencement functional, that as long as it continues in this state it is capable of cure or of relief by various means."

His chemist colleagues, Bostock, Barlow, and Rees, further softened the sting of albuminuria by their careful analyses, demanding that laboratory data necessary for a diagnosis of Bright's disease include other tests on urine, such as the nitric acid ring test, in addition to the heat test. While confirming its general importance as pointed out by Bright, they noted cases in which albuminuria was "so trifling in nature as to render it almost a constant occurrence."

MODERN SIGNIFICANCE OF ALBUMINURIA

The development of modern tests of kidney function has extended knowledge of the diseases and disturbances of kidneys so that the finding of albumin in the urine is no longer interpreted as the equivalent of Bright's disease. It is merely a signpost pointing to any one of several different conditions. It constitutes the most readily detected aberration of normal renal function. While it is thus usually the earliest sign of renal disturbance, functional or organic, it may occur in persons who in other respects are apparently entirely normal, or it may be initiated by any one of many conditions that can disturb kidney function, disturbances which are frequently not great enough to warrant the term "nephritis." However, when albumin does appear, it generally indicates a kidney whose function is embarrassed due to some change, slight or great, temporary or permanent, in its cells.

Albumin is a simple protein found in nearly all animal and many vegetable tissues. It is soluble in water and coagulates as egg white (albumin) does on heating. It is formed by the dissolution of dead tissue cells, either of food or from the body, including red and white blood cells. Digested foods form proteins, which are absorbed and circulate in blood to be used in human growth. About two thirds of this blood protein is in the form of albumin. As already noted, healthy kidneys do not allow this useful substance, food albumin, to pass out from the circulation into the kidney tubes and be lost in urine. Hence, the liquid that passes through the small filters of the kidney is normally free of protein or albumin.

There are two additional sources from which albumin may arise to appear in the urine. When tissue cells of the body die, instead of becoming food protein, they occur in the blood as waste protein. Other forms of waste or foreign protein may arise from impure foods or injected proteins. The kidney filters do not try to keep them back, but allow them to pass into the urine as waste in the form of albumin to be excreted. Albumin in urine must come, therefore, either from food or waste proteins in the blood passing through the kidneys or from the breaking down of cells in the kidney itself or along the urinary passages. The loss of food proteins is accidental, that of waste proteins is purposeful.

Because urine from healthy persons is practically free of protein, albuminuria should always be considered an abnormality, even though its significance is exceedingly variable. Found in the course of an examination for life insurance, it serves as the starting point for other than a routine examination.

INCIDENCE

The incidence of albuminuria in a large group of healthy people is approximately 5 per cent. Certain tests demonstrate albumin more readily than others. Various workers using the nitric acid test found an incidence of albuminuria on a single test ranging from 3 to 16 per cent, with 5 to 7 per cent most commonly reported. Albuminuria was noted in about 5 per cent of 60,000 healthy soldiers (MacLean) and in a similar proportion of 5,000 healthy students (Lee). In another series of 20,000 young men (Diehl-McKinlay), 5.3 per cent showed albuminuria on the first examination. In 66 per cent of these the albuminuria was transient, discovered only once; it was occasionally present in

13 per cent, and persistent in 12 per cent, without any other evidence indicating kidney damage. In only 6.5 per cent of those with albuminuria were there other signs indicating probable renal disease. About 3 per cent of 100,924 male life insurance policyholders showed definite albumin in the urine, while slight traces were found in about 19 per cent more (Sydenstricker and Britten). Sudden increases in its incidence may be noted, as in the "epidemics" of albuminuria seen in healthy West Point cadets (Ashburn).

It is found much more frequently in those who are sick or who consider themselves sick and consult physicians. At a large clinic, albumin was detected in the first specimen in 39 per cent of 663 patients seen consecutively (Sanford, Conner, Magath, and Heck). When three different methods were used, albumin was indicated by one or more tests in more than half (59 per cent) of those studied. Further investigations, however, revealed definite kidney disease in less than half (40 per cent) of the 39 per cent in whose urine albumin was found.

Albuminuria bears a definite relationship to age (Calvin, Isaacs and Meyer, Sydenstricker and Britten). Its incidence increases from childhood up to sixteen years of age. From this peak, there is a rapid decline to between thirty and forty years of age, after which a progressive increase again occurs up to seventy years and more.

TYPES OF ALBUMINURIA

When albumin leaks into urine through or from the kidneys, the condition is "renal albuminuria"; when albumin is added to urine in the lower part of the urinary passages below the kidneys, the condition is called "nonrenal" or "postrenal" albuminuria.

Renal albuminuria may be caused by imperfect working of normal kidneys or by actual disease of the kidneys. It occurs (1) when there is disease primarily in the kidneys or when, in a general disease of the body, renal disease constitutes a major part of the disability; (2) from disease primarily arising in other organs but definitely affecting the kidneys and (3) with certain states in which the working of the kidneys is disturbed, thus causing benign albuminuria without other signs indicating disease.

Most important is the first condition when there is true kidney disease affecting either the kidneys themselves, or some other part of the body, with subsequent enhancement of the primary kidney disease. Generally, but with certain exceptions, albuminuria in these conditions is associated with the presence in the urine of casts (plugs of material washed out of the tubules) and sometimes red blood corpuscles but no pus cells and with variations in the amount and composition of urine. There is also a variety of signs and symptoms due to changes in the blood and other organs in addition to the kidneys. The main examples are the various forms of true, acute, and chronic Bright's disease (diffuse bilateral nephritis), cysts or tumors of the kidney, disease of kidneys in pregnancy and in chronic gout, plugging of blood vessels (thrombi) to or in kidneys, and disease caused by the presence of renal stones, tuberculosis, or obstruction to urinary flow. Strangely enough, cases of severe kidney disease without albuminuria are occasionally seen, and then the diagnosis rests on other findings.

Secondly, a large variety of diseases in other regions may affect the kidneys to an extent that albumin appears in urine. Other definite urinary abnormalities are generally not evident. Varying degrees of disturbed kidney function, however, may result. Transient albuminuria may appear in children after a trivial illness, a cold or bronchitis; marked anemia or jaundice may induce it. This type of renal albuminuria may result from almost any febrile condition, especially scarlet fever, diphtheria, malaria, erysipelas, smallpox, and pneumonia; less frequently, from certain drugs, anesthetic agents (ether or chloroform), poisoning with lead, mercury, arsenic, or phosphorus, from alcoholism, burns, toxic goiter, acute gout, from certain diseases of the blood and blood-forming organs and from parasitic infestations and severe burns. It also occurs with disturbances of circulation ensuing from diseases of the heart with heart failure, and with certain vasomotor conditions producing spasm of blood vessels. Many of these conditions produce degeneration of kidney cells, causing a type of kidney involvement, which may ultimately clear up.

The third variety of renal albuminuria is that often called "physiologic" or "benign" albuminuria, arising from a number of conditions producing alterations in the general circulation and corresponding changes in the normal rate and flow of blood in kidneys. They generally result from certain physical or functional states whose influence on the kidney is reflected by a transient, sometimes a rather persistent, albuminuria without additional evidence of renal impairment. The disability produced may be harmless and insufficient to justify the term "nephritis." Thus various amounts of albumin may appear in urine after strenuous exercise, such as rowing, boxing, and running, after sunburn and so forth and in emotional states and malnutrition. This form appears in adolescence, often without apparent cause. It may occur after a cold shower or exposure to cold, in students cramming for examinations, and in football players after a game. Its relation to malnutrition is shown by the fact that more than 60 per cent of poor children had albuminuria, while only 15 per cent of an equal number of children under the best hygienic care demonstrated it.

Some of these benign forms of albuminuria appear only when the person is in the erect position, and hence are called postural orthostatic (cyclic or intermittent) forms of albuminuria. A curious variety, the lordotic type of orthostatic albuminuria, is found occasionally in healthy young persons who have an exaggerated curve in the small of the back. Under these conditions, considerable albumin may be present in urine passed in daytime, but that formed at night while the person is in a reclining position or passed when the person arises in the morning shows none. When the person is up and about again, it reappears. It is thought to be due to pressure of abdominal organs on the vein of the left kidney, causing interference with adequate circulation when the body is upright. As body growth is completed, the condition usually disappears and the patient remains healthy. Some investigators consider it to be caused by mild but persistent kidney damage from an unknown cause.

NONRENAL OR POSTRENAL ALBUMINURIA

Albumin forms on the dissolution of any tissue cells. In the lower part of the urinary tract cellular debris may give origin to small quantities of albumin that are added to urine after its formation in the kidney and its passage into the tubules. The presence of spermatozoa in the male genital tract or of cells from the vagina in women may account for mild albuminuria, because of contamination of an otherwise normal urine. Catheterized specimens are, therefore, sometimes necessary when women are examined. Urine passed by a woman during the menstrual period may be contaminated by large numbers of red blood cells, which invariably give a strong positive reaction for albumin. When inflammation occurs with formation of pus in the urinary tract below the kidneys, such cells may dissolve in varying quantities. Nonrenal albuminuria may thus arise in cystitis (inflammation of the bladder), pyelitis (inflammation of the kidney pelvis), prostatitis, or from stones in the bladder, ureters, or kidneys.

CHEMICAL TYPES OF ALBUMINURIA

The term "albuminuria" is not strictly accurate, for the coagulable protein of urine consists generally of a mixture made up not only of albumin but also of globulin, mucin, and other proteins. In benign albuminuria proteins besides albumin derived from blood serum are prominently present, such as globulin, nucleo-albumin, and mucin. In true nephritis most of the urinary protein consists of serum albumin and globulin, which may be derived from the food proteins in the blood leaking through damaged glomeruli. Occasionally part of the albuminuria comes from proteins other than those normally circulating in blood; one of these is Bence-Jones protein, which will be discussed later. Some evidence indicates that, in the early stages of diffuse bilateral renal disease, at least part of the urinary albumin comes from degenerated liver cells. Later, protein may be liberated from degenerating kidney cells. These, becoming more permeable, then permit the loss of large amounts of serum albumin. Although methods of easily differentiating these chemical types of albumin are as yet not perfected, studies with the microcentrifuge and electrophoresis of proteins have progressed to the point that, before long, these questions, many of which are at present controversial, will be fully elucidated.

CONCLUSIONS REGARDING ALBUMINURIA

Albuminuria has been discussed in some detail because of the importance popularly attached to it. Obviously to determine the type of albuminuria present, a doctor is necessary and not just a microscope or laboratory, as the differentiation between significant and insignificant forms can be made only after a careful history has been taken and physical examination made in addition to chemical studies. It is particularly important to recognize benign, postural, and other forms of functional albuminuria to prevent persons so affected from being limited by unwarranted fears and by needless restrictions in diet and activity, as occurs when such conditions are confused with true nephritis. In such instances the psychic harm from a dreaded diagnosis may be much greater than the physical harm afforded by the condition itself. Thus are created "renal neurotics." It has been said that "frequently the 'disease' occurs only in the physician's test tube and in the mind of the patient" (Calvin, Isaacs, and Meyer).

To the fearful patient, the discovery of albuminuria may be a rude awakening, arousing unduly great concern. Yet even when significant, albuminuria sometimes constitutes a positive advantage, a beneficent warning to slow up, thereby preventing serious illness. From this viewpoint, a great physician once wrote a paper with the paradoxic title, "On the Advantage of a Trace of Albumin and a Few Casts in the Urine of Men over Fifty."

In general, albuminuria in older persons usually represents some organic disease of variable degree, while that in the young is often functional. In many cases either one may be entirely consistent with the prospect of a healthy and active life. When doubts are entertained, prolonged but not too anxious observation is justified, using such supplementary examinations over a period of several months as seem necessary.

The fallacy of placing much reliance on periodic urinalyses without an accompanying history and physical examination seems evident. Of themselves, such analyses are of little value and may do more harm than good. It has been rightfully said that a physical examination with a urinalysis once a year is of far greater value than a urinalysis alone once a week. Yet a mail-order house some years ago offered such service for a short time. The service was catalogued between a bathtub mat and a bottle of milk of magnesia, and an "analysis covering twenty-nine chemical and microscopical tests" was promised.

A woman presented to a great English physician of the seventeenth century a specimen of her husband's urine, requesting a diagnosis and prescription. "Where is he?" asked the doctor, to which she replied, "Sick in bed four miles off." "What is he?" "A boot-maker." Throwing out the urine and substituting a fresh sample, the doctor said, "Take this home with you, and if your husband will undertake to fit me with a pair of boots by its inspection, I will diagnose and treat him by a similar examination."

Shakespeare commented similarly when to Falstaff's inquiry, "What says the doctor to my water?" the page replies, "He said, sir, the water itself was a good healthy water, but for the party that owned it he might have more diseases than he knows for." A modern counterpart is the inelegant but pertinent tale of the canny gentleman who, on receiving a favorable report from a single, but mixed, specimen sent to a laboratory, happily said, "Good! Mama's well, papa's well, the whole family's well."

MODERN METHODS OF EXAMINING THE KIDNEYS

As Bright found more than one test useful, indeed necessary, so benefits are derived by that scientific ingenuity which has provided a number of ways for study of the condition of the kidneys. A routine urinalysis constitutes the first test to be used and affords the chief point of departure, indicating whether other tests are necessary. While it is true that occasional cases of severe nephritis have been found in which the urine was apparently normal, not even containing albumin, generally some abnormality is present. Ordinarily urine is examined for its alkaline or acid reaction, its specific gravity, the presence of albumin, sugar, pus or blood cells, sediment, and casts. The odor and sediment of urine of a normal person can be altered in several ways; by the kind and amount of food eaten, amount of water drunk, length of time the urine has stood, time of day it was passed, and so forth. Odoriferous or cloudy urine, therefore, does not of itself indicate nephritis, nor is clear urine a sure token of healthy kidneys. Casual inspection is valueless and, indeed, may be misleading.

Casts, as has been said, are small masses of protein, cylindric in structure and taking the shape of the kidney tubule. They are of various types. Those most frequently found are the pale, transparent, "hyaline" casts. Others with cellular debris attached to them are called granular, fatty, waxy, epithelial, or blood casts. Their origin is not perfectly understood. Normal persons may pass small numbers of hyaline casts that arise from the same conditions producing albuminuria. When hyaline casts are numerous or when other types of casts are present, the fact usually signifies inflammation or degeneration from renal disease.

The ability of the kidneys to excrete a large amount of waste in a small amount of fluid—in other words, to elaborate a thick or concentrated urine—is one of their most important functions. By the water-dilution and water-concentration tests, it can be determined whether their diluting and concentrating powers are being maintained. On one day a patient is given solid, dry food only; no fluids are permitted. The urine is collected at certain intervals; normally it should become thick and highly colored, with a specific gravity of 1.020 or greater. On another day 7½ glasses (3 pints) of water are given to the fasting patient within a period of one half hour. At least 75 per cent of this water should be passed normally within the next four hours; the urine becomes thin and watery, with a specific gravity as low as 1.002. When the kidney function is seriously impaired, this concentrating and diluting ability is lost and the specific gravity becomes relatively fixed around 1.010. As long as this ability is partially preserved, maximal renal damage has not yet occurred.

The size, shape, and position of the kidney usually can be faintly but unmistakably outlined in an ordinary X-ray picture of the abdomen. The size and shape of the pelvic cavity inside the kidney can be studied also by special means. One of medicine's recent triumphs is the utilization of a harmless substance which, injected by vein, finds its way to the kidneys and becomes concentrated sufficiently to cast a shadow on X-ray plates, thereby in some cases avoiding the discomfort of the cystoscope. This test is termed the "excretory urogram." By means of the cystoscope and ureteral catheters, certain liquids opaque to the X-ray can be made to flow gently up the ureters to fill the renal pelvis, outlining it sharply in the X-ray picture, like a glove with many projecting fingers (a pyelogram). If disease has destroyed part of the kidney substance or its tubular projections, or if a stone is present, blocking all or part of the pelvis or ureter, characteristic alterations from the normal shadow are produced which help the trained eye in diagnosis.

The excretory ability of the kidneys can be tested by injecting into the muscles or veins certain harmless dyes (phenolsulfonphthalein, indigo carmine, or methylene blue) to see how rapidly and completely they are eliminated in the urine. Eight to ten minutes after injection, the dye begins to appear in the urine, and 40 to 60 per cent of the amount injected should appear within the following hour. Disease of the kidneys or any block to the free passage of urine below the kidneys in the tubes or bladder (from stone, adjacent tumors, or enlarged prostate) causes a definite reduction in the amount of dye recovered. Since it is not known just which cells, glomeruli, or tubules have most to do with the excretion of dyes, retention of dye does not imply specifically localizable damage.

By means of dyes and the cystoscope, a trained physician can often determine whether one or both kidneys are diseased and how much. By passage of small ureteral catheters or collecting tubes into each ureter as it enters the bladder, it can be ascertained, in the samples of urine collected separately from each kidney, whether blood, pus, or germs (such as tubercle bacilli) are coming from one or both sides. The importance of this test can be imagined when it is deemed necessary to remove one kidney. The function of the other must be adequately gauged.

Finer details concerning excretory capacity can be determined by giving orally or injecting into veins not foreign dyes but measured amounts of those products which the kidneys naturally handle (urea, uric acid, or creatinine), then studying their concentration in blood and urine and the speed of their elimination. These are called "clearance" or "concentration" tests.

When kidney function is appreciably impaired, waste substances accumulate in the blood so that their concentration may increase from ten to fifty times (urea 40 to 700 mg. per 100 cc.; uric acid 2 to 30 mg.; creatinine 1 to 20 mg. or more, and sulfates from 2 to 40 mg. or more). Since inorganic sulfates are excreted by the normal kidney with maximal difficulty, when the kidneys are disturbed, sulfates are one of the first substances to increase in blood. Urea and uric acid are excreted fairly readily, and the estimation of concentration of urea in blood is the most important and common test of renal function next to a urinalysis. Since creatinine is excreted with great ease, it is an extremely sick kidney that cannot still rid the blood of it; hence it is the last substance to increase. When it increases appreciably and constantly, it is generally an omen of impending death, indicating a kidney too disturbed even to carry on this, its simplest function. Thus it can be appreciated that blood analyses may give information of great value.

As waste substances accumulate in the blood, they begin to adulterate all body tissues and to appear in abnormal amounts in such fluids as saliva, breast milk, bile, and the fluids that bathe the brain, spinal cord, heart, lungs, and joints. They even accumulate in fluids of the eyeballs and are present excessively in tears. Dr. Philip S. Hench showed that when blood tests are inconvenient or impossible because people have small veins or swollen, edematous extremities, a simple estimation of the amount of urea in saliva gives a satisfactory index of nitrogen retention in the body. When disease is serious, nitrogenous waste products and associated poisons are eliminated excessively in sweat and by the bowels and may cause small ulcers of the skin or bowel. In such cases "uremia" is present, a condition to be described later.

The kidneys are not isolated structures, and their disturbances may affect distant organs and systems, especially the heart-blood vessel (cardiovascular) system. Therefore the doctor examines the heart, the blood pressure, the blood vessels in the arms, and, particularly, the smaller vessels in the eye, where at times certain disturbances may be clearly seen with an ophthalmoscope.

KNOWLEDGE DERIVED FROM KIDNEY TESTS

Physicians have gone far—some say too far—from the simple test for albumin in finding ways of diagnosing nephritis. However, no one test tells the whole tale of a kidney's woe. Nor is an elaborate array of expensive tests ordinarily necessary. The intelligent use of four or five (urinalysis, dye test or estimation of urea, water dilution and concentration test, and blood count), along with the patient's story and a physical examination, will give most of the necessary information, at least in so-called medical nephritis. When pus and blood are present or when stones and other surgical conditions are suspected, advantage should be taken of certain additional tests. In many cases the physician from such studies can with remarkable exactness tell the cause and extent of the disease and the exact parts of the kidney affected. He may venture a prophecy on whether or not the patient will recover, and if not how long he may live. Sometimes the information gained from such examinations is limited. While they show approximately how badly the kidneys are diseased, it cannot always be stated that "only the tubules are involved" or "the glomeruli are alone concerned." The kidney filters and tubules work together essentially as units, and when one part is diseased the other part is apt to become disturbed also. Often when the kidney is "sick," it is like the boy with the toothache, "sick all over." At other times, when one part of the kidney is too disturbed to carry on its function, that work is apparently taken over by another part (a compensatory mechanism). Furthermore, invisible lesions are sometimes present that cannot be demonstrated by means of the microscope and test tube.

While the doctor cannot see how the kidneys look, he can determine how they are working and act accordingly.

GENERAL CAUSES OF KIDNEY DISEASE

Bright's disease, as the term is used inclusively, is "the response of the kidney to any alteration in its environment, especially to the irritation of toxic substances." As these toxic substances may be numerous, so the causes of nephritis are many. Nephritis may result from (1) invasion of the kidneys by germs (bacteria) of many kinds; (2) poisons either manufactured by bacteria or formed in infected tissues; (3) toxins not of bacterial origin, such as from metals or chemical poisons; (4) infections and intoxications from mechanical interference to the normal passage of urine produced by obstruction (such as from stones or an enlarged prostate gland); (5) abnormalities of growth, such as cysts and benign or malignant tumors, producing interference in the kidneys' function, and (6) by impairment of the blood supply to the kidney as a result of a disease process in the blood vessels themselves.

A large variety of bacteria may be brought to the kidneys and there set up infections that may localize in the kidneys alone or invade surrounding tissues and the lower part of the urinary passages. The commonest bacteria found in such infections are the colon bacillus (the constant inhabitant of the normal intestinal tract), staphylococci, and streptococci. The tubercle bacillus is also an important invader. Some of the bacteria present a curious consistency in the "geography" of their invasion. Thus the colon bacillus usually attacks the interior part of the kidney, its pelvis and urinary tubes, while the cocci fight their battles in the outer part, the cortex and fatty tissues about the kidney. Some bacteria are especially prone to cause precipitation of matter that forms stones. The various bacteria reach the kidney by several routes: through blood vessels (an infected blood stream), along infected lymph channels, or from infected urine dammed back by any interference with urinary flow, such as may be produced by a stone, kink in a ureter, or an enlarged prostate gland. Bacteria that reach the kidneys through the blood arise from an infected focus elsewhere in the body—small collections of bacteria in infected teeth, tonsils, ears, or other organs.

Some bacteria do not themselves invade the kidneys, but, from a distance, liberate toxins or poisons that injure kidney cells. Toxins may arise in distant infected regions from dying infected cells and injure the kidney tissues as they are being excreted from the blood. Many poisons not of bacterial origin may produce nephritis. Some of them have been mentioned: certain metals, such as mercury, uranium, and lead, and poisons resulting from burns, goiter, gout, and pregnancy.

Some disturbing agents arouse rather individualistic reactions and special types of cellular disturbance identified by signs and symptoms fairly peculiar unto themselves. Such, for example, are tuberculous infections or the manifestation of stones. The majority of such agents, however, initiate changes in function and structure that, at least in the beginning, arouse in their victims more or less identical complaints.

GENERAL SYMPTOMS AND SIGNS OF KIDNEY DISEASE

In the mildest forms there may be no symptoms, and the patient only accidentally learns about his trouble at the time of an examination for life insurance or for some other purpose. The blood pressure may be a little too high, the heart may be a little inadequate, or the urine test may betray its guilty secret—any of these may introduce the unexpected, brutal revelation of the presence of kidney disease. Some patients are aware of vague discomfort; they feel "out of sorts," or "off color," without knowing why. They may complain of an unaccustomed listlessness, unexplainable fatigue, dull headaches, slight puffiness about the eyes, or a poor appetite. Careful parents especially will be alert to such insidious complaints in their children.

As the kidneys become further diseased, a more or less identical train of events often occurs without regard to cause. Slight disturbances of vision may be noted, such as occasional blurring or spots in front of the eyes. There may be disturbances of sleep because of the desire to void urine at night. Wetting of the bed, however, does not necessarily signify nephritis, as it may be caused by a variety of conditions.[7] Dryness of the mouth may appear, with thirst necessitating frequent drinking of water. There may be loss of weight, or if water-logging of tissues (edema) occurs, the patient may gain weight as if he were healthy, and thus attain a sense of false security. When stones, abscesses, or inflammations with pus in the lower part of the urinary passages are present, pain may be present, often accompanied by chills and fever. In the majority of kidney diseases, however, pain is not a feature and may be entirely absent. The well-known advertisement illustrating a man slightly stooped with his hand on a painful flank is greatly misleading, inferring, as it does, that pain in this region generally means kidney disease, for which the advertiser has a wonderful medicine for so much a bottle. Most patients who have chronic pain in the flanks are not suffering from nephritis at all, but from some other disease, often some form of rheumatism in the muscles or joints of the spinal column.

As kidney disease progresses, other organs may become disturbed, and a variety of symptoms may arise, such as dizziness, nausea, vomiting, perhaps diarrhea, severe headache, shortness of breath, swelling of feet and arms, enlargement of the abdomen from fluid, and symptoms of congestion in lungs and liver. As the nephritis approaches its most serious phase, unconsciousness may arise from uremic coma, and convulsions may occur.

The general signs of kidney disease may be local or constitutional. Local signs pertain to alterations in quantity, appearance, and quality of the urine.

---

[7]Paulus Aegineta (A. D. 625–690) recommended the following for incontinence of urine (bed-wetting): "Burn the crop of a cock, and give to the patient to drink in tepid water when fasting, or the flowers of the white ox-eye (chrysanthemum) in like manner" (Vol. I, p. 548).

The urine may be pale and thin and voided frequently or in large amounts. In other cases it is dark, cloudy, and markedly diminished in amount. Tests will show alterations in the urine and changes in the amounts of blood wastes present. Signs that reflect constitutional disturbances in association with nephritis may be: increase in blood pressure, an enlarged heart, fluid in the lungs, small hemorrhages in the skin or in the back of the eyeballs, and especially a pale, pasty complexion and anemia. Sick kidneys are truly versatile in the range and scope of their symptomatology.

UREMIA

If both kidneys are removed or both ureters blocked, death results in a few days, as a result of formation and retention of poisons in the blood and tissues of the body. This toxic state is called "uremia," the main characteristic of which is a period of drowsiness interrupted perhaps by convulsions. A similar intoxication may occur in cases of acute or chronic kidney insufficiency. Its first manifestations are often itching of the skin, headache, and cramps or twitchings in muscles. Then intense nausea, vomiting, and shortness of breath may occur. If the condition persists, it may be distressingly punctuated by convulsive or epileptiform seizures, or the patient may lapse into a drowsy state ending in coma and death. There is no more complete nor accurate description of the uremic state to be found in the medical literature than the eloquent words of Richard Bright, written in 1836, to define the characteristics and progress of this unfortunate and pathetic train of events: "Again the patient is restored to tolerable health; again he enters on his active duties; or he is perhaps, less fortunate;—the swelling increases, the urine becomes scanty, the powers of life seem to yield, the lungs become oedematous, and, in a state of asphyxia or coma, he sinks into the grave; or a sudden effusion of serum into the glottis closes the passages of the air, and brings on a more sudden dissolution. Should he, however, have resumed the avocations of life, he is usually subject to constant recurrence of his symptoms; or again, almost dismissing the recollection of his ailment, he is suddenly seized with an acute attack of pericarditis, or with a still more acute attack of peritonitis, which, without any renewed warning, deprives him, in eight and forty hours, of his life. Should he escape this danger likewise, other perils await him; his headaches have been observed to become more frequent; his stomach more deranged; his vision indistinct; his hearing depraved: he is suddenly seized with a convulsive fit, and becomes blind. He struggles through the attack; but again and again it returns; and before a day or week has elapsed, worn out by convulsions, or overwhelmed by coma, the painful history of his disease is closed."

Uremia is not entirely dependent on the duration or amount of kidney disturbance. It may appear as a tragic surprise early in the course of acute and seemingly moderate kidney inadequacy, or it may be postponed for long periods in a patient whose kidneys are known to be hardly functioning at all. It may attack with sudden fury a person in active and apparently healthy life, unaware of impending catastrophe. Nor is uremia dependent on the amount of urea dammed back in the blood, for a marked excess may be long present yet the patient escape its symptoms. It may occur in nephrosis, that form of kidney disease characterized by water and salt retention, when the ability of the kidneys to eliminate toxic waste products fails, whereas it occurs in its most violent form in nephritis without dropsy.

The exact substance responsible for uremic poisoning is not known. When his colleague Babington first noted an increase of urea in the blood of nephritic patients, Bright used the term "uremia," considering urea to be a toxic substance. Recent studies seem to indicate that urea is not sufficiently toxic to account for this profound upset. While various minor disturbances can be produced in the body by feeding excess urea, Hewlett and others noted only slight muscular fatigue, drowsiness, and lassitude after taking sufficiently large amounts of urea to raise its concentration in the blood for several hours to almost ten times the normal amount. The conclusions of such feeding experiments have only a limited application, however, just as symptoms of acute drunkenness cannot be compared to those in the chronic poisoning of habitual alcoholism.

In some illuminating experiments the physiologists, Bollman and Mann, transplanted the ureters of animals into the bowel, thereby causing at least part of the urinary substances to be reabsorbed through the intestine into the blood. The amazing concentration of more than 1,600 mg. of urea for each 100 cc. of blood was reached (at least fifty times as much as is normally present), yet the animals continued to live with no noticeable effect whatever. This seems to present indisputable evidence that urea is not toxic, and physicians must therefore seek to discover and eliminate some far more potent poison.

When uremia begins to occur, that is, when an appreciable and prolonged increase of urea and other waste products in the blood takes place, great caution must be exercised to prevent serious, perhaps fatal, toxicity. A sudden increase of headaches or muscular pains, a rapid increase of blood pressure or blood urea, should warn of impending danger and prompt the physician to initiate the necessary additions to treatment. Unfortunately, in cases of progressively failing kidneys the physician's efforts often only postpone an inevitable tragedy but they do make its coming more bearable.

AIMS IN THE TREATMENT OF KIDNEY DISEASE AND KIDNEY FAILURE

Special treatment is required for such forms of kidney trouble as tuberculosis, tumors, infections, stones, the kidney poisoning that occasionally occurs in pregnancy, and that caused by obstruction from an enlarged prostate gland producing a backflow of urine. What the doctor tries to do in the treatment of nephritis and of renal insufficiency or kidney failure of other types can be discussed together briefly.

There are two aims in treatment: (1) Where possible, to discover and remove the cause of the kidney trouble and (2) to lighten the burden on the diseased kidney while it is damaged. The commonest known causes of nephritis are bacterial and chemical poisons. In nephritis of youth and middle age any chronic source of infection should if possible be removed. If this is impossible, local treatment should be provided for disease such as may exist in tonsils, the middle ears and sinuses, especially in children, the teeth, the prostate gland, and occasionally about the female organs. The time for removal or treatment must be carefully chosen. The habitual use, by susceptible persons, of certain medicines is occasionally found to be a causal factor. "Cleansing mercury douches," for example, may seriously irritate the kidneys, and for this reason their use is to be condemned.

A physician of antiquity (Galen) wrote that "the offices of the kidneys and bladder being incessant, these parts, if diseased, having no rest, can scarcely get well." It has been found, however, that the kidneys as a whole do not work incessantly. Only certain units in a kidney are working at any one time, but when working they do so at full speed. Richards, a physiologist, has proved this by watching, through a special microscope, the glomeruli of a frog's kidney actually working. The glomeruli did not all work continuously but in shifts, some taking time off. Through this wise provision of nature the vitality of these delicate but energetic units is conserved.

The units of a sick kidney need even more rest. For them rest is the great restorer of health and life. It is the one measure that may tide them over until such time as they can recuperate fully, or may conserve their energies so they can carry on as long as possible. The kidneys can be rested in several ways: by not adding to their burdens, by shifting part of their work to other organs, and by helping them carry on such work as is unavoidable. During physical activity body tissues are forming wastes that the kidneys must handle. Rest in bed during the acute stage of nephritis is therefore advisable to prevent avoidable and unnecessary formation of body wastes. Some wastes are excreted through sweat and by bowels. Years ago it was felt that the kidney could be spared considerable work by stimulating the skin and intestines to greater activity. This was accomplished in some cases by the repeated use of mild or strong laxatives, frequent enemas, daily warm baths, and, in some instances, hot packs applied to the entire body to induce sweating. Such measures, for the most part, in recent years have been discarded because of their weakening effect on the patient and because the amounts of waste products eliminated by such means are infinitesimally small. There are, however, three procedures by means of which urea and other waste products can be eliminated from the body across membranes other than the glomerular filter in patients whose kidneys are so damaged that the filtering apparatus is inadequate for this function.

In the first of these methods a tube is introduced by way of the mouth or nose, past the stomach and into the small intestine (intestinal lavage). Introduction of a special solution into the tube causes waste products from the blood to be filtered across the wall of the intestine to be eliminated in the stools. The second method (peritoneal lavage) involves the introduction of tubes through the abdominal wall and filling the abdominal cavity with a special solution of various salts and water, which, as in the former method, causes waste products to be filtered across the peritoneal membrane into the abdominal cavity, from whence they are removed by suction. In the third method (artificial kidney) the patient's blood containing waste products in high concentrations is passed through coils of cellophane tubing immersed in a bath of a specially prepared solution. As the blood passes through the coils of cellophane, waste products are filtered across the cellophane wall into the bath, and the "purified blood" is returned to the patient's body. These three methods of "extrarenal" excretion have rather definite indications for use and have been found to be of great value—indeed, in some instances, life-saving—particularly in patients whose kidney damage is acute, transient, or reversible in nature, when nature will repair the kidney damage present if the functional load on the kidney can be lightened for several days or weeks to allow such repair to take place. However, it must be stated that none of these measures are without some degree of risk, and their use in patients who have far advanced, chronic, irreversible damage to kidney function is debatable if not contraindicated.

Catching cold or the "flu" may add a serious burden to the kidney, and protection from prevalent infections should be afforded, such as avoidance of crowds, keeping away from sick relatives, and so forth.

One of the most important measures is a carefully selected diet. A milk diet is by no means universally adequate. In some types of kidney disease such a diet may provide too much fluid; in another type it may contain too much protein or salt. A proper diet for each patient can be planned only by a physician who has carried out the indicated number of laboratory procedures previously mentioned. Those who have found this necessity irksome will sympathize with Bill Nye. "I have just been sent to the hospital. My physician did it. He did it with an analysis. Anybody who amounts to anything nowadays gets analyzed. Sometimes you find casts, sometimes you find maple sugar and sometimes acids, oxides, paints, oils, varnish, white lead, borax, albumin, lime, hair and cement. In these cases the patient should be placed on a strict diet or he will in the course of his life become a corpse. . . . An analysis today shows more casts, fibrin, gelatin and some zinc and copper. The chemist also discovers that in 1853 I fell from an apple tree and tore my pants in two places. He says I will be unhappy with my third wife. She will be unhappy also."

The important features of diet concern the amounts of salt, water, and protein permissible. When dropsy is present or impending, the amount of salt and fluid allowed must be carefully estimated. When retention of urea and other wastes occurs in the blood, it has long seemed best to restrict the ingestion of proteins. Recently some physicians, as the result of certain experiments, have become more lax, allowing rather generous amounts of protein. Until the effects of such diets are better known, moderate restrictions in meats, eggs, and other proteins seem indicated. A certain amount of fluids and of protein, however, is vitally necessary, and complete abstinence is rarely required. In a form of nephritis known as nephrosis, in which the kidney is adequately able to eliminate urea and other waste products from the body, but in which the content of protein in the blood is below normal, a diet that provides much protein but little salt is called for. There is no essential difference between so-called red meats and white meats as far as nephritis is concerned.

The elimination of wastes by the kidneys can be increased by use of a variety of diuretics, substances which cause these wastes to pass through the kidneys in added amounts.[8] Water itself is a diuretic, and some persons after drinking a quart of water will within a short time eliminate perhaps a quart and a half of urine. Concentrated solution of glucose, coffee, tea, certain mineral waters, beer, and a number of drugs will promote an augmented flow of urine. Some of these diuretics are indicated when dropsy occurs without the increase of wastes in the tissues. Choice of a proper diuretic is important, as the wrong one may irritate the kidneys and add to their embarrassment, thus causing further damage.

The treatment of kidney disease has been made much more successful by the recent discovery of several new and more efficient diuretics. Contemplating the ease of their administration and their efficacy, one can be thankful to live in modern times. Only about two centuries ago an esteemed physician wrote (Pechey cited by Hewitt): "Put washed worms into a curcurbit [flask] so well stoppered that nothing can exhale. Place it to digest either in sea water or in the heat of the sun, that the worms may putrefy and ferment. This fermentation is sometimes so very great that it breaks the glass. The fermentation being over, the earthy part sinks to the bottom, and the skins swim on top, the spiritous liquor is in the middle. Separate this and distill it, and it will yield a spirit; this spirit is an excellent diuretic."

Dropsy or waterlogging of tissues occurs in some cases where too much common salt (sodium chloride) is eaten. However, when a different salt is used (ammonium chloride, ammonium nitrate, potassium nitrate, or potassium chloride), dropsy may be relieved. In cases of nephritis in which dropsy is associated with a decreased amount of protein in the circulating blood (nephrosis), certain substances called "plasma volume expanders" are valuable in promoting flow of urine and reduction of dropsical fluid in the tissues. Acacia, solutions of gelatin, a special preparation of concentrated blood serum, and more recently a substance called "dextran," all have a similar action. In some instances one substance works more effectively than others. In Bright's time mercury in certain forms was used but often was found to

---

[8]"Diuresis" means "to urinate through"; a diuretic is a substance that increases the secretion of urine.

be harmful. Newer mercury preparations are now available that are less harmful and often almost miraculous in ridding the body of great quantities of dropsical fluid rapidly. When necessary, such preparations have been given by injection repeatedly almost weekly for five years without harm. However, mercury in any form must be used with caution in patients suffering from kidney disease, lest the drug, whose effectiveness lies in its property as a mild irritant to the kidney, produce further kidney damage.

If ascites, the accumulation of fluid in the abdomen, is present and cannot be relieved by the use of diuretics, the abdominal cavity may have to be tapped and the fluid removed through a tube (paracentesis). An eighteenth-century physician (Mead) cited the "remarkable case of Lady Page who in seventy-seven months was tapped seventy-six times and had taken away two hundred and forty gallons of water without ever repining at her case, or ever fearing the operation." Fortunately, modern diets and diuretics have largely done away with the necessity for this procedure.

When uremia occurs, drastic measures may be necessary to prevent convulsions and unconsciousness, or even death. Then the resources of the physician are taxed indeed, but sometimes by injections of fluid, transfusions of blood, and other procedures a new lease on life, or at least some comfort, may be provided.

Quack remedies for kidney diseases abound in great numbers. In a recent circular are advertised fifty different "kidney tablets," fifty-one "kidney remedies," and one hundred and twenty-seven "kidney pills," as well as various "kidney-tonics, bitters, cordials, capsules, drops, medicines, treatments and herb teas." Many of them are called "kidney and backache remedies," fostering the classic falsehood of the quacks regarding urinary sediments and pain in the back. The charlatan often recommends a nostrum indiscriminately for nephritis and diabetes, making no distinction between these utterly different types of disease. Scores of them have been analyzed by government and national medical laboratories. Most of them contain drugs that tend to increase the quantity of urine but not the amount of waste excreted. In some cases this is done in a particularly vicious way by including a powerful irritant to the kidney which, though it increases the amount of urine, may cause serious damage. Others are harmless but quite useless. One used to "cure Bright's disease, gravel, all urinary troubles and pain in the back or groin from kidney trouble" was found to contain white sugar exclusively! One widely advertised backache and kidney pill that sells for seventy-five cents for a box of forty pills, and which has been estimated as costing one cent a box to make, was found to contain one harmless and one equally useless but irritating substance. Another well-known diuretic pill, also ineffective, was advertised as worth five dollars a box, sells for twenty-five cents for a box of thirty-five pills, and has been estimated as costing about a quarter of a cent for a full box! Certainly there is no place for alleged cures for the self-treatment of such a potentially dangerous condition as kidney disease.

CLASSIFICATION OF KIDNEY DISEASES: SYNOPSIS OF CHIEF FORMS

None of the many classifications of kidney diseases is entirely satisfactory. Were the cause of each known it would be simple to designate them accordingly, "tuberculous nephritis," "mercurial nephritis," and so on. In many instances the cause is obscure, and classifications are based on the part of the kidney chiefly involved, on what the microscope shows after death: "glomerular nephritis," "tubular nephritis." Others are named from the chief symptoms and signs they produce (or from the main functional derangement): "chronic nephritis with edema," "salt and water nephritis." This presentation permits only a brief mention of the chief forms of kidney disturbance.

They can be divided into four groups. Group I constitutes those diseases which affect primarily the kidneys alone or in which the kidney disturbance becomes the chief cause of ill health. Group II includes different types of toxic or diseased states in which the kidneys are disturbed on account of disease elsewhere and become a secondary cause of ill health. Group III involves certain conditions in which nephritis is absent (the kidneys are relatively unaffected), but in which alterations in the quality or quantity of urine afford important signs in diagnosis. Group IV includes disturbances of kidneys dependent on maldevelopment.

GROUP I. DISEASES IN WHICH NEPHRITIS BECOMES THE
CHIEF CAUSE OF ILL HEALTH

The kidneys do not live to or for themselves alone, and nephritis is rarely if ever strictly a disease solely of the kidneys. They become diseased from poisons and bacteria brought to them from some distant site; as a result of the subsequent nephritis, other tissues in turn become involved. The blood vessels of the kidneys may participate with those of other organs in a systemic disease affecting vessels throughout the body. One organ may suffer more than others; when the kidney does so, the nephritis becomes the chief cause of ill health. Kidney damage associated with essential hypertension (high blood pressure) may be an example of the former; acute and chronic glomerulonephritis are examples of the latter. The small blood vessels of many organs, such as heart, brain, muscles, eyes, and liver, are diseased, but the difficulty in the kidney dominates the picture. It is, for example, as if all the pipes in a house become clogged; damage to those in the kitchen where food must be prepared would cause a greater disturbance than to those in the parlor radiator or the bath.

Kidney Disease Secondary to High Blood Pressure

While the blood pressure increases with or as a result of certain forms of nephritis, some types of increased blood pressure (so-called essential hypertension) come at first without nephritis and indeed may never be associated with significant kidney disturbance. As, however, thickening occurs in the walls of the tiny blood vessels in the kidneys (afferent arterioles) as part of the generalized thickening of blood vessel walls throughout the entire body, circulation to the kidney is diminished, and the function of these organs is thereby impaired. By constricting the renal artery, one investigator (Goldblatt) has produced high blood pressure in animals similar to that seen in humans. When the constriction is removed, the blood pressure returns to normal or near normal limits. By wrapping the kidney of an animal in a non-elastic envelope (cellophane), thereby interfering with the normal circulation of blood through the kidney, two other investigators (Page and Corcoran) have found that the blood pressure increases. They have found also that in animals in which high blood pressure has been thus produced, a chemical substance is released into the blood. Blood containing this chemical substance, when injected into a normal animal, causes the blood pressure to increase.

Chronic Renal Arteriosclerosis

Chronic renal arteriosclerosis may occur in elderly persons (more than forty-five or fifty years of age) who have hardening of large arteries elsewhere, at the "temples," wrists, and so on. The condition is often discovered by chance during a yearly checkup or from urinalysis in the course of an examination for life insurance. The larger, not the small, vessels of the kidney are chiefly diseased; hence, a degree of accommodation takes place whereby the patient may not be noticeably incapacitated. The blood pressure increases to force blood through the stiffened vessels. Dropsy is rare. Some anemia may occur, and there may be a lag in ridding the blood of wastes. As a rule, no special cause for alarm need be felt. Under supervision the patient may lead a comparatively comfortable and useful existence for a number of years. Plenty of fluids are required to rid the body of wastes, but because excretion of water is slowed, fluids should be taken mostly before supper to avoid the necessity of arising during the night for urination.

Acute Glomerulonephritis (Acute Bright's Disease)

Acute glomerulonephritis is usually a disease of young people. During World War I it affected many soldiers and acquired the term "war" or "trench" nephritis. Its cause is unknown, but is thought to be due to bacterial infection or to the effect of bacterial poisons on the glomeruli; sometimes it disappears after a focus of infection is removed. The urine is cloudy, dark, and scanty, and contains albumin, casts, and red blood cells and sometimes even visible blood. Wastes do not often accumulate markedly in the blood. Dropsy occurs, and the blood pressure increases. The death rate is low, perhaps 3 per cent. It often clears entirely in a few weeks. Occasionally it progresses into chronic glomerulonephritis.

Chronic Glomerulonephritis (Chronic Bright's Disease)

Chronic glomerulonephritis is perhaps the most serious of all forms of nephritis. It is that form first described by Bright and from which arose the erroneous idea that all nephritis was extremely serious. Its onset is usually before forty years of age and may be insidious or may follow acute glomerulonephritis. It is often part of a general disease of blood vessels. The patient may pass thin watery urine at frequent intervals during the day and night, a total of two or three quarts or more. The urine contains albumin and casts. Dropsy is usually absent or not marked. The blood pressure increases, and the complexion becomes pasty because of anemia. Wastes accumulate in the blood. The heart enlarges and weakens. Vessels in the brain may be affected. Thus death may result from heart failure, a stroke, or from uremia. Some patients live several years, but as chronic invalids. Others are able to lead moderately active lives for many years.

Chronic Glomerulonephritis with Nephrotic Features (Chronic Bright's Disease with Dropsy)

This disease is characterized by marked albuminuria and dropsy, and the presence of peculiar fatty or lipoid bodies in the urine. Anemia, high blood pressure, and involvement of the heart and eyes are not present as early in this disease as they are in the dry form of chronic glomerulonephritis. Kidney function is adequate except for excretion of salt and water, and diets must be arranged accordingly. Diuretics are especially useful in this condition. The edema may clear, and the danger to life may not be great for a long period, although the patient's resistance to infections seems lowered. Health may return, but albuminuria as a rule continues more or less persistently. In many cases a "mixed nephritis" follows, however, in which the symptoms and signs of the dry form of Bright's disease described above are superimposed on the nephrotic picture. This train of events usually is progressive, and the outlook is less favorable.

Conditions Affecting the Renal Tubules (Nephroses)

There are many conditions that produce in kidneys a toxic state affecting chiefly the renal tubules, nephrosis, which affords a secondary cause of ill health. In nephrosis there is usually marked albuminuria, but no increase in blood pressure or generally of waste products in the blood. In some forms dropsy is absent, in others much dropsy occurs. Chemical nephrosis may be caused by certain metals, drugs, anesthetic agents, or food poisons, such as from meat, fish, or mushrooms. The commonest causes are mercury and arsenic. Other responsible substances are phosphorus, chromates, lead, bismuth, uranium, zinc, turpentine, tar, cresol, carbolic acid, certain alcohols, chloroform, carbon tetrachloride, and ether. Toxic nephrosis may be caused, in the absence of fever, by such conditions as jaundice, intestinal obstruction, burns, pernicious anemia, diabetes mellitus, syphilis, and thyroid disease, or by a variety of infectious diseases with fever. Febrile nephroses (febrile albuminuria) may result from pneumonia, malaria, yellow fever, typhoid fever, diphtheria, empyema, blood poisoning, peritonitis, gangrene, or injections of foreign protein. Lipoid nephrosis is a special rare form of tubular disease, the cause of which is unknown.

Mercurial Nephrosis: Excesses of mercury produce serious kidney trouble. The acute form is encountered when tablets of bichloride of mercury are taken by mistake or with suicidal intent. The urine becomes loaded with albumin, casts, and red blood cells. Complete suspension of kidney function with suppression of urine for several days may follow the extensive tubular damage present. Uremia and death may ensue, or slow recovery may follow prompt and vigorous treatment. While the physician is awaited, the patient should be given several raw eggs in milk. Chronic mercurial poisoning is an industrial hazard for the makers of thermometers, barometers, felt hats, and other products necessitating the use of the metal or salts of mercury.

Acute Tubular Insufficiency (Lower Nephron Nephrosis): Mercurial nephrosis, together with tubular damage as a result of several other causative agents, may be classed under the heading of lower nephron nephrosis, or, more correctly, acute tubular insufficiency. This condition is characterized by failure of the kidneys to secrete urine in any appreciable amounts, if at all, progressive retention of waste products in the blood, uremia, and death. It may occur secondarily to any of the systemic conditions already listed, to shock and prolonged decrease in blood pressure associated with hemorrhage or surgical procedures, to transfusion with incompatible blood, and to numerous other situations. The "crush injury" syndrome, frequently encountered in battle and civilian casualties during World War II, is an example. Fortunately, the damage to the kidneys in many of these conditions is self-limiting, reversible, and capable of repair. It is in this group of patients that the three methods of extrarenal excretion described previously (intestinal lavage, peritoneal lavage, and artificial kidney) find their greatest usefulness.

Pyelonephritis

Acute pyelonephritis is caused by bacteria invading the kidneys in the course of infection of the blood stream, or by an infection secondary to obstruction of urinary flow by stones or an enlarged prostate blocking the ureters. Chills, fever, vomiting, and sweating occur, and there may be severe pain and tenderness or merely a dull ache in the kidney region. The urine contains pus, red blood cells, albumin, and bacteria. Wastes accumulate in the blood, but dropsy and high blood pressure are uncommon. When the infection is apparently confined chiefly to the pelvis of the kidney, it is called pyelitis, a condition not uncommon in infants and in pregnant women. It usually clears completely, but sometimes progresses to chronic pyelonephritis and even uremia. When scar tissue forms as the result of chronic pyelonephritis, the kidney often gradually shrinks in size. As this shrinkage occurs, the blood pressure may gradually increase.

[Most infections of the kidney are now treated successfully with sulphonamides, mandelic acid, or one of the antibiotic drugs.—Ed.]

Perinephritic abscess, another form of "pus kidney," is a localized purulent infection in pads of fat about the kidney, usually only on one side. Severe pain in the flanks, chills, and fever are present. An operation to drain the abscess is necessary.

GROUP II. DISEASES IN WHICH THE KIDNEYS ARE DISTURBED BY DISEASE ELSEWHERE AND BECOME A SECONDARY CAUSE OF ILL HEALTH

Renal Lithiasis

A stone in the kidney (renal lithiasis) may give no symptoms, or may produce kidney colic, one of the most agonizing pains known to man. Pain is produced only when a stone tries to pass out of the kidney into the narrow ureter. Small stones traversing the ureters may cause great suffering unless, and until, they pass out into the bladder. Some pass spontaneously or can be removed by instruments. Others must be removed by operation or they may cause obstruction to the flow of urine with resulting pyelonephritis or even complete destruction of kidneys. No known medicines or mineral waters have any effect whatsoever on dissolving stones, the multitudinous promises of quacks, ancient and modern, to the contrary. Stones are of various types, most of which (though not all) cast shadows in X-ray pictures. They consist of urinary salts and albuminous substances precipitated together. The reasons why these salts, normally kept in solution, become precipitated is not known, but such an event is probably induced by chemical alterations and bacterial infections.

Kidney Disturbances During Pregnancy

Most women are able to complete pregnancy with little or no real kidney trouble. In the last three or four months of pregnancy the womb may so crowd the bladder and ureters that free passage of urine is interfered with. When slowing of urinary flow results, a mild bacterial infection of bladder urine often occurs. Occasionally more serious trouble arises, which was formerly called "kidney of pregnancy" or "nephritis of pregnancy" and believed to be essentially one form of kidney disease. Now it is recognized that this term really includes several different disturbances: pyelitis, pyelonephritis, acute or chronic glomerulonephritis, acute nephrosis, pre-eclampsia, or eclampsia. Glomerulonephritis or nephrosis, existing prior to pregnancy but so mild as to go unrecognized, may flare up acutely under the stress of childbearing. More serious are those conditions called eclampsia and pre-eclamptic toxemia, manifestations of a poisoning caused presumably by toxic products thrown out from the uterus or from the growing baby. The manifestations of such a poisoning are headache, disturbances of vision, nausea, vomiting, dizziness, restlessness, dropsy, albuminuria, and high blood pressure. Without convulsions, they indicate pre-eclampsia. "Eclampsia" means convulsions and represents the most serious phenomenon of this condition. It arises more frequently in first pregnancies (about 1 in every 250) and only about once in every 1,200 later pregnancies. In all it occurs only about once for every 500 or 600 births. Generally it is noted during the last three months of pregnancy. Degeneration of the liver and the kidney tubules may be present, and a special form of glomerulonephritis may result. Under appropriate treatment, the pregnancy may occasionally be completed. Sometimes interruption of pregnancy is necessary to spare the patient's life. Thereafter kidney function may be remarkably restored. Obviously it is most important for an expectant mother to co-operate with her physician in routine and repeated examination of urine and blood pressure. It is equally important for a mother, who has experienced eclampsia with a previous pregnancy, to seek competent evaluation of heart and kidney function and advice before attempting further pregnancy.

Tuberculosis of Kidneys

Tuberculosis of kidneys is always secondary to tuberculosis elsewhere—in lungs, lymph nodes, bones or joints. Usually involving both kidneys to a degree at least, it invades one kidney especially and may destroy it entirely. The urine contains albumin, blood, pus, and tubercle bacilli. The latter may be difficult to find, and tests utilizing guinea pigs may be necessary. Tuberculosis in kidneys practically never heals spontaneously, and if the kidney is not removed the disease may invade other tissues and endanger the other kidney. The operation is generally quite safe and the outcome hopeful. Half of a group of patients studied by Wildbolz were found to be apparently completely relieved ten years after operation.

Kidney Disease from Enlarged Prostate Gland

For some unknown reason the prostate gland frequently enlarges in men more than fifty years of age. This may cause difficulty in starting urination, frequent urination, and dribbling due to partial blockage of the urethra. If free flow is not re-established, infection (pyelitis or pyelonephritis) and destruction of kidney tissue may ensue. Ureters and pelvis may be ballooned out with urine (hydroureter and hydronephrosis). Wastes accumulate in the blood and uremia may result. If appreciable urinary retention is present, careful drainage of the bladder and surgical removal of the prostate gland or of a portion of it are generally necessary, despite long-winded and long-distance radio advice otherwise.

Gouty Nephritis (Gouty Bright's Disease)

Years ago a German physician (Hahn) found that when a patient who had gout took small quantities of turpentine, the odor of violets present in the urine of normal persons after taking turpentine was absent. This was one of the earliest tests of renal function. The exact relationship between gout and nephritis is not known, but in chronic gout there is often disturbed kidney function. A mild form of chronic nephritis with manifestations somewhat like those of renal arteriosclerosis may be present. Kidney stones of uric acid salts are not infrequent, and occasionally the actual precipitation of crystals of uric acid salts occurs in kidney tissue.

Scarlatinal Nephritis

In the course of scarlet fever there is usually some albuminuria with no other signs of renal disease. In about 10 per cent of cases, however, definite nephritis develops about the second or third week. If mild, it is signalized by transient dropsy, with albumin, casts, and a few red blood cells in the urine. In other cases considerable dropsy may develop, and the signs of nephritis may last a number of weeks or so and then gradually disappear. In a few patients typical acute glomerulonephritis occurs, which temporarily, at least, may be severe and accompanied by uremia. More or less complete recovery usually follows, but chronic nephritis occasionally results. It is said to occur, however, in only about twenty out of five thousand cases.

Bence-Jones Proteinuria ("White Urine")

Ordinary albumin is invisible in cold urine but becomes apparent as a white cloud after urine is heated. In multiple myeloma, a disease of bones, a special kind of albumin called "Bence-Jones protein" may appear. A patient may pass white urine when voiding outdoors in the cold. The white cloud disappears on heating the urine and reappears on cooling. Early in the disease the kidneys themselves are normal, merely excreting the abnormal substance. However, as the disease progresses, the renal tubules may become blocked with casts of Bence-Jones protein, and renal function may gradually fail, causing progressive accumulation of waste products in the blood, secondary elevation of blood pressure, and death from uremia.

GROUP III. CONDITIONS IN WHICH THE URINE IS ABNORMAL BUT NO NEPHRITIS IS PRESENT

There is a group of diseases in which abnormal substances are present in urine but in which no nephritis exists. The kidneys are merely excreting material present abnormally or in unusual amounts. Alterations in the quality or quantity of urine occur, but renal function is normal.

Diabetes Mellitus

In *diabetes mellitus,*[9] a disease of the pancreas, or human sweetbread, the first symptom generally noted by the patient is the passage of large amounts of urine, usually three to six quarts, sometimes ten quarts or more, daily. In

[9]"Diabetes" means "to go through."

mild cases the output of urine is normal, but in any event sugar is present therein. It has been noted that when blood contains the usual amounts of sugar, the kidneys are able to hold it back and its loss in urine is prevented. When the blood sugar is highly concentrated, as in diabetes mellitus, the excess spills over into urine. Other cardinal symptoms of diabetes mellitus are increasing thirst and consumption of large quantities of water, increased appetite, loss of weight, and itching.

Renal Diabetes

In *renal diabetes* there exists an unusual permeability of the kidney to even normal amounts of circulating blood sugar, such that, even without diabetes mellitus being present, sugar (glucose) appears in the urine. The patients are not sick, and no diet or other treatment is necessary except, of course, sufficient observation to make sure that true diabetes mellitus is not present. It is an uncommon condition, and the cause is unknown.

Diabetes Insipidus

In *diabetes insipidus* there is no sugar in the urine and no disease of the pancreas or kidneys, yet the patient passes large amounts of urine that is normal except for its low specific gravity. As a rule, four to ten quarts are passed each day; in severe cases the output may reach from twenty to thirty or more quarts a day. I recall a sixteen-year-old boy who passed thirty-three quarts of urine every twenty-four hours; in forty hours the weight of urine was equivalent to his own body weight. Ten years later he was still passing these enormous amounts. A case is recorded of a twenty-four-year-old man who passed about forty-three quarts in twenty-four hours (Trousseau). Diabetes insipidus is a rather rare disease and usually afflicts children or young adults, probably as a result of disease of the pituitary gland after infection or injury to the brain. It causes intense thirst constantly day and night. Injection of pituitary extract or inhalation of powdered pituitary extract may control the excessive thirst and urination.

"Black Urine"

A curious and rare urinary disturbance is that presented by certain persons who have an inherited anomaly of nutrition producing "alkaptonuria." The infant's urine may stain its linen brown or black. The urine turns dark when exposed to air. In itself the condition is a trifling matter, inconvenient rather than harmful (Garrod). In rare instances the cartilages of the ears and joints also turn dark. There are no symptoms and no treatment is necessary.

GROUP IV. DISTURBANCES OF THE KIDNEY DEPENDENT ON MALFORMATION

This includes such conditions as "single," "horseshoe," "floating," and "polycystic" kidney and certain anomalies of the ureters, such as double ureter and absent ureter. About 1 in 1,800 persons is born with only one kidney. Persons who have this anomaly are unaware of it and there are no symptoms. The kidney present is usually enlarged to compensate for the absent one. The chief importance of this condition is that when the only kidney is diseased, danger to life is great. A diagnosis of single kidney is, of course, of vital importance when considering kidney removal for any surgical condition.

A bridge of renal tissue may extend across from one kidney to the other, generally at the lower pole, connecting them to form a horseshoe kidney. Such a condition is symptomless and is recognized almost exclusively by means of a pyelogram, an X-ray of the inside of the kidney. When disease is present in one side of a horseshoe kidney, it may spread to the other readily, and thus the union is dangerous to health and life. It may complicate or prevent operation when renal tuberculosis or abscesses are present, and therefore its recognition is important.

The normal kidney can move up and down about an inch, and, as has been noted, the right kidney is lower and more readily felt than the left. Such a palpable kidney is entirely normal. When the kidney moves excessively owing to weakness of its supporting structures, it is then known as a "wandering," "movable," or "floating" kidney and may be felt low in the abdomen or even in the pelvis. It is found low in women six times as often as in men, and generally on the right side in thin individuals. It usually gives no symptoms. Sometimes a dull ache in the flank is present, or, when it moves enough to cause kinking of the ureter, severe pain may result. Operation to secure the kidney should be done only when exercises to strengthen abdominal muscles, the use of supporting belts, and sometimes rest in bed and nutritious diets to replace fat about the kidney have proved unsuccessful.

Certain abnormalities occur in the ureters also, chief of which is the presence of an extra one on either or both sides. These occur in about 1 per cent of people, and when disease is present therein may cause trouble in diagnosis. Special X-rays will reveal their presence.

Polycystic Kidneys

Polycystic kidneys represent a curious congenital anomaly recognized as present in about 1 in every 3,500 patients (Braasch). Often unrecognized, the condition occurs actually much more frequently than this, being found in about 1 of every 1,000 post-mortem examinations. The cause is unknown, but is thought to be related to inadequate fusion of constituent parts of the kidney units during the time the body is developing in the mother's womb. The kidneys swell to various sizes, forming abdominal tumors that are sometimes enormous. A forty-year-old man was found to have such kidneys, each weighing about seventeen pounds! (Normal weight of each is about one third of a pound.) Although both kidneys become enlarged, one is usually felt earlier than the other. The enlargement is due to the accumulation of small and large masses of watery or semigelatinous material in multitudinous pockets or cysts. Symptoms rarely arise before thirty or forty years of age. Weakness appears and a dull ache may be present in the flank. Sometimes blood appears in the urine. A slowly progressive type of uremia develops, and the patient may live several years in relative comfort, even when two to three times the normal amount of wastes are present in the blood.

CONCLUSION

The advice of a fifteenth-century physician (Arderne) on "the governance of nephritics" included the admonition that such patients "should put away anger and all strenuous business and intense occupation and all manner of things that disturb the soul or move it in any way save only joy." Easy words those, but in that day the joyous state of mind must have been indeed difficult of adoption. Today, as a result of the enormous advances of the past century, or even of the past twenty years, it has become possible to remove from many the soul-disturbing fear of nephritis. It has become possible to send many nephritic patients back to their strenuous business. To others more seriously ill, it has become the physician's happy lot to bring a degree of physical comfort undreamed of heretofore.

CHAPTER XVII

The Blood and Its Diseases

KARL SINGER, M.D.

B LOOD IS THE red fluid which, driven by the pumping action of the heart, circulates through the blood vessels to all parts of the body. The various body organs (liver, muscles, glands, brain, lungs, etc.) depend upon each other for their proper functioning. They may be visualized as "factories" which require a constant supply of raw materials for turning out their special products, which, in turn, are in demand by other organs. There is also some waste material of the production processes which has to be eliminated. The blood vessels represent a well-developed network of highways and smaller roads connecting the different "factories." The vehicle which transports the raw material, the various end products, and the waste on these highways from and to the various organs is the blood.

COMPOSITION OF THE BLOOD. THE MEANING OF A "BLOOD TEST"

Blood consists of three types of structures called the red cells, the white cells, and the platelets; these are suspended in a pale-yellow liquid called the plasma. The plasma also carries the blood proteins, blood sugar, blood fat, various salts, and many other substances which are needed in the well-planned economy of the body.

In health the composition of the blood is kept remarkably constant. This stability is maintained because anything that is "used up" or "taken away" from the blood is immediately replaced. Because of this constant composition, the doctor knows the normal amounts of the various types of cells and substances present in the blood. When, however, an organ becomes involved in a disease, it may turn out either an increased or decreased amount of its regular products, or some abnormal factors may appear in the blood. The composition of the blood may thus become quite different from that of a healthy person, and the doctor may learn from such alterations which organ is diseased and to what extent.

Obviously there is no such thing as a single "blood test." There are many different blood tests, each for a special factor. When you speak of a "blood test," you must really know what has been examined specifically. Thus blood is tested for its increased content of sugar in patients with diabetes; for "uric acid" in instances of suspected gout; or blood is examined for the presence of specific "antibodies" which develop when a previous infection has occurred. When this infection is syphilis, the test for such "antibodies" is called the "Wassermann" or "Kahn" test. A "positive Wassermann" indicates that a person most likely has had a syphilitic infection in the past, and that some time later in his or her life, there probably will develop severe damage to the heart, the nervous system, or other parts of the body if the hidden syphilis is not vigorously treated. Most states in the United States now require pre-marriage blood (Wassermann) tests in order to discover slumbering syphilis in the prospective parents, since this disease may also seriously affect the health of future babies. By energetic treatment of the syphilitic bride or bride-groom with penicillin, this danger to the child can be prevented, and a cure or at least an improvement of the sick adult achieved.

Commonly, the expression "blood test" or "blood count" is used when the doctor wants to know about changes that may have occurred in the number or quality of the red or white cells or platelets. Disorders in which altera-tions in these particular constituents of the blood are the outstanding feature are frequently called "blood diseases." This is not a good term, since changes concerning the blood cells rather express changes in either their production or destruction.

RED BLOOD CELLS

The human red cell is a biconcave disk filled with a red-colored matter named "hemoglobin." The cell's diameter is about .0003 of an inch. Normally, women have about 4½ million, and men about 5 million of such red cells in one cubic millimeter of blood. One cubic millimeter is about a .000034 part of one ounce. The red cells are manufactured in the bone marrow which is located in the interior of the bones. In infants the marrow of all bones pro-duces red cells, whereas in adults only the marrow of the smaller bones (the vertebrae, ribs, breastbone, and the bones of the skull) takes part in this process. The red cells ripen in the marrow and only when fully matured are they discharged into the circulating blood. There they remain for about 120 days before they begin to fall apart. Almost any cell which breaks up is immediately replaced by a new one from the bone marrow. In this way the number of red cells in the blood always remains the same.

When the physician wants to know whether the bone marrow functions properly, he can insert a needle into the cavity of the bone and suck out some particles from the marrow. This procedure is called "bone marrow puncture" and most commonly the breastbone is used for this purpose. Since the skin and the bone are made insensitive by an injection of Novocain prior to the puncture, this little operation is not painful. The marrow particles obtained by such a puncture are then spread out on thin glass plates, stained by special dyes, and examined under the microscope. A specialist can thus obtain considerable information about the composition of the marrow in various disease processes.

The main function of the red cells is to carry the hemoglobin. This red substance contains iron, which is built into a very complex chemical structure and has the ability to combine with oxygen from the air within the lungs. From the lungs, the hemoglobin within the red cells transports the oxygen to the various organs which are in great need of this particular chemical and take it up eagerly. Without oxygen no organs can function properly, and therefore an adequate oxygen supply is essential for life. When the number of red cells, or their hemoglobin content, is appreciably diminished, anemia results.

WHITE BLOOD CELLS

Normally the number of white cells in one cubic millimeter of blood amounts to 5,000 to 10,000. Some of the white cells, named granulocytes, are, like the red cells, manufactured in the bone marrow, but others, called lymphocytes, are produced in the spleen and in the lymph modes. In contradistinction to the red cells, the white cells can actively leave the blood stream and wander into the tissues. These cells are able to digest bacteria which have been successful in invading the body. The white cells act, therefore, as the scavengers of the highway system as well as of the various factories of the body. When bacteria become lodged in an organ and begin to multiply there, the white cells move to this location and attempt to defend the body against a further spread of the invasion. They first surround the bacteria, and then attack them and, by engulfing and digesting them, try to kill them. Many infectious diseases, therefore, show an increase of the white blood cell count, because many more of these cells are mobilized under these circumstances and sent rapidly through the highway system of the body (i.e., the blood vessels) to the endangered area. The physician, by taking a white blood cell count, may thus get information that such an inflamed area exists somewhere in the body. This is of great diagnostic significance, since the symptoms of some harmless belly ache caused, for instance, by gas, may be quite similar to those caused by a bacterial inflammation. The finding of an elevated white cell count in infection is also an important demonstration that this particular defense mechanism of the body is in good working order.

BLOOD PLATELETS

The platelet is a minute particle of protoplasm (the basic material of cells) which is much smaller than the red blood cell. There are about 300,000 to 800,000 platelets in one cubic millimeter of normal blood. One of the functions of the platelets is to maintain the texture of the smallest blood vessels (the so-called capillaries) in proper condition. In the absence of platelets, red cells often leak out from the capillaries, and tiny bleeding points resembling flea bites may then be seen in the skin and mucous membranes. Furthermore, platelets seal openings which occur in the wall of the capillaries due to injuries. When such a small blood vessel is injured, the platelets clump together and plug the hole. At the same time they release a substance which contracts the capillaries, and this also aids in stopping the bleeding. Patients who have not enough platelets, or poorly constructed ones, will require a much longer time than do normal persons to cease bleeding from a needle puncture. This test is called the determination of the bleeding time and is best performed at the lobe of the ear.

When larger blood vessels are injured, the platelets are incapable of plugging a bigger hole. In these instances the vessels contract and the rent in the wall is closed by means of a clot. In order to produce such a clot, the platelets release a substance which acts on a specific protein present in the plasma. From this interaction, a new factor, called thromboplastin, results, which initiates the formation of a clot in collaboration with several other proteins also present in the plasma. One of the substances activated by thromboplastin is called prothrombin. When the amount of prothrombin in the blood is diminished, clot formation is decreased and delayed. The physician can measure the amount of prothrombin present by means of a complicated test called the determination of the prothrombin time.

Clot formation represents a defense mechanism of the body against blood loss from injured vessels. However, clot formation may also take place in a blood vessel which has been damaged by a disease process. Then the clot may grow within the vessel to such an extent that it completely obstructs it and interferes with the blood supply to this particular region of the body. To make things worse, such a clot frequently becomes dislodged and travels in the veins toward the lungs, where it then may plug the vital lung vessels and cause sudden death. Recently a drug named dicoumarol has been discovered which depresses the amount of prothrombin in the blood and thus counteracts the tendency to undesirable clot formation in certain diseases. The history of the discovery of this drug is quite interesting. It was observed that cattle, when fed spoiled sweet clover, began to bleed profusely. From this spoiled clover, dicoumarol was extracted and chemically analyzed; it was found to have a composition similar to aspirin. Dicoumarol is now regularly given to patients who have a small blood clot within one of the vitally important blood vessels which supply the heart (the coronary arteries), and in this manner further growth of such a clot may be prevented. Thanks to this new treatment, fewer people die now from this all too frequent heart condition.

THE SYMPTOMS OF ANEMIA

When insufficient hemoglobin is present in the blood, either because the red cells contain too little hemoglobin, or because the number of red cells is diminished, an insufficient supply of oxygen is carried to all organs of the body. In such a state the heart will attempt to circulate the blood at a faster rate in order to make up for the lack of red coloring matter. Thus the first sign of anemia in a patient may be a feeling that his heart beats faster than usual, and he may experience a thumping in the chest. When such a person exerts himself, he may readily become short of breath, may pant on climbing stairs, and may think that he has a weakened heart, although his heart is normal. When the anemia is more severe and cannot be compensated by the increased activity of the heart, practically all organs send out danger signals that they have not obtained enough oxygen. The brain will react with headaches, dizziness, a feeling of faintness, loss of memory, nervousness, irritability, and even drowsiness. Many people experience insomnia (lack of sleep), and numbness, and tingling in the fingers and toes. There may be ringing in the ears, and black spots in front of the eyes. The muscles fatigue easily and the patients feel quite weak. There is loss of appetite, the stomach may rebel, and there may be nausea, vomiting, and gas pains. Because anemic persons do not eat properly, there may be loss of weight. The shortness of breath may get progressively worse. When the kidneys become involved there may be swelling of the legs and frequent urination during the night. There may be pallor of the face, and the skin may take on a waxy color. However, it should be remembered that some healthy people always look pale and sometimes it is hard to tell the difference between the naturally sallow complexion of a person who lives mostly indoors and the pallor of anemia. Many of these various danger signals of the organs in anemia may, however, also be caused by disturbances of a quite different nature, and only the blood count will objectively reveal the presence and severity of the lack of hemoglobin.

THE CAUSES OF ANEMIA

Anemia is never a disease in itself, but is always caused by other factors which the physician must recognize in order to institute proper treatment. Sometimes the cause of the anemia is quite obvious, whereas in other instances it may be difficult to find and require many special laboratory studies.

1. *Acute Blood Loss.* When a patient loses a large amount of blood, for instance, by being injured in an accident, or by extensive bleeding from the nose, or from a stomach ulcer, or from hemorrhoids, or by excessive bleeding from the womb or any other organ, a sudden anemia may develop. The body will then immediately throw its reserves of red cells from the bone marrow into the circulation to counteract this loss. When the bleeding is quite extensive, the patient may go into shock and must then be treated with blood transfusions.

2. *Anemia Due to Lack of Iron.* Hemoglobin contains iron as a necessary building stone. When there is a lack of iron, not enough hemoglobin can be formed. The number of red cells in the blood is then relatively little diminished,

but the amount of hemoglobin in the single red cell may be only one half or less of that found in a healthy person. Lack of iron in the body results when the intake of iron is poor due to a deficient diet and simultaneously there exists a slow, but appreciable, loss of blood over a longer period of time. Then the iron reserves of the body become exhausted, and an "iron deficiency anemia" results. In a normal person the iron from the red cells which fall apart is re-used over and over again in the body for the formation of new hemoglobin. But when bleeding occurs, this iron from the red cells is permanently lost for re-utilization. Women who lose much blood with the menstrual flow and with pregnancies are particularly prone to develop iron deficiency anemia. In pregnancy not only must iron be supplied by the mother for the growing child, but blood is also lost with the delivery of the baby. Thus pregnant women should have a diet rich in iron, and should also get some iron medication. Foodstuffs rich in iron are liver, kidney, meat, eggs, bread, cereals, chocolate, fruits, and all green vegetables, whereas only a little iron is found in chicken, fish, milk, and milk products.

3. *The Anemia of Chronic Infections.* In chronic infections, caused, for example, by the tubercle bacillus, or by other types of bacteria, a similar type of anemia develops as is seen in iron deficiency. Poisonous products, released by the bacteria, interfere with the "building-in" of iron into the hemoglobin structure. Contrary to iron deficiency anemia, this type of anemia will not respond to iron medication, but will disappear only when the causative bacterial disease is successfully treated.

A similar type of anemia is noted in chronic kidney disturbances, in which the body has great difficulties in getting rid of certain waste materials. When these waste products accumulate, they often interfere with the proper functioning of the bone marrow.

4. *Mediterranean Anemia.* In some families who live in the southern parts of Italy or in Greece—countries which lie on the Mediterranean Sea—an anemia is found in which the red cells contain little hemoglobin and are thinner than normal ones. Iron treatment is not effective. This disease is caused by an inability of the body to build up normal hemoglobin. Mediterranean anemia is a hereditary disease (transmitted from the parents to the child), and in the United States it may be found in native-born Americans of Italian or Greek ancestry. This disorder was first discovered not in Italy, but in Detroit, Michigan, a city which has a large population of Italian stock. This variety of anemia is also often called—after its discoverer—"Cooley's" anemia. Blood transfusions may bring some improvement.

5. *Pernicious Anemia.* In this type of anemia the red cells are larger than normal, oval-shaped, and well filled with hemoglobin. However, the bone marrow has great difficulties in manufacturing these red cells because it lacks a certain substance necessary for the ripening of normal red cells. This important substance has, therefore, been called the "maturation factor." Patients with pernicious anemia do not secrete normal gastric juice, and the lining of

their stomachs becomes thinned. In the normal gastric juice is a substance called the "intrinsic factor" which permits the body to absorb the "maturation (extrinsic) factor" present in the food. In patients with pernicious anemia the stomach does not secrete the "intrinsic" factor. Thus this anemia is really caused by a primary disease of the stomach and develops secondarily to the deficient stomach secretion.

Until 1926 treatment was not available for this anemia, and it was the most "pernicious" of the many types of anemia known because it always led to death. Then it was discovered that the "maturation factor" is stored in the liver. When the liver of animals was fed to patients with pernicious anemia, their bone marrow could take up again the production of normal red cells, and such patients recovered completely. To obtain such an effect and to maintain it, however, every day about one pound of almost raw liver had to be eaten by the patient. This is a diet hard to endure for a long time, even if one knows that one's life depends upon it. Fortunately, however, extracts were soon prepared from mashed beef or pork livers, and small amounts of these extracts, when injected into the muscles of patients with pernicious anemia, produced the same miraculous results as did the eating of large helpings of liver.

The true nature of the active principle in the liver extract remained unknown for many years. Recently it was found that certain bacteria also need this liver extract principle for growth. It was possible, by testing out the effects of the various chemicals in the liver extract, upon the growth of these bacteria, to isolate the "maturation factor." The latter is now known to be a vitamin and goes under the name of vitamin B_{12}. It is of a reddish-purple color and, surprisingly, contains small amounts of the metal cobalt. Astonishingly, vitamin B_{12} is also produced by certain fungi (yeastlike plants) which also release the powerful drug streptomycin employed in the treatment of tuberculosis and other infections. Since these fungi are now grown commercially on a larger scale to obtain streptomycin, vitamin B_{12} has become a valuable by-product in this industry and is now on the market at a relatively cheap price.

Frequently pernicious anemia causes severe involvement of the nervous system. The patient may be unable to walk with his eyes closed, he may have a staggering gait and a feeling of "pins and needles" in his hands and feet. He may be unable to feed himself because of muscular weakness, and severe bladder disturbances may develop. In some patients the signs pointing to a disorder of the nervous system are much more pronounced than is the anemia, whereas in others the anemia may be severe, but the nervous manifestations are hardly noticeable. When treated with liver extract or vitamin B_{12}, the anemia responds rather rapidly and the patient may regain an almost normal blood count within a few weeks; however, the healing of the damage to the nervous system requires a much longer time, and it is sometimes necessary to administer treatment daily for half a year until improvement becomes manifest. Because of these nervous complications, an early diagnosis and rapid institution of treatment are most important in pernicious anemia.

6. *Aplastic Anemia.* Occasionally the bone marrow stops almost entirely its production of all cells; this condition is called "aplasia" of the marrow. A severe anemia develops, and the number of white cells and of platelets in the blood is likewise markedly decreased. Such a damage to the marrow may follow exposure to some chemicals (benzine and others), or when certain otherwise useful drugs are taken for a long time. Aplastic anemia may also be observed after extensive uncontrolled radiation with X-rays or other powerful physical agents. It was quite frequently noticed to develop in the Japanese who escaped immediate death after the atom bombing during the last war. Sometimes an obvious cause can not be detected in patients with aplastic anemia. Specific treatment is not available for such a damaged bone marrow, but the life of such patients may be maintained for many years by numerous blood transfusions. These persons live on borrowed blood.

7. *Hereditary Spherocytosis or Familial Hemolytic Jaundice.* In this hereditary condition the red cells are smaller and thicker than normal ones since their shapes changed from a disk to a sphere. These "spherocytes" do not stay for the usual 120 days within the circulation, but only for about 20 to 30 days. They are trapped by the spleen and destroyed there. The disease can, therefore, be cured by removal of the spleen. Contrary to popular superstition, the spleen is not an organ necessary for life, and people without a spleen are not especially susceptible to infections and may live as long as any normal person. In hereditary spherocytosis the spleen is usually enlarged and the patients show slight jaundice; that is, a yellow coloring of the eyeballs and the skin. This jaundice develops because some part of the hemoglobin structure is transformed, to a much greater extent than in normal people, to an orange-yellow dye called "bilirubin." This bilirubin is then deposited in the skin and eyes and stains them. The anemia that occurs in hereditary spherocytosis is called hemolytic because this term refers to a very rapid destruction of red cells, regardless of the mechanisms which are responsible for their destruction.

8. *Acquired (non-hereditary) "Hemolytic" Anemia.* In some people, for unknown reasons, the body develops a red cell destroying factor, and then an anemia results which is quite similar to that found in hereditary spherocytosis. The red cells assume a round shape, and jaundice develops. Removal of the spleen may or may not have any curative effect. Recently treatment with the hormone cortisone has been successful in stopping the production of this red cell destroying factor.

9. *Sickle Cell Anemia.* This disease occurs almost exclusively in Negroes. The red cells assume a sickle shape, and in the severe form of the disease they break up much more rapidly than do normal cells. As many as 8 per cent of the 15 million Negroes in the United States have a hereditary tendency to develop these abnormally shaped cells. In most of the Negroes the disorder is mild, and anemia is absent. However, if two people with this tendency marry, some of their children will develop the severe form which is called sickle cell anemia. The sickle shape of the red cells is caused by an abnormal type of

hemoglobin. A cure for this disease is not known at present, and removal of the spleen is not effective. Before marriage Negroes should have their blood examined for these sickled cells, and if both bride and bridegroom show this tendency to produce sickle-shaped red cells, they should be forewarned that some of their children may become afflicted with the severe form of sickle cell disease. When sickle cell anemia occurs in white people, which is extremely rare, there is always some admixture of Negro blood in their ancestry.

10. *The Anemia of Cancer.* When cancer is present, the patient may become anemic, because the malignant cancer tissue may cause bleeding, or because the food intake (and, therefore, the iron and vitamin supply) is poor due to the loss of appetite, or because the cancer invades the bone marrow and destroys it. Many cancer patients, however, do not have anemia, and the presence of anemia is by no means in itself a sign of cancer. As with any other disease, a complete and careful study of the patient is required to establish the correct diagnosis in order that proper treatment can be administered.

TREATMENT OF ANEMIA

Since so many different types of anemia exist, no general single remedy will counteract the lack of red blood cells or of hemoglobin. Iron will work only when the body needs and can use iron. There are many iron preparations on the market in which iron is combined with vitamins or other remedies. These patent medicines will only be effective in combating iron deficiency anemia due to their iron content, and are, in this respect, no better than simple iron pills, although their price is much higher. Many patients, when taking iron, complain of nausea, stomach pain, and either constipation or diarrhea. These side effects can be avoided if the iron pills are never taken on an empty stomach, but either during or immediately after meals. Because iron tablets are sugar-coated, they are occasionally eaten like candy by very young children, and then they may cause great harm in such babies by injuring the delicate lining of their stomachs. Parents should put such iron tablets—like any other medicine—out of reach of their babies.

Liver and vitamin B_{12} injections should be given only to patients with pernicious anemia, since in the other types of anemia they are without effect. Some people may be allergic to one brand of liver extract and may get hives and fainting spells from such an injection. Then the experienced physician will try another brand.

Recently a drug called "folic acid" has been developed. This folic acid is present in many foodstuffs and is necessary for the normal growth and function of many organs. Folic acid has been found to be effective in pernicious anemia, but does not influence the nervous manifestations of this disease. In this respect, it is inferior to liver extract.

Whether removal of the spleen or whether the hormone cortisone may be of benefit in certain anemias requires the expert knowledge of a specialist.

BLOOD TRANSFUSIONS

When the loss of blood in a patient has been particularly severe, transfusion of blood from another person may be lifesaving. To give blood transfusions has now become almost a routine procedure in any hospital. Before such a transfusion is given, a sample of the blood of the donor must be mixed with that of the patient in order to see that the two bloods, when mixed, do not cause clumping of the red blood cells; since such clumps would block the small blood vessels of the recipient. All human beings belong to one of four main blood groups, named A, B, AB, and O, and only certain groups do not clump the red cells of other groups on mixing. Before giving a transfusion one must also be sure that the donor is healthy, that he has not had an infectious liver disease or syphilis. The Wassermann test of the donor must always be negative before his blood can be used for transfusion. Because blood should be given immediately in emergencies, most hospitals now have "blood banks" in which blood of various types is stored in the refrigerator, ready for use. Blood may be stored in a suitable refrigerator for more than two weeks without harming the red cells. In some patients only the red cells are transfused, the plasma having been separated from the cells; other patients may require only a plasma transfusion. With modern laboratory techniques the water of the plasma may be evaporated, and a powder results which can be redissolved in water before use. Dry, powdered plasma is particularly important for use on the battlefield for wounded soldiers, since the transportation of the dry plasma preparations does not present as great a problem as the transportation of bottles containing whole blood.

THE RHESUS (RH) FACTOR AND THE HEMOLYTIC DISEASE OF THE NEWBORN

The observation was made when a person received several blood transfusions from a donor with the same blood group as the patient's, that the first transfusion was well tolerated, but the second and third caused severe side reactions. Then it was discovered that another "blood group" exists besides the four already mentioned. This new blood group system was demonstrated to be identical with a blood factor occurring in the Rhesus monkey, and therefore has been called the "Rh factor." About 85 per cent of all human beings have this Rh factor within their red cells, but 15 per cent do not. When red cells containing the Rh factor are transfused into a recipient whose blood does not contain this factor, the body of the recipient develops an "anti-Rh" substance which clumps the foreign transfused cells. It is, therefore, not sufficient to type blood only for the A-B-O groups, but this also must be done for the Rh factor. Recipients whose red cells do not contain the Rh factor are called "Rh negative," and they should receive only transfusions of Rh negative blood. Since Rh negative blood is relatively rare—only 15 per cent of the donated blood will be Rh negative—any blood bank needs a great number of blood donations to be well equipped for an emergency.

The discovery of the Rh factor has also led to an understanding of a severe anemia which may develop in newborn infants. When the mother is Rh negative, but the embryo produces Rh positive blood cells, blood from the embryo may leak out during pregnancy into the body of the mother, and there stimulate the formation of the "anti-Rh factor." This anti-Rh factor may then flow back into the circulation of the embryo, and cause there severe damage to his red cells. Such infants, when born, show all the signs of rapid blood destruction, and therefore this disease is called hemolytic anemia of the newborn. For this disease to develop in the baby, there must be some leakage from the blood of the Rh positive embryo into the system of the Rh negative mother. Such a leakage does not take place in all Rh negative mothers, and therefore the occurrence of hemolytic disease of the newborn is relatively rare. Only about 5 per cent of the Rh negative mothers may give birth to such a sick child.

In the milder cases treatment of the sick baby consists of giving blood transfusions with Rh negative blood, since the latter cannot be attacked by the anti-Rh factor. In the severely sick infant, however, when a large amount of anti-Rh factor has entered from the mother into the body of the baby, almost all its red cells may be damaged. In such cases the blood of the child may have to be completely exchanged with Rh negative blood. This time-consuming procedure, which often lasts for several hours, has been named exchange transfusion and has rescued the life of many infants. The discovery of the Rh factor has not only made blood transfusions a much safer procedure, but has also led to the correct and effective treatment of the hemolytic anemia of the newborn. This discovery represents, therefore, one of the truly great steps in the progress of modern medicine.

POLYCYTHEMIA

"Polycythemia" means that there is an abnormally high number of red cells in the blood; as many as 8 to 10 million in one cubic millimeter may be found instead of the usual 5 million. Not only is the red cell count per cubic millimeter increased, but also the quantity of blood in the circulation, which is normally about 5 quarts, may increase to as much as 8 to 10 quarts. The blood is of a much thicker consistency than normally, and the heart has much more work to do to keep the blood circulating. All tissues are overfilled with blood, and the movement of the blood within the organs is considerably slowed down. There is a kind of traffic jam in the highway system (blood vessels) of the body. Such patients have a ruddy complexion and look quite healthy, but they have symptoms similar to those of patients with anemia. There are complaints of headache, nervousness, numbness, and tingling in hands and feet. The liver and spleen may become enlarged, since these organs even normally contain much more blood than others. About 8 per cent of the patients have a stomach ulcer, which will not readily heal if the polycythemia is not properly treated.

Polycythemia is caused by an uninhibited manufacture of red cells, but no one knows as yet why the bone marrow steps up the production.

Treatment includes either removal of the surplus blood by frequent blood-lettings, or some destruction of the bone marrow by means of X-ray radiation. The best results have been obtained by injecting small amounts of radioactive phosphorus. Phosphorus is one of the building stones of bones, and, when radioactive, it sends out its rays directly into the marrow located within the bones, and thus cuts down red cell production. However, even if the production is sufficiently stopped by the radioactive phosphorus, it will take several weeks until the red cells which are already in the circulation will fall apart. Thus the best treatment for polycythemia is to remove the surplus blood from the patient by blood-lettings and, at the same time, to inject radioactive phosphorus to cut down the increased formation of red cells.

In some patients with certain diseases of the heart or the lungs the hemoglobin has great difficulties in taking up the oxygen from the air. In order to improve this situation, the body responds by increasing the number of red cells. When the heart or lung disease improves sufficiently, the increased number of red cells diminishes spontaneously.

People who live in high altitudes (above 10,000 ft.) also have an increased number of red cells because the amount of oxygen in the air at this altitude is decreased, and therefore the body again reacts with increased red cell production. When such people move to countries of a lower altitude, their polycythemia disappears. Sudden exposure to high altitudes in persons not used to it may bring on the so-called "mountain sickness" with symptoms similar to those of sudden anemia due to extensive and rapid blood loss. These symptoms are not caused by a lack of hemoglobin or of red cells, but by the inadequate uptake of oxygen from the rarefied thin air. To avoid mountain sickness, the approach to high altitudes should be rather slow in order to permit the body to adapt itself to the changed environmental conditions. High altitude sickness is avoided in high-flying airplanes by artificially increasing the oxygen content of the air within the cabin of the plane from special tanks in which this vital gas is stored under pressure. Therefore patients with anemia or with heart disease who are particularly liable to get the symptoms of mountain sickness may travel in such pressurized planes without any danger to their lives.

LEUKOPENIA AND AGRANULOCYTOSIS

When the number of white cells in the blood is below 5,000 per cubic millimeter, a state of leukopenia, which means not enough white cells in the blood stream, exists. Some infectious diseases, typhoid, undulant fever, influenza, and others, almost regularly show leukopenia. Leukopenia is also almost regularly seen when an enlargement of the spleen is present. Since the spleen probably controls the discharge of the white cells from the bone marrow, a scarcity of white cells may occur, caused by increased splenic function (hypersplenism).

In such cases removal of the spleen may again provide the body with enough white cells, and thus strengthen its defense power against bacteria.

Complete disappearance of those white cells which are produced in the bone marrow and are called granulocytes may develop within a few hours in persons who become hypersensitive to certain drugs. Because there are no granulocytes, this allergic reaction has been called agranulocytosis. Such patients with agranulocytosis develop sudden chills, high fever, pneumonia, and other signs of blood poisoning, since the bacteria overwhelm the body, unchecked by the usual defense activity of the white cells. Before penicillin and the other powerful anti-bacterial drugs were available, this blood poisoning often led to death. Since agranulocytosis is most commonly caused by an abnormal reaction to drugs, any medicine taken prior to the onset of the disease has to be omitted immediately in such patients. The surprising feature of drug allergy causing agranulocytosis is that a patient may have taken a certain drug for many years without any harm and then suddenly reacts so violently to it. Medicines which are apparently quite harmless may turn out not to be so on closer inspection. Thus it was discovered several years ago, that pyramidon (aminopyrene), which was widely used in Europe as an excellent painkiller similar to aspirin, may cause agranulocytosis. In Denmark with a population of 3½ million, about 350 deaths due to agranulocytosis were observed within one year. When the sale of pyramidon was prohibited, almost no agranulocytosis was seen in the following year.

Although the number of people who may develop such a hypersensitivity reaction is small, the potential danger of any drug must be realized. Many of the new, powerful remedies may occasionally cause agranulocytosis, and the physician must always be on the alert for such a possible complication.

LEUKEMIA

The term leukemia means white blood. In this condition the white blood cells may increase in number to such an extent that they influence the color of the blood. The production of white cells in the bone marrow as well as in the spleen and lymph nodes increases tremendously, and the white cells wander into various organs and spread there. Because the bone marrow is so busy producing white cells, the manufacture of the other cells of the blood, the red cells and the platelets, may become severely handicapped, and anemia and a severe bleeding tendency may occur. The spleen, which in an adult weighs normally about 5 oz., may become much enlarged up to a weight of 1 to 3 lbs., or more. The lymph nodes and the liver also enlarge. Many of the white cells in the blood and the organs are not fully ripened, and leukemia signifies not only an increased formation, but also a disturbance in the maturation of the white blood cells.

The symptoms of a patient with chronic leukemia are caused by the anemia and the bleeding tendency as well as by the disturbance of the function of many other organs which are loaded with white cells. These patients usually feel very weak, may have high fever and pain in the abdomen due to the enlargement of the liver and spleen which press upon the stomach and the bowels. Often the patients suffer from a terrible itching of the skin. In some instances, particularly in children, the disease may strike quite suddenly and show a rapid course leading to death. Why the various organs which manufacture white blood cells step up the production of immature cells so tremendously is not definitely known. Leukemia may represent a condition similar to cancerous growth arising in other organs. In the chronic type of leukemia one may attempt to inhibit the increased white cell production by radiating the spleen or the whole body with X-ray, or by damaging the white cell producing organs with certain chemicals, such as aminopterin or nitrogen mustards.

A true cure has not yet been found for leukemia. However, in the chronic cases the course of the disease may be slowed down by proper treatment and the suffering of the patient be greatly relieved. Not infrequently chronic leukemia may last for many years, and the patient will learn to live with his disease and be relatively comfortable.

The number of white cells in the blood does not necessarily indicate the severity of the disease, since the disturbance in body economy results from the accumulation of white cells in the organs and not within the blood stream. One may have severe damage to vital factories, but the traffic on the highway system may not always reflect these damages. Thus in some patients with leukemia the organs are loaded with white blood cells, but the number of these cells in the circulation is not always greatly increased. This state of leukemia without associated white blood has been called aleukemic leukemia.

In the acute type of leukemia, particularly in children, a significant improvement can sometimes be achieved by the use of the hormone cortisone or by aminopterin. This latter drug counteracts the activity of folic acid, which is a cell-growth promoting agent. Unfortunately, the improvement in patients with acute leukemia is almost always relatively short-lived; after a few months to one year, the disease recurs despite continued treatment, and the patients die from bleeding into the heart or into the brain. The mere fact, however, that such temporary miraculous improvements have been accomplished recently may indeed raise some hope that with strenuous research leukemia may become a curable disease in the not too distant future.

ENLARGEMENT OF THE LYMPH NODES

The lymph glands or lymph nodes are small structures which are scattered throughout the body, especially in the neck, the armpits, the groins, and around the lungs and intestines. They produce a particular type of white cells, called lymphocytes, which they discharge into the blood stream. They also act as a sieve, filtering out bacteria which may try to enter the blood stream. Thus if one cuts his finger and bacteria enter the tissue below the skin through this wound, the lymph nodes of the arm and the armpit will swell and become inflamed as a result of their strenuous efforts to combat the invasion by trapping the bacteria. The tonsils are also lymph nodes, and frequently they become inflamed because bacteria are always present in the mouth and often try to invade the body. Sometimes the defense power of the tonsils becomes weakened and then they may house live bacteria and represent an outpost of the enemy rather than a defense organ of the body. In such instances removal of the tonsils will be quite beneficial.

In some diseases the lymph nodes are the site of the diseases themselves. A cancer-like growth may develop from them and spread all over the body. Such malignant diseases of the lymph nodes are called lymphomas (tumor of the lymph node). Hodgkin's disease represents a special variety of such a lymphoma. The diagnosis of lymphoma, in many patients, can only be made by having a surgeon remove an affected lymph node and then examine it under the microscope after suitable preparation. Some of the lymphomas disappear rapidly when treated with X-rays, whereas others are rather resistant to such treatment. The malignant diseases of the lymph nodes may, like any other cancerous growth, invade other organs and finally lead to death. When a lymphoma no longer responds to X-ray radiation, injection of nitrogen mustard may still occasionally prolong the life of the patient for one to two years.

INFECTIOUS MONONUCLEOSIS

Sometimes tiny living elements called viruses invade the body and produce swelling of the lymph nodes and the spleen, thus simulating either leukemia or lymphoma. However, this disease, called infectious mononucleosis, or glandular fever, is usually quite harmless and can readily be recognized by the peculiarly shaped, large lymphocytes which are found in the blood stream. Furthermore, the blood plasma in this disease contains a peculiar factor which is capable of agglutinating (clumping) the red cells of sheep. This so-called heterophil agglutination test is quite specific for glandular fever. In any patient who has swelling of the lymph nodes and spleen together with fever, one must always consider infectious mononucleosis; this is a rather harmless disease and must be distinguished from leukemia, an incurable disease.

ENLARGEMENT OF THE SPLEEN

The spleen may be considered as the lymph node of the blood, and its particular function, together with the white blood cells, is the cleansing of the blood of foreign matter, dead cells, and bacteria which may have entered the blood stream. When the spleen is removed, no serious weakening of the body results, however, since other cleaners of the blood similar to the spleen (the liver and also parts of the bone marrow) take over; in the absence of the spleen, these cleansing stations work overtime.

Sometimes the spleen enlarges tremendously because it retains some disease-causing organisms which enter the spleen through the blood. Furthermore, the damaged red cells, white cells, and platelets, when they begin to fall apart, are also held back in the spleen. This organ, therefore, has been called the grave-yard of the body.

In some patients the spleen actively destroys the blood cells and thus becomes the slaughterhouse for these cells, causing severe anemia, or bleeding, due to lack of platelets. In rare instances the spleen swells because it produces some fatty material. Such disorders have been called after their discoverers "Gaucher's disease," and "Niemann-Pick's disease," and occur quite often in persons of the Jewish race. Enlargement of the spleen is also encountered in many infectious diseases, particularly in malaria which is the most common disease in the world, although, fortunately, rare in the United States, it is widespread in the tropics. Sometimes the spleen may become distended to such an extent that it ruptures, and the patient, when not immediately operated upon, may die from an internal hemorrhage. It is interesting that in the wars between the primitive tribes of the uncivilized tropical countries, in which almost everyone has a large spleen due to malaria, the warriors try to hit the enemy in the region of the spleen in order to produce such a rupture.

When a physician finds an enlarged spleen in a patient, he must always attempt to find the cause of this enlargement. This is sometimes difficult. One may insert a needle through the abdominal wall into such an enlarged spleen and suck out some material which can be examined under the microscope. In the hands of a trained specialist, such a splenic puncture may give valuable information and may lead to the correct diagnosis of the ailment responsible for the enlargement of the spleen. If no adequate cause for the splenic enlargement is found after intensive study of the patient, the surgeon should remove such a big spleen, since sometimes a lymphoma may originate there and be responsible for the increased size of this organ.

DISEASES WITH AN ABNORMAL BLEEDING TENDENCY

Bleeding into the skin or from one of the openings of the body (mouth, nose, rectum, womb) frequently brings the patient to the physician. In most instances such bleeding is caused by a local disease which leads to the rupture of a blood vessel. There are, however, disorders in which the compositions of the blood is changed, and such patients have either a spontaneous bleeding tendency, or they react to a slight injury with an extremely massive hemorrhage. If the physician does not find any local cause for the hemorrhage, he must always consider that the patient may have such an abnormal bleeding tendency.

1. *Hemophilia.* In hemophilia the blood will not form a clot for hours after removal from the body. This disease is hereditary and manifests itself only in the male sex, but is exclusively transmitted by women. Such women, the daughters of a patient with hemophilia, are called carriers or conductors, because they transmit the disease but do not show it themselves. Some sons of such a conductor may be normal, but others may be hemophiliacs, and also

some of the daughters of such a conductor may again be conductors, but others may not. The sons of a man with hemophilia will always be normal, but all daughters will show the tendency to transmit hemophilia to some of their sons.

Patients with hemophilia have normal platelets and therefore do not bleed from a tiny cut; such injuries to the small blood vessels can be taken care of by the clumping of the platelets at the site of the trauma. However, if a larger vessel is injured, almost uncontrollable hemorrhage may follow, since clot formation is only achieved with the greatest difficulties. Frequently hemophiliacs bleed into the joints if somewhat larger vessels are injured by a sudden twist of the body, and then the joint may become severely damaged by the hemorrhage and stiff for the rest of the patient's life. Patients with hemophilia must refrain from all athletic exercises and should lead a protected life. If they have a hemorrhage, blood transfusions will supply the clotting factor which the hemophiliac is unable to produce. Thanks to safe blood transfusions, surgery, if necessary, can be performed on hemophiliacs when they have obtained sufficient normal blood plasma prior to the operation to tide them over the danger period. Some hemophiliacs have been kept free from bleeding symptoms by giving them weekly or semiweekly small blood transfusions for a long period of time. Such a treatment, however, is not practical in the majority of patients. The plasma factor which helps in hemophilia has been isolated and called the antihemophilic globulin. Unfortunately, this substance is not yet available commercially. When injected in sufficient amounts, it may permit almost normal clot formation in a hemophiliac for one to two days.

2. *Purpura Due to the Absence of Platelets.* In this condition, which may have many causes, the skin shows many tiny bleeding spots which may also be seen in the eyelids and in the mucous membranes of the mouth and other organs. Besides, the skin may also show black-and-blue marks identical with the bruises seen in a normal person after an injury. However, in such patients trauma cannot be made responsible for these bruises. When the blood from such patients is examined, it often shows a diminution or complete absence of the blood platelets. What causes the platelets to disappear is not entirely known. Sometimes the platelets disappear when certain drugs are taken. Sometimes the spleen produces an anti-platelet factor which destroys the platelets. In other patients the production of platelets in the bone marrow is inhibited, or there may be leukemia or cancer responsible for the decreased platelet count.

Regardless of the cause, the symptoms mentioned are called purpura. When purpura is present, a careful study is necessary to determine what may be responsible for the disappearance of the platelets. Research has shown great benefit in many cases following the use of ACTH and/or cortisone. Removal of the spleen may be lifesaving, and the platelet count may return to normal within a few days after the operation.

3. *Vascular Purpura. Scurvy.* In other patients with purpura the platelet count is quite normal, and in such persons the blood vessels are at fault. The normal texture of the blood vessels may be damaged when there is an absence

of vitamin C, and this condition is called scurvy. Vitamin C is present in great amounts in all citrus fruits, and the American habit of drinking orange or other fruit juices at breakfast is an excellent preventive of scurvy. Nowadays, scurvy is quite rare and only seen in some food faddists, or in bachelors who do not care for fruits and vegetables and have an inadequate diet. Scurvy occurs also in young children whose main food consists of milk, which is relatively poor in vitamin C. Purpura due to some damage of the blood vessels ("vascular purpura") also occurs frequently in patients with high blood pressure or with diabetes. It may also be seen, without any apparent cause, in women at the time of the menopause, and is then called devil's pinches. This is not a dangerous condition and the patient should be told so. Since there is an hereditary tendency in many cases of vascular purpura, the physician will inquire whether there is any bleeder in the family. Operations can be performed without any danger on a patient who has the harmless type of vascular purpura.

CHAPTER XVIII

Deficiency Diseases

RUSSELL M. WILDER, M.D., and HUGH R. BUTT, M.D.

M OST DISEASES are due to the presence in the body of abnormal factors such as result from infection by germs, from intoxication or poisoning of some sort, or from the growth of tumors, or from accidents. More recently, doctors, chemists, and biologists have been studying a group of diseases known as "deficiency diseases." These are abnormal conditions or diseases due to the absence of certain necessary substances usually found in food. Their discovery has depended on finding in food certain factors which are essential for health. It has long been known that proteins, fats, carbohydrates, salts, and water are necessary for life. More recently, however, another group of substances, known as the vitamins, has been found. These are just as necessary for the maintenance of health as the other food factors just noted. Both from experience with human beings and laboratory research, it has been established that the body not only requires these substances for the preservation of health, but that a well selected diet furnishes them in adequate amounts.

Fats and carbohydrates, which are used chiefly as fuel in the food of man and animals, are found in almost all food substances. The relative ease of interchangeable use of these substances in the body makes the development of diseases due to their deficiency unusual. The protein of a mixed diet is rarely inadequate. Although deficiencies of certain salts such as those of iron, iodine, and lime will produce disease, the term deficiency disease is usually restricted to deficiency of one or more of the vitamins. The vitamins probably act to speed up or to initiate certain chemical reactions in the body. They do not serve directly as fuel or builders of tissue. They are, therefore, necessary in small quantities only. The separation of man from his natural environment, which has occurred with the development of civilization, has made the procurement of adequate natural foods steadily more difficult. The preparation of food in highly concentrated and purified form, such as flour, prepared oils, sugar and foods "ready to serve," while it has many benefits, has also limited the amount of food taken in the natural or fresh state. Although properly canned vegetables and fruits are equally wholesome, it is in the natural state that foods are richest in vitamin value.

The beginning of knowledge concerning vitamins is more the product of development than of any isolated discovery. Much of this development came before the first use of the word "vitamin." Eijkman, Hopkins, Funk, Osborne and Mendel, and McCollum and Davis are names which stand out prominently in the investigation and development of present conceptions of deficiency diseases: (1) Animals on a diet of purified foods furnishing adequate proteins, fats, carbohydrates, salts and water, fail to secure normal growth until given some natural food such as milk, butter, or fish oil. (2) Certain diseases of man can be cured by adding to the diet certain natural foodstuffs.

Diseases which are today recognized as being due to vitamin deficiency have occurred for hundred of years. A summary of the vitamins and the deficiency diseases produced by their absence may be found in the table at the end of this article.

With the exception of rickets and pellagra, the United States is relatively free of dietary-deficiency diseases. It must be added immediately, however, that we may not be free of vitamin-deficiency states. In this connection, McCollum and Simmonds said:

> We appreciate the existence of many grades of malnutrition. It is becoming constantly more evident that even a slight departure from the optimum in the composition of food may lead to states of nutritional instability which become contributing factors to physical breakdown when hygienic factors are unfavorable or when infectious processes are operative.

In order to produce a deficiency disease recognizable by its symptoms, the deficiency of a vitamin must be considerable. It is probable that deficiency states exist in which the food is not devoid of sufficient vitamin to produce a recognizable deficiency disease and yet is insufficient for normal nutritional needs. Perhaps such a state might more properly be called not a deficient state but one of failure of enrichment of diet by the vitamin. In the words of Sherman, who is an authority on the subject:

> It seems to be true of vitamin B, as also of vitamins A and C, that the optimal amount is much higher than the minimal ("actual") requirement: in other words, that the body is able to make good use of a much more liberal intake than can be proved to be absolutely necessary.

That is, there is a zone between the merely adequate and the optimal in nutrition. This is a relatively new and exceedingly important conception. Although we may be getting enough vitamin to give us "passable" health, we may not be getting enough for "buoyant" health. It seems reasonable that in the future in this country we shall be concerned more with this idea than with the occurrence of actual deficiency diseases. Indeed, we may go even further and eventually discover, as suggested by Sherman:

Just as a lack of this factor [vitamin B] brings about a condition of malnutrition which may contribute to premature senility, so a liberal intake of vitamin B contributes to a better than average nutritional condition and thus to what McCollum and Simmonds have aptly termed "the preservation of the characteristics of youth."

Possibly other vitamins in optimal amounts may not only lead to buoyant health but also to the preservation of the characteristics of youth. We are certain of one thing, and that is our incomplete knowledge. As Hess said:

We are only at the threshold of an understanding of the nutritional values of the foods and combinations of foods which enter into our dietaries.

Although diseases produced by deficiency of vitamins are distinct among themselves when clear cut, in the earlier stages and in those states between passable and buoyant health it may be impossible to determine clearly which vitamin is deficient. As a rule, all deficiency states at first lead to failure to gain weight, or loss of weight, exhaustion, lassitude, and weakness.

The knowledge of deficiency diseases gained through animal experiments has been indispensable in our understanding of their nature, prevention, and treatment. The dependability with which such disorders develop among certain animals on suitable diets, and the relative ease with which these experiments allow study of the various dietary-deficiency conditions, has advanced our knowledge further in proportion than in the case of many other diseases. If we were able to produce other diseases experimentally as readily as we do dietary deficiencies, the knowledge gained and the suffering saved would be priceless.

The average American dietary is adequate to prevent the development of dietary-deficiency diseases. It may not be adequate in all cases to maintain buoyant health. It is only under unusual circumstances in this country, such as war, famine, floods, and other deprivations, that actual deficiencies are likely to develop, with the possible exception of rickets (and pellagra in the South). There are other factors which must be thought of in a consideration of the elements which enter into the development of deficiency diseases, such as differences or disturbances in the assimilation of vitamins from the digestive tract, due to disease, or variability in storage of a vitamin in the body.

The most gratifying feature about deficiency diseases, both to the physician and to the patient, is that these conditions are not only curable but preventable. From the individual standpoint, therefore, their control is easy. From the standpoint of the community, the state, and the nation, the problem is one of public health and economics, and one cannot but hope that the day of deficiency diseases throughout the world will eventually be past. That still greater benefit than eradication of deficiency diseases is available may be surmised from the following expression of Sherman:

One of the most impressive features in recent discoveries regarding the relation of food to health and vitality is that the benefit of better feeding usually becomes fully apparent only when it is continued throughout a large part of the life cycle, and often the benefit is greater to the second generation than to the first.

Vitamin A Deficiency and Xerophthalmia

The most readily appreciated symptoms of vitamin A deficiency are changes occurring in the eyes. In previous years vitamin A deficiency has been considered to be manifested chiefly, if not entirely, in this way. The characteristic abnormality is a dryness of the eyes, so the disease has been known as xerophthalmia (dryness of the eyes). Vitamin A has been called the anti-xerophthalmic or anti-ophthalmic vitamin, since it prevented the occurrence of this condition. In the last few years, however, our knowledge of the function of this vitamin has increased tremendously. We now know that it serves an exceedingly useful and essential purpose in maintaining the skin and other coverings of the body in a healthy state. Because the onset of many infections depends on loss of integrity of these body coverings, and since vitamin A maintains these in a healthy state and is therefore indirectly partially responsible for preventing such infection, the vitamin has also become known as the "anti-infective vitamin." Since it is essential to growth, it has also been called the "growth-promoting vitamin."

HISTORY

It has been known for hundreds of years that certain diseases of the eyes developed after long fasts or after the use of improper foods. It was not until 1913 that we began to understand why they occurred. Osborne and Mendel, and McCollum and Davis, in that year reported that experimental animals such as rats, fed on food mixtures alike in all other respects, would continue to grow and thrive, or would soon cease to grow and shortly thereafter sicken and die, according as the fat in these mixtures was butter fat, cod-liver oil, egg yolk, or lard. Animals having lard as fat failed to grow, were unhealthy, and disease of the eyes developed; those with one of the other three fatty foods mentioned were healthy. This demonstrated that egg yolk, cod-liver oil, and butter contained an essential substance lacking in such a fat as lard; this substance we know as vitamin A.

Bloch, in Denmark, during World War I, suspected a relationship between a condition of malnutrition and eye trouble of children with insufficient amounts of fat in the diet and inadvertently made a remarkable experiment. In 1919, in an institution in Copenhagen he divided thirty-two healthy children, aged from one to four years, into two groups. One group received whole milk or butter with their food; the other, vegetable fat. In eight cases in the second group (those on vegetable fats) dryness of the eyes (xerophthalmia) developed subsequently and was relieved by cod-liver oil, whereas, in the group given whole milk, trouble did not develop. This showed conclusively that butter fat contained some substance essential for the maintenance of the eyes in a healthy state. Widmark, also in Denmark, was able to show a direct relationship between the amount of butter used and the occurrence of xerophthalmia among children.

A great deal of our knowledge concerning the effects of vitamin A deficiency has been obtained from the Orient, where xerophthalmia has been prevalent, and from experiments on animals.

Infants and children, just as young animals, are more susceptible to such deficiency than adults. In the first place, vitamin A is essential for adequate growth of the infant and child; also because its deprivation leads to lessening of resistance to infections, children are subject to severe and perhaps fatal infections if deficiency of vitamin A persists for a considerable length of time.

In the second place, vitamin A is essential for the maintenance in a healthy state of the tissues which serve as a covering for the body, such as the skin and the membranes covering the eyes, digestive tract, urinary tract, respiratory tract, and their associated glands. These covering tissues are known as the epithelial tissues. The essential change, in vitamin A deficiency, in these tissues is a drying, hardening, and thickening, so that they become much more susceptible to the occurrence of infection.

The manifestations in the eyes of vitamin A deficiency are xerophthalmia, or dryness, and night blindness. The xerophthalmia is manifested by drying of the tissues which cover the eye, resulting in dimness of vision and eventually infection, with partial or complete blindness if the disorder has been allowed to continue. This condition is a frequent cause of blindness in the Orient. Night blindness, or inability to see clearly in dusky light, is frequently due to vitamin A deficiency and is a result of disturbance in the delicately balanced mechanism of vision. Sometimes it is the first symptom of vitamin A deficiency to develop.

In cases of vitamin A deficiency, bronchopneumonia is the chief manifestation of infections in the organs of respiration. The effects on the digestive system are as yet uncertain. Possibly such deficiency may be significant in the occurrence of some types of stones in the bladder and kidneys, but such a definite relationship in man cannot as yet be absolutely established, although it is likely to occur among certain animals. The skin of people with vitamin A deficiency is frequently dry, scaly, shriveled, and pigmented.

At present the greatest interest in the importance of vitamin A is in connection with its relationship to infections. Does a normal supply of vitamin A give a person greater resistance to infections than an inadequate supply? More important, does an excessive supply increase the resistance to infection of the person concerned over that of the normal? It is as yet impossible to answer definitely these important questions. Evidence has been offered which would indicate that this vitamin is not only important in increasing the resistance of the body to infection, but that it is of importance in combating infections once they have occurred. However, conservatism leads one to say that at present vitamin A is to be considered as a substance protecting against infection by virtue of the fact that it maintains the integrity of the epithelial linings (coverings) of the various tracts, digestive, respiratory, and urinary, and of the skin, but its anti-infective power, that is, its ability to cure infections when the barrier of these coverings has been passed, or to prevent or cure infections in the blood stream, is questionable. Attempts have been made to show that this vitamin is important in the prevention of the common cold and childbed fever, but such evidence is not as yet convincing.

SOURCE, NATURE, AND ACTION OF VITAMIN A

Vitamin A, formerly known as fat-soluble A (and before its distinction from vitamin D known also as the anti-rachitic vitamin), is generally considered to occur in the fatty foods of animal origin, such as milk, butter, cod-liver oil, and egg yolk. It is now known, however, that the chemical predecessor or precursor of vitamin A is the yellow pigment, carotene, which gives the color to green or yellow vegetables, such as carrots, sweet potatoes, yellow corn, and green beans. This substance, carotene, which can be extracted in the chemical laboratory, is exceedingly potent and is converted in the animal body into what we know as vitamin A. Consequently, vitamin A may be obtained from either animal or vegetable sources. The way in which vitamin A acts on the tissues after its formation is unknown. The liver stores large quantities of it, a supply sufficient to last several months. This explains why liver oil is such a rich source of the vitamin. The liver of the cod is particularly rich in the vitamin, but more recently it has been found that liver oil from the halibut is many times richer in vitamin A and, in fact, is almost pure vitamin A.

PREVENTION AND TREATMENT

The prevention and treatment of the vitamin A deficiency states are exceedingly simple and depend on an adequate intake of foods containing vitamin A, which include milk, butter, eggs, and fresh vegetables containing the green and yellow pigments. Various concentrated preparations of vitamin A are also available.

THE VITAMIN B COMPLEX

All the water-soluble vitamins found in yeast were once called B vitamins, but the rapid advances in chemical knowledge have led to the isolation of many of these factors and very recently their rôle in human metabolism has been established. All the members of this large group are associated closely in nature and it is perhaps for this reason that deficiency of one of this large group is likely to bring about deficiency of several components of the vitamin B complex. There are many known factors in this complex but vitamin B_1 (thiamine), nicotinic acid, riboflavin, pyridoxine (vitamin B_6), pantothenic acid and vitamin B_{12} are the only substances which are known to be of usefulness in human nutrition. Within a few years many more substances undoubtedly will be added to this already long list of essential nutrients.

THIAMINE OR VITAMIN B₁ DEFICIENCY

Vitamin B_1 is distributed widely in the plant world and occurs most abundantly in yeast, rice bran, whole grain flour, meat, dried beans and peas. It has now been identified as a chemical compound called thiamine.

Although it was first thought that there was no deficiency of vitamin B_1 in American diets, it is now recognized that widespread deficiency may result from eating highly refined grains. In normal human subjects fed diets lacking in vitamin B_1 for periods of several months, fatigue, depression, irritability, multiple neurasthenic complaints, fall in blood pressure, loss of appetite, constipation and loss of weight develop. These abnormalities are all corrected quickly when vitamin B_1 is added again to the diet. This and many other studies lead one to believe that a borderline adequacy of a vitamin or mineral is likely to lead to poor health.

The importance of adequate intake of vitamin B_1 to national health has been recognized recently by the "enrichment" of white flour with vitamin and mineral supplements. Through the leadership of the Food and Nutrition Board of the National Research Council, "enriched flour" containing thiamine, nicotinic acid and iron in prescribed amounts is now available to the public at no extra cost. "Enriched bread" prepared from this flour or by the use by the baker of the enriching ingredients is of great importance to our national health standard.

Beriberi was thought once to be a tropical disease resulting purely from vitamin B_1 deficiency. It is characterized by swelling of the limbs, a weak heart, painful legs and finally paralysis of the nerves. We later learned that this disease occurred fairly frequently, in the United States, in cases of pregnancy, as well as in alcoholism and other diseases. This disease is not, apparently, the result of deficiency of vitamin B_1 alone but is the result of multiple deficiencies of the vitamin B complex.

NIACIN DEFICIENCY

Niacin is found in liver, lean meats and whole cereal grains. It is effective in the treatment of pellagra in human beings. When human beings have pellagra, the giving of niacin will lead to a disappearance of the disturbances of digestion and of the skin which are characteristic of the disease. Moreover, some of the mental symptoms which do not represent complete degeneration of the tissues of the nervous system will also improve. However, like most diseases resulting from deficiency of a member of the vitamin B complex, pellagra responds best to the administration of niacin plus other members of the B complex.

In addition to its specific value in the treatment of pellagra, niacin also is useful in the treatment of a formerly highly fatal syndrome involving the nervous system. This syndrome is characterized by clouding of the consciousness, delirium and other nerve changes and may occur either with or without manifestations of any deficiency disease. This disease is thought to represent an acute, complete lack of niacin, in contrast to pellagra, which is considered as a chronic deficiency of niacin and other B vitamins.

RIBOFLAVIN DEFICIENCY (*Ariboflavinosis*)

Animal liver and kidneys, milk and yeast are rich sources of riboflavin. Pure deficiency of this vitamin in the human subject results in a pallor of the mucosa in the angles of the mouth which in a few days becomes macerated and transverse superficial cracks or fissures appear. At the same time the lips become red and a fine, scaly, greasy desquamation (like dandruff) appears at the openings of the nostrils and on the side of the nose, in the ears and sometimes on the cheeks and forehead. In addition the tongue becomes magenta colored (in contrast to the beefy red tongue of pellagra), the eyes are red and bright lights will cause them to water and burn. All these symptoms disappear dramatically within a few days when riboflavin is added again to the diet.

OTHER VITAMIN B FACTORS

Pyridoxine (vitamin B_6), pantothenic acid and choline have been recognized and identified by the fact that they are necessary for the maintenance of health of animals, but it is not yet established definitely whether they are necessary for normal health of human beings.

Pyridoxine appears to be of value in the treatment of certain nervous manifestations that occur in cases of pellagra.

Studies on pantothenic acid indicate that it is perhaps essential in human nutrition and that its function is associated closely with that of riboflavin. Although choline may be of some value in preventing accumulation of fat in the liver under certain circumstances, its use in human beings is uncertain and nothing is known of the proper dosage.

From liver extract a crystalline cobalt containing a substance known as vitamin B_{12} has been isolated. The clinical results from the use of adequate amounts of vitamin B_{12} for pernicious anemia alone appear to be equal in every way to those obtained from a potent liver extract. It is also reported that this vitamin is effective in the treatment of fish tape worm anemia and in certain types of anemia seen following total removal of the stomach.

Folic acid was isolated in 1943 and has proven to be an essential factor for blood formation in man, monkeys and other species. This substance is not a complete treatment for pernicious anemia but in the treatment of certain anemias of pregnancy and anemia associated with intestinal disease such as strictures and fistulas and in nutritional macrocytic anemia of the tropics the use of folic acid brings results and prompt recovery.

SCURVY, OR VITAMIN C DEFICIENCY

Scurvy is a disease produced as a result of deficiency of ascorbic acid in the diet. It is characterized chiefly by serious weakness, bleeding into the tissues, and softening of the bones. The occurrence of scurvy in times of deprivation of food, and particularly among sailors, is a matter of common knowledge. At present the occurrence of well-developed scurvy among adult persons is rare.

SYMPTOMS

Scurvy does not develop immediately on the deprivation of foods containing vitamin C. As a rule, from four to seven months are required before such deprivation leads to the development of symptoms of scurvy. This period is known as the depletion period and corresponds roughly to the incubation period of infectious diseases.

The number, situation, and amount of the hemorrhages into the tissues decide, in large part, the symptoms of which the patient will complain. The bleeding probably is not due to changes in the blood but to alterations in the substances which help to hold together the cells which compose the walls of the blood vessels. Areas in which hemorrhages occur are the gums, skin, muscles, bones, and nose. The gums swell and become red and spongy or fungus-like.

COURSE

It is amazing to consider the rapidity with which persons with scurvy recover as soon as the diet becomes adequate. Just a few days may be required, unless permanent injury has been done.

Interest among physicians considering scurvy at the present time is chiefly concerned with scurvy in infants. Infantile scurvy is not seen, as a rule, before the child is aged six months. It is usually manifested by some of the following symptoms: swelling and bleeding of the gums, tenderness of the legs due to bleeding into the muscles or beneath the periosteum (tissue covering the bones), anemia, dental decay, susceptibility to infection, and cessation of growth. It has recently been claimed that dental caries (decay of teeth) is the result of vitamin C deficiency. This may be of the greatest significance, for if consumption of adequate amounts of vitamin C will in part prevent the development of such dental decay, its importance can hardly be overestimated.

X-ray studies of the bones help to establish the diagnosis of scurvy if hemorrhages in the bones are present.

TREATMENT

The treatment of scurvy is simple and consists in giving a diet rich in foods containing vitamin C. Oranges, lemons, limes, germinating seeds and fresh fruits, especially tomatoes, and vegetables are the most abundant sources of this element.

Heating is detrimental if not destructive to vitamin C. This apparently explained the insufficiency of pasteurized or boiled milk, canned and cooked foods, as substances useful against scurvy until Hess pointed out that it was not the actual heat which destroyed the vitamin, but oxidation. Consequently, the preparation of canned foods has been fitted to this fact.

CONTRIBUTION OF SELECTED SERVINGS OF A FEW FOODS AS PERCENTAGES
OF ADULT MALE ALLOWANCE (5000 INTERNATIONAL UNITS (I.U.))

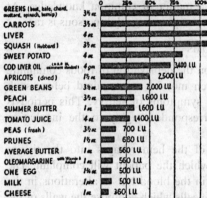

CONTRIBUTION OF SELECTED SERVINGS OF A FEW FOODS AS
PERCENTAGES OF ADULT MALE ALLOWANCE (1.8 MILLIGRAMS)

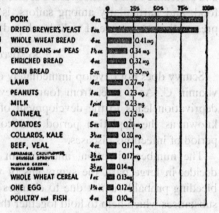

Fig. 31. Foods as sources of Vitamin A. Green, leafy, and yellow vegetables are outstanding sources. Dairy products, eggs and liver (and fish liver oils) are the important animal sources. Vitamin A is well conserved in cooking.

Fig. 32. Foods as sources of Thiamine (Vitamin B₁). Except for pork, common foods supply only small amounts of thiamine, the best sources being nutritionally unimpaired cereals and meats; some thiamine may be lost in cooking, either through destruction by heat or extraction by water.

CONTRIBUTION OF SELECTED SERVINGS OF A FEW FOODS AS
PERCENTAGES OF ADULT MALE ALLOWANCE (75 MILLIGRAMS)

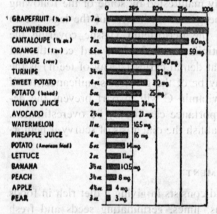

CONTRIBUTION OF SELECTED SERVINGS OF A FEW FOODS AS
PERCENTAGES OF ADULT MALE ALLOWANCE (27 MILLIGRAMS)

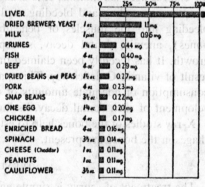

Fig. 33. Foods as sources of Ascorbic Acid (Vitamin C). In addition to citrus fruits and tomatoes many common fruits and vegetables supply significant amounts of ascorbic acid, especially if eaten raw. This vitamin is readily destroyed by heat and it is extracted by water.

Fig. 34. Foods as sources of Riboflavin (Vitamin G). Milk is the most important common source of riboflavin. This vitamin is not readily destroyed by heat but it may be lost by extraction in water during cooking and by prolonged exposure to light.

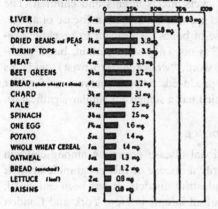

CONTRIBUTION OF SELECTED SERVINGS OF A FEW FOODS AS
PERCENTAGES OF ADULT MALE ALLOWANCE (12 MILLIGRAMS)

LIVER	4 oz	93 mg
OYSTERS	3½ oz	5.8 mg
DRIED BEANS and PEAS	½ oz	3.8 mg
TURNIP TOPS	3½ oz	3.5 mg
MEAT	4 oz	3.3 mg
BEET GREENS	3½ oz	3.2 mg
BREAD (whole wheat) (4 slices)	4 oz	3.2 mg
CHARD	3½ oz	3.1 mg
KALE	3½ oz	2.5 mg
SPINACH	3½ oz	2.5 mg
ONE EGG	1¾ oz	1.6 mg
POTATO	5 oz	1.4 mg
WHOLE WHEAT CEREAL	1 oz	1.4 mg
OATMEAL	1 oz	1.3 mg
BREAD (enriched)	4 oz	1.2 mg
LETTUCE (leaf)	2 oz	0.8 mg
RAISINS	1 oz	0.8 mg

Fig. 35. Foods as sources of Iron.
Beans, meats, the green leafy vegetables
and nutritionally unimpaired cereals
are the best common sources of iron

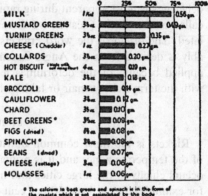

CONTRIBUTION OF SELECTED SERVINGS OF A FEW FOODS AS
PERCENTAGES OF ADULT MALE ALLOWANCE (0.8 GRAM)

MILK	1 Pint	0.56 gm
MUSTARD GREENS	3½ oz	0.49 gm
TURNIP GREENS	3½ oz	0.35 gm
CHEESE (Cheddar)	1 oz	0.27 gm
COLLARDS	3½ oz	0.20 gm
HOT BISCUIT (made with 4 oz	0.19 gm
KALE	3½ oz	0.18 gm
BROCCOLI	3½ oz	0.14 gm
CAULIFLOWER	3½ oz	0.12 gm
CHARD	3½ oz	0.10 gm
BEET GREENS*	3½ oz	0.09 gm
FIGS (dried)	1¾ oz	0.08 gm
SPINACH*	3½ oz	0.08 gm
BEANS (dried)	1 oz	0.07 gm
CHEESE (cottage)	3 oz	0.06 gm
MOLASSES	1 oz	0.06 gm

* The calcium in beet greens and spinach is in the form of
the oxalate which is not assimilated by the body

Fig. 36. Foods as sources of Calcium.
Milk is the most important common
source of calcium.

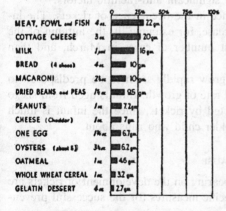

CONTRIBUTION OF SELECTED SERVINGS OF A FEW FOODS
AS PERCENTAGES OF ADULT MALE ALLOWANCE (70 GRAMS)

MEAT, FOWL and FISH	4 oz	22 gm
COTTAGE CHEESE	3 oz	20 gm
MILK	1 pint	16 gm
BREAD (4 slices)	4 oz	10 gm
MACARONI	2½ oz	10 gm
DRIED BEANS and PEAS	½ oz	9.5 gm
PEANUTS	1 oz	7.2 gm
CHEESE (Cheddar)	1 oz	7 gm
ONE EGG	1¾ oz	6.7 gm
OYSTERS (about 8)	3½ oz	6.2 gm
OATMEAL	1 oz	4.6 gm
WHOLE WHEAT CEREAL	1 oz	3.2 gm
GELATIN DESSERT	4 oz	2.7 gm

Fig. 37. Foods as sources of Protein.
Animal foods are the best sources of
good quality protein.

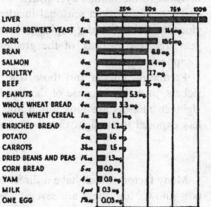

CONTRIBUTION OF SELECTED SERVINGS OF A FEW FOODS AS
PERCENTAGES OF ADULT MALE ALLOWANCE (18 MILLIGRAMS)

LIVER	4 oz	
DRIED BREWER'S YEAST	1 oz	14 mg
PORK	4 oz	10.6 mg
BRAN	1 oz	8.8 mg
SALMON	4 oz	8.4 mg
POULTRY	4 oz	7.7 mg
BEEF	4 oz	7.5 mg
PEANUTS	1 oz	5.3 mg
WHOLE WHEAT BREAD	4 oz	3.3 mg
WHOLE WHEAT CEREAL	1 oz	1.8 mg
ENRICHED BREAD	4 oz	1.7 mg
POTATO	5 oz	1.6 mg
CARROTS	3½ oz	1.5 mg
DRIED BEANS AND PEAS	1½ oz	1.3 mg
CORN BREAD	5 oz	0.9 mg
YAM	4 oz	0.9 mg
MILK	1 pint	0.3 mg
ONE EGG	1¾ oz	0.03 mg

Fig. 38. Foods as sources of Niacin
(Nicotinic Acid). Meats are the most
important sources of this vitamin.

RICKETS: A VITAMIN D DEFICIENCY

Rickets is a chronic nutritional disorder of infants and children, producing alterations chiefly in the bones, and considered by many to be a deficiency disease due to a lack of vitamin D. Rickets affects infants and children. The deficiency is most apparent during rapid growth, but a similar disease of adults, called osteomalacia (destructive disease of bones) is thought to be closely related. The origin of the word "rickets" is not known for certain, but it probably is derived from the Anglo-Saxon word, "wrickken" (to twist), and was applied because of the deformities it produced. Almost everyone is familiar with the term rickety chair or table, which has a somewhat similar significance.

INCIDENCE

Rickets is the most common nutritional disease occurring among children of the temperate zone, and it is primarily a disease of this geographic area. It occurs chiefly in the large cities and industrial districts. It has been estimated, for example, that at least 50 per cent of all infants in New York and London have rickets. It must be remembered, however, that this does not mean severe rickets, as was known in previous centuries and still exists, in the minds of many laymen. The disorder is frequently so mild in the present day as to be unrecognized except by experts.

The intensity and incidence or rickets throughout the world corresponds fairly closely to the amount of sunshine present. It is the sun's untraviolet rays, invisible to the human eye, which are significant anti-rachitic factors.

There is a distinct seasonal incidence in the occurrence of rickets. The incidence of the disorder begins to increase, for example, in the autumn of the year, reaches its peak of the greatest number of cases in March, and then disappears rapidly.

Premature infants and those who grow rapidly seem to be predisposed to rickets, probably because of the rapid rate of growth. Infants aged from six to eighteen months are most often affected by rickets, since the infant is much less exposed to sunlight than is the older child who runs about.

CAUSE

Many factors which have a direct bearing on the development of rickets are now known, and there are several specific measures for the successful prevention and treatment of the disease.

The diet and condition of the mother before birth of her child probably have some effect on the subsequent development of rickets. Bottle-fed babies are much more likely to develop rickets than are breast-fed babies, but the latter do sometimes have rickets.

The distinguishing characteristic of rickets is that the bone which is formed is not of normal composition, since it is improperly and inadequately calcified (hardened). The result is that the bone is abnormally soft, and deformity, bending, and twisting occur. Naturally, the more abundant the growth of bone, the more likely is the hardening to be insufficient, which explains the increasing frequency of rickets in the more rapidly growing and well-nourished child.

The greatest recent advance in the study of rickets has been in the understanding of the precise nature of the effect of sunlight on the disease. It has been established that the ultraviolet rays of the sunlight are the significant factors. It is remarkable that these rays of invisible light are of such great importance in the hardening of bone. It is still more remarkable, and certainly beyond our present comprehension, that only those ultraviolet waves of a certain length (290 to 313 millimicrons) are effective, and that a difference of as little as from ten to twenty millionths of a millimeter (25 mm. to an inch) is sufficient to render ultraviolet light effective or ineffective in curing or preventing rickets. During the winter months the absorption of these ultraviolet waves by moisture, dust, smoke, and other foreign substances in the air makes their quantity reaching the skin of the well-covered infant extremely small, even though the child is out of doors. Direct sunlight is not essential, since it has been shown that the so-called skyshine, light reflected from the sky, clouds, and so forth, possesses approximately from half to two thirds the anti-rachitic effect of sunshine. This is an extremely important observation. An infant obtains considerable ultraviolet irradiation without being in the direct sunlight. Ordinary window glass removes the ultraviolet rays, so that sunshine which passes through a window pane is ineffective against rickets. Special kinds of glass are made which do not remove these rays.

The exact mechanism of action of the ultraviolet waves in hardening bone is unknown. Probably the ultraviolet light acts by producing chemical changes in the traces of ergosterol (one of the fatty materials) of the skin, with the production of a substance known as vitamin D. Ultraviolet waves from artificial sources, for example, mercury vapor lamps, are quite as effective, if not more so, against rickets when properly given than is direct sunlight.

The factor leading to the hardening (calcification) of the bones may be obtained not only by the action of sunlight on the skin but by the ingestion of certain foods (anti-rachitic) such as cod-liver oil, egg yolk, foods which have been treated with ultraviolet light (irradiated foods), to some extent breast milk, and irradiated ergosterol (viosterol). These substances all contain vitamin D.

SYMPTOMS

The earliest signs of rickets are restlessness, irritability, and sweating of the head. These signs are, however, only suggestive and not conclusive; they also occur under other circumstances. In the bones will be found definite evidence of rickets, which shows itself by enlargement of the ends of the bones (epiphysial areas) and by softening. The most reliable early sign is thickening or beading of the ends of the ribs about the nipple line, at the points where the bony and cartilaginous ribs join. This swelling or beading is known as the "rachitic rosary." There is also enlargement of the bones, particularly about the wrist and the knee, squaring of the head, failure of the soft areas (fontanels) in the head to close at the proper time, and softness of the bones of the head. These symptoms are not all necessarily present in one case. Subsequently, enlargement of the abdomen, grooving in of the lower ribs (Harrison's groove), squaring of the head, and bowlegs or knock knees may develop. The muscles become soft and flabby; the physical development is poor, so that rachitic children usually are slow in sitting and walking; the eruption of the teeth is tardy, and occasionally curvature of the spine occurs. The importance of rickets as a factor in causing delay in the development and eruption of the teeth and in the subsequent development of dental decay is as yet unknown, but the relationship seems significant.

The diagnosis of rickets is easily made in a classical, well-developed case. In the early stages, it may be necessary to resort to laboratory measures, such as X-ray examinations of the bones, and studies of the phosphorus content of the blood, which is generally below normal.

The outlook for recovery of the rachitic infant is excellent, especially if treatment is given. As a rule, the mild condition recovers spontaneously during the summer. Occasionally deformities persist if the condition remains too long untreated; rickets is readily cured by adequate treatment.

PREVENTION AND TREATMENT

Rickets can be prevented. People are so rapidly becoming educated in the matter of prevention and cure of rickets that the disease becomes less serious and perhaps less common as time goes on.

The prevention and treatment of rickets are unique; it is the only disease for which there are several specific methods of cure. These are the use of cod-liver oil, ultraviolet light, irradiated foods (foods treated with ultraviolet light), and irradiated ergosterol. The efficacy of cod-liver oil has been definitely established within the last few years, and its effectiveness definitely shown on experimental animals with rickets.

The amount of cod-liver oil to be used in preventing or treating rickets is variable and depends on the age of the patient, the severity of the disease, the vitamin D and anti-rachitic value of the cod-liver oil, as well as the associated treatment applied. It is difficult to make a general statement concerning the matter, and this should be left to the discretion of the physician in a given case. The Council on Pharmacy and Chemistry of the American Medical Association has decided that a dosage of 3 teaspoonfuls (12 c.c., 3 fluid drachms) daily may tentatively be set as the standard optimal dosage of standard cod-liver oil for the average infant aged three months.

For preventive measures, administration of cod-liver oil should be started early and should reach the full dose certainly by the end of the second month of life. It is well to remember that in the active treatment of rickets, milk containing vitamin D does not exhibit sufficient activity to end the disease abruptly. Premature infants may need ten to twenty times as much vitamin D to prevent rickets as does a normal infant.

Sunlight or ultraviolet light artificially produced, as for instance by the mercury vapor lamp, is perhaps as effective as any other measure in the prevention and treatment of rickets. Sunlight and skyshine, as mentioned, should be more generally used, especially in cities, than they are at present.

Irradiated ergosterol (viosterol), which is highly specific for rickets, should be used only under the direct supervision of a physician. The tremendous anti-rachitic power of irradiated ergosterol can be seen from the fact that 5 mg. ($\frac{5}{1000}$ of a gram) of this substance is estimated to be equivalent to one quart of cod-liver oil. Excessive doses of this potent substance are known to have produced undesirable effects.

It should be remembered, also, that breast milk, although not a specific for rickets itself, is one of the most valuable measures for combating the disease.

Within the past few years it has been shown that the administration by injection of large doses of vitamin D to children who have rickets (including premature infants) is followed by uniformly rapid healing and complete absence of clinical evidence of any toxicity. This large dose of vitamin D is given as a single dose and the method seems to be now well established.

PELLAGRA

The name "pellagra" is probably derived from the Italian words *pelle,* for skin, and *agra,* for rough, since roughened skin is one of the most frequently observed symptoms in this disease.

Probably pellagra occurred occasionally in the United States during the nineteenth century, but scientific reports of its occurrence in this country were almost lacking until 1907, when an investigator named Searcy made the first report. Perhaps previous failure of recognition in the United States was due to the fact that pellagra was considered a disease of the tropics or of Europe only, and therefore it received practically no recognition in medical textbooks published in this country before that time. However, knowledge of the disease spread rapidly throughout the southern part of the United States, and numerous reports of cases and of epidemics were recorded; thus a great deal of knowledge has been acquired concerning pellagra since 1907.

CAUSE

Dr. J. Goldberger showed that most, if not all, cases of pellagra are closely associated with a deficiency in the intake of food. Goldberger said:

Indeed it may be stated that our knowledge of the nature of the dietary deficiency has now been sufficiently clarified to warrant placing pellagra in a category closely related to, if not identical with, that of beriberi and scurvy.

Several vitamins are lacking in most cases of pellagra; especially important is lack of nicotinic acid.

INCIDENCE

Pellagra is endemic in the South; that is, it is constantly occurring, chiefly in the spring and summer months. There also seems to be a close relationship between the number of cases and economic depression. Individuals who are victims of pellagra usually fall into three groups: (1) those with simple deficiencies of diet; (2) those with deficiencies of food due to prolonged use of large amounts of alcohol, and (3) those with deficiencies because of organic disease of the digestive system.

SYMPTOMS

For many years medical students have been taught that the great triad of symptoms in pellagra was "the three D's," dermatitis, dementia, and diarrhea; that is, inflammation of the skin, abnormal mental symptoms, and looseness of the bowels, but there are few existing diseases which are more variable in nature than is pellagra. The occurrence of these three symptoms together, or in the same patient, is found only in the severest cases and usually means that the outlook is bad. The skin, the digestive tract, and the nervous system are, however, the three parts of the body which are particularly affected when pellagra occurs. Goldberger said:

> The eruption is the most characteristic telltale of the disease and the main reliance in its recognition. When the eruption first shows itself it may look much like, and frequently is mistaken for, a sunburn. The sunburned appearance soon changes and in many cases the reddened skin turns to a somewhat dirty brown and frequently acquires a parchment-like appearance, then quickly becomes rough and scaly, or cracks and peels. . . . Among the most distinctive peculiarities of the eruption is its preference for certain parts of the body surface. The backs of the hands, forearms, and the backs of the feet are its favorite sites. [It also occurs on the face, neck, trunk, and legs.] Another marked peculiarity of the eruption is its tendency to appear at about the same time and to cover similar areas, both as to extent and peculiarities of outline, on both sides of the body.

The skin may peel and become dark. Eventually, as the disease is overcome, the eruption on the skin may entirely disappear or the area affected may remain dark. The symptoms related to the skin in themselves are rarely serious, but as a result of them the patient may look old and scrawny.

The digestive symptoms include burning in mouth and throat, excessive gas in the stomach and in the bowels, loss of appetite, vague distress in the abdomen, and constipation or diarrhea. Loss of appetite is less common. Diarrhea is common late in the disease and is usually difficult to control. Blood in the material excreted indicates a more severe condition. There is usually a lack of hydrochloric acid in the content of the stomach.

The effects on the nervous system which are first noted are exhaustion, lassitude, insomnia, and subsequently, in the severe cases, hallucinations, and finally insanity. Only a small proportion of cases go on to this condition, from which recovery is infrequent.

COURSE

The course of pellagra is variable. At times it may begin without any notice save for a little burning of the hands or feet, a sense of heat in the pit of the stomach, and a little nervousness and restlessness at night. In other cases the skin changes only will be present and, because of frequent resemblance to sunburn, may not be particularly noted by the patient. In the absence of skin symptoms, the diagnosis of the disease can only be made by an expert.

Although the disease is frequently completely overcome by patients, it may remain chronic, with flare-ups each spring and summer.

Underhill stated: "In general, pellagra seems no more dangerous than measles." Death occurs in about 3 per cent of the cases of pellagra, although in certain types of cases this incidence may be considerably higher.

TREATMENT

As once stated by Goldberger, the keystone in considering pellagra should be prevention. Although a patient may have placed before him an adequate amount of food containing substances which will prevent pellagra, it is to be remembered that individual eccentricities of taste may make the actual vitamin content of food consumed inadequate for his needs. This at times explains the occurrence of pellagra in the well-to-do person who has apparently sufficient food. It has now been well established that the administration of niacin in doses of 200 to 500 mg. a day by mouth will result, within a few days, in a disappearance of most of the signs and symptoms of this disease.

As mentioned before under the vitamin B complex, in addition to administering niacin, it is often necessary to administer foods such as liver, yeast and meats which are rich in all members of the vitamin B complex. To treat a patient who has pellagra with niacin alone is not sufficient.

VITAMIN E

Vitamin E, which has been discovered more recently than the other vitamins, has been shown to be necessary for normal reproduction in certain animals. It has also been demonstrated recently that deficiency of this substance in certain animals produces certain neuromuscular changes. [Research has proposed the use of vitamin E for habitual abortion; for several forms of sclerosis of the spinal cord, and for degenerative changes in the heart muscle. When the results have been reinvestigated, the research has failed to support the original claims. Even tocopherol, an active principle derived from vitamin E, has not been found specifically useful in any human disease. The addition of vitamin E to mixtures of vitamins does not seem to be warranted since claims of benefit from it cannot be sustained.—Ed.]

RÉSUMÉ OF THE KNOWN VITAMINS, THEIR NAMES, SOURCES, PURPOSES, AND DEFICIENCIES

Vitamin	Other Names	Sources Fair	Sources Good	Sources Excellent	Excellent Purposes	Deficiency Leads to
A	Anti-ophthalmic Anti-infective Growth promoting Fat soluble A Carotene or pro-vitamin A	Fruits	Tomatoes Whole yellow corn Hen's eggs Ordinary green vegetables	Butter Cod-liver oil Other liver oils Spinach Kale Turnip greens	Maintains integrity of epithelial (covering) tissues, thereby helping in part to prevent infections Promotes growth and vigor Essential for reproduction	Lowered resistance to infection of many organs, especially of the eyes (xerophthalmia) Failure of growth of children Loss of vigor Night blindness
B	B_1 Anti-neuritic Anti-beriberi Thiamine chloride	Green vegetables Dried beans Soya beans	Heart, liver, kidney, eggs, milk Whole cereals Lean muscle meat	Wheat germ Yeast	Promotes appetite and digestion Stimulates body activity Overcomes some forms of neuritis	Loss of tone of digestive tract Fatigue Depression Loss of appetite Forms of neuritis
	B_2 Riboflavin	Whole wheat Dried beans Soya beans	Wheat germ Meat Green vegetables	Dried yeast Milk Eggs Heart Kidney	Extrinsic factor in pernicious anemia (Castle)? Necessary for normal growth Development of cells	Disorders of growth Digestive disturbances Nervous weakness Infection
	Nicotinic acid	Milk Wheat germ Lean meats	Green vegetables Beans	Yeast	Prevention of features of pellagra	Nerve, skin and intestinal disturbances

C Anti-scorbutic Ascorbic acid Cevitamic acid	Fresh apples and onions	Bananas Pineapple Collards Green peas	Green peppers Tomatoes Grapefruit Lemons Oranges Tomato juice Cabbage	Protects body from scurvy Required for proper formation of bones and teeth	Scurvy Softening of bones Decay of teeth Loss of muscle strength Hemorrhage
D Anti-rachitic Irradiated ergosterol Viosterol	Milk or butter	Eggs	Cod-liver oil Sunlight Artificial ultra-violet lights Irradiated ergosterol (viosterol)	Proper calcification (hardening) of bones Prevents rickets	Rickets Bone deformities Defects and caries of teeth General muscular weakness
E Anti-sterility	Whole cereals	Whole wheat Lettuce Watercress	Wheat germ	Necessary for reproduction in animals and man?	Sterility (noted in animals only) Failure of reproduction (noted in animals only)
K Anti-hemorrhagic vitamin	Grass	Alfalfa	Concentrates	Prevention of hemorrhage by maintaining concentration of prothrombin in blood	Tendency to bleed, in newborn infants and in patients who have jaundice
Vitamin B Complex Vitamin B complex includes also filtrate factor; vitamin B_2 $_{49}$ $_{59}$ and	These factors are known particularly for effects in absence in animals but have been related to complications of pellagra and similar disturbances in human beings. Pantothenic acid (filtrate factor) is related to graying of hair in human beings. Vitamin B_6 (pyridoxine) is related to some chronic nervous disturbances.				

Vitamin K Deficiency

HISTORY

Vitamin K was first discovered by Henrik Dam in Copenhagen. He found that this vitamin would prevent abnormal bleeding in young chicks. Soon it was found in this country that this substance would also prevent and cure the bleeding which sometimes occurs among patients who have jaundice. Later, it was discovered that this vitamin would prevent bleeding that occurred in certain intestinal diseases and in newborn infants.

SOURCE, NATURE, AND ACTION

This vitamin is distributed widely in nature and is found abundantly in the green leaves of certain plants such as alfalfa, kale, spinach, and so forth. It is soluble in fat and, therefore, bile for digestion of fat is necessary for its absorption from the intestines. When vitamin K is not absorbed the pro-thrombin (a substance in the blood necessary to cause clotting) of the blood decreases to such levels that the blood will not clot, and, therefore, any operation on such a person results frequently in fatal hemorrhage. It is not known exactly how vitamin K acts in man, but it is associated intimately with and necessary for the production of prothrombin and for this to take place one must have an intact liver or else the vitamin does not work.

CONDITIONS IN WHICH VITAMIN K IS USEFUL

In patients who have jaundice normal secretion of bile does not enter the intestine and, therefore, vitamin K is not absorbed properly from the food. In these patients the symptom of vitamin K deficiency, which is bleeding, may develop. Bleeding may occur from the mouth and nose, intestinal tract or bladder.

Patients who have severe diarrhea or those who because of some disease vomit or have to have their stomach contents drawn out during some surgical operation also fail to absorb vitamin K properly and a bleeding tendency may develop.

It has been known for a long time that certain newborn infants bleed to death for no apparent cause. It has now been established that most of these fatal hemorrhages are the result of a deficiency of prothrombin in the blood and that this deficiency can be corrected by the administration of vitamin K. It is now thought that vitamin K should be given to all newborn infants at birth or else that vitamin K should be given to the mother during the last week of pregnancy or at the time of labor. It is felt that this simple procedure might prevent many deaths from hemorrhage among the newborn and even may prevent some of the instances of cerebral hemorrhage which result in terrible paralytic birth injuries.

PREVENTION AND TREATMENT

[The doctor can make a prothrombin determination in the laboratory. Reduction to 20 per cent of normal means increased bleeding. Failure of vitamin K to be absorbed or damage to the liver means lessened prothrombin. Many diseases, such as scurvy, allergic purpura, or lowered blood platelets give hemorrhagic symptoms without lessened prothrombin.

The doctor can prescribe vitamin K, called menadione, as tablets or by injection. The drug may also be needed to overcome excessive bleeding after using some of the anticoagulants like dicumarol or heparin or tromexan.—Ed.]

CHAPTER XIX

Allergy

INCLUDING: HAY FEVER, ASTHMA, ALLERGIC RHINITIS, HIVES,
SKIN ALLERGY, CONTACT DERMATITIS, MIGRAINE,
GASTRO-INTESTINAL ALLERGY, ETC.

LEO H. CRIEP, M.D.

INTRODUCTION

TREMENDOUS ADVANCES *have been made in the field of allergy since 1940. Because allergic manifestations are common and because symptoms of allergy have a tendency to be persistent, people need to have an intelligent understanding of the whys and wherefores of this group of diseases.*

INCIDENCE OF ALLERGY

About 10 per cent of the population suffer from major allergic disorders such as bronchial asthma, hay fever, nasal allergy, hives, and allergic eczema. Approximately 40 to 60 per cent of the population have minor allergies, such as intolerance and idiosyncrasy to certain foods, and other substances. It is thus seen that allergic diseases involve many patients. Furthermore, the symptoms of allergy are persistent.

WHAT IS ALLERGY?

A person is said to be allergic if he reacts to a substance in a manner different from the ordinary or normal person. Thus to most of us an egg is harmless and wholesome food—yet in certain persons even a small amount of egg may produce such symptoms as swelling of the lips, a skin rash, or even severe asthma. Such persons may be normal in every other respect except for this peculiarity or idiosyncrasy, and so we say of such persons that they are hypersensitive to egg protein or, in medical parlance, that they are allergic.

HEREDITY AND ALLERGY

The tendency to develop some types of allergy is in many instances hereditary, being handed down from parent to child. Such transmission, of course, cannot be prevented any more than could blue eyes or red hair. It follows, therefore, that the stronger the hereditary factor, the more likely it is that the offspring will show some form of allergic manifestation. All that can be done from a preventive point of view is to keep such children in the best of possible health and to treat any suspicious symptoms of allergy as soon as they appear. Although asthma and some allergic skin disorders are hereditary, none of these conditions is contagious or "catching," so there need be no fear of people coming into intimate contact with such cases.

HISTORY OF ALLERGY

The earliest mention of allergy is by Hippocrates, who comments on the appearance of a skin rash which no doubt was hives as a result of the ingestion of certain foods. In the second century, A.D., Galen mentioned the development of nasal symptoms from exposure to roses. A physician by the name of Bostock described in 1819 his own seasonal nasal symptoms, which he thought were due to heat and cold as well as to certain particles which he inhaled. He recognized these symptoms in himself and described them as hay fever, a term which came to be adopted in standard medical nomenclature. Sometime later Salter realized that he must be sensitive to cat hair because when playing with cats he developed wheals or welts at the point where he was scratched by the cat. In 1890, Koch, while working with tuberculosis, realized that patients and animals developed a sensitivity to tuberculin, the product of the tuberculosis germ. At present allergy is on a sound scientific basis, even though there are many things about the subject which remain to be learned.

HOW IS ALLERGY PRODUCED?

RÔLE OF CONTACT

Previous contact with or to a substance is necessary in order for a person to develop allergy to that substance. Such contact is not always easily demonstrable. For example, one may question the occurrence of previous contact in the case of a baby who develops hives, eczema, or asthma upon ingesting cow milk for the first time. However, it may be demonstrated that the contact which produced sensitivity occurred before the baby was born and was caused by enough of the protein from cow milk ingested by the mother, reaching the baby through the placental circulation. That contact plays a rôle in the development of allergy is demonstrated by the fact that allergic individuals living in Europe where there is no ragweed pollen never develop sensitivity to this pollen. In the same way there is no sensitivity to poison ivy among Eskimos who are not exposed to poison ivy.

The next question is, how does such contact bring about allergy? This may be explained on the basis of an immunological reaction. Exposure to a given substance in a person who is predisposed to allergy causes certain tissues and organs—namely, the lymph glands, spleen, and bone marrow—to produce certain substances which are referred to as antibodies. These antibodies usually protect the person from the harmful effects of a second exposure to the same substance. For example, vaccination or infection with typhoid germs brings about the development of certain antibodies against typhoid. As long as these antibodies are present in the blood and tissues, additional exposure or infection with typhoid will bring about only mild if any symptoms at all, because the antibodies tend to neutralize or destroy the typhoid germs. So it is with many other infectious agents. However, in the case of non-living agents such as proteins, the story is quite different. An allergic person will develop antibodies against some of the proteins to which he is exposed. If, at any later date, he meets the same proteins, a union occurs between this protein or antigen and the antibodies which have been previously produced by the same protein. This union or interaction between the protein, dusts, foods, animal danders, etc., and the specifically related antibody in the tissue is thought to liberate, at least in some instances, a chemical substance which is related to histamine. This chemical substance acts upon the tissues producing the symptoms of allergy. The action largely consists of spasm of muscle and dilatation of blood vessels. When this action occurs in the skin, dilatation of the blood vessels brings about oozing of the watery portion of the blood under the skin, so that there are localized welts, and hives result; if the interaction of antigen and antibody takes place in the mucous membrane of the nose, then the water comes out of the dilated blood vessels and swells up this lining membrane so that the nasal airway is reduced and there is nasal stuffiness and nasal watery discharge and sneezing. When this interaction occurs in the lung, the lining membrane of the tubes of the lungs, the bronchi, becomes swollen, and the openings of these tubes are reduced or may even be occluded. This narrowing is also contributed to by the spasm of the muscles of the walls of the bronchi and by the outpouring of mucus in the tubes; the patient, therefore, has breathing difficulty referred to commonly as asthma. The type of symptoms produced will depend entirely on the selective sensitiveness of the particular part of the body where the antigen antibody reaction occurs. It would appear, therefore, that although the symptoms are varied, the fundamental basis for the allergic condition is the same; that is, a swelling occurring in the sensitized tissue of the allergic patient. Some allergic reactions are somewhat differently characterized by inflammatory and connective tissue changes, but in general the basis is the same. These symptoms may occur, therefore, in various parts of the body, that is, in the nose, the bronchi, the gastro-intestinal tract, or the skin. It is natural, then, for the allergic patient to seek relief by consulting various specialists, not realizing that while the manifestations are different, the cause is the same. Thus the person who has an asthmatic attack when he comes in contact with a cat, dog, or horse, and another who gets hives from eating strawberries really have the same trouble—both are allergic.

AGE OF ONSET

Allergy may develop at any age—in the young and in the old. The reason for this is not known. Of two allergic patients living in the same climate and area and exposed to the same vegetation and pollen, one may show signs of hay fever at the age of five, and the other may develop hay fever at the age of thirty-five.

DURATION

Once developed, an allergy, if untreated, usually lasts for many years. Occasionally complete disappearance may occur; this is called a spontaneous loss of sensitivity. Most frequently, though, complete loss of allergic symptoms is due to the fact that the patient no longer is exposed to the substances which produce his symptoms.

RELATION OF ALLERGY TO ADRENAL GLANDS

The adrenal glands are located one on each side at the upper pole of the kidney. These small glands produce certain substances referred to as hormones. The adrenal hormones, as discussed in the chapter on glands, have many important functions. Among these may be mentioned the regulation of water balance in the body, the metabolism of sugar and proteins, and finally the growth of certain white cells in the blood and some immunologic properties. The adrenal hormones have a profound effect on allergic conditions. The exact nature of this effect is not as yet altogether clear. At any rate, the administration of these hormones, namely cortisone, is beneficial in the treatment of allergy. In the same way ACTH, a hormone produced by the pituitary gland, which stimulates the production of the cortisone, has the same beneficial value.

CAUSES OF ALLERGY

In general, the causes of allergy may be grouped by the manner in which they become introduced into the body, that is, as inhalants, ingestants, contactants, injectants, and infectants.

INHALANTS

A large number of substances reach the body through breathing or inhalation. The fact that they are introduced through inhalation does not necessarily indicate that the symptoms will be only respiratory; for example, inhaled substances can produce hives, and conversely foods may cause asthma. Air-borne pollen and molds produce seasonal hay fever. House dust is a very important inhalant antigen. Animal hairs are frequent offenders, and for this reason allergic patients should avoid contact with or exposure to animals regardless as to whether they are skin sensitive to their hair. Contact with horses, especially riding behind a horse, or using horse blankets or being in the company of people who wear riding habits may produce severe allergic symptoms. A little boy, a physician's child, was sensitive, among other things, to horse dander and had severe asthma. With treatment his condition improved. On two separate occasions, however, the child had severe asthma. Once he attended a children's party at which one or two of the children were dressed as Indians, wrapped up in horse blankets. The second time he was feeling well. He and his mother were walking along the street when they met some friends who had just returned from horseback riding and were in an automobile. The car was stopped, the window was lowered while the conversation was carried on. A brief period of exposure to these people and their riding habits contaminated by horse dander brought about severe asthma. A social worker was also allergic to horses. Her asthma did not respond to treatment. Investigation into the possible causes of failure of therapy indicated that though this intelligent patient had been warned not to go horseback riding or come in contact with horses, she did not realize that the horse saddle which she kept under the bed in her small apartment bedroom was sufficient exposure to cause her to develop asthma, especially at night.

Infinitesimally small quantities of a substance can produce symptoms in an allergic patient. An egg-sensitive patient may develop symptoms if he uses a knife or fork that had previously been contaminated with egg and not washed properly. A child who was sensitive to potatoes could not enter the house without developing asthma if potatoes were being peeled. Another sensitive to sardines would get severe hives if present when a can of sardines was opened, and still another would get severe sneezing and asthma if present when fish was being cooked. House dust is a potent inhalant antigen. This accounts for the fact that so many allergic people sneeze and cough and develop other symptoms when they are exposed to house dust either through cleaning or sweeping. If a patient is sensitive to basement or attic dust, we suspect mold allergy. Feathers, especially old feathers, similarly are important in these conditions. Rabbit hair may be found in stuffed toys and cushions, and in various furs. Mohair contains goat hair, also a frequent offender. Until recently most cosmetics contained orris root, an ingredient which is seldom, if ever, used now in commercial cosmetics; it is no longer necessary to resort to specially high-priced so-called non-allergenic cosmetics in order to avoid orris root. Janitors are frequently sensitive to insecticides, the most common ingredient of which is pyrethrum. Among inhalants are insect emanations. This includes the caddis fly, moth, butterfly, mayfly, bee, and others. These insects give off certain hairs to which some people may be consistently sensitive. It is not uncommon, therefore, to find that there are people who develop manifestations in areas where sand flies predominate.

INGESTANTS (FOODS)

People may be sensitive to single or to multiple foods. Here again are some foods which are botanically related, so that if a patient is sensitive to one food in this group, he is sensitive to the others. Examples of this may be cited in the case of cabbage, Brussels sprouts, and cauliflower. Many of the sea foods and fresh water fish are thus similarly related; so that if a patient is sensitive to one type of fresh water fish, he is likely sensitive to the others. The most frequent allergy-producing foods are common foods, namely, milk, eggs and wheat, fish and nuts. It is unfortunate that this is the case because these are also essential foods, and this avoidance becomes a serious problem in undernourished people and in children or infants. When a patient is definitely sensitive to one or two foods only, it is not difficult for him to realize it himself. The difficulty arises, however, when he is allergic to many foods. Under these circumstances he is likely to become confused and then he needs a physician's help. Allergy to a food may be of various degrees of severity. Symptoms of asthma or hives may not arise if only one food is eaten if the sensitivity is mild. However, if a number of such foods are ingested at one time, the symptoms may be pronounced. Another factor which is important in connection with the production of symptoms is the readiness with which a food is absorbed from the gastro-intestinal tract. The quicker the absorption, the more rapid will the symptoms develop after eating.

In the case of sensitivity to eggs, the allergy, as a rule, is to the egg white and not to the egg yolk. Heating destroys, in many instances, the active part of the egg white by coagulating it. For this reason some people who are allergic to eggs may find it possible to eat hard-boiled eggs without developing symptoms. The same is true in the case of milk because heat destroys certain active principles in the milk and under given circumstances, some allergic people may find it possible to drink boiled milk. Patients who are sensitive to egg or milk or wheat find it impossible to take any foods which contain these various ingredients. The name of a proprietary food does not always indicate the presence of these substances; thus eggs are found in mayonnaise, waffles, ice cream, meringue icing, covering for bonbons, and bread. Certain vaccines, like the influenza vaccine, are prepared on egg media and should be avoided by such patients.

Similarly, milk-sensitive patients should avoid milk-containing foods: custards, candy, cake, cheese, and bread; nor can such people drink powdered or evaporated milk.

Cereals include many substances to which one may be sensitive. These are corn, rice, oats, rye, buckwheat, wheat, and others. Wheat is found in a large variety of foods: sauces, macaroni, spaghetti, noodles, bread, coffee substitutes such as postum, and many others. Corn may be used in the preparation of beer or whiskey. It is found in corn muffins, corn mush, or corn bread. Rice and rye go into the preparation of breakfast foods and many other foods.

Fish is a strong antigen because it usually produces severe symptoms. Some patients may develop asthma if they are exposed even to the odor of fish that is being cooked. The same is true of nuts. A variety of symptoms may result from the eating of nuts. These may include asthma, nose allergy, hives, or headaches. A physician, upon eating nuts, developed an eye condition which led to blindness in one eye as a result of a small hive occurring in the delicate structures of the eye. The same patient developed migraine headaches from the ingestion of peanut butter. This patient was extremely sensitive to peanuts (actually a legume, not a nut). Even the oils from nuts may contain sufficient nut protein to give symptoms, and this should be kept in mind because peanut oil is used in cooking and in the preparation of many products (candy, etc.).

Among the spices, perhaps mustard is the most frequent offender. Wieners and certain spiced meats contain mustard. Oil of wintergreen is another such agent. One patient developed severe asthma after eating a popular brand of candy bar. Then, it was discovered that this candy contained wintergreen oil. When a drop of diluted wintergreen oil was placed under the tip of the tongue of the patient, he developed severe asthma and hives. Allergy to seeds is not uncommon. This includes cottonseed and beans. A large group of asthmatic patients lived in the vicinity of a castor bean factory in Toledo; smoke from this factory contained sufficient castor bean dust to sensitize many of these people.

CONTACTANTS

These are substances with which the person comes in contact by touching or by external physical contact. A wide variety of such substances will be discussed later. These include various cosmetics, such as shampoos, face lotions, shaving lotions, mascara, and many others. Poison ivy is also a good example. Ointments which are prescribed for the relief of certain skin conditions may produce skin rashes.

INJECTANTS

Various drugs are injected into patients. These substances may elicit allergic reactions. A classical example is horse serum which has been used for a long time as a carrier for certain antitoxins and other immunity-producing agents. Not uncommonly people receiving such injections develop a reaction which is due to an allergy to the horse serum. Insect bites may also be classed under this heading. Patients may become sensitive to the proteins in the serum injected by bees, flies, or bedbugs. I saw an instance of severe hives in a nurse, thought at first to be due to foods; however, it was found later that this patient suffered with hives only when she slept in a rooming house where she boarded. She never had this difficulty when she went home. Further investigation revealed that she had severe allergy to bedbugs, with which her rooming house was infested.

PHYSICAL AGENTS

These include heat, cold, and sunlight. Severe skin reactions and other allergic manifestations may be produced by such agents.

BACTERIA AND FUNGI

Bacteria and fungi are known to be frequent sources of allergy. Infection in the nose may produce nose allergy or asthma. Intestinal parasites may similarly cause these conditions.

How Is Allergy Diagnosed?

Many people who suffer with bizarre symptoms, or with conditions that have not responded to ordinary treatment, suspect that their condition may be allergic. The purpose of an allergic diagnosis is to indicate the specific causes of a patient's allergic symptoms. However, before doing this it becomes necessary to determine that the patient's condition is allergic in nature. In this way one may avoid disillusionment and unnecessary medical handling. We know in a general way that certain diseases are allergic; for example, we know that bronchial asthma, hay fever, hives, certain forms of eczema, skin rashes, and headaches are frequently allergic in origin. We also know that certain other diseases —for example, heart disease, cancer, or acne—are not allergic. Furthermore, allergic persons as a rule present a family history of some allergic disease; they present a past or present personal history of other allergic involvement. They frequently state that they have noticed that when they eat certain things, or when they are exposed to animals or to dust, they develop symptoms; and finally they respond in a characteristic manner to certain anti-allergic drugs. On examination of the blood, many of these patients will show characteristic cells (eosinophiles), which cells may suggest the possibility of allergic disease.

HISTORY

Of all the forms of investigation to which an allergic person is submitted, none is more useful than the story told by the person himself. This frequently reveals all-important clues to the diagnosis. For this reason it is important for the patient to become acquainted with the manifestations of allergy, so that he can become more observant about the relation between his environment, his occupation, food, and habits to his symptoms. For this reason patients are encouraged to read reliable information about allergy. Much time is consumed by history taking. The history includes a detailed analysis of the various symptoms. One inquires into the date of onset, course, and severity of the condition. The occupation of the patient may shed an important light; janitors are found to be sensitive to insect powder; florists to flowers; bakers to bakery sweepings; stablemen to horses; pharmacists, in some instances, to drugs, furriers to furs. Some times symptoms are related to the acquisition of new furniture such as upholstered chairs, or new carpets, or new bedding. Children may be found sensitive to stuffed toys; some people react to cosmetics, so that they develop bronchial asthma or nose allergy when they attend movies or go to church or are in crowds in confined places. Some patients are better at work, others at home, which suggests environmental factors. A husband may be sensitive to the cosmetics used by his wife. This has been called conjugal allergy. Allergic diagnosis sometimes requires actual detective work, and much patience on the part of both the physician and his patient. A business executive had an intractable rash on his forearms. Various tests revealed little, until one day the diagnosis was finally made. On walking into the examining room and turning the doorknob, the physician commented on the fact that the wax which was used in shining the door found its way to the doorknob. The patient, who was seated in the examining room, commented casually that in his office building they used the same wax for shining the desk tops; subsequently the dermatitis with which he was severely troubled for a long time was found to be due to this wax. The patient worked with his sleeves rolled up, and contact with the wax caused the rash.

PHYSICAL EXAMINATION

Every allergic person, especially those suffering with asthma, is entitled to a careful physical examination. This is important to make sure that the condition is not due to some disease with which allergy may be confused. Frequently nasal infection produces symptoms of nasal allergy. A careful examination of the nose will reveal the presence of such an infection and the necessity of combating it by adequate treatment. Similarly, not everything that wheezes is asthma. And so it becomes necessary to determine whether the patient has tuberculosis, tumor of the lung, or heart disease, or even a foreign body in the lung, of which conditions may well produce symptoms which are indistinguishable from those of bronchial asthma. Furthermore, a skin condition which may be thought to be allergic may actually be scabies or some other non-allergic condition.

SENSITIZATION TESTS

Sensitization tests include skin tests, eye and nose tests. Unfortunately, many people, including even many physicians, believe an allergic diagnosis is synonymous with skin tests. Actually, they form only a part of the allergic survey. Furthermore, certain types of skin tests are valuable and diagnostic only for given allergic conditions, and useless and misleading in others. The materials— or extracts, as they are called—which are employed for the performance of skin tests must be active and reliable. In addition, the interpretation of the results of skin testing is equally important. Hence these tests should be read by competent physicians. It is silly to test patients with substances they never eat or to which they will never be exposed. It serves little or no purpose, for example, to test a laborer to caviar, or a shop girl to sable. The number of skin tests to be carried out will depend on the conditions surrounding the situation with which the patient is confronted. When these tests are properly performed and critically and correctly interpreted, they are an important link in the chain of evidence which may unearth the cause of the allergy. The fact that a person has had skin tests without receiving much benefit casts no reflection on skin tests themselves as a procedure. This may indicate merely that the skin tests were probably not properly performed or interpreted.

TYPE OF TESTS

In conditions in which the agent producing allergy is introduced into the body, such as through eating or inhalation, skin tests are performed by means of scratching the material into the skin or by injecting a small amount of the extract into the skin. After waiting for a period of five to ten minutes, one "reads" the reaction. The appearance of a localized swelling, wheal, or welt at the point of the scratch or injection surrounded by an area of redness indicates a positive skin test. Such a positive reaction merely indicates skin sensitivity and does not always mean that the patient cannot eat or inhale the substance. (Plate XVIII.)

When a person is sensitive through contact, the test of choice is a so-called patch test. For example, if we suspect a patient to be sensitive by contact to nail polish, it would serve no purpose to inject the nail polish with a needle; the proper procedure in such a case, or similarly in the case of poison ivy, is to apply a drop of the suspected material to the surface of the skin. After covering it with a small square of cellophane, it is held in place for forty-eight hours with adhesive. At the end of this period the material is removed; if an area of dermatitis or skin rash appears at the point of contact, we say that the patient is in all likelihood sensitive to the substance to which he was patch tested. (Plate XVIII.)

None of these tests are particularly painful. If properly performed they certainly are not dangerous. Infants as a rule do not have a very reactive skin; for this reason skin testing should be postponed until later in childhood.

Occasionally it may be useful to test for sensitivity of the lining membrane of the eyes or of the nose. In these cases a drop of a suitable liquid extract is introduced into the eye or nose. At the end of a waiting period of ten minutes, if the reaction is positive, the membranes become red and congested. Local symptoms appear—that is, watering and itching of eyes and nose—and we say that the patient is sensitive to that substance.

Another useful test in instances of suspected food allergy is the elimination diet or trial diet test. The patient is given a limited diet consisting of four or five foods for a period of five to seven days. The effect of such restriction on his symptoms is noted. Various items of food are then added to the diet every few days.

LABORATORY AND SPECIAL EXAMINATION

It frequently becomes necessary to expose the patient to additional medical studies; these may include an examination of the urine and of the blood; in cases of asthma the sputum is frequently examined for the presence of tuberculosis or of mold infection. X-rays of the chest are necessary to eliminate coexisting or other diseases. In cases of heart disease an electrocardiogram is helpful. Various tests which determine the functional capacity of the lung may also be employed. Since infections of the nose are of great importance in connection with allergy of the respiratory tract, nasal secretions are examined carefully and X-ray studies are made of the sinuses.

CONSTITUTIONAL REACTIONS

Every allergic patient and his physician must appreciate that an occasional reaction of variable severity may occur following testing or treatment with allergenic extracts. As a rule, in competent hands such reactions are rare and relatively easily controlled. They occur because the patient has been exposed to too strong a dose of extract. Patients are kept waiting in the physician's office for about half an hour following testing or treatment in order to detect a reaction as soon as it occurs, because the effect of the treatment for a reaction depends entirely on the promptness with which it is instituted. The reaction may come on within a few minutes or a few hours. When it occurs more than a half hour or an hour after treatment, it is usually not severe and not a source of worry. The sooner it occurs, the more severe is it likely to be. At first the patient experiences the itchiness of the palms of the hands, the lips, the roof of the mouth and the nose. The patient's face is flushed; hives may appear; the nose may become stuffed and begin to run. There is a choking sensation accompanied by wheezing and choking. When treatment is instituted promptly, it is effective and all of these symptoms disappear in a matter of a half hour. It is well for the patient to carry with him capsules containing ephedrine and some antihistamine so that he may take one or two such capsules should he develop a reaction after he leaves the physician's office and before he has had a chance to contact him. Unfortunately, some patients have had unfavorable experiences with such reactions and have come to the conclusion that the treatment is worse than the disease. However, such experiences are usually avoidable and easily treated if necessary.

HAY FEVER

The term hay fever is a misnomer because the condition is not due to hay nor is it associated with fever. Constant usage, however, justifies its adoption. The symptoms are well known, including usually obstruction to nasal breathing, sneezing, lacrimation, itching of the eyes and nose, and a watery nasal discharge. Occasionally these patients may have asthma. Because the symptoms result from sensitivity to pollen, they will be seasonal and will coincide with the pollination dates in a given area, because pollen surveys indicate what pollens are prevalent in various areas. This information is of great value since patients have been known to leave the eastern seaboard, for example, and go to California, Florida, or Texas in order to avoid hay fever. They may, however, leave their home when the hay fever season is about over and reach their destination at the beginning of the pollinating season in that region of the country. Of course, in order for a pollen to be hay fever producing it is necessary for it to fulfil certain requirements; the pollen must grow in abundance in the given district; it must be light and wind-borne, and must be sufficiently widely distributed. Pollen that is heavy is carried by the wind with difficulty, and since it is not found in the air it will not produce hay fever. Goldenrod is an example. This pollen is conspicuous because of its color and because it is found in the neighborhood of ragweed, a common hay fever producing plant. Because of these reasons the patient frequently blames goldenrod as a cause of his trouble. Prevailing climatic conditions also control the abundance of pollen in the air and, therefore, the severity of the patient's symptoms. For example, heavy rain preceding the hay fever season naturally aids in the growth of vegetation and increases the supply of pollen. Sunshine in the early morning hours helps to dry the pollen and in this way renders it lighter for wind distribution. Heavy winds further help to distribute pollen and increase its concentration in the air. Some parts of the country are pollen free. These are usually areas in the northern parts of Canada. Pollen can be carried by the wind for a hundred miles or even more. Seasonal hay fever symptoms may be due not only to sensitivity to pollens, but also to sensitivity to the spores of certain molds and fungi which may be found in the air during certain seasons. (Plate XIX.)

In spite of the fact that the symptoms of a hay fever patient are a source of great entertainment to non-hay-fever sufferers, hay fever patients are frequently quite miserable. Their symptoms may interfere with their happiness, with their ability to do their work, and to lead a normal life for several weeks or months out of the year. Just how seriously this condition may interfere with one's life may be gathered from reading a biography of Daniel Webster—a hay fever sufferer.

DIAGNOSIS OF HAY FEVER

The history as to the date of onset and the date of termination of symptoms is highly suggestive of the cause, because we know the date of pollination for the given areas. Skin tests are performed with dilutions of these various pollens to confirm the diagnosis. Occasionally eye or "sniff" tests are made.

TREATMENT OF HAY FEVER

Much can be done for the hay fever patient. The most rational and the most dependable form of treatment is still the "desensitization" treatment. This involves the injection of increasing doses of pollen extracts at variable intervals. The treatment is begun sufficiently before the beginning of the season so that the patient may receive a maximum dose at this time. The injections are spaced from three to seven days apart; each subsequent dose is increased in strength, provided the patient's arm does not swell and become sore as a result of the previous dose. After reaching the top dose, treatment is then continued at monthly intervals throughout the entire year. The responsibility of carrying out and adhering to this schedule is the patient's. Treatments may not be given at intervals longer than four weeks. Unless this is remembered, a constitutional reaction may follow, for there is a tendency for a patient to lose his tolerance for a given dose under these circumstances. This form of treatment is not only effective in ridding the patient of symptoms and making life more pleasant for him, but it is also helpful in avoiding the extension of the patient's hay fever symptoms into his chest and the development of asthma. As a result of lessening the hay fever symptoms, treated patients are less likely to develop sinusitis and other undesirable complications of hay fever.

The hay fever sufferer will do well to avoid drafts and winds. He should not travel through the country. Ventilation for his bedroom should be provided with a partly opened window in the next room. If it is necessary that the bedroom window be opened, a damp sheet should be stretched across it so as to catch the incoming dust and pollens. The use of a damp gauze mask or any of the other available masks may be helpful. Change of climate is effective provided it is definitely known that the offending pollen is not found at the patient's intended destination. Many resorts widely advertise that they are pollen-free, but on investigation are found to be no better than the patient's home town. The seashore offers relief only on days when the wind blows from the sea inland.

In addition, these patients are helped by certain drugs such as antihistamines, nose drops, and by ephedrine.

The treatment as outlined is a long cry from that used during the life and time of Oliver Wendell Holmes, a hay fever sufferer himself, who said the only effective treatment for this condition was six feet of gravel.

PERENNIAL NASAL ALLERGY (ALLERGIC RHINITIS)

Nasal allergy is a condition associated with symptoms referable to the nose. These are obstruction to nasal breathing, stuffiness of the nose, sneezing, and a nasal discharge which is usually watery. Unlike hay fever which is seasonal, this condition is present throughout the year. It is frequently confused with the common cold.

THE DIAGNOSIS

If a person has frequent colds which last for a variable period of time, maybe a few hours to a few days, and recur again and again, one should suspect allergy involving the nasal membrane. This diagnosis may be corroborated by the examination of the nose and its secretions. It must be differentiated from sinusitis, which in reality is not an allergy but an infection. Nasal allergy may become complicated, if untreated, by sinusitis.

THE TREATMENT

This includes avoidance of causative agents, diet, and injection treatment or so-called desensitization. Correction of nasal deformity which blocks off the nasal passages may be necessary. If sinusitis is present, the condition is treated as though there were no allergy present, and then allergic treatment follows.

Emotional factors should also be attended to. A man had typical nasal allergy. Because of his difficulty in proper breathing, he used nose drops constantly and this actually made him worse; he could not attend a dinner party or business conference without using his nose drops. He had just changed jobs and there was considerable insecurity in his new position. This instability made his nasal condition unbearable until it was remedied.

Nasal mucous membrane constrictors, while giving the patient relief for a few minutes, invariably cause the condition to become worse later because of the secondary swelling or congestion that follows. For this reason patients with nasal allergy should not use nose drops to excess. In instances in which emotional factors play an important contributory rôle, psychotherapy—that is, discussion of the patient's problems with him—in addition to allergic treatment is helpful. Antihistamine drugs are also valuable in the treatment of these conditions. People with allergic rhinitis should not sleep in a room the temperature of which falls below seventy, because chilling of various parts of the body produces nasal congestion.

PROGNOSIS (OUTLOOK)

In most instances of nasal allergy the outlook is fairly good; especially if the condition has not reached the irreversible stage in which there are various complications, and especially if nasal infection is absent. Because these complications occur so frequently, nasal allergy should be treated early.

BRONCHIAL ASTHMA

Bronchial asthma is a form of allergy which involves the lungs and its tubes —the bronchi. It is characterized by spells of coughing, wheezing, choking, and shortness of breath. In children the only manifestation may be an intractable, recurrent cough which is of unknown cause and which does not respond to ordinary treatment.

FACTORS AFFECTING ASTHMA

Climate seems to affect the asthmatic patient. This is particularly true of climate characterized by great variations of temperature and increased humidity. Under these circumstances an increased incidence of respiratory tract infections occurs, and these in turn precipitate asthma. Seasonal variations are present particularly in instances of pollen or mold sensitivity. The patient's occupation may play a very important role. Glandular disturbances such as accompany pregnancy, menstruation, and menopause may contribute to the severity of the asthmatic attack. Many patients are free or relatively free of asthma during pregnancy and are invariably worse during the menstrual cycle. Emotional factors are quite important in this connection; they affect all allergic patients to a great extent. Pungent and irritating odors, such as turpentine, gasoline, smoke, and fog, have a bad effect on the asthmatic symptoms.

An allergic patient should be studied carefully from a medical as well as an allergic point of view. This is necessary because wheezing, choking, and shortness of breath may be caused by conditions which are not allergic. Heart disease, tuberculosis, tumor of the lung, foreign bodies, and many other conditions may cause symptoms which are indistinguishable from those of bronchial asthma. A young man had severe asthmatic manifestations for three years. He had various studies, including allergic studies followed by treatment which proved ineffective. It developed that he had a small foreign body at the base of the right lung. This was later removed by bronchoscopic treatment. Shortly before the onset of his asthma, the patient was in a brawl in one of the local night clubs. He was bounced out of the night club unceremoniously, and during this procedure he had several teeth knocked out. He aspirated one of these which was attached by a small metal clip. Following bronchoscopic removal of the tooth, the patient's condition improved.

TREATMENT OF ASTHMA

Treatment of bronchial asthma includes removal of the offending substance from the patient's environment, desensitization, and the administration of certain drugs.

"DESENSITIZATION"

Increasing doses of extracts of the substance to which the patient is sensitive are administered. Most of these patients are allergic to house dust. Some of them are sensitive to molds. Suitable mixtures of these may be prepared, including also other inhalants which the patient finds impossible to avoid; the patient is then treated with such extracts in a manner similar to that adopted in the treatment of the hay fever.

Asthmatics are suspectible to frequent colds, and because they usually have an associated bronchitis, they also receive suitable help toward controlling these conditions.

DRUGS

Medicinal treatment includes the use of many drugs; perhaps the most important of these is epinephrin, or, as it is sometimes called, adrenalin. There are now available adrenalin preparations which may be used by inhalation with a nebulizer as well as by injection, in accordance with the following directions: Remove stopper from throat tube and drop solution in as directed in the instructions with nebulizer. Place throat tube inside teeth and inhale deeply while compressing the bulb. Do not press bulb while exhaling. Only press on bulb three to five times at each treatment, and only use nebulizer about every three hours. Replace stopper after each use so that solution does not spoil, and return nebulizer to box. Add solutions only when necessary. Clean instrument according to instructions which are inclosed. A clean nebulizer and knowledge of how to use it are essential for maximum benefit. Ephedrine capsules and iodides are also helpful in loosening up the secretions which clog the bronchi.

In instances in which the asthmatic attack does not respond to such treatment, it may be necessary for the patient to be hospitalized. It is amazing to see how quickly improvement takes place under those circumstances. Oxygen as well as ACTH and cortisone may also be given if necessary.

Antibiotics are employed if infection is present.

NASAL INFECTION AND ASTHMA

Nasal infection should be treated conservatively at first and by surgery if necessary.

BRONCHIAL ASTHMA AS A SURGICAL RISK

As a rule, it is safe to proceed with any surgery during the period between asthmatic attacks. Precaution should be observed with regard to the anesthetic and drugs employed.

PROGNOSIS (OUTLOOK)

The results from treatment are usually dramatic in patients who have asthma due to one or two substances. It is comparatively easy for these patients to avoid these offending agents. If there are no complicating factors, the results are even better. This is especially true in children. However, when there are complications such as infection and changes in the structure of the lung, the outlook is not quite as good. Even in these cases proper and prolonged treatment accompanied by co-operation on the patient's part is helpful. The asthmatic person must realize that the condition from which he has been suffering for a period of many years cannot disappear overnight; and that a great deal of effort, co-operation, and painstaking treatment is necessary to bring about desirable results. Fortunately, death occurs but rarely from asthma. The younger the patient, the better is the outlook. As the patient's condition lasts longer, certain complications result; these include infection in the lungs (bronchitis and bronchiectasis) and pulmonary fibrosis.

SKIN ALLERGY

The incidence of skin allergy is high. There are many different kinds of skin allergy. These may be divided into allergic skin conditions due to sensitivity to substances which reach the body through contact from without and those which produce allergy as a result of distribution following eating or inhaling of certain other foods or material. The skin is an important organ of the body; it takes a great deal of punishment. It is exposed constantly to all sorts of changes in temperature and humidity, to pressure, pull, tear, rubbing, infection and many mechanical and chemical factors.

CONTACT DERMATITIS

The outstanding example of contact dermatitis is poison ivy dermatitis, which affects a large segment of the population. This type of skin rash is due to an allergy or sensitivity to the oily fraction in the poison ivy plant; since symptoms are produced by contact, the dermatitis or rash occurs on the exposed surfaces of the body. However, it is not unusual to find these manifestations also on covered parts of the body. The explanation for this is that the material to which the person is sensitive is carried by the fingers to these areas. To indicate the frequency with which this type of mechanism can play a rôle in contact dermatitis, Dr. Sulzberger, some time ago, carried out the following experiment: He painted fluorescein on the fingers of a number of his patients and instructed them not to wash their hands or to take a bath for twenty-four hours. At the end of this time he exposed these patients, in the nude in a dark room, to ultraviolet rays. Now ultraviolet rays cause this material to fluoresce. This took place not only on the previously painted fingers, but also on various parts of the body that were covered.

CAUSES OF CONTACT DERMATITIS

There are many substances that produce contact dermatitis. I have already mentioned plant oils. Occasionally there are people who develop a contact dermatitis during certain seasons of the year. Closer investigation reveals that these people are sensitive to oily fraction of seasonal pollens and plants. Contact dermatitis may also be due to occupational substances such as chemicals, furs, dyes, leather, cosmetics, and many drugs.

When confronted with a condition that is suspected as being contact dermatitis, we try to find out as much information as possible to shed light upon the possible causes.

In the case of factory workers sensitive to given substances, certain preventative measures must be employed. These include forced circulation which gets rid of the dust to which the person may be sensitive, compulsory showers, protective clothing, gloves, etc. In some instances it may be necessary for the person to change his occupation. In these instances the amount of local application which is intended to relieve the itching is reduced to a minimum. At first these local applications do give the patient some relief, but eventually in many instances they may make him worse, because he may actually become allergic to the ointment which is prescribed for his relief.

In some instances treatment with the offending agent is employed, such as in the case of poison ivy dermatitis where the patient is given increasing doses of a poison ivy extract in the hope of increasing tolerance to this material. One must exercise care in such treatment for fear of distributing and aggravating the condition.

COSMETICS

Among cosmetics, nail polish and mascara are a frequent cause of contact dermatitis. Nail polish contains tin oxide and some abrasive powder. It may be colorless when used for men, or it may be slightly tinted. Nail enamel or liquid nail polish contains a large variety of ingredients. Dermatitis in these instances does not necessarily occur on the hands, but usually occurs on the face, especially on the eyelids because of the habit of some people to rub their eyelids with the back of their fingers. Various preparations which are applied to the face or to the hair may produce contact dermatitis, among which two of the most important are hair dyes and permanent wave preparations. Hair lacquer shellac is a frequent offender. It would, therefore, seem desirable to test people for sensitivity to the substances when they have dermatitis of unknown origin. Certainly no one who has a tendency to contact dermatitis should use hair dyes without first making sure that he is not sensitive to these dyes. A woman who was emotionally unstable dyed her hair. She had dyed her hair some years previously and following this second experience she developed a severe dermatitis of the entire scalp, face, and neck; the itching and subsequent nervous manifestations became so serious that in her despondency she committed suicide.

Other causes of such psychodermatitis are perspiration detergents and deodorants. In men, after-shaving lotions, shaving creams, and shaving soaps may produce dermatitis of the face. Plastics have been known to be a frequent offender in this connection, and of course numberless articles contain plastics. Artificial teeth, telephone receivers, cigar holders, varnishes, cheap jewelry, stockings, steering wheels, dishes, water containers, and other devices are made of plastic.

INFANTILE ECZEMA (ATOPIC DERMATITIS)

Skin eruptions which may occur at any time in life but which usually are found in infants and children may be eczema. The condition at first appears on the face and on the back of the wrists. Later in childhood it may be found in the bends of the elbows and the region back of the knees. At first the skin becomes red. Later small blobs or vesicles appear. As a result of scratching, these break open and oozing takes place. There is severe itchiness, and this constitutes the most disturbing feature of the disease. Allergic factors play a rather important rôle in this dermatitis. Most of these people have a family history of allergy. They may present other allergic manifestations, such as hay fever or asthma. Indeed, in some instances it is realized that the infant or child cannot tolerate certain foods or is sensitive to certain substances in his environment. One two-year-old boy had eczema on the inner surface of the elbows and back of the knees. The child would lose his voice following the ingestion of potatoes, peas, chicken, and eggs. Playing with stuffed toys produced paroxysms of asthma. He was quite sensitive to spices. Once while in the kitchen, he got hold of several boxes of spices which he emptied into a pot and pretended he was going to bake a cake for his father. He immediately developed a severe attack of asthma and a severe flare-up in his eczema. There is also evidence which emphasizes that nervous influences play an equally important role in the causation of this disease. If the cause of infantile eczema is not recognized and treated properly and early, there may occur, as a result of continuous scratching and skin injury, certain secondary changes in the skin. The skin becomes thick and leathery, and fissured or infected.

Because the skin of infants is not suitable for skin testing, it is important to arrive at a diagnosis by trial and elimination. As a rule, it is best to study such cases in the hospital. By so doing, the patient is most likely to be removed from the environmental sources of his difficulty; these factors may be dust, household inhalants, and many other substances which are present in his home, and to which he may be allergic. Elimination diets are tried.

LOCAL TREATMENT OF ALLERGIC DERMATITIS

Most persons who suffer with allergic dermatitis have accumulated numberless lotions, salves, ointments, and other local preparations. These have either been prescribed for them or suggested to them by their family or friends. For the most part, the effects of these long-continued local applications is to further irritate and traumatize the skin, so that in the end more harm than good is done. First take away all these various drugs and prescribe only such bland preparations as are least likely to injure the skin. These must be cautiously and carefully applied, observing their changing effect. Indeed, at times it is necessary to use the preparation of one area of the skin only, such as one arm or one leg, and observe the difference between the dermatitis on that area and on the area of the body where no preparation has been used. Furthermore, an allergy may develop to the very preparation or substance that has been prescribed for the alleviation of the patient's disturbing itch. All local irritants must be avoided. The most important of these is soap. The patient is urged to employ a non-irritating cleansing substance, of which there are many on the market, such as Lowella Cake or Phisoderm Basis Soap. The patient must, of course, avoid washing dishes. If that is absolutely essential, she should use thin white cotton gloves over which may be worn thin rubber gloves. One avoids the use of rubber gloves directly on the skin because the heat and the sweat which is thus generated may macerate and further hurt the skin.

In the case of infants it must be remembered that the severe itchiness disturbs the child and renders him sleepless and fussy, causing him to lose weight. As a result of scratching, secondary infection appears, and this requires special treatment. In view of the fact that the mother's emotional attitude so frequently reflects itself on the child's reaction to his condition, it is often necessary to direct one's effort toward the proper handling of the mother. She must be reassured that the child's skin condition is not infectious and contagious and that it will in no way affect the infant's general health. The mother must learn to be more patient and less anxious about the child's condition. With older children it is important to take time out to discuss the nature of the condition and give some hope and encouragement as to the final outcome.

One should, of course, avoid the irritating effects of rough clothing and blankets, particularly wool. Feather pillows should be covered, or, better still, rubber foam pillows should be procured. If the child comes in direct contact with the mother, she should avoid the use of irritating and allergenic cosmetics and perfumes. The room should be kept at a steady temperature because constant changes in temperature will affect the skin also. Excitement should be avoided insofar as possible. Digestive disturbances and the effects of irritating fumes and odors should be eliminated. Diapers should be boiled in boric acid in order to remove traces of soap. This also helps to counteract the irritating effects of ammoniacal urine. In infants it is frequently necessary to immobilize the arms, especially at night, in order to avoid scratching. This is done by placing cardboard cylinders around the elbows. The nails are filed and the fingers are taped. If the baby has an intolerance to milk, boiled skimmed milk or, better still, goat milk should be given. One should watch for such symptoms as diarrhea and loss of weight and evidence of infection, which conditions should be treated as soon as they appear. At times it is necessary to give the child some form of sedation which the doctor will prescribe.

Urticaria and Angioedema (Hives)

Hives consist of wheals and welts of various sizes occurring throughout the entire body. These are accompanied by severe itching. At times these may be massive so that the swelling may involve the lips or the eyes. Indeed, the eyes may become shut, or the tongue may become swollen. A glue-sensitive patient developed tremendous swelling of the tongue after licking stamps so that he had difficulty getting his tongue back in his mouth. These swellings may occur in the throat so that the patient may have difficulty in swallowing or difficulty in breathing. When this occurs one may have to deal with a serious emergency. A young college student was found sensitive to sulfa drugs. In spite of being warned about this, he chose to chew some sulfa gum when he thought he was developing a sore throat. Soon after that he developed edema or swelling of the throat and uvula so that he began to choke. He was brought to the emergency room where the condition was found to be so critical that the intern did not take the time to take him to the operating room, but immediately performed a tracheotomy—that is, made a hole in the patient's windpipe in order to permit him to breathe and thus dramatically saved his life.

In about one third or one half of all cases of hives, some form of allergy may be demonstrated. Once the cause is found, treatment becomes rather simple. It consists largely in avoidance. Careful dietetic treatment is often necessary. In addition, the patient is frequently relieved by the administration of the antihistamine drugs. These should be taken only as prescribed by the physician.

SERUM DISEASE

There are occasions when it is necessary to treat patients with serum obtained from some animal, usually horses. These horses are immunized against certain diseases, and their serum contains the specific antibody which will help fight the disease in the patient. However, serum injection may lead to a train of symptoms referred to as serum reaction. This is a form of allergy. Two to twelve days following the administration of serum, the patient develops hives, a slight elevation of temperature, joint symptoms, and nausea and vomiting. As a rule, however, these symptoms are easily treated with antihistamines and adrenalin, and in a few days the patient is well. There is nothing dangerous about this type of reaction.

Rarely, however, a patient who has had serum before may, upon receiving serum for the second time, develop much more serious reactions. For this reason asthmatic patients, especially those who give a history of sensitivity or allergy to horses, must avoid such serums.

ALLERGY TO DRUGS

A similar type of reaction to that which occurs following the administration of horse serum may also occur following certain drugs. Almost any kind of skin rash may develop as a result of drug allergy; or the patient may develop asthma or hay fever. Whenever a patient develops a skin rash or unexplainable symptoms during the course of some illness, keep in mind the possibility that these symptoms are produced by a drug which the patient is receiving. Not infrequently the elimination of these drugs will cause a sudden disappearance of the symptoms. Sulfa drugs, aspirin, coal-tar products, iodine, bromine, belladonna, antibiotics such as penicillin, insulin, liver extract, and many others are frequent offenders in this connection. These reactions are so common that the question arising now during the course of treatment is not what drug to prescribe, but which drug to omit.

PHYSICAL ALLERGY

Some persons, when exposed to changes in temperature such as cold or heat or when exposed to sudden effort or sunlight, may develop allergic manifestations, such as asthma, hay fever, or hives. In these instances the cold or heat acts as an antigen, much the same as milk or pollen may produce allergy. The demonstration of the presence of such sensitivity requires special tests. In the case of a patient sensitive to cold one tests the patient by attaching a small tube containing ice water to the skin of the arm. The tube is held in place with adhesive. Sensitivity to cold is determined by the appearance of a large welt or hive at the point of contact. A similar test may be carried out with hot water. Undoubtedly, under this classification of allergy are also included those patients who when exposed to a draft or a cold breeze develop nasal symptoms followed by severe so-called sinus headaches.

Physical allergy is relatively not serious. Under unusual circumstances it may prove to be serious. Some instances are reported in which a child, after diving into a swimming pool, died suddenly. Examination after death did not reveal water in the lungs. Obviously the child did not drown. He was a good swimmer. There was no history of pre-existing heart disease or other conditions which might explain such a sudden death. Death in these cases is usually due to asphyxia, brought about by the sudden swelling or hivelike formation in the throat, shutting off the air passages so that the patient cannot breathe. These hives or swellings are produced by sensitivity to cold. The change in temperature brought about by the sudden diving into the cold water is responsible for symptoms in cold-sensitive patients.

Similarly other patients develop hives or certain forms of skin rashes upon exposure to a small amount of sunlight. This type of skin reaction is unusually severe. It occurs upon minimal exposure as compared with the sunburn which most people develop upon prolonged sunlight exposure. A directress of nurses was sensitive to sunlight. She sought a position in one of the Pittsburgh hospitals because she had heard that Pittsburgh has little sunlight. A few days after her arrival in Pittsburgh she found out otherwise. She continued to develop severe dermatitis on exposed surfaces, in spite of the fact that she protected herself by wearing a large picture hat, and using newspapers or a parasol when walking during the daytime from the nurses' home to the main hospital building.

There is no specific and effective treatment against physical allergy. Antihistamines are of some help. However, such patients must be taught to protect themselves against exposure. Sometimes a tolerance may be developed by continued exposure to small doses of cold, heat, or sunlight, whichever the offending agent may be.

ALLERGIC HEADACHE

Certain types of headache are allergic in origin. In these cases patients develop headaches of variable severity when exposed to substances to which they are allergic. These may be food or inhalants. The symptoms vary with the person. As a rule, the pain is deep and sometimes throbbing, or it may acquire the characteristics of so-called sick headache or migraine. Not all instances of migraine are allergic in nature. When one realizes that chronic headaches interfere with the patient's happiness and productivity, a serious effort must be made in each case to discover its cause. It must by no means be assumed that every case of headache is allergic, because most frequently the cause of headache is something other than allergy. In the case of chronic recurrent headache one must always rule out some serious systemic condition like kidney disease, anemia, infection, or brain tumor.

As a rule, sick headaches are accompanied by pain which is located on one side of the face and head. The patient may be sick at the stomach, and the very thought or odor of food nauseates him. He usually cannot tolerate light and prefers to be lying down. He does not want to be disturbed. He does not invite sympathy. A young physician would invariably get these sick headaches on holidays. Not until he had an allergic survey was it discovered that he was very sensitive to chicken. These two facts were then correlated. There was usually a family dinner on holidays, and chicken was invariably served at these functions. As a matter of fact, this patient could not eat any soup which had chicken stock in it, nor could he eat any food which had been cooked in pots that had previously contained chicken unless they were thoroughly scrubbed. By scrupulously avoiding chicken, he managed to reduce the frequency and severity of his headaches. The patient's "nerves" may also have a bearing on the occurrence of his headaches. Most of these persons have a characteristic personality. They are usually perfectionists. They burn the candle at both ends and usually also in the middle. They demand a lot from themselves, as well as from those by whom they are surrounded. They have tremendous drive. Treatment involves, in addition to allergic management and improvement in general health, an attempt at change in the patient's philosophy of living and attitude toward his environment. He must learn to take things a bit easier. He must learn to enjoy leisure time. Conflicts and the cause of emotional upsets must be resolved. Some form of psychotherapy is often helpful. Those who suffer with chronic recurrent intractable headaches are miserable. There is no class of more grateful people than these—if they experience relief from their distressing symptoms; hence they are entitled to every bit of help they can get.

BACTERIAL ALLERGY

A person may be allergic not only to foods and inhalants, but also to the bacteria or germs which may infect him. Particularly is this true of bacteria which produce infection in the nasal sinuses, so that one may well develop asthma or nose symptoms as a result of such bacterial allergy. Indeed, it is thought that rheumatic fever symptoms are produced by an allergy to the germ that is found associated with this condition. Another example of bacterial allergy is tuberculosis. Symptoms of tuberculosis have been shown to develop from allergy to the products of the tuberculosis germ, namely tuberculin. For this reason present or past tuberculous infection may be demonstrated by skin testing with tuberculin.

ALLERGY OF THE EYES

Many eye conditions are possibly due to an allergy. This includes not only involvement of the eyelids—that is, both the inner and outer surface of the eyelids—but also of the eyeball and of some of the delicate structures within the eye. An elderly physician experienced a "blind spot" in one eye and swelling of the fingers after eating fish. Contact dermatitis of the eyelids is not uncommon. Eye symptoms are frequent in hay fever.

ALLERGIC DIZZINESS

Many are the causes of dizziness. However, if a person is otherwise allergic and after a careful examination no other causes are found for his dizziness, then it is well to think of the possibility that this condition is produced by allergy. There may or may not be associated ringing in the ears and various degrees of loss of hearing. In certain conditions a person may break out in a cold sweat; the duration of the condition may vary from a few minutes to a few hours. There may be vomiting. When due to allergy, dizziness is caused by hives or swelling of the delicate structures of the internal ears. A clerk developed these symptoms for the first time after he was engaged in licking stamps and envelope flaps on a large number of items that were to be mailed. Subsequently it was found that this patient was sensitive to sweet potatoes, and we discovered that stamp glue is made from sweet potatoes. Absorption of this material into the blood produced ear involvement and the resulting dizziness. A civil engineer was found sensitive among other things to garlic. After he received his report and on thinking it over, it occurred to him that he had been having many of his attacks of dizziness after his evening meal. Further inquiry revealed the interesting information that they were using garlic in a shaker for seasoning foods at the table. Doing away with the garlic shaker, his evening attacks of dizziness almost completely disappeared.

GASTRO-INTESTINAL ALLERGY

Gastric symptoms often follow the ingestion of certain foods. Children are particularly prone to develop vomiting and abdominal pain from foods to which they are allergic. If the food is an essential one like milk or eggs, and one does not realize that the child is allergic, the parents are likely to insist that the child continue to drink milk or eat eggs in spite of these symptoms. As a result, the child continues to become worse. The manifestation of such allergy may be only gastro-intestinal—namely, nausea, vomiting, cramps, and diarrhea. There may be skin lesions about the mouth, namely, eczema; or there may be ulcerations in the mouth, in the throat, or of the stomach or the intestines. Any or all parts of the gastro-intestinal tract may be involved. Mucous colitis is frequently due to an allergic condition. The elimination of the offending foods frequently brings about an almost miraculous change in the patient's condition. Skin tests, careful history, and trial and elimination diets are frequently helpful.

URINARY BLADDER SYMPTOMS

Urinary bladder symptoms may on occasion be produced as a result of allergy. Careful examination fails to reveal any evidence of disease, and yet the patient has serious local symptoms; eliminating the offending factors may bring about almost immediate relief.

MENSTRUAL DISTURBANCES

Many reports indicate that on occasion menstrual disturbances are due to allergic factors. In this connection, occasionally, when a constitutional reaction is obtained in a female patient, due to an overdose of treatment, menstrual cramps may develop.

JOINT INVOLVEMENT

Swelling and pain in the joints may occur because of an allergy to foods or other substances. Joint involvement is a frequent accompaniment of allergy to serums and to drugs. Similar symptoms may also be found after ingestion of foods. The wife of a physician had severe hives at various times in her life. The last attack of hives was associated with excruciating pain in the region of the back of the neck. The patient had severe pain in the neck and limitation of motion. X-ray and other examinations of this region failed to reveal any evidence of disease. The patient was anxious, restless, and sleepless. Because of this it was thought at first that these were nervous manifestations, and the patient was diagnosed as a psychoneurotic. An allergy survey revealed that she was sensitive to several foods and particularly to grapes. On several occasions she noticed that drinking champagne, or grape wine, brought about an attack of hives as well as an attack of pain in the neck. Proper allergic treatment gave her complete relief from all of these disturbing symptoms.

EPILEPSY

Several instances are on record of convulsions which have been relieved by removal of offending foods from the patient's diet. These instances are rare. The epileptic patient who is otherwise allergic, and has a family history of allergy, is entitled to an allergic survey and allergic management in the hope that such investigation may bring about some improvement in the condition.

ALLERGY IN CHILDREN

The importance of an early diagnosis of allergy cannot be overemphasized. This diagnosis should be made in infancy or early childhood. This involves not only recognition that the condition affecting the child is allergic, but also a serious attempt at discovering the cause of the allergy. In doing this, however, one meets frequently with a great deal of resistance by the mother because she does not want to see the child hurt, or because she somehow has a vague suspicion that skin testing endangers the child's health. The mother must understand the importance of such an early diagnosis. She must realize that delay is equivalent to neglect, and that neglect needlessly exposes the child to the dangers of complications which may result from an untreated allergy. When handled early, it is comparatively easy to diagnose and treat effectively a case of hay fever or a case of asthma in a child. After a few years, however, this condition becomes complicated by nasal infection or by bronchitis, or by changes in the tissues of the lungs. These changes become refractory to treatment, so that even if the allergy is discovered, treatment of complications becomes difficult if not impossible. The mother must also understand that skin testing, if properly done, is not dangerous and does not affect the child's physical condition.

Bronchial asthma is frequently preceded in infants and in children by an unexplainable persistent cough which occurs in spasms and does not respond to ordinary treatment; furthermore, because asthma in infants and children is frequently associated with fever, the condition is misdiagnosed as due to pneumonia. If a child has frequent unexplained cough accompanied by wheezing and high fever, he probably does not have pneumonia, but has bronchial asthma. If the child's nasal or chest symptoms are seasonal, always suspect that he is sensitive to pollen or to seasonal molds. These patients are not uncommonly said to suffer with frequent so-called summer colds, when in reality they are allergic. A little girl had attacks of asthma especially severe in the early summer when she was taken to the lake where her parents had a cottage. Investigation revealed her to be sensitive not only to certain foods, but also to dust and to fungi. The cottage was closed during the winter and became dusty and mildewed due to increased humidity and to lack of ventilation. Her allergy to these molds found in the cottage was responsible for her summer asthma.

Furthermore, infants are frequently sensitive to many foods. Many different ingredients are included in the numerous proprietary baby foods. In the case of breast-fed babies the infant may be sensitive to some food ingested by the mother and passed into mother's milk in quantities sufficient to produce symptoms in the baby. Nasal allergy is common in children. The child experiences considerable itchiness of the nose. His delicate nasal membranes are swollen, and he finds it difficult to breathe through the nose; the child makes an attempt at scratching the tip of the nose with the palm of his hand, pushing the tip of the nose upward and backward, in that way spreading the nasal walls apart so that he can also breathe more easily. Nose rubbing and nose wrinkling are some of the common mannerisms developed by these children, and have been dubbed "the allergic salute." (Plate XXI.)

Because little was known about allergy some twenty years ago, it was not an uncommon practice for physicians to dismiss an allergic infant or child with the remark, "The child will outgrow his condition." On rare occasions spontaneous recovery does result. Most frequently, however, when recovery results, it is because of a fortuitous coincidental removal of the patient from environmental substances to which he is allergic. As a rule, in spite of wishful thinking and endless temporizing, if untreated, the allergic child continues to suffer, and as a result of this neglect he frequently develops complications and secondary changes which make difficult the solution of a problem which was comparatively simple in the beginning. For this reason the parents of allergic children have a direct and immediate responsibility, to seek competent and adequate attention for their allergic children.

In the case of children suffering from allergic skin conditions do not attempt to vaccinate the child during the active phase of the skin condition because such a procedure may lead to a widespread involvement and aggravation of the skin condition.

IMMUNIZATION PROCEDURES IN CHILDREN

Children must be vaccinated against smallpox, diphtheria, and tetanus. In certain regions of the country typhoid vaccination is indicated. A tuberculin test should always be done. Rabies vaccine should be used when necessary. Tetanus toxoid should be given to children who have been previously immunized against tetanus when exposure demands it. Immunization procedures are essential, necessary, and effective. They carry with them no danger whatever. In many instances they are, indeed, lifesaving.

Vaccination against smallpox should be carried out between the ages of three and twelve months. This vaccination should be repeated between the ages of seven and eleven years, especially if there is an epidemic or if the patient is to leave for another country. Tuberculin tests should be performed at the age of three years, and later if needed. Possible combined vaccines are being used successfully now against diphtheria, tetanus, and pertussis, starting at the age of three months.

A Schick test is done between the ages of eighteen and twenty-four months in order to determine whether the child has developed immunity against diphtheria. Re-immunization should be performed if needed. Tetanus toxoid may be given at any period, although booster doses are repeated every one to three years. Typhoid fever vaccine is administered if the child is to travel to areas where there is typhoid fever or there is a possible danger of such exposure.

TREATMENT OF ALLERGY

The general principles of allergic treatment are somewhat similar for all allergic diseases. Every allergic patient should have an understanding of what this treatment implies. Following the completion of the diagnostic procedures, the patient is given to understand that his complete co-operation is essential. Unless he is willing to help, any effort at allergic management is bound to lead to disappointment. The nature and duration of the patient's condition itself indicates the necessity of prolonged and careful treatment.

GENERAL PROCEDURES

The patient's health is cared for. There must be a sufficient amount of rest. Foci of infection, such as diseased teeth and tonsils, are removed. If the patient is anemic, an attempt is made to correct this condition.

PSYCHOTHERAPY AND PSYCHOSOMATIC APPROACH

There is little doubt that emotional factors have a profound effect upon an allergic condition. The reverse is also true, allergic diseases affect the patient emotionally. A patient who suffers with a long-standing chronic condition like asthma, or a patient whose normal life is seriously interfered with during a good portion of the year because of hay fever, is bound to become nervous and upset. These patients develop emotional disturbances which in turn contribute to or aggravate their condition. The person who has been the subject of repeated asthmatic paroxysms, or one who experiences continuous itching from an allergic skin condition, naturally becomes disturbed, irritable, and nervous. The more severe the condition, the more profound are the emotional changes which are brought about in that particular patient. If the disorder starts early in life, the child's personality may become definitely affected. He may become submissive or introverted and lead the life of an invalid, demanding a great deal of attention and sympathy from his family and refusing to partake of his normal responsibility; or, the child may overcompensate and become extroverted and aggressive.

There are many instances which indicate that emotional upheavals have had either an indirect or even a direct effect upon the patient's allergic condition. The power of suggestion may bring about allergic symptoms. This is exemplified by the instance of the hay fever patient, sensitive to ragweed, who began to sneeze violently in the winter when shown a ragweed plant framed under a glass cover. Every physician has seen patients develop severe attacks of asthma under severe emotional strain, or patients with allergic eczema whose dermatitis flares up under similar circumstances. Under the impact of fear, anxiety, or some other emotional explosion, the patient's wheezing, cough, and shortness of breath, or his itching may become unbearable. The patient becomes dissatisfied with life and discouraged. He loses sleep, his appetite is poor, and he loses weight. All these symptoms may contribute to and make worse his already existing allergic symptoms. Real improvement may result following psychotherapy, that is an attempt to discuss the patient's condition with him and give him an opportunity to express himself. Everyone knows that emotions may affect certain normal bodily functions. Examples of this are palpitation, vomiting, blushing, sweating, diarrhea, and insomnia, all of which normal functions may be exaggerated and brought about by nervous influences. However, in some patients various conflicts, frustrations, anxieties, and other nervous states may lead to maladjustment and contribute to and emphasize the allergic symptoms. These patients do not respond to medical treatment unless the nervous condition is also properly cared for. Physicians find it increasingly necessary to devote more and more time to careful discussion with the patient so that an understanding may be obtained of the patient's personality and of his domestic, social, and business problems. A realization of such problems and such conflicts will influence profoundly the clinical course and the outcome of treatment. The person who is maladjusted cannot be well and happy, and an unhappy person will not respond to even the most effective form of medical treatment. At the same time it is unwise to assume that just because an asthmatic patient is nervous, his asthma is due to his emotional difficulties.

ASTHMA DUE TO FOREIGN BODIES

A patient had severe asthma which did not respond to usual medical treatment. It was of three years duration and occurred in a relatively young man. The physician who knew him well brought up the possibility of psychosomatic factors playing an important part in producing the asthma. The patient showed emotional instability and was poorly adjusted. His family was wealthy. He had never followed a definite line of work. He took up drinking. Attempts at rehabilitation were unsuccessful. Obviously strong psychogenic influences were at work. Since all examinations inducted at one of the clinics failed to show a cause for the asthmatic condition, psychoanalysis was suggested and adopted. The results were poor. He was re-examined. Bronchoscopy was advised. This examination revealed nothing of note, although it was not satisfactory because the patient jumped off the table before the bronchoscope was introduced. The chest X-ray was repeated and at this time closer examination of the film showed a small metal clip at the base of the right lung. The mere presence of emotional conflicts and psychosomatic problems in an asthmatic patient is no proof that these factors are always the important causative factor in producing his condition.

AVOIDANCE OF CAUSATIVE FACTORS

The prime and basic principle of allergic treatment is to avoid the cause of the allergy. Allergic treatment cannot be carried out without an accurate allergic diagnosis. This may frequently involve a visit to the patient's home in order to discover whether there are many factors in the home which produce the allergy. People who are sensitive to goat hair may have their symptoms as a result of exposure to mohair furniture. The person's occupation should be carefully investigated. Allergic people are frequently sensitive to house dust and this makes it desirable to render the living room and bedroom dust-free, if possible.

INSTRUCTIONS FOR PREPARATION AND MAINTENANCE OF A DUST-FREE ROOM

In order to avoid house dust, an allergen of particular importance in respiratory allergy, the patient is given a list of directions which will help him as much as possible in ridding his house of dust. A suggested set of directions follows:

The bedroom should be entered seldom by others. Cleaning should be done only when the patient is out of the room. Remove all hangings, carpets, and extra furnishings from the sleeping room, as they are dust catchers. There should be no overstuffed (upholstered) furniture in the room. Clean the walls and ceilings. Scrub the woodwork (floors, baseboards, closets, etc.); scrubbing should be repeated each week. Scrub the bedsteads and all open coil springs at least once each month. A scrubbed wooden or metal chair may be used. Use cotton rag rugs and plain light curtains, and wash them weekly. Window shades (blinds) of the pull type are desirable. Mattresses, pillows, and up-holstered box springs are inclosed in dustproof covers. Use only washable blankets and washable cotton bedspreads (use no chenille or tufted candlewick type); blankets should be washed at least once each month. (For woolen blankets this washing may be done in the bathtub in a simple manner. The use of "Dreft" suds is recommended, as they remove fiber dusts rapidly.) If there is sensitivity to wool, ordinary cotton blankets may be put into sheets (old, soft, well laundered) before being brought into the room. These sheets should be changed only outside the room.

Do not store household objects or outer clothing such as shoes and overcoats in the clothes closets. When possible, the ventilation is to be obtained from out-doors. A suitable ventilator with a filter should be installed in the window. All doors leading to other rooms should be kept closed. If furnace heat outlets exist, a dust filter must be installed and changed frequently.

GENERAL AVOIDANCE INSTRUCTIONS

General directions are given to each patient emphasizing certain avoidance advice as follows: Use no insect powder in any part of the house without specific permission. This includes fly sprays, roach and ant powders, dog flea powders, and certain other types of mothproofing preparations. As far as it is possible, none of the substances to which the patient is sensitive should be found in his home.

The patient should avoid exposure to inhalants, particularly animal hairs and insecticides. This necessitates an understanding of the various toys, hats, furs, carpets, that may contain such hairs. Foods to which the patient is sensitive should also be eliminated. In this connection, and especially in the case of children, keep in mind the possibility of the development of de-ficiency diseases because certain minerals and certain vital vitamins may have been eliminated from the diet. Therefore, allergic treatment sometimes must be supplemented by the administration of vitamins and a proper com-bination of the various constituents of a healthy diet. The weight should be carefully watched. An asthmatic woman spoke English with difficulty. She was definitely food sensitive. Treatment therefore included some dietary re-strictions. She was instructed to report to the clinic at intervals of two weeks, so that her diet might be properly adjusted. However, her asthma disappeared. She properly attributed this to her dietary treatment and of her own will pro-ceeded to restrict her food intake further. Though asthma-free, she continued to lose weight and finally was hospitalized with pellagra.

No fresh or artificial (dust catcher) flowers should be kept in the house. Use only washable toys (remove all stuffed or hair fabric toys). Avoid contact with irritating odors from leaking stoves and electric refrigerators, kero-sene lamps, fresh paint, tobacco smoke, camphor, tar, etc. Do not keep any animal pets in your home unless specifically permitted. Do not indulge in any physical exertion which makes you short of breath or causes you to become overheated. Do not hurry; walk slowly and stop occasionally. Protect yourself against exposure to changes in weather so that you do not catch colds. Do not use mustard plasters or flaxseed poultices. Take drugs only when prescribed, for harmless medicine may be injurious to you. Avoid perfumes, face powders, sachet, and scented talcum powders, shaving and shampoo soaps, toothpaste, toilet water, and scented soaps. Many of these contain orris root and rice powder. Use only those specifically recommended. Avoid all dusty and musty places (basements, storerooms, attics, etc.). Avoid all contacts and foods listed for you. Avoid swimming unless specifically permitted. Do not over-load your stomach with heavy meals. Avoid carbonated waters, such as seltzer, cola, pop, ginger ale, etc. Consult your physician if troubled by constipation. Use no condiments, spices, peppers, sauces, mustards, pickles, or any other highly seasoned foods.

DESENSITIZATION

Desensitization is an accepted form of treatment, in which doses of the substance to which the patient is sensitive are injected. In this manner, an increased tolerance to this substance is frequently produced. Such treatment is usually effective, and carries little danger if properly carried out. The method is employed in hay fever, asthma, etc. Patients are "desensitized" to dust, pollen, molds, etc.

DRUG TREATMENT

Many drugs are used in the treatment of allergy. Since histamine seems to be at the bottom of all allergic reactions, medical scientists searched for a long time for a chemical which could destroy histamine, hoping that in such a drug would be found the final answer to the treatment of the allergic patient.

For the past ten years intensive research has centered on work with many such drugs, commonly referred to as histamine antagonists. In 1937 certain substances such as histadine, cystine, and arginine were found which seemed to inhibit to some extent the action of histamine on animals. However, these could not be used in man because of their poisonous action. In 1942 a new series of related chemical compounds were discovered which proved effective against histamine and yet not too toxic in man. This investigation was carried on first by several Frenchmen working in their laboratories in France, then by a twenty-six-year-old chemist in Cincinnati and finally by several pharma-cologists in other parts of the United States. Many chemicals were studied by rearranging their molecular structure, and each of these seemed to have certain advantages over the other until a final compound was discovered which seemed to meet all objections. The drug appeared to be the answer to the long struggle and search for a suitable antihistamine chemical. This substance is called beta dimethylamino-ethyl-benzhydryl-ether-hydrochloride, and is named "Benadryl." Another drug which serves practically the same purpose but has a slightly different chemical composition is "Pyribenzamine." Both drugs have been used extensively in the laboratory and in medical practice. Experimentally, they will protect sensitive guinea pigs against the shock produced by injecting them with the proteins to which they are sensitive. In other words, if one administers to an animal a small amount of Benadryl or Pyribenzamine and then injects the animal with either the protein to which it is sensitive or with histamine itself, the animal will be found protected by the administration of the drug. These new chemicals in some way interfere with the action of histamine on certain cells and tissues of the body, both in animals and in man, and in that way prevent the usual histamine effect. They bring about satisfactory results in the palliative treatment of certain allergic conditions particularly hives and nasal allergic disorders, such as hay fever. The patient obtains relief from his sneezing, nasal obstruction, or from his itching. The effect of the drug, however, is only transitory so that it must be taken continually. It has no effect on the basic allergic condition or in reducing the patient's sensitivity to pollen, dust, foods, or other substances to which he is allergic. As soon as the medication is stopped the symptoms recur.

Antihistamine agents are effective in connection with the treatment of nose allergy and hives and are ineffective in asthma. These drugs unfortunately have some side effects, namely, nausea, vomiting, dizziness, and drowsiness. The drowsiness may lead to serious accidents in industry or in persons driving a car while under the influence of the drug. A young lady took a capsule of "Benadryl" after dinner for the first time for the control of her hay fever symptoms. By the time her "date" showed up an hour later to take her to the theater, she was so sleepy that she insisted they abandon their plans to go out and remained at home for the evening. Some of these drugs are more effective than others. They should be taken only on a physician's prescription. They must not be used as a substitute for proper allergic diagnosis and effective rational treatment. Some of the present available antihistamine drugs are "Neohetramine," "Benadryl," "Pyribenzamine," "Histadyl," and "Chlortrimeton." These may be had in capsules, pills, or liquid form. Their effect is transitory. Patients also become used to them so that after a while the drugs are ineffective and a change is made to another antihistamine.

A milestone has been reached in the fight against allergy with chemicals. These discoveries may well forecast the development of a new era in the approach to the management of the allergic patient. However, these drugs are effective only as palliative, transient, and temporary measures, and then only for some and not all allergic disorders. Epinephrin or adrenalin is a useful drug in the treatment of many allergic disorders. It is used in asthma extensively, by injection under the skin or by inhalation through a nebulizer. It may be used as nose drops in nose allergy. Occasionally it is administered mixed with gelatin or oil by injection because it is more slowly absorbed and has a longer lasting effect. Its prolonged use has not been shown to produce heart damage. The drug has an immediate beneficial effect. However, it has a tendency to produce side reactions such as palpitation, nervousness, insomnia, blanching of the skin, and other disturbing symptoms. Since it may exaggerate or precipitate heart pain in already existing heart disease, it must be employed with caution in such instances.

Ephedrine has much the same effect as adrenalin. It has the added advantage of being more stable and can be taken by mouth in the form of capsules. Because it has powerful side effects, especially because it produces nervousness and sleeplessness, it is given in conjunction with one of the sedative drugs. There are, in addition, a host of other drugs related or derived from adrenalin and ephedrine. These may also be used as drops or by injection. A few are "Neosynephrin," "Propadrine," "Privine," "Paredrine," "Benzedrine" and others. These are marketed in various strengths and are supplied occasionally mixed with antibiotics such as penicillin and others to be used intranasally when there is local associated infection. These should be used sparingly and always only on the prescription of a physician.

ACTH and cortisone are valuable additions to the drug armamentarium. They are employed in acute emergencies, such as severe asthma and allergic dermatitis that has not responded to usual treatment. These hormones should not be taken routinely. Careful examination is necessary before their administration. The presence of stomach ulcer, tuberculosis, acne, furunculosis, and certain mental and emotional disorders contraindicates the prescribing of these products. Since certain side reactions may occur and since some of these may be serious, the person is kept under observation while ACTH or cortisone are given. The patient's weight, blood pressure, blood, and other studies are followed. After such a period of observation, these hormones may be taken at home as maintenance treatment. In many instances these drugs are lifesaving and will tide the patient over an acute fulminating stage of the disease. They are, however, not a substitute for careful and adequate investigation of the allergic patient.

Sedatives are frequently necessary. The choice of the proper drug is important in this connection. "Aminophyllin" is occasionally prescribed in the form of rectal suppositories and is useful in the treatment of asthma. Iodides form the basis for an old and useful remedy in the treatment of asthma. The drug helps in loosening of the cough and aids in liquefying the sputum so the patient has less difficulty in bringing it up. Oxygen may be necessary in severe asthma. If infection is present in the nose or chest, the physician may wish to give the patient antibiotics. Some of these may produce allergic and other undesirable symptoms. Many other drugs are used with various success in the treatment of allergic symptoms. They are employed, however, only as adjuncts and only to help tide the patient over the acute manifestations of his allergy. The basic and most useful form of treatment consists in discovering the source of the patient's allergy and removing it as thoroughly as possible from the patient's environment.

Many so-called cures, many quackeries and nostrums have been advocated and promoted to the public, from time to time. These, for the most part, are advanced by unscrupulous money-seeking agents. The medical profession can only warn the patient that most of these products are not only useless and ineffective, but are actually harmful because they give patients a false sense of security. Furthermore, they invariably and inevitably lead to disillusionment and the neglect of early proper treatment, neglect which breeds needless complications and structural irreversible changes in the affected organs.

CHAPTER XX

Endocrinology

ELMER L. SEVRINGHAUS, M.D.

INTRODUCTION

MEDICAL SCIENCE *has accumulated more and more information about the glands and the manner in which they and their secretions affect the general condition of the body. When it first began to be realized how important were the functions of such tissues as the thyroid, the pituitary, the parathyroid, the pancreas, the adrenals and other glandular organs, philosopher-physicians began to develop all sorts of interesting theories as to the importance of these tissues to the human body.*

By removing glands from animals and observing the subsequent changes, investigators were able to determine the activities of each of the glands. For instance, the glands known as the adrenals, which lie just above the kidneys, are sometimes destroyed by serious disease. When this occurs, the person is likely to develop a condition known as Addison's disease, in which there is usually great weakness, dizziness, shortness of breath, loss of weight, and gradual breaking down of the human body. Usually the skin becomes pigmented and turns to a sort of bronze color. In the absence of the secretion of the adrenal glands, the person is likely to die.

The pituitary is a small gland lying near the brain. Its overgrowth may be associated with peculiar changes in the structure of the body. Giantism and dwarfism are not infrequent in relation to changes in this gland. We know that it supplies hormones which affect the thyroid, adrenals, and sex glands. The pancreas secretes the substance that is important in the handling of sugar by the body. Destruction of portions of the cells of the pancreas results in diabetes. Goiter is an enlargement of the thyroid gland. Changes in the secretions of the sex glands may result in anomalies being developed which are of great interest. The extracts of these glands have important effects on several parts of the body.

So much has been learned in the years since 1930 that a whole new science of glands called endocrinology has been created. The hormones from the pituitary and from the cortex of the adrenal are able to influence profoundly the constitution of an individual. Extracts from these glands called ACTH and cortisone are potent agents used in treating rheumatoid arthritis, rheumatic fever, allergies, addictions, and many other conditions. They act also against depressive states, by producing a sense of well-being.

The human tissues are built for a life cycle of seventy years, including twenty years of growth, thirty years of maturity, and twenty years of degeneration and decay. It has not yet been established by any scientific investigation that the administration of glandular extracts seriously modifies this process, and it is safe to say that rejuvenation is not yet even in sight.

Man's search for the elixir of youth is eternal. Since the first announcement by Voronoff and by Steinach that their methods would rejuvenate the elderly, hundreds of experiments have been made to control their claims, but none of these experiments has confirmed their notions.

It is interesting to have the views of the pathologist Warthin on this subject. An investigation of human bodies postmortem indicates that few men over fifty-five years of age have the power of reproduction, and that certainly the stories of reproductive ability much later in life are to be viewed with skepticism. It is interesting to have the view of the distinguished pathologist as to the possibilities of rejuvenation. He says:

"What philosophy then may we draw from this? Is old age inevitable? Yes, escape from it is possible only for those who meet a premature pathologic death.

"For those who live to their biologic limit, age cannot be escaped. Nor can it be deferred. Nor is rejuvenescence possible. The deferring of old age, the rejuvenating of the senescent individual is but idle and foolish talk, and we have had much of this in the last decade.

"What modern medicine has accomplished along the lines of hygiene and prevention of disease has been only to increase the number of human individuals, both the fit and unfit—unfortunately too many of the latter kind— who come to maturity and to the period of senescence.

"More individuals will achieve their biologic life limit; and this means what?—ultimately a much greater increase in the number of senile, more or less useless, human beings in the age decades of the eighties and the nineties.

"There will be some increase in the number who will reach the age of one hundred years or even pass it, due to their own family inheritance, but this number will not be greatly increased in the present period of evolution."

M. F.

Both the structure and activities of the human body are highly complicated. Among the simplest chemical events connected with any of our foods is the series of processes by which starch is digested into a simple sugar, dextrose, and this sugar is absorbed, stored in the liver as glycogen; later it is used as fuel for heat and the work of the muscles. All such chemical events are made possible by the facilitating activity of a number of enzymes. Obviously these processes must be arranged in an orderly fashion. One of the greatest marvels of the body is the careful coördination of processes and adaptation of structures to make a harmonious whole. Among the mechanisms providing this coördination is the action of a group of organs known as *glands of internal secretion* or *endocrine glands*. The products of these glands, known as *hor-*

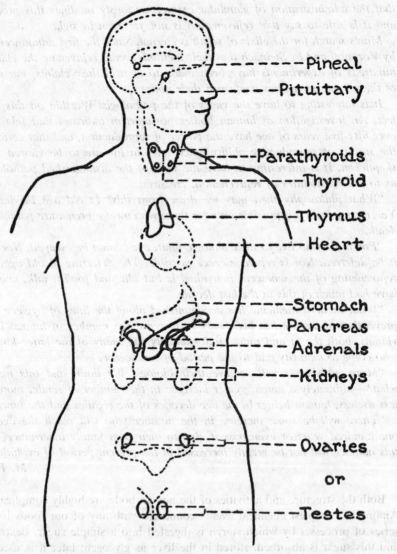

Fig. 39. Location of various important glands in the human body.

mones, are distributed by the blood to all parts of the body. Thus the hormones are able to communicate chemical messages or impulses to any tissue which can respond. By the continued supply of such hormones it becomes possible for a gland to correlate the activities of several parts of the body, remote from each other, for an orderly achievement of some biological purpose.

THE NERVOUS SYSTEM AND THE GLANDS

When communication of impulses and correlation of processes is considered, the nervous system usually comes first to mind. The accomplishment of these ends by action of the nervous system differs from that by endocrine gland secretion in several ways. First, nervous action begins and ends instantaneously, and often is limited to brief periods. Gland action begins and ends more gradually, and is best adapted to long-sustained effects. Again, nervous impulses are directed to a few places at one time, limiting the results to certain parts of the body. Gland secretions are distributed to all tissues alike, and the responses depend on the capacities of various tissues to act under such stimulation. Third, the nervous impulses may set in motion processes which were previously dormant, or stop completely action which had been going on. Endocrine secretions act merely to accelerate or to slow down processes which are already going on, but they never start new processes. This accelerating type of action is known to chemists as *catalysis.* In some respects it may be compared to lubrication of machinery so that it will run more swiftly and easily. Both nerves and glands are involved in the processes of communicating impulses and of correlating processes for an orderly life, and each system has its advantages and special functions.

A natural question concerns the connections between the two systems, by which their separate functions may be made to fit appropriately together. There are only a few such connections well understood at present. The glandular secretions are concerned with the more primitive biological processes, such as keeping warm, mustering reserves to meet emergencies for defense, and making sure of the reproduction of the species, in addition to the controls on the use of sugar, protein, and fat foods, and the balance of salts and water in the body. Since our mental states depend to such a large extent on our comfort, sense of security, and the satisfactions of our several appetites, the activity of the endocrine glands has important, even though indirect, consequences in mental and emotional life.

Such concepts of the significance of the glands of internal secretion have developed rather recently. This understanding began about the middle of the nineteenth century, progressed slowly until 1890 when the first human patient was treated with animal thyroid glands, and has been gaining momentum in the present century. Progress has become more rapid because of the increasingly close coöperation in research between medical men and biologists and chemists. So rapid has been this progress that within the present century chemists have discovered how to make artificially six of these hormones, which are identical with the secretions produced by such glands as the thyroid, adrenals, ovaries and testes. The chemical complexity of the products from the pituitary, parathyroids, and pancreas has resisted the efforts of chemists to duplicate them up to the present.

Sometimes there is confusion as to the significance of the term *gland*. Three meanings must be distinguished. The structures which serve to remove from the lymphatic stream the poisonous materials from infections have been called lymphatic glands. These often become enlarged to the point where they can be felt, as with the glands in the neck during an attack of tonsillitis. Such structures should be termed *lymph nodes,* not glands. The glands of *external* secretion serve several purposes. The simplest of these are sweat glands in the skin, which deliver their secretion, sweat, through tiny ducts or tubes onto the surface of the skin. Digestive glands are also of this type. The glands of *internal* secretion produce secretions which pass directly back into the blood, and circulate throughout the body. The recognized endocrine glands are the thyroid, parathyroids, pancreas, adrenals, ovaries, testes, and the pituitary.

THE THYROID

The thyroid lies in the lower front portion of the neck, extending across the bottom and up either side of the cartilages which enclose the larynx, recognized as the Adam's apple. The normal thyroid is small enough to fit into this space without being seen as an enlargement. It can be felt by an experienced physician only where it crosses the cartilages in the middle of the neck. Whenever the thyroid becomes enlarged so that it causes a visible fullness in the neck, and can be felt more readily, it is called a *goiter*. There are several types of goiter, depending on different causes and having different significance for health. The existence of a goiter, or enlarged thyroid, should lead one to seek medical examination, to determine the cause, and to decide whether treatment is necessary.

SIMPLE GOITER

The commonest cause for enlargement of the thyroid or *simple goiter* is a deficient supply of iodine in the food and drink of children and youths. Iodine is one of the indispensable elements used by the thyroid in the manufacture of the hormone which this gland produces. The thyroid requires not more than 0.05 milligram of iodine per day for the purpose. (A drop of water weights 1300 times this much.) In most parts of the world the water and food will provide more than this small amount of iodine, and goiter is infrequent in such regions. In those areas where for long periods melting snow has extracted iodine from the soil and carried it down into the sea, the soil is depleted of iodine. In these regions surface or well water, as well as locally grown plant and animal food, will be almost entirely free of iodine.

Thus many mountainous regions and the extensively glaciated area about the Great Lakes of North America are lacking in iodine and goiter occurs with high frequency in the populations of these areas.

Since this relationship was recognized it has become possible to prevent most of this type of goiter simply by furnishing iodine to the school children. At first this was done by use of tablets or solutions providing the iodine as a medicine for a few days twice each year. The thyroid is able to store iodine for periods of weeks to months, and to draw on this reservoir as needed. Other methods have been tried, such as introducing iodine into the municipal water supply and into table salt. The use of the water supply has been abandoned because it is not economical; most municipal water is not used for drinking. Iodized table salt as a source of supply has a number of features to recommend it: it is used principally for human food; it is used by almost everyone; the iodine content of the salt can be determined with ease and the cost is very small. Until the recent introduction of highly refined salt, the use of sea salt or of mined salt provided iodine as one of the "impurities" in table salt used by most of the human race. Due to the lack of iodine in modern refined salt, goiter may be termed to some extent a disease of "civilization."

There is standardization in the iodine content of iodized salt as prepared and sold in the United States. Control has been provided. An amount commonly used is one part of potassium iodide in 2000 to 5000 parts of common salt, sodium chloride. At first there was some apprehension that such an amount of iodine might be harmful. This fear has been almost entirely dispelled. More recently there has been some suspicion that the iodine supplied in this way might be inadequate, especially for infants or children who add no salt voluntarily to their food. Recent tests have indicated that when so-called "iodized salt" is used in the home, the infants and children will receive enough iodine in their food to prevent goiter. Only iodized salt should be used in those geographic areas where goiter is known to be common. This constitutes a safe and effective way to prevent most of the common types of goiter.

During periods of rapid growth of the body it appears that the thyroid requires more than the usual amount of iodine. Such an increased need may exist also at other times, as after severe infections, or during pregnancy. Under such circumstances it may be wise for the physician to prescribe some form of iodine to meet the temporarily increased need.

In many communities in the United States iodine is still being administered to school children. The commonest way is by use of chocolate-coated tablets of combinations of iodine with fatty substances which will render the iodine tasteless and prevent its evaporation. The method is effective, safe, and not expensive. The disadvantages are that it does not reach pre-school children, adults, or those who happen to be absent from school on the days the tablets are distributed. Use of iodized salt by all the population will make this method unnecessary. Ultimately there may be governmental control of the amount of iodine in salt, as a part of the supervision of the nutrition of the citizens.

If goiter has occurred because of lack of iodine, it is still possible to make up for the lack during the years of childhood or of early adolescence, and to cause the goiter to become much smaller. This is often sufficient to make the enlarged thyroid decrease to a point where it is no longer a visible mass in the neck. Such a type of treatment with iodine must be undertaken only under supervision of a physician. The effect of iodine on any particular goiter is not easy to predict. Medical guidance is of importance for adequate dosage, discrimination as to which person should be treated, and decision as to other treatment which may also be helpful.

Besides being unsightly, a goiter may become large enough to cause discomfort by the fit of clothing, or by pressure on other structures in the neck. More important than these consequences are the tendencies to complicated types of goiter later in life. By a succession of changes the simple type of soft goiter already described may become a sort of tumor, called an *adenoma*, which will accentuate the above-mentioned difficulties. There are two further risks of the adenoma type of goiter: possibility of the development of cancer or the gradual appearance of the condition known as toxic goiter. Cancer of the thyroid is not extremely frequent, but since it occurs more often in adenomas than otherwise, such goiter merits careful medical attention. The damage from toxic goiter comes on so insidiously, usually in middle life, that it may cause permanent changes in the heart before the condition has been recognized. For these reasons it is often considered wise to have thyroid adenomas removed surgically as a precautionary measure. Such operative treatment should be reserved for surgeons who have been especially trained in the methods of preparation for this operation and the aftercare of these patients, as well as in the operative technique.

Exophthalmic Goiter—Thyrotoxicosis

Perhaps the most damaging type of goiter is the relatively small gland with rapidly developing evidences of toxicity. This disorder has been called by several names: *exophthalmic goiter,* because of the frequent, though not universal, association of prominence of the eyeballs; *hyperthyroidism,* because of the fact that most of the trouble is the same as can be produced by administering an excessively large dose of thyroid daily to a healthy individual; *thyrotoxicosis,* because the disease is due to poisoning with thyroid secretion; "inward goiter," because the enlargement of the gland is not obvious in many patients, and some people believed that the gland enlarged toward the inside of the neck and chest cavity. The disease has also been called by the names of the men in various countries who first recognized its nature.

This toxic form of thyroid disorder is most common between the ages of 15 and 40, and it is often associated with the existence of a nervous and emotional make-up which can be easily disturbed. Often the thyroid disease and the unstable nervous system are hard to distinguish and the physician must use great care in making the diagnosis and planning the treatment. The care of patients with toxic goiter is highly important. If not adequately treated there may be serious damage to the heart, the nervous system, or to certain other glands. The simplest, most certain way to treat patients with thyrotoxicosis is by surgical removal of about nine tenths of the thyroid gland. The rest of the gland is usually adequate to continue the necessary functions.

During the past decade it has been found possible to use any one of several drugs, most commonly propylthiouracil, in order to suppress excessive activity of the thyroid, thereby inducing a remission of thyrotoxicosis. Sometimes this remission may be maintained by such medical means; at other times it allows sufficient improvement to permit surgical removal as mentioned with little risk. Such drugs are occasionally toxic, and they must be used only under the continued observation of a physician. Another interesting and important method of treating thyrotoxicosis is based upon administration of iodine which has been made radioactive. Since iodine is quickly collected in the thyroid gland after it has been given, the radioactive iodine delivers a destructive dose of radiation to the thyroid cells. By careful measurement of the dose of such iodine, an overactive gland may be reduced to one with a normal amount of activity. Although these non-surgical methods of treatment have been studied intensively for a few years, it is not yet certain that they can always replace operative removal of a large part of an overactive thyroid gland.

HYPOTHYROIDISM

In a small proportion of cases even after operation there may be a recurrence of the trouble, since the thyroid, like other glands, has the ability to increase in size and it may again become too active. Sometimes a second operation may be required. At times the surgeon may find it necessary to remove so much of the gland that the remainder is inadequate for the body's needs. In such a case there develops very gradually a condition known as *hypothyroidism,* a deficiency of thyroid secretion. This can be treated easily by the use of a daily ration of tablets made from the thyroids of slaughterhouse animals. Such a treatment must be continued throughout life.

Hypothyroidism may also occur spontaneously. If it occurs before birth, the infant will be retarded in development and growth, and will be a feeble-minded dwarf of the type known as a *cretin.* If the deficiency begins later in life, after the earlier development has been normal, the condition of hypothyroidism is called *myxedema.* This term refers to a curious accumulation beneath the skin and elsewhere of an abnormal tissue which gives a swollen appearance to the face, arms, and legs resembling in some respects edema (dropsy).

The one specific treatment for any of these forms of hypothyroidism is the daily administration of tablets of thyroid. Fortunately the hormone produced by the thyroid gland is not destroyed in the digestive tract, and the tablets lose none of their potency when taken by mouth. Their effects occur slowly and the results of a daily dose become increasingly evident for the succeeding months of continued treatment. The physician can estimate the appropriate doses of thyroid and the need for any change in such treatment by the use of the *basal metabolism test*.

BASAL METABOLISM TESTS

The basal metabolism test is merely a method for measuring how much oxygen the individual uses per hour. Tests are usually carried on for 8 or 10 minute periods, during which the subject breathes through a rubber mouthpiece from a tank containing a measured amount of air. The carbon dioxide and excess moisture are absorbed as they are exhaled into the apparatus, and the decrease in the amount of air in the tank is due to the oxygen used up by the subject. When the thyroid hormone supply is inadequate for normal health the rate of oxygen use is reduced, and the basal metabolism may be found as much as 40 per cent below the normal for the age, height and weight of the subject. Anyone using thyroid tablets regularly ought to have the treatment checked by a physician at intervals of not more than a few months. The most satisfactory check on such treatment includes a basal metabolism test.

This same test is used to detect the smaller deviations of thyroid function from normal when the other evidence is not adequate to make the diagnosis obvious to the physician. Basal metabolism is increased when a goiter is toxic, and the increase is a fair measure of the gravity of the illness. The test is also of importance in determining the extent of improvement following any type of treatment for such goiter. The basal metabolism test is not infallible, for it is subject to distortion by excitement of the subject, or by any one of several errors in the preparation for the test or the conduct of the measurement. Such tests should be conducted by trained persons, and only after careful explanation to the patient of the way in which his coöperation is required.

Many people, including entirely too many physicians, have come to believe that an abnormally low basal metabolism is the cause of obesity. This is rarely true. Associated with this belief has been the use of thyroid as a means to reduce excessive weight. Such treatment seldom produces significant weight loss unless the doses of thyroid are so high that the individual is made definitely ill. Nevertheless a number of "reducing remedies" sold without prescription are mixtures containing thyroid. Use of such preparations is to be avoided for at least three reasons. First, these remedies are usually of no help, hence they are wasteful expenditures. Second, if the doses of such drugs are large enough to cause definite effects genuine illness is apt to be produced. Finally, excessive weight may come from any one of several causes. Appropriate dietary schemes and exercise for the needs of the individual patient require the advice of a physician who has been adequately trained in the problems involved. Obesity is a sufficient reason for requesting medical advice. There is no simple and safe way to reduce excessive weight except by the time-honored use of less food and more work. The details of such a program need to be prescribed just as definitely as do medicines for other diseases.

THE PANCREAS

Just one year before thyroid deficiency was first treated by the feeding of animal thyroid gland, two German investigators proved that removal of the pancreas from dogs caused the animals to become diabetic. Not until 33 years later was it possible for the Canadians, the late Dr. F. G. Banting and Dr. C. H. Best, to prepare from the pancreas of animals an extract which would counteract diabetes in human patients. This extract contains the hormone made by the pancreas, to which the name *insulin* has been applied. This name is derived from a Latin term for islands, since the part of the pancreas which makes insulin is a group of specialized cells collected into small "islands" distributed throughout the pancreas. The larger part of the pancreas is a gland of external secretion, which produces an important digestive juice for use in the upper part of the intestine. The pancreas is therefore two glands in one. In certain fish these two glands occur in separate parts of the body, which makes these fish a convenient source of pure insulin. This hormone must be injected, for if it is given by mouth the digestive juices destroy most of it.

Insulin is a substance whose structure is still a puzzle to chemists in spite of almost 30 years of intensive study. It can be prepared in a high degree of purity, and it has been made available for use by diabetic patients in all countries of the world. The cost for enough to maintain excellent health in a human with even the most severe type of diabetes seldom exceeds 25 cents per day. Since there are over one million diabetics in the United States alone, and since more than half of these patients must use insulin daily, it is easy to realize what an important contribution this advance in medicine has been. Probably no other single step in endocrine research has been of equal significance.

The action of insulin cannot be described with great exactness in chemical terms. This hormone is necessary if the body is to make prompt and thorough use of sugar in the several ways which are involved in normal life processes. Deficiency of insulin, leading to impaired ability to use sugar, handicaps the brain, heart, liver, kidneys, and the muscles. In fact long-continued diabetes if untreated is apt to lead to disturbances in any body structure one examines. This is merely another way of saying that every tissue in the body requires sugar in some fashion. If the utilization of sugar is interfered with, other fuels are consumed in greater amounts than usual. This leads to the burning of stores of fat, with consequent loss of weight, and to destruction of protein from living tissues, with eventual weakness. When the disease is very severe the attempt of the body to use fats as fuel is so extensive that there is an accumulation of a dangerously large amount of acid materials, which causes acidosis. This process may become so overwhelming that death follows within a matter of a few days. All these disturbances can be corrected with promptness and certainty by the injection of appropriate doses of insulin.

Diabetes mellitus, the proper term for this disease which is sometimes called "sugar diabetes," received its name because the body appeared to melt down into urine and flow away, and because the urine was found to contain sugar. This latter feature is one of the least important things about the disease, except that it is so frequently the means for detecting the trouble, and that the absence of sugar in the urine of one who is known to have diabetes is one of the best evidences that he is keeping his difficulty under control. The presence of sugar in the urine of the diabetic is the consequence of his inability to use sugar. The unused sugar accumulates in the blood. In order to prevent dangerous excess of sugar in the blood, the kidneys remove the sugar when it rises above a certain level, i.e., approximately twice the normal level of blood sugar. Therefore, the physician can detect diabetes more certainly and in milder degrees by determining the amount of sugar in the blood than by testing for sugar in the urine.

It seems obvious that such a disturbance might be met by merely restricting the intake of sugar and other carbohydrates (sugar-forming foods). An increased amount of fat might be used to make up the deficit in calories. This method is a satisfactory one for many diabetics. Until the discovery of insulin it was the best method available. But when diabetes is very severe the method is not adequate. If the body cannot use sugar in even the small amounts which are absolutely essential, the liver will make sugar from such sources as protein even though there is already an excess of sugar in the blood. Therefore the blood sugar of the severe diabetic remains abnormally high, without any carbohydrate food. The only remedy for this situation is the daily hypodermic injection of insulin. Lacking this treatment, the severe diabetic will gradually lose weight and strength, and eventually die. Therefore, it will be evident that dietary management is adequate for some diabetics, whereas others require insulin.

At first it was hoped that the use of insulin would make diet limitation entirely unnecessary for diabetics. This hope has not been realized. On the contrary, it is probably more important to use careful diets with the injection of insulin than without. This is not due to any inability of insulin to accomplish desired results. The difficulty is that the isulin once injected continues to have an effect, stimulating the body to use sugar rapidly. If there is not a sufficient supply of sugar coming from the food, its concentration in the blood will fall and the brain will be deprived of sugar. The consequences of a shortage of sugar supply to the brain will be first hunger and nervous irritability, which should serve the diabetic as a warning to procure food. If this warning is not understood or heeded, still further brain disturbances may occur, with sweating, trembling, and lack of coördination of muscles. The individual may act as if ill or intoxicated with alcohol. If relief is not obtained the brain activity may be suppressed to the point of unconsciousness. The remedy for all these brain disorders is a quick supply of sugar. If the results have been allowed to proceed to a point where the patient can no longer take food by mouth, a physician may have to inject a solution of pure dextrose into a vein. Under these circumstances recovery is dramatically prompt.

The consequence of these discoveries is that diabetic patients are trained to weigh or at least to estimate carefully their food regularly so that they may eat uniform amounts of carbohydrate food daily. The amount of insulin is then adjusted to the point where the blood sugar concentration is very nearly normal, but care is taken to avoid unduly low blood sugar levels. The diabetic orders his life between two limits: too little blood sugar, which can produce the reaction described, or too much blood sugar, which will be followed by loss of some sugar in the urine, and a tendency to increasingly severe diabetes. If the amount of food is adjusted to maintain proper weight of the body, this routine of carefully limited diet and hypodermic injection of insulin is only a slight inconvenience. By following these directions the diabetic may remain otherwise in excellent health, pursue his usual occupation, and expect to live a few years longer than if he had not become a diabetic. This increased life expectancy is probably because of his careful attention to many matters of hygiene.

Originally insulin had to be given two to four times daily. This followed from the very rapid but brief activity of the material injected. If a whole day's supply was given at one time the results would be too intense within the first few hours, and would have disappeared before the day had passed. A few years later it was found possible to combine insulin with a protein called protamine and with zinc in small amounts. This preparation of *protamine zinc insulin* is not soluble in water, but is used in a milky suspension which can be injected hypodermically. Under the skin the insulin is slowly dissolved and absorbed, so that it becomes available at just about the rate required throughout the day. By the use of this type of insulin it has become possible to give only one injection per 24 hours to most diabetics. In some patients, especially those who use large amounts of carbohydrate, it is still the practice to use both the older and quick-acting insulin plus the newer and slow-acting variety. Recently it has been found possible to prepare protamine zinc insulin according to a method which allows it to act like a mixture of the slow and quick acting types. This is called NPH insulin, and is coming into wide use for the more convenient and adequate treatment of many diabetics.

The discovery of insulin and the understanding of the consequences of the injection of an excessive amount of insulin led to the recognition of a condition which had not been previously suspected. This is the occurrence of unduly low blood sugar concentrations in persons who do not have diabetes. It was suspected that some of these individuals who frequently had extremely low levels of sugar in their blood might be found to have tumors in the pancreas. This has been proved in only a few patients, but when such tumors have been removed the patients have been cured of very distressing conditions, which resembled epilepsy or other brain disturbances.

Far more important has been the realization that a large number of otherwise healthy persons have temporarily excessive reductions in the amount of circulating sugar. This is especially true from 2 to 4 hours after a meal which was rich in sugar and starch. When such food is being absorbed from the digestive tract the amount of sugar in the blood is sharply increased. The immediate reaction of the pancreas is to secrete more insulin into the blood, to facilitate the use and storage of this sugar. The production of insulin under these conditions is generous, and may be slightly in excess of the needs. Under these circumstances the body may withdraw sugar from the blood more rapidly than the new supply can enter from the intestine. If this produces a slight deficit of sugar in the blood, hunger follows, and if the process goes a bit farther the individual may become irritable, nervous, or even feel temporarily weak. This process will be accentuated if vigorous exercise is being undertaken. Such a chain of events is especially common in children, and is responsible for the need of frequent feedings. Adults, too, who respond in this way to sweet food will find they are more comfortable with several small meals per day. Another alternative is the use of meals with very small portions of carbohydrate food, and larger amounts of the protein and fat foods which are more slowly digested. The presence of these latter materials in the bowel prevents too rapid absorption of sugar and avoids the rapid changes in blood sugar.

It is not infrequently found that the occurrence of this hunger between conventional meal times is the cause for lunching, and for use of sweet and rich foods at every opportunity. The obvious result in many such individuals is a steady gain in weight. When obesity results from this exaggeration of normal reactions to use of sugar it is easy to plan a reducing diet along the lines just mentioned. The person who follows such a diet is able not only to lose weight, but actually to be less hungry on less food than he was eating before. Such a result is due to limiting the amount of sweet food in each meal.

ADRENAL GLANDS

The adrenal glands are a pair of small structures placed just on top of the kidneys, and made up of two different types of tissue. The outer layers of these glands are so important that life will not continue for more than a few days if they are destroyed or removed. The inner portion of the same glands is less vitally necessary, but it has highly specialized functions to perform. This inner part, called the *medulla,* is really a part of the sympathetic nervous system. When impulses pass down the sympathetic nerves, as during any emotional experience, the medulla of the adrenal gland is stimulated and the response is a secretion of the hormone, called epinephrine or adrenin. (One widely known commercial product of this hormone is known as adrenalin.) When epinephrine (or adrenalin) circulates through the body it causes a series of results which are essentially preparations to meet various emergencies. Included are increases in heart rate, in breathing, in blood pressure, in the amount of sugar in the blood, in the speed with which blood will clot in a cut, and in the strength which can be exerted by the muscles. These rather striking phenomena are to be viewed as adaptations by which the primitive man, when frightened or enraged or endangered, could summon greater strength for combat and better avoid death from blood loss if wounded. In the relatively quiet existence of modern civilized life this mechanism is seldom of vital importance. The tendency of emotional reactions to increase blood-sugar concentration, however, is frequently helpful. When blood sugar decreases for any reason a slight stimulation of the sympathetic nerves results, and the epinephrine secreted by the adrenal glands causes the liver to release some of the sugar stored there as glycogen. This probably happens daily in such smoothly adjusted fashion that most people never know of the reaction. It is an example of the nicely balanced forces with which the body is equipped to maintain stable conditions from hour to hour. A further result of the production of increased amounts of epinephrine is stimulation of great activity in the adrenal cortex (see below). As a consequence further reserve capacities of the body are made available during several succeeding hours.

One medical use of epinephrine is based on the ability of this hormone to cause puckering of the tiny blood vessels in any region where it is applied, thereby limiting the oozing of blood from wounds. Another important value of the hormone is its capacity to relax the muscles in the bronchial tubes, in this way relieving patients who are suffering from asthma. But there is no established use for this hormone as a substitute for deficient secretion by the adrenal glands. In fact physicians do not recognize any condition which can be considered as lack of secretion by the adrenal medulla.

The situation is far different in the case of the outer portion of the same glands, called the *cortex*. This vitally important tissue constantly secretes one or more hormone substances. Although chemists have identified at least 28 compounds in extracts prepared from adrenal glands of animals, it is probable that there are not more than 3 or 4 real hormones acting in the body. It is still not decided which of these numerous compounds is the genuine adrenal cortex hormone. These hormones enable the body to retain a sufficient supply of salt, and therefore of water also, to maintain the normal fluid conditions within the cells as well as the blood, and to maintain a proper blood pressure. Another important function of this secretion is to make it possible for the liver to change protein food into sugar when there is more protein or less sugar than the body needs. It is less easy to explain why these glands are a part of the means by which the body resists the attack of certain infections and poisons. This group of responsibilities is so fundamental to health that when the adrenal glands are seriously damaged or destroyed fatal disease occurs. This difficulty is called adrenal deficiency, usually spoken of as *Addison's disease*. Of course there are various degrees of severity of the disease. The less severe forms predispose to suddenly exaggerated attacks due to minor infections or overwork, or loss of a great deal of salt from the body.

Within only the last few years it has become possible to prepare extracts which contain this life-maintaining material from animal adrenal glands, with little or no epinephrine. The latter hormone, derived from the less necessary medullary portion of the glands, is a disadvantage in such extracts because of effects it would have if injected in large amounts. With such purified adrenal cortex extracts physicians can now save the lives of patients suffering from even the severe forms of Addison's disease, and can often restore their health to a considerable degree. Unfortunately many of these people suffer from Addison's disease because of tuberculosis involving the adrenal glands as well as some other portions of the body. In such patients it is often not possible to secure healing of the tuberculosis, which is ultimately fatal. There is some ground for hope that continuous and thorough treatment of patients with Addison's disease, if begun early, may help in arresting the tuberculosis and obtaining a permanent improvement or partial cure. Combining this with use of treatment for tuberculosis such as streptomycin, para-aminosalicylic acid, and the more recent isonizide drugs may well make possible a brighter outlook for even this group of patients.

The work of several chemists has resulted in identifying 28 compounds which are to be found in extracts made from the adrenal glands. Some of these have properties resembling the whole extract, but no one is an adequate and complete substitute for the solutions made from the animal glands. One of the group of compounds, known as desoxycorticosterone has been made synthetically, i.e., from other sources than the extracts of the glands. This material can be injected under the skin and its use has been life-saving for many patients suffering from Addison's disease. Two more of the compounds, cortisone and dihydrocortisone, have been made more recently in amounts large enough to allow extensive treatment trials in a great many diseases. Preparations with 4 or 5 times the potency of cortisone are known as prednisone and prednisolone. Dramatic improvement has been achieved in rheumatic fever, rheumatoid arthritis, lupus erythematosus, severe asthmatic seizures, and other illnesses. These compounds have powerful effects and must be used with great caution.

Small pellets of desoxycorticosterone can be made, and implanted under the skin. From this place they will be slowly dissolved and used by the body over a period of a few months. By such a technique it is possible to give the treatment two to four times a year, instead of as many times per day with the gland extracts. Aldosterone isolated from the adrenal in 1954 is the hormone that controls salt and water balance.

Whereas this treatment with adrenal cortex hormones sounds simple, it is associated with a number of difficulties. The adrenal cortex has much to do with the ability of the body to hold salt and water, and the capacity of the kidneys to excrete these substances. When the patient with Addison's disease is being treated with either adrenal gland extracts or with desoxycorticosterone it is essential to control his use of salt with care. Too little salt will increase the amount of the hormone required; too much will lead to accumulation of fluid in undesirable places which may cause serious consequences for the heart. The details of such treatment are being constantly refined by the medical specialists who have had experience with the materials used. Improved results are being achieved by use of carefully adjusted mixtures of desoxycorticosterone and the newer compounds E and F. The best results are obtained by use of extracts made from the glands of animals. It is to be expected that the future will have better methods for the management of Addison's disease as chemists and medical men discover more about the glands and their products.

Usually there are cases of overactivity of glands of internal secretion as well as of underactivity. In the case of the adrenal medulla the only type of overactivity known is of a rare sort of tumor which produces epinephrine by spurts, and therefore tends to make the individual have sudden surges of high blood pressure. When this condition is recognized, removal of the tumor surgically will produce a cure. This is also rarely found to be true in patients who have steadily increased blood pressure, a disorder usually due to entirely different causes.

Overactivity of the adrenal cortex is a puzzle only beginning to be solved. It is apparent that one type of overactivity of the adrenal glands in women will lead to a growth of hair on the face and body in those regions where it is normally seen only in men. There are other reasons for thinking that this unfortunate condition is not due to a mere excess of adrenal hormone so much as to some abnormal type of chemical produced by these glands. Certainly there are some women with excessive hair and other evidences of decreased feminine constitution who have diseased adrenal glands. Still others with similar trouble have disturbances in the pituitary or in the ovaries. Finally there are many women with increased hair on the face, arms and legs, but with no other discoverable abnormality. It is entirely erroneous to assume that there is always a connection between the adrenal glands and too much hair in women. At present, women who are disturbed about too much hair need the advice of physicians trained in care of the skin. When there is a marked tendency to development of excess hair in a woman not previously so afflicted, there are usually other evidences of trouble which will suggest disorder in the adrenals or the other glands mentioned. In the latter case the attention of specialists in endocrine study is important.

Among the undesired effects following use of excessive amounts of cortisone (or of ACTH, mentioned in the chapter on the Pituitary) in women are excessive growth of hair, deepening of the voice, and disturbances in the skin, in fat distribution, and in the strength of structural tissues including the bones.

THE PARATHYROIDS

At the edges of the thyroid gland are found four small bodies which are entirely different, called parathyroid glands from their location. Their task is to control the amount of calcium and phosphorus which circulates in the blood. The decrease in activity of these glands is followed by a decrease in blood calcium but an increase in phosphorus. Under such circumstances muscles become more easily stimulated, and when the change is marked enough certain muscles begin to contract or exhibit spasms spontaneously. This is called *tetany* (not to be confused with tetanus, which is the result of a specific infection). In tetany the commonest spasms are of the hands, arms, legs and feet, but the most dangerous contractions can occur in the muscles of the larynx, closing the passage through which the breath passes. This emergency can be relieved quickly by the injection into a vein of a solution of calcium salts. The decreased amount of circulating calcium is the cause of the increased irritability of the muscles. Tetany may occur spontaneously from disease of the parathyroids, but this is uncommon. Most cases are the result of destruction or removal of the glands during the operative treatment for goiter. Surgeons are careful to avoid these small glands during thyroid operations, but the parathyroids are small, difficult to identify during an operation, and are occasionally removed unintentionally by even the most experienced surgeons.

The treatment of tetany by means of extracts of animal parathyroids became possible in 1925, when this potent material was discovered simultaneously by two investigators. Unfortunately the continuous use of even the best of the extracts is not satisfactory, since the treatment gradually loses its efficacy after a number of months. Several other measures help make the relief of tetany effective. If the diet is selected so that there is a minimum of phosphorus, if calcium salts are added in frequent doses, and if vitamin D is used liberally, many patients with tetany can get along well enough. Vitamin D increases the body's ability to absorb calcium from the digestive tract. A few years ago a chemist was able to prepare an artificial vitamin D derivative which is especially potent in keeping up the calcium and assisting the kidneys to eliminate phosphorus. This is named dihydrotachysterol. It is now recognized that pure vitamin D is equally useful. It can be taken by mouth in small doses every day or two, whereas the parathyroid hormone must be injected hypodermically. Fortunately the use of dihydrotachysterol does not become less beneficial as time goes on, and this is coming to be the preferred method of treating tetany. The synthetic vitamin is superior to the extracts of the animal glands. The reason is not known, but it is believed to be due to impurities in the gland extracts as they have so far been made.

OVERACTIVE PARATHYROID AND BRITTLE BONES

In some persons the parathyroid glands develop into tumors, or become *overactive*, secreting an excessive amount of the hormone. The consequence is removal of too much phosphorus from the blood by the kidneys, following which the bones act as a reservoir of phosphorus and replace the blood's supply. In doing so the bones lose not only phosphorus but also calcium into the blood, and the amount of blood calcium may be significantly increased.

This gradually weakens the bones of the entire body. Sometimes the dissolving of calcium and phosphorus occurs in spotty fashion, and the X-rays of these bones look as though local excavations had been made. Such weakened bones are broken by trivial injuries. Healing is apt to follow with deformity unless great precaution is taken. Repeated fractures of several bones is a common result of the disease. The X-rays of bones, taken as a guide to the treatment of any fracture, will show evidences of this disease if it is present, and give warning to the surgeon of the further treatment needed in addition to proper setting.

EFFECTS ON KIDNEYS OF OVERACTIVE PARATHYROIDS

The long-continued excretion through the kidneys of the excess of phosphorus and calcium causes damage to these organs and a slowly progressive type of inflammation of the kidneys occurs. This may become fatal, as does any extensive damage to the kidneys' ability to excrete waste materials. In this case the outlook is more hopeful than in other types of nephritis, for the overactivity of the parathyroids can usually be cured and then the kidneys may regain healthy function if the disease has been diagnosed before damage is too extensive. Cure of this parathyroid disturbance is based on surgical removal of the tumors. If there are no distinct tumors, the surgeon must remove one, two, or even three of the four parathyroid glands. Since they are so difficult to identify, it will be evident that this is a task for a surgeon who has made a special study of the field. It is often not easy to make a certain diagnosis of overactivity of these glands, and here again it is important, when such trouble is suspected, that a competent physician carry out studies of such patients in hospitals equipped for special chemical investigations of this type.

THE TESTES OR MALE SEX GLANDS

Among the first structures to be suspected of secreting hormones were the testes or male sex glands. The striking change induced in young men who were deprived of these organs was the basis of this belief. The first experimental evidence was secured a hundred years ago, but it has been only within the past two decades that any great certainty has been achieved. The testes produce at least one hormone, known as *testosterone*, which has been studied so extensively that its chemical nature is known and it can be made synthetically by the chemist without the use of animal glands. Some investigators believe there is at least one further hormone made by testicular tissue, but the evidence for this is still uncertain.

The activity of testosterone is seen in many different parts of the body. As might be expected, this hormone is first produced in significant amounts as a boy approaches puberty, and the hormone is the stimulus which makes the external reproductive organs grow to their adult proportions. It is also the factor which leads to the growth of the prostate gland, situated at the bottom of the bladder. But effects of testosterone are found also in every kind of tissue of the body. The bones of adult men are heavier and stronger than those of boys because of this stimulus. The muscular development of men is brought about, in part, by this hormone. Growth of the cartilages in the larynx is accelerated by this factor, as a consequence of which the vocal cords become longer, and the voice achieves a lower pitch. Testosterone stimulates the growth of hair on the face and on those body areas which have come to be known as typically hairy in adult men. There are well-marked effects of testosterone on mental and emotional life also. The obvious increase in sex interest, leading ultimately to marriage and reproduction, is the most direct expansion of the effect of the hormone on behavior. But there are less obvious although just as real effects in the complicated group of ambitions, interests, and personality traits which teachers and parents recognize as the evidence of developing adult character. In summary, it may be said that testosterone is the hormone which is required to stimulate development from boyhood to manhood, and to maintain typically manly qualities thereafter.

Lack of testosterone for any reason is followed by failure to achieve this development or by a regression from adult type to a less virile and active physique and mental status. Individuals with sub-normally active testes, or who have lost these glands, suffer not only physical handicaps, as suggested above, but may have psychological difficulties associated with their consciousness of being different from others. It has become possible to inject solutions of testosterone into such men, and thereby to replace much of the lacking testicular secretion. Most of the features of adolescent development and adult interest can be induced in this way, so long as the treatment is maintained. Of course this type of treatment cannot substitute for the activity of healthy testes in producing the sperm cells, which are the essential testicular product for the fertilization of the ovum of the female, necessary for reproduction.

Much interest has been shown in the possible results of administering testosterone to the female. Such treatment produces rather curious results. In some ways the female is made to appear masculinized, as to changes in hair distribution, amount of muscles, and size of the cartilages in the larynx. The activity of the female sex organs is suppressed. The individual is neither typically male nor female. These results are maintained only so long as treatment is continued. It is possible that studies of this type, carried out on experimental animals, may give the explanation as to how certain unfortunate individuals are born with part of the sex equipment of the male, part of the female type. It is hoped also that investigations in this field will help to explain the curious behavior of some individuals who have been classed as homosexual, that is, attracted to others of the same sex. The solutions of these difficult problems remain for further study.

It is certainly rare that testes produce so much testosterone that an individual can be termed over-sexed. Probably this term, as applied to conduct, indicates merely a lack of intelligent self-discipline or too much thinking about sexual matters. Tumors do occur in the testes, but their dangers are due to factors other than overproduction of the hormone. By analogy with the overactivity of other glands of internal secretion, overactivity of testes might be expected. Perhaps this is prevented by the striking balanced action between these glands and the *pituitary* gland, which stimulates the testes to grow and secrete. The hormone of the testes, when injected in large amounts, will cause a decrease in that hormone of the pituitary which stimulates the testicular secretion. It appears that we have here another example of an automatic control which is set to prevent oversecretion of testicular hormone, for such an excess becomes promptly the inhibitor, or damper, on the process which leads to its own formation. On the other hand, it is certain that in some boys with delayed development of adolescence the fault is not the absence of testes, but inadequate secretion of the pituitary hormones, which must stimulate the testes into adolescent activity. This matter will be explained further in connection with other actions of the pituitary which apply to both sexes.

THE OVARIES

The ovaries have a dual task, as do the testes: they produce ova, or egg cells, and secrete hormones. The ovaries are now known to produce two types of hormone, both of them available in chemically pure form as a consequence of the intensive work of many investigators during the last 30 years. The first and best known of these hormones has been called the "female sex hormone" and is known technically as *estradiol* or *dihydrotheelin*. There are several chemical compounds related to this hormone which occur in the body, and are excreted in the urine. A few of these are so nearly like estradiol that they serve as substitutes for the real hormone in experimental work or in treatment of women who need the hormone as medicine. Estradiol is the most powerful of all the naturally occurring female hormones, and is probably the original and fundamental one in healthy ovarian action. A second ovarian hormone, chemically distinct, and having entirely different functions, is called *progesterone,* to be mentioned again below.

During adolescence the ovaries produce increasing amounts of both these hormones, and this process continues until the occurrence of the *menopause.* The physiological effects of the hormone called estradiol are varied: it causes growth of the uterus and development of the lining of the vagina to their adult types, stimulates the growth of the external genital parts to adult proportions, brings about the growth of hair in the armpits and about the genital organs, and stimulates the growth of the duct or tube system in the breasts. Besides these physical features of the directly reproductive apparatus, this hormone causes the development of the typically feminine figure, with narrow shoulders, broad hips and pelvic bones, and the deposition of fat under the skin which covers the bones and contributes to the graceful lines of the young adult female figure. Furthermore, this hormone is apparently the one which is responsible for that psychological development of ambitions and interests characterizing the adolescent young woman as contrasted to the girl.

One of the very important tasks apparently assigned to estradiol is the development of enormous numbers of glands in the lining of the uterus. This is a partial preparation for the reception of a fertilized egg. But before such an egg can become implanted in the uterus, it is also required that the second hormone, progesterone, shall have been available for a few days. Progesterone induces a change in these numerous uterine glands, enabling them to secrete into the uterus protein and carbohydrate material, which can serve as food for the egg cell, if this arrives. Without this latter step pregnancy cannot occur. Progesterone has been named for this feature, i.e., it is in behalf of (*pro*) pregnancy or *gestation*. Progesterone has a few other effects, such as reducing the muscular contractions of the uterus, and especially making secreting glands develop in the breasts. It is evident, therefore, that these two hormones of the ovaries are concerned with the direct and indirect provisions for reproduction of the race.

The production of estradiol is almost continuous from near the beginning of the second decade of life to near the end of the fifth decade. There are variations in the amounts secreted from week to week. The usual cycle of events in human ovaries is the liberation of an ovum from the ovary about once in four weeks. Not until this has occurred does the ovary begin to produce progesterone. This latter hormone is secreted for only a week or ten days at most. If the egg is not fertilized and implanted within this time, the secretion of progesterone subsides and a few days later the highly developed lining of the uterus is washed away, together with some bloody discharge. This flow of a blood-stained secretion is termed menstruation (because it occurs about once per month). Following this flow, which lasts a few days only, the cycle of events is repeated again and again.

If a fertilized egg cell is implanted in the lining of the properly prepared uterus, a different chain of events begins. The ovary is caused to continue the secretion of progesterone, in order that the egg may continue to have its nutrient material. Very soon the egg develops into an embryo, and forms a specialized structure called the *placenta*. This resembles a root system, which brings the circulation of the embryo into intimate contact with that of the mother, in the wall of the uterus. The placenta also produces a special hormone (*chorionic gonadotropin*) for the purpose of maintaining progesterone secretion in the ovary, and also of preventing the ovaries from liberating more ova. Later the placenta develops its own supply of progesterone, and then the ovaries are quiescent during the remainder of the pregnancy. There is a production of these two hormones, and estradiol, also, in this interesting placental structure throughout the nine months of pregnancy. At the end of this period changes in the proportions of these hormones occur, which are probably connected in some way with the onset of the muscular activity in the uterus which brings about the birth of the baby.

During pregnancy the increased supply of estradiol and progesterone brings about an increase in the number of glands in the breasts. The beginning of actual secretion of milk is dependent upon a special hormone from the pituitary, but this is counteracted during pregnancy by the ovarian hormones. Within a day or two after the birth of the child and the removal of the placenta, the sudden withdrawal of the supply of this placental hormone allows the pituitary hormone to produce the secretion of milk. This continues under the stimulation of suckling, but fails rapidly if the mechanical stimulus is absent.

Except during pregnancies the ovaries continue the cycles of producing ova and the accompanying secretions until in the fifth decade as a rule. Then a gradual decrease in the intensity of ovarian secretion occurs, eventually ova fail to be liberated, and no progesterone is formed. Still later estradiol is formed in smaller and smaller amounts, ultimately no hormone being produced. With such a change the menstrual rhythm is subject to a variety of alterations. Flows may become irregular in rhythm, may occur more or less frequently than once a month, may become more scant or more profuse, or may have any combination of such alterations. Such alterations as compared with the usually experienced routine should make the menopause the first consideration for any woman who has reached the fifth decade of life. Unfortunately, any of these same changes may occur at earlier ages, as evidences of disturbance in the endocrine activity of the ovaries. Also altered characteristics of menstruation, especially in the fourth and fifth decades, are often the first signal of the growth of fibroid or other types of tumors in the uterus. Therefore it is important that whenever women note any shift from their usual routine of menstruation they should report promptly for medical examination, to determine whether the change is due to a tumor, or to an endocrine change, and if the latter, whether it is the menopause or some other disturbance.

If menstrual regularity is altered, or if there are certain disturbances in glandular action, it may be possible to correct the condition by the use of pituitary gland extracts, but as these are still only in the stage of experimental use, other means for correction of such irregularity must be relied upon. Often a skilled physician can accomplish much in treating women who have irregularity of menstrual rhythm, if treatment is not delayed too long. If the flows are becoming irregular due to the menopause, there is no need to attempt to change this course of events. For a great many women there is little other evidence of a shift in the activity of the ovaries. But often women find that parallel to these objective changes there are a number of disturbing sensations, such as surges of heat, followed by sudden sweating and coolness, feelings of tenseness, headaches, consciousness of heart action and difficulty with breathing, dizziness, numbness and odd sensations on the skin. Also such women are frequently found to be more easily disturbed by minor vexations, with weeping, worrying, and periods of feeling depressed. Difficulty in sleeping soundly is a very common complaint. Women who undergo these symptoms, when they have had good health previously and have had no obvious illness to explain their discomforts, may begin to think their mental stability is disappearing. Yet nothing more than the subsiding activity of the ovaries may explain it all. It is not safe to make this assumption without medical advice, however, for any or all these complaints may be associated with other types of illness. Therefore whenever any of these bothersome symptoms become noticeable to a woman she owes it to herself and her family to give her physician the opportunity for a careful medical examination. Incidentally, this is usually at a time of life when several diseases occur more frequently, and such a health examination will serve to detect, or, still better, disprove the existence of such other disease.

One of the most widely applied benefits of research in the field of hormones has been the relief of all these complaints associated with the menopause. After it became possible, beginning in 1927, to prepare ovarian extracts of purity and definite strength, these were administered to women who were thought to need such hormones. It did not take long to convince both physician and patient that a new "specific" had been found. This term refers to a drug which is adapted with unusual exactness to the treatment of a given disorder. When the dose of ovarian hormone is adequate in size and in frequency, all the unpleasant symptoms of the period of "change of life" can be relieved. If the doses are large enough the uterus can be made to produce menstrual flows again. There is no advantage in this latter feature, however. Fortunately it is almost always possible to secure relief from the subjective difficulties without using a dose large enough to restore flowing. At first the treatment was given by hypodermic injections, but it was soon shown that this hormone can be administered by mouth. There is a rather prompt destruction of the hormone by the liver, immediately after absorption, but if the doses are large enough, and especially if they are given 2 or 3 times daily, oral treatment is entirely satisfactory. The choice of dosage, frequency with which it should be taken, most advantageous preparation for use, duration of treatment, and other variations are matters upon which every woman will need professional advice. For these reasons it is unwise for any woman to attempt to purchase ovarian materials for treating herself for such complaints, except on a physician's prescription. When the ovaries have been removed surgically, or when radium or X-ray treatment has been applied to the pelvic organs, similar symptoms are as apt to occur as during the menopause which develops spontaneously. Treatment is just as helpful under these circumstances.

At first it was thought that use of ovarian hormone treatment for relief of the symptoms of the menopause should be stopped as soon as it was no longer needed for the comfort of the woman. Now it is becoming apparent that longer continued use of hormone treatment may be of great value to bone strength, to healthy joints, and to the skin. Other benefits are being sought and the proper doses of the hormone for continued use will have to be determined by extended study over the next few years.

There is an old tradition that removal or inactivation of the ovaries will make a woman gain weight. The same thing has been said of the menopause. This is not true in all cases, and therefore we may be assured that it is not a necessary result of this change in ovarian secretion. Also it is very certain that treatment with the hormones of the ovary will not prevent or cure obesity. The frequent tendency to obesity in middle life has several factors which may contribute to the one result. Those who tend to gain need to revise their habits of eating and of exercise, again under medical advice. For those women who follow sound rules of hygiene, using medical treatment when really necessary, the passing of the menopause usually means reaching a period of greater stability of health and comfort than before.

THE PITUITARY

Mention has been made in several places of the relationship of the pituitary to other endocrine glands. The activity of the pituitary body, also known as the hypophysis, is more complicated than that of any other gland. In the first place one should speak of two, or possibly more, distinct portions of this gland. The *posterior pituitary* has to do with the retention of water by the kidneys, preventing dehydration of the body. It may have some functions connected with the muscular activity of the blood vessels, the intestines, and the uterus. These matters will be described in greater detail later. The *anterior pituitary* is a larger and entirely distinct part of the organ, which has far more important responsibilities. Although it is not known how many separate hormones the anterior pituitary secretes, it is certain that they include substances which stimulate the growth and activity of the thyroid, the pancreas, the adrenal cortex, the breasts, and the testes and ovaries. Also there are effects on growth, on the use of sugar and of fat, and possibly on the organs which manufacture blood cells. It is difficult to believe that there is a separate hormone for each of these effects, and equally hard to conceive of all these actions being carried on by only one hormone. But it is too soon to determine just how many separate pituitary hormones are produced.

The stimulation of growth by the anterior pituitary is one of its best known functions, though the manner of this action is still veiled in mystery. If the growth hormone is inadequately supplied the child will grow too slowly, but will have a well-proportioned body and average intelligence. If there is no other abnormality in physiology the individual will remain dwarfed throughout life. If, on the other hand, the growth hormone is supplied by the pituitary in greater than usual amounts, the stature will increase faster than the average, and the adult will be usually tall, or even a "giant." When this overactivity of the gland does not begin until after adult years have been reached, the stature cannot be increased because the bones no longer have a capacity for growing longer. The bones may grow thicker, and the head, hand, and foot sizes larger. The features become very coarse, the tongue large, and all the internal organs increase in size. This rare condition is called *acromegaly*. It is usually due to a tumor in the anterior pituitary. Sometimes this has to be removed surgically, but in other patients it is possible to stop the process with powerful X-ray treatments. Such pituitary tumors have another important feature: they are immediately in contact with the nerves passing from the eyes to the brain. A tumor (i.e., an enlargement) of the pituitary is therefore in danger of pressing on these nerves and damaging vision. It is for this reason especially that pituitary tumors deserve prompt and very expert treatment.

Growth of bones usually ceases by the age of 25 at the latest. As a rule, actual changes in stature stop before 20. Yet there is a continued production of the growth hormone throughout most of the remaining years of adult life. The use which the body makes of this hormone after the growing years is still a subject of investigation. It seems probable that this hormone has an importance in several ways, but almost the only evidence of this is that when the anterior pituitary gland is destroyed, the individual tends to become weak, underweight, and unusually susceptible to a variety of illnesses.

One of the most remarkable features of the growth mechanism is that the pituitary stimulates this process through the first 10 to 15 years of life, and then the same gland begins to stimulate the action of the testes or ovaries. When these latter glands have achieved something like adult secretion of their hormones, no more growth in height can be produced by the pituitary growth hormone. This is another one of the automatically balanced control systems which keep the human body in what we call normal condition. The explanation of this curious balance is of importance to those who are concerned with the growth and development of children. The growth of the long bones in the arms and legs determines the body's eventual stature more than other factors. These bones grow at both ends, by means of at least two centers of bone formation. Such centers are attached to the shaft of the bone by actively growing cartilages, in which the bone is being made. The pituitary growth hormone stimulates this bone-building process. Ultimately these growing centers become larger and the growing center and the bone unite with each other. After this union has occurred there is no cartilage in which further bone may be produced to elongate the bone. The enlargement of these centers of bone growth and their union with the shafts of bone is stimulated by two hormones, produced by the thyroid and the sex glands, testes or ovaries. The sex glands are especially important in increasing the speed with which the growing centers unite with the shaft. Thus it is that during adolescence the marked increase in secretion of testosterone or estradiol brings about this step in the maturity of bones and thus determines adult stature for the individual. It is of prime importance that the pituitary should stimulate growth to nearly adult proportions before the same gland begins to stimulate the typically adult functions of the reproductive organs. The way in which this sequence of affairs is regulated is still a profound mystery.

From these facts it will be evident that if any treatment is to be directed toward altering the growth process it must be undertaken in the years before adolescence is completed. Within recent years the growth hormone has been prepared in partially purified form, such that it can be given to children whose growth is going on more slowly than in the average child. The extracts must be given by injections, since there is no good evidence that they accomplish anything when fed. The effects appear slowly, and the treatment must be continued for many months if accomplishments are to be significant. It has been possible to induce more rapid growth in some children by this means, thereby avoiding what seemed certain to be abnormally short stature. Obviously that treatment needs to be carried out by a physician who knows what to expect of the procedure, and when it should be stopped. The use of X-ray pictures of the bones in the thigh is of value in determining when growth can still be expected. This bone is one of the last bones to complete its growth in length.

Unfortunately the increases in growth rate have so often been disappointing when pituitary extracts have been used that other methods have been tried. In a number of instances very gratifying results have followed careful use of combinations of thyroid with the sex hormones. This method has disadvantages which make it essential that the treatment be carried out only under the most careful medical supervision.

The normal supply of anterior pituitary hormones to stimulate the reproductive system begins gradually and comes to full intensity by the early years of the second decade of life. The development of testes and ovaries to fully adult activity requires a few years to be completed. The transformation in physical type as well as emotional attitudes and intellectual interests continues at a pace which seems rapid to the parent, often slow to the youth. It is probably well for the health of both body and mind that the process does not go on more rapidly. In fact there are some individuals who develop so rapidly that the coördination of processes is temporarily imperfect. It is common in this adolescent period to find awkwardness of muscles, instability of emotions, and minor disorders of the skin such as acne, or of the nervous system, such as sweating or irregular and fast heart action. Usually these matters are only evidences of a temporary imbalance, but medical supervision of such children is wise to make certain there are no disease processes concerned. Unusual leanness or excessive weight is frequently encountered at such periods, and these may necessitate instruction in appropriate habits of eating and of exercise.

In a few youths there is evidently a distinctly inadequate supply of the pituitary sex-stimulating hormones. If the evidences of adolescence are not seen by the age of 15 this is commonly thought to be abnormally delayed development. One needs to inquire about the time of maturity of the parents, for there may be a family tendency to early or late adolescence, which must be taken into account. If there is no inherited tendency to late adolescence, and no disease which serves as a handicap to either the pituitary or the sex organs, it may be wise to use special types of pituitary extract to augment the inadequate supply of the youth's own gland. This type of pituitary extract is of relatively recent origin, and is still being used chiefly by specialists in endocrinology, so that the rules for its successful use are not yet widely known. It is becoming evident that much can be accomplished by careful endocrinologists for some young people who are developing too slowly or incompletely.

A very similar treatment is used for adults whose fertility is reduced, when there is evidence of underactive testes or ovaries. Such use of pituitary gland extracts is of no value if the sex glands have been damaged by infections, such as mumps or gonorrhea, which leave permanent scars in the glands. Especially among women there are several types of partial deficiency in the secretion of pituitary or ovarian hormones, which interfere with achieving a pregnancy. During recent years, working with the partially purified pituitary materials available, physicians have been able to correct these deficiencies in a number of cases, helping women to become pregnant. It is probable that the accomplishments of endocrine treatment in the near future will be far better, when more highly purified pituitary hormone extracts have been prepared.

Another function of the pituitary is to stimulate the adrenal cortex tissue to greater activity. The hormone which is involved is called ACTH, since these are the initials of the words Adreno-Cortico-Trophic Hormone, which define the activity. It is fortunate that the adrenal cortex can continue to produce at least enough of its special hormone to support life even though the pituitary is inactive or even absent (as after an accident or surgical removal because of a tumor). But without ACTH stimulation the adrenal cortex does not produce enough hormone for good health. The production of ACTH varies widely from day to day, depending upon the stresses placed upon the body by emotions, great exertion, exposure to cold, the occurrence of infection, etc. Within very recent years an increased effort has been put forth to produce large supplies of ACTH from animal glands, since this hormone has been found to be very helpful in almost the same way as described for compound E, cortisone, of the adrenal cortex. So, for example, the use of appropriate doses of ACTH will give quick relief to sufferers from rheumatoid arthritis, lupus erythematosus, periarteritis nodosum, severe asthma or extensive hives, and it may interrupt dangerously high fevers. To date all efforts to prepare ACTH in really pure form have been unsuccessful, and of course the hormone cannot be made synthetically. The activity of these hormone containing extracts is measured by three different tests, based upon the effects on the adrenal glands of laboratory animals. Since these three tests do not always agree in the potency indicated, some investigators think there may be two or more compounds included in the term ACTH, and that these compounds exert distinct effects upon the adrenal glands.

As is the case with all active hormones, the use of too large doses can cause undesired effects. The body apparently requires only minute amounts for normal operation. Since the discovery of the benefits obtainable from treatment with ACTH it has been discovered that use of large amounts of ACTH, or of cortisone, will interfere with the usual method by which the tissues use sugar. As a consequence the pancreas is subjected to greatly increased demands for production of insulin. If this situation persists for many days the production of insulin is inadequate, or in other words diabetes mellitus appears. This is only temporary if the difficulty is recognized and use of ACTH or of cortisone is reduced. But if the treatment is not altered soon enough the diabetes may become permanent. This discovery has given a new understanding of the possible mechanism by which some cases of diabetes may result from overproduction of ACTH by the pituitary gland of the diabetic himself. One further result of this intensive study of ACTH treatment has been to demonstrate that the diseases which are ameliorated by use of ACTH cannot be considered as hormone deficiencies of either ACTH or of adrenal cortex hormones. The hormones are used as very powerful drugs to help the body recover from diseases caused by a variety of harmful agents. It is obvious that such treatment calls not only for medical skill, but that since experience in this field is recent, much remains to be learned about the best use to be made of these hormones.

The *posterior pituitary* is supplied with a large number of nerve fibers, originating in a part of the brain which is concerned with the unconscious regulation of temperature, weight, water retention, sleep, and muscular co-ordination, as well as of emotional activity. If these nerve fibers are severed the posterior pituitary will atrophy and be inactive. In this case, or if the posterior pituitary is destroyed by a tumor or injury, there follows a condition called *diabetes insipidus*. The name was used because of the passage of large amounts of urine. The word *insipidus* refers to the fact that the urine contains no sugar, therefore lacks the sweet taste of urine voided by a diabetic of the mellitus type. The posterior pituitary secretes a hormone which stimulates the kidneys to conserve water by the formation of more concentrated urine. The supply of this hormone is increased whenever the blood begins to become concentrated by the loss of water. In the person with diabetes insipidus this regulatory mechanism is inadequate. The kidneys continue to excrete water until the blood is seriously concentrated, making it more viscous and difficult to circulate. Before genuine danger occurs a second line of defense is set into motion: conscious thirst appears and compels the individual to secure more water. Of course this avoids damage to the body, but at the expense of unusually frequent drinking and unduly frequent voiding of urine. The process may cause disturbance of sleep, and thereby, and from the embarrassment of the frequent voiding, may cause more or less nervous difficulty.

Diabetes insipidus can be kept under control by the use of extracts of the posterior pituitary, which may be injected hypodermically from one to four times daily as required to avoid frequent passage of urine. Fortunately this hormone may also be absorbed through the lining of the nose, although it is destroyed if swallowed. The purified extract need not be used. Pituitary glands that have been dried and ground to a fine powder may be used as a snuff a few times a day to give easy and comfortable control of the loss of water. This treatment is not a cure, but must be continued indefinitely.

This extract of the posterior pituitary will also cause contraction of the muscular coats in the walls of the arteries, of the intestine, and of the uterus just at or after the birth of a baby.

Under special conditions extracts can be prepared from the pituitary which will cause changes in the distribution of the coloring matter of frogs and some species of fish. This has led to the belief that there is a relationship between pituitary hormones and some of the abnormalities of pigmentation in human skin.

OTHER GLANDS

The pineal, a small structure attached to the upper surface of the brain, and the thymus, occurring in the upper portion of the chest, just in front of the trachea, have long been suspected of being glands which produce internal secretions. The evidence is so little and so lacking in consistency that these structures merit no further consideration as endocrine organs. The fact that in many patients who have a progressive disease called myasthenia gravis the thymus has been enlarged, or more commonly found to contain a tumor, led to suspicion that the myasthenia resulted from an excess of secretion of some unidentified hormone by the thymus. This does not appear probable. In many cases surgical removal of the thymus or of the tumor has been carried out. The results do not convince most students of this subject that the thymus is responsible for the disease, or that the operation should be advised.

The thymus has been a cause of great concern because in infants it is often large enough to cause some pressure on the trachea and possibly to interfere with breathing. It has been suspected at times of being connected with sudden death in infancy from trivial injuries or infections. The thymus becomes smaller as the child grows older.

In the digestive tract there are several hormones produced during the processes of digesting food. One of these stimulates the flow of pancreatic juice when food leaves the stomach with the acid from the gastric juice. Another hormone derived from the lining of the bowel stimulates contraction of the gall bladder, forcing out some of the stored bile. A third hormone from the bowel serves to reduce the activity of the stomach. This is probably a factor in slowing down the emptying of the stomach, thereby extending the time available for digestion in both the stomach and the bowel. These digestive hormones seem different from most of the others already described in that they have only local actions in the stomach, bowel, and gall bladder.

CHAPTER XXI

Diabetes

ELLIOTT P. JOSLIN, M.D.

INTRODUCTION

DEATHS FROM DIABETES *in the United States have risen to nearly three times that of the rate in 1900. In the United States, for example, the rate per 100,000 population in 1900 was 9.7. In 1950, it was 29.7. Perhaps even more serious is the fact that more women have been dying of diabetes than men. The death rates for men and women were about the same until about 1905. Then the rate among women began to rise more rapidly, so that by 1932 about twice as many women as men died of diabetes. Sound conclusions regarding diabetes, however, cannot be drawn, because insulin was introduced around 1923, and diagnosis has become more frequent.*

A part of the reason for the greater number of cases found among women in recent years has been the improvement in diagnosis and the fact that women are being examined more frequently and regularly than they were in an earlier day. At present it would appear that diabetes is no more common among single women of any age than among men. Not all the people who have diabetes get an early diagnosis. Moreover, a laboratory examination is required to make a positive diagnosis. This, and the fact that women are appearing more frequently in positions requiring physical examinations, explain some of the increase in diabetes as found in women. Another reason is the aging of the population. Thus in 1901 the expectancy of life for white men was 48.2 years and for women 51.1 years, but in 1949 for men it was 65.9 years and for women 71.5 years. This growing older of the population increases the number of liabilities, because two thirds of all the cases begin after forty years of age.

A remarkable change has been brought about by the use of insulin in the causes of death of diabetics. Formerly, people who died of diabetes died from coma—a form of unconsciousness which resulted from chemical changes in the body. Today the number of deaths from this cause has decreased greatly. For instance, from 1897–1914 to 1944–51 the number of diabetic deaths due to coma dropped from 63.8 to 1.8 per cent in one large clinical group. At the same time there was a rise from 17.5 to 70.8 per cent in the deaths from diabetes associated with changes in the heart, the blood vessels, the brain, and the kidneys; but it is encouraging that gangrene resulting from poor circulation in the blood vessels of the lower extremities has decreased from 8.0 to 1.1 per cent between 1922–32 and 1950–52 as a cause of death.

Persons who have diabetes live much longer nowadays than those in former years. This explains why diabetics die of other conditions.

It must be realized that the person who develops diabetes has a lifelong problem. He must watch his condition carefully if he is to gain the maximum benefit from methods of treatment. It is known that in some cases the changes that have taken place in the body resulting from diabetes are hereditary. By use of insulin, children with diabetes—which used to be especially fatal to youngsters—now live and are likely to have children. Hence the question of heredity in diabetes will, in the future, be an increasingly important problem.

In the attack on diabetes in the United States, one of the most important contributors has been Dr. E. P. Joslin, whose article follows. He is author of a popular handbook on the subject, as well as of a scientific text widely used by physicians throughout the world. In the article which follows he clarifies the subject for the average reader and indicates at the same time the manner in which those with it may co-operate with the physician to the best advantage of their health. While recognizing that the average person may be competent to regulate his own diet under the advice of the doctor and also to administer remedies to himself, Dr. Joslin does not suggest either self-diagnosis or self-treatment as safe for anyone suffering from this disorder.

M. F.

THE INCREASING NUMBER OF DIABETICS AND THEIR LENGTHENING LIVES

It is hard work to keep up with the modern story of diabetes, and no wonder: first, because the number of cases increases so fast, and, second, because the treatment improves so much from year to year. In the closing twenty years of the last century the death rate from diabetes in the registration area of the United States trebled, rising from 2.8 per 100,000 in 1880 to 9.7 in 1900, but it took forty-nine years of this century for it to treble again, reaching 29.7 per 100,000 in 1949. During 1948, in New York City, the mortality was 48.2 per 100,000; in Cleveland, 39.6; and in Boston, 37.6. But this is only part of the story.

Fifty years ago my diabetic patients lived on the average a scant five years. Today diabetic patients expect to live indefinitely and, in fact, many live longer with the disease than, from insurance tables, one would expect them to live without it. I believe mine are living on the average three times as long, and, for those developing the disease under forty years of age, the average duration, based on the length of life of fatal cases, is twenty years, and indeed for all ages 30 per cent reach this duration.

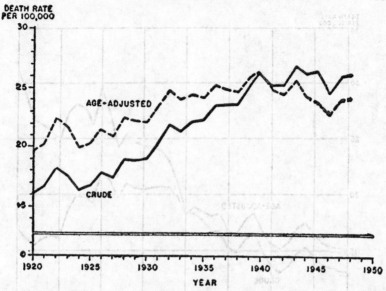

Fig. 40. Crude and age-adjusted death rates from diabetes United States Registration Area, 1920–1948.

(Courtesy of the Public Health Service, National Office of Vital Statistics)

The trend of the death rate from diabetes in the United States is shown in Fig. 40. The rate rose steadily up to 1940, but thereafter changed little, as is shown by the solid line of the diagram. However, the trend shown by this line is affected by changes in the age composition of the population because death rates from diabetes are much higher after forty years of age than under forty years, and the number of older people and their proportion to the total population of the country have increased. Adjusted death rates which make allowance for this change in the make-up of the population are shown in the broken line of the diagram. These are the rates which would have been recorded if the age distribution of the population had been constant over the period covered in the chart. These figures show a fall in the level of diabetes mortality since 1940. A similar diagram (Fig. 41), representing the death rate from diabetes among policyholders of the Metropolitan Life Insurance Company, shows this even more strikingly.

In 1946 the United States Public Health Service pushed ahead our knowledge of the frequency of diabetes by examining the urine and blood of most of the people in a community to find out the number of existing cases of diabetes, instead of depending on hearsay evidence by a house-to-house canvass. They chose a country town, Oxford, in Worcester County, Massachusetts, for their first research. This town of some 5,000 inhabitants was diabetically minded and medically minded, because it was the birthplace of Clara Barton, the founder of the Red Cross, and also because at her birthplace was a camp for diabetic girls, whom the townspeople often saw on their streets in the sum-

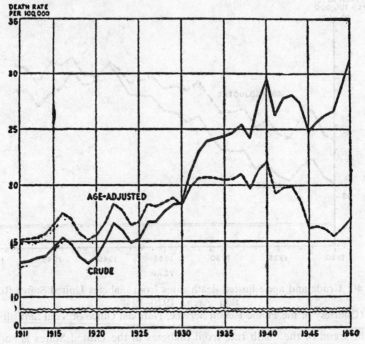

Fig. 41. Diabetes—crude and adjusted death rates 1911–1950.
(Courtesy of the Metropolitan Life Insurance Company)

mertime. As a result, Dr. H. C. L. Wilkerson, Chief of the Diabetic Section of the United States Public Health Service, found, first, that already there were known to the doctors in the town forty cases of diabetes, or a little less than one for each hundred; but, of far more importance, he discovered, by tests of urine and blood, thirty additional cases hitherto unrecognized.

The final results indicated that if all the 5,000 inhabitants had been examined, instead of 3,500 of the 5,000, there was one *unknown* diabetic for each *known*. Applying the results of this investigation and other similar surveys to the whole population in the United States, because Oxford, Massachusetts, is a representative community, one is justified in concluding that at least one in one hundred of all the inhabitants has known diabetes. I think today we should not say that another one in one hundred is unrecognized because doctors and people generally are more alert to discover it and because in those under forty years of age the signs and symptoms of diabetes are so striking it is more often and more easily recognized.

Years ago Dr. Priscilla White found that among the relatives of our diabetic children the disease was seven times as common as among non-relatives, and more recently the United States Public Health Service has found in Florida that it was four or five times as common among the relatives of known diabetics. This shows the importance of heredity, of which more later.

I believe diabetes is universal. In Arizona, where the mortality was reported to be 10 per 100,000—in contrast to New York and Rhode Island, where the mortality was around 40 per 100,000—I found in 1939 that actually, when I interviewed the doctors in every town of 3,000 inhabitants or over in the state, the doctors were treating just as many cases as in the northeastern states. Furthermore, among the Indians of Arizona I learned from examinations of their blood and urine that it was just as common as elsewhere when one allowed for age, sex, availability and accuracy of statistics. The rich Pima tribe of Indians, who rented their lands, showed the most, and the poorer wandering Navajos the least cases.

Studies of the American Diabetes Association in its diabetic programs have disclosed many cases, directly by tests of urine and blood of thousands, and indirectly by urging doctors to hunt for new cases, particularly among the obese and the relatives of diabetics.

Early detection and diagnosis of diabetes is of the greatest importance, just as we all recognize the importance of the early discovery of tuberculosis if one wishes to arrest the disease. Cases detected by insurance examinations are usually unknown and thus early cases, and it has been proved that these are the ones who do the best.

The known frequency of diabetes differs in different states of the United States and in various countries. We have seen reasons for this by comparing Arizona with New York, Rhode Island, Massachusetts, and other states. One cannot as easily explain why it is twice as great in Norway (13.6 per 100,000) as in Sweden (5.3); in Denmark (19.8) as in the Netherlands (8.5). At the meeting of the First International Congress of the International Diabetes Foundation, a vote was passed requesting the World Health Organization in Geneva to explain these differences. Obviously, stepping over the boundaries between Sweden and Norway, or the Netherlands and Denmark, will not double the incidence. Probably the explanation is connected with differences in the way the disease is reported by the doctors in these countries on the death certificates. Thus, we know in the United States by the methods of the *Fifth* Revision of the United States Census that the death rate was estimated at 29.1 per 100,000 for 1949, but by the *Sixth* Revision, in which doctors reported the actual cause of the diabetic's death and not diabetes alone, it was 16.9 per 100,000. The Sixth Revision of the Census prescribed methods nearer like those employed in England and Wales, where the rate was 8.4 in 1950.

Diabetes is far more important as a cause of death now than in 1920. This is due to the lowering of death rates from infectious diseases and diseases of childhood. In 1900 diabetes ranked 27th, but now is exceeded by the three diseases of the blood vessels in the heart, kidneys, and brain, by cancer and by tuberculosis and pneumonia, although in many states it surpasses the latter two. Diabetics are prone to diseases of the blood vessels. Every time we post-pone or prevent such a death from hardening of the arteries in a diabetic, we are also helping to prevent it in a non-diabetic. The diabetics are the guinea pigs who may teach the whole world how to live longer and in better health. Diabetics are useful members of the community.

Table 1. Chief Causes of Death (1) in the United States and (2) among the Policyholders of the Metropolitan Life Insurance Company per 100,000 for 1949.

Causes of Death	United States	Metropolitan Life Insurance Company
Heart disease	349	217
Cancer	139	114
Cerebral hemorrhage	101	57
Accidents and violence	61	48
Certain diseases of early infancy	43	—
Influenza and pneumonia	30	18[1]
Tuberculosis	26	24
Kidney disease	20	31
Diabetes mellitus	17	25

[1]Pneumonia all forms.

Table 1 shows the chief causes of death both for the United States and for the policyholders of the Metropolitan Life Insurance Company for 1949. In both lists the first four causes are the same: heart disease, cancer, cerebral hemorrhage (shock), and accidents. For the United States, certain diseases of children were fifth, but this does not hold for the insurance company because it insures comparatively few children. Influenza and pneumonia and tubercu-losis rank sixth and seventh for the country as a whole, but they are less prominent for the Metropolitan Life Insurance Company, perhaps because the policyholders receive better medical care. Kidney disease ranks eighth for the country, but fifth in the Metropolitan Life Insurance Company, thus leaving diabetes ninth in rank for the whole United States and sixth for insurance policyholders.

WHAT IS DIABETES?

Diabetes is a chronic disease. It is controllable not curable. It is a disease in which the patient fails to get the benefit of the food which he eats, particu-larly the sugar and starch (carbohydrate foods), and to a lesser degree of the meat, fish, eggs, and cheese (protein foods), and even of the fatty foods such as the fat on meat, cream, butter, oil, and the fat in nuts. The diabetic fails to get the full nutritive value of these foods because the pancreas, commonly known as the sweetbread and situated behind the stomach, produces an in-sufficient quantity of a substance named insulin. As a result of this lack of insulin, much of the food, including most of the carbohydrate, a notable quan-tity of the protein, but only a small portion of the fat, changes to sugar, and this sugar accumulates to excess in the blood and tissues. In normal people this sugar is quickly removed from the blood by insulin and stored in the liver, muscles, and skin, changed to fat or burned up to keep the body warm or furnish energy. In diabetes this normal routine is broken, and the sugar spills over and passes out of the body through the kidneys, escaping with the urine.

Years ago it was noticed that the urine of a diabetic was sweet, as sweet as honey, and so the disease was called *diabetes mellitus,* in contrast to a much rarer disease, *diabetes insipidus,* in which the urine is simply watery. The sugar is thus lost to the body, and from this fact anyone can imagine what most of the symptoms of diabetes must be. The untreated patient loses weight, because he loses the sugar in his urine. This sugar may amount to as much as one pound or even more in a day. He is thirsty because he must excrete the sugar in soluble form, and to do this he drinks large quantities of water. As a result he voids large quantities of urine. Of course he is thirsty, of course he loses weight, of course he becomes weak and debilitated, and years ago, when treatment was unsatisfactory, he became a prey to almost any disease. But now all this is changed, and, thanks to a better knowledge of diet and the discovery and use of insulin, the diabetic patient can live indefinitely. There are many times as many diabetics as fifty years ago, but this is largely because the treatment has correspondingly improved and kept alive those who have it for years—children fifteen times as long, and all patients on the average at least three times as long. A goodly percentage live longer with the disease than they were expected to live without it, because of their following the rules and living a more hygienic life.

Diabetes is not a bad disease, because it is clean and not contagious, and the patient who learns the rules of treatment and follows them can keep it largely under control. Many of the most celebrated people in the world have had diabetes. There is some ground for the belief that the diabetic is born more capable than the usual person. Be that as it may, certainly, through the training of his mind to control his condition, he acquires character. Therefore the diabetic should be encouraged. There may be compensations. With courage and persistence he can prove himself to be the master of his fate.

PREVENTION OF DIABETES

BLAMABLE DIABETICS (INFLUENCE OF OVERWEIGHT)

My friend Richard Wagner, formerly of Vienna, who has had many diabetic children to treat and has written an excellent book with Richard Priesel on the disease,[1] divides diabetics into two classes according to the origin of the disease: the blameless diabetics and the blamable diabetics. Let us consider the blamable diabetics first.

If a man gets smallpox today, we say he is to be blamed for it; he is blamable. If he gets drunk and has an accident, we blame him; if he is an adult and gets typhoid fever, we say he could have avoided it, he is blamable. No

[1] *Die Zuckerkrankheit und ihre Behandlung im Kindesalter,* George Thieme, Leipzig.

man needs to get smallpox, needs to get drunk, needs to get typhoid fever, because he can be vaccinated against smallpox, leave alcohol alone, and be immunized against typhoid. So it is with a large group of diabetics. Needless overweight precedes their diabetes. Most of those who have diabetes in middle life have overeaten and were fat before they got it. Take any group of diabetics of the age of fifty years or more, and the highest weights of most any ten of them before they developed the disease would have added up to a ton. Over and over again I have demonstrated this to my classes of patients, and this is what we can call blamable diabetes, because one cannot escape the conclusion that in the vast majority of instances, if obesity had been avoided, diabetes quite probably might have been prevented.

It was a common occurrence years ago to assemble at our diabetes classes ten diabetics whose maximum weights totaled a ton, but now I think fat people are less common. In Holland this summer I saw few obese individuals. Perhaps this is because most everyone there rides a bicycle. This fat type of diabetes contrasts sharply with *blameless* diabetes, in which overweight is insignificant and the chief factor is heredity. Overweight should be avoided particularly by relatives of diabetics, among whom diabetes is much more apt to occur. Overweight at all ages above the second decade predisposes to diabetes, but it is of little account among those who develop it until middle life. Eighty per cent of diabetics with onset above twenty years of age are overweight. In Jewish adults the figures are still higher, and among Jewish women reach no less than 94 per cent. Of my diabetics with onset between fifty-one and sixty years of age, only one in 1,000 gave a history of always having been underweight. Diabetic children are overheight rather than overweight, and the contrast shows from the earliest years of onset. When I see a diabetic who, I suspect, is overweight, I look up the age, weight, and height table and, if overweight is present, I make a large red cross on the history sheet along with the pounds in excess to attract his and my attention. I always weigh the relative of a diabetic coming to the office, if overweight seems probable, as a warning.

Table 2. Variation from Normal of Maximum Weights at or Prior to Onset of 1000 Cases of True Diabetes, Calculated for Height, Age and Sex

Age, Years	Number of Cases	Percentage in Normal Average Zone (+5 to -5 Per Cent)	Percentage of Each Decade	
			Below Standard Weight	Above Standard Weight
0 to 10	43	37	44	19
11 to 20	84	39	29	32
21 to 30	112	19	10	71
31 to 40	172	6	5	89
41 to 50	244	12	3	85
51 to 60	252	12	1	87
61 to 70	79	10	6	84
71 to 80	14	14	7	79

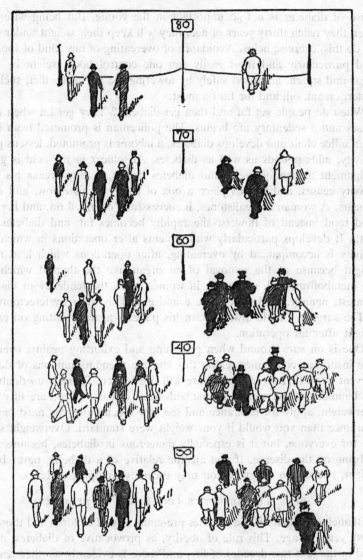

Fig. 42. How 10 fat and 10 lean men fare as they walk through life.
(Reproduced by permission of Lea & Febiger, from *Diabetic
Manual*, 8th Ed., by Dr. Elliott P. Joslin.)

Wise people, and particularly the wise relatives of a diabetic, remembering
the frequency of diabetes among the fat and the possibility of heredity, will
strive to keep their weight under control. If they are under the age of thirty-
five, they should not try to be underweight, because the young man or
young woman who is underweight has a shorter expectancy of life than the
one of normal weight or slightly above, and, furthermore, overweight as a

cause of diabetes is not so important in the young. But being wise people, when they reach thirty years of age, they will keep their weight under control. To do this, exercise helps. Avoidance of overeating of any kind of food helps. And particularly and most easily can one control body weight by limiting sugar and starch, and most safely by lowering the fat in the diet, such as the butter, cream, oil, and the fat on meat.

When do people get fat and then get diabetes? They get fat when exercise ceases and a sedentary life begins. The policeman is promoted from his beat to an office chair and develops diabetes; a laborer is promoted, lessens physical activity, adds pounds as well as diabetes. An officer in the field is given an assignment at headquarters, and diabetes begins. A boy breaks his leg, his activity ceases, and friends place a box of candy at his elbow, and diabetes appears. A woman has gallstones, is successfully operated on, and her friends send food instead of flowers; she rapidly becomes fat, and diabetes breaks forth. It develops particularly with patients after operations in which under-activity is accompanied by overeating, after operations which lead to over-weight because of the removal of an organ like the thyroid which lowers the metabolism; and, above all, in women when the tendency to diabetes is greatest, namely, at the menopause and especially after hysterectomy.

The surgeon should always warn his patients against putting on excessive weight after an operation.

One is on sure ground when preaching and exhorting against overweight. The insurance companies realize this and are spending millions of dollars to prevent it, so that those they insure will live longer. There is no doubt about the handicap of overweight to one with heart disease. If you are fifty pounds overweight, apply for insurance and see how much more you must pay to get insurance than you would if your weight were standard. Overweight shortens life for everyone, but it is especially dangerous in diabetes, because it helps to bring on the disease. If you are the relative of a diabetic, never be over-weight, because in this way you may escape developing diabetes.

BLAMELESS DIABETICS (INFLUENCE OF HEREDITY)

Blameless diabetes is the diabetes pre-eminently of children and those under thirty years of age. This rule of obesity, as provocative of diabetes, does not hold in the first two decades of life, and there is evidently another reason for the breaking out of diabetes in the young. Blameless diabetes is the diabetes, then, of the child, and why is his diabetes blameless and that of the poor old man or woman blamable? The diabetic child could not follow Oliver Wendell Holmes's rule and pick out his parents. Although Naunyn suspected and recognized heredity as the cause of diabetes, it is only recently that the proof of its influence has arrived. At first heredity did not seem to be of great importance, because in only 20 per cent of our cases in children could we trace a relative who had the disease. We did not realize years ago that this was simply because the children only lived a year or two and so we lost track of them. Their families were so sad at the death of their children that one did not feel justified in seeking information in after years about the later appearance of the disease in the parents or other members of the family. But today we have a sufficiently large group of diabetic children for statistical purposes who have already lived twenty years. And now we find that, instead of one child in five, or 20 per cent, having a relative with the disease, today, according to Dr. Priscilla White, every other child (actually 55 per cent) has a diabetic relative. As the parents of many of our diabetic children are still young, they have hardly entered the diabetic zone of fifty years, the year in which diabetes is most common, and therefore it is probable that still more may show it before they die. Dr. Priscilla White has studied this most carefully in association with Dr. Gregory Pincus, formerly of the Biological Department of Harvard University, now of the Worcester Foundation for Experimental Biology.

Table 3. Incidence of Diabetes in the Families of Diabetics. Percentage of Cases Reporting Hereditary and/or Familial Types of Family History. Recent Clinical Experiences.

	No. of Cases	Per Cent with Family History of Diabetes
Joslin, 1920–1928	4831	25.6
Joslin, 1941. Hospital Cases	1619	41.0
Joslin, total children, 1946	2191	35.0
Joslin, 1946. Children of 20 or more years' duration	249	55.0

The diabetic child is born with a tendency to diabetes. The facts correspond with the theory. Consequently, if you do not want diabetes, first of all pick out non-diabetic parents. The tendency to diabetes appears to be transmitted as a so-called recessive characteristic. If the tendency is strong, the disease comes on soon after birth; if the tendency is slight, it takes some secondary cause to make it develop, and of these secondary causes obesity stands first. Perhaps, after all, our fat friend is not so blamable as we may have thought: he may have been born with a tendency to diabetes. However, if he had kept thin, perhaps he could have avoided it.

The rules, therefore, for the prevention of diabetes as far as heredity is concerned are quite definite and can be summarized as follows:

To prevent the transmission of the disease to the offspring:

1. Two diabetics should not marry and have children, because theoretically all their children would have their disease.

2. If a diabetic marries a non-diabetic, but in whose family there is a close diabetic relative, half of the children are liable to have diabetes.

3. If two individuals marry who do not have diabetes, but in whose families the disease exists, the chances are that one in four of the children will develop the disease.

4. If a diabetic marries a non-diabetic who is of a non-diabetic family, no diabetic children should be expected, although their children could transmit the tendency.

For *practical* purposes, the liability of the offspring of diabetics to diabetes is not quite so strong as indicated above. It is only about *half the theoretical,* because those born of diabetics, like those of non-diabetic parents, die from other causes before the time arrives at which they would develop diabetes. Thus we know that only one diabetic in three develops the disease under forty years of age, one in three between forty and fifty-five, and the remaining one in three between fifty-five and one hundred years.

A diabetic child, therefore, is always a blameless diabetic. It is rather the parents who may be blamable. But the parents of a diabetic child are not always blamable, because they may not have been aware of the extent of diabetes in their families and may not ever have heard that diabetes is hereditary.

If you want to dodge diabetes, therefore, pick out your ancestors, don't get fat, and keep active; and if you have diabetes, or if it is in your family and you do not want to hand it down, fall in love with someone who does not have the disease or whose family is free from it. Of course, this may be a hardship, because you may not find anyone to marry who is as nice and bright as a diabetic, but still there are compensations, because your grandchildren may rise up and call you blessed. Remember there are 156,000,000 people in the United States, and only one fourth of them have a diabetic tendency. So there are left some 117,000,000 for you to choose from.

Every once in a while a diabetic discovers diabetes in a relative, and, contrary to his expectations, he is rewarded by finding that his relative does better with treatment than he himself. The reason may be that he has discovered the relative's disease at an earlier stage than that at which his own was recognized, and so treatment was started early, which is always a help. Furthermore, any diabetic who picks up the disease in a relative can be encouraged, because the treatment of diabetes is improving so rapidly that his relative, who develops it a few years after his own disease began, will be able to begin the treatment under improved conditions and so will do particularly well. I have seen this occur in various families where a second child has come down with the disease, and recently it was a great comfort to me to note the attitude of the parents when they found out that their second child had diabetes. They were sorry but not overwhelmed, because from their experience with their older boy they were confident they could keep the disease under control. This is about the best confirmatory evidence of improvement in the treatment of diabetes that I have.

The diabetic, if he is fond of his family, will not only point out to his relatives the dangers of being fat, but will go a step farther and along with the tests which he makes of his own urine he will make similar tests for the rest of the family whenever their birthdays occur.

Today the diabetic children are the pathfinders for the diabetic adults. Every honest diabetic day which a child lives teaches a lesson which helps a feeble old diabetic man or woman to live more comfortably. Children are exploring unknown diabetic regions. When I began practice I used to keep a record of the days a diabetic child lived, so as to see if the next diabetic child would live a day or two longer. Gradually little improvements in treatment occurred, and I could measure the life of a child by months, but up until the discovery of insulin the span of life of the diabetic child was less than two years. Today, the younger the child the longer can be the length of his life, and instead of saying, as we used to do, the older you are the milder the diabetes, now all agree the younger you are the greater the diabetic life expectancy.

THE ORGAN IN THE BODY RESPONSIBLE FOR DIABETES IS THE PANCREAS

Diabetes centers around the pancreas. This is commonly known as the sweetbread and lies behind the stomach and just in front of the backbone. It was not until 1889 that the discovery was made by Minkowsi and von Mering that by removing this gland from a dog diabetes developed. In the pancreas are groups of cells called islands of Langerhans. Their work was described by a young German doctor in 1869 and given his name, but no one appreciated what they were for until in 1901 Opie and Ssobolew discovered that when they were destroyed diabetes was present. It is not the whole pancreas but these collections of cells in it, which weigh not more than two and a half to five grams, or the weight of a dime or a nickel, that are responsible for diabetes. In them, insulin is made; and when we do not have insulin, diabetes exists. But there are other glands which influence the secretion of the Langerhans islands which make insulin. The most important is perhaps the pituitary gland situated in the center of the head and protected by a bony case. This is a tiny gland, the master gland of the body, which makes many hormones. It controls growth and sexual development and has many other functions. Inject an extract of it into a sound animal and diabetes will eventually appear, because it destroys the insulin-producing cells of the islands of Langerhans. Remove it and the diabetes gets milder.

Another gland situated on the upper pole of each kidney also influences the secretion of insulin. One of its powers is to interfere with the secretion of insulin, another is to accelerate the rapid breakdown of glycogen (animal starch) and protein in the liver and thus increase their change to sugar, thus making the diabetes more severe, providing insulin is not available to control the rate of change.

The thyroid gland in the neck, if overactive as in that type of goiter which is manifest by rapid pulse, protruding eyes, sweating and tremor, and rapid consumption of body tissue—increased metabolism—is another gland which affects the diabetes and makes it much more severe. Fortunately, by its partial removal this unfavorable action can be eliminated.

The liver is the storehouse of animal starch—glycogen—and is the factory where this can be broken down into sugar for the body to use or be con-

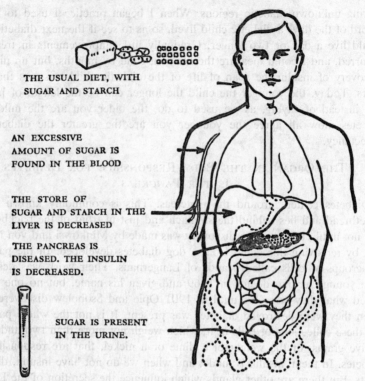

THE USUAL DIET, WITH
SUGAR AND STARCH

AN EXCESSIVE
AMOUNT OF SUGAR IS
FOUND IN THE BLOOD

THE STORE OF
SUGAR AND STARCH IN THE
LIVER IS DECREASED

THE PANCREAS IS
DISEASED. THE INSULIN
IS DECREASED.

SUGAR IS PRESENT
IN THE URINE.

Fig. 43. A diabetic patient untreated. The pancreas of a person with diabetes makes so little insulin that an excess of sugar is left in the body.

verted into fat and then either stored in the liver or transported for storage to other parts of the body. The liver is very important in diabetes because in it one kind of food is interchanged with another. We need to know much more about its many activities.

EXPERIMENTAL DIABETES

Dunn, in Scotland, while experimenting to learn the cause of shock, was so observant as to note that when alloxan, one of the many chemicals he was testing, was injected into an animal the islands of Langerhans were singled out and destroyed almost immediately, leaving the remainder of the body uninjured. He deserves great credit for having observed this, because grossly there was no change in the pancreas and it was disclosed only by microscopical examination. Alloxan is a derivative of uric acid, which is a common component of the body. If it were true that alloxan and uric acid were found in excess in diabetes, then we would be a step nearer to an explanation of its cause. However, this is not the case; for as yet alloxan has not been found in human beings, although studies revolving around it have taught us much.

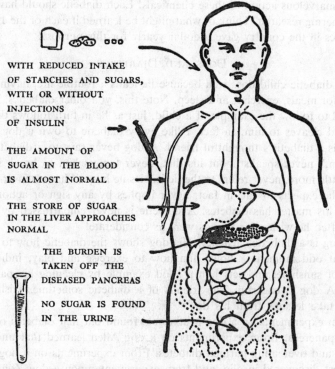

WITH REDUCED INTAKE
OF STARCHES AND SUGARS,
WITH OR WITHOUT
INJECTIONS
OF INSULIN

THE AMOUNT OF
SUGAR IN THE BLOOD
IS ALMOST NORMAL

THE STORE OF SUGAR
IN THE LIVER APPROACHES
NORMAL

THE BURDEN IS
TAKEN OFF THE
DISEASED PANCREAS

NO SUGAR IS FOUND
IN THE URINE

Fig. 44. A diabetic patient adequately treated. Before each meal, the
patient with severe diabetes must supplement his small supply of insulin with an extra amount obtained from an animal.

In Chile it was discovered that if glutathione was injected five minutes before
the alloxan, the effect of alloxan was abolished. Unfortunately, we do not
have glutathione in abundance in human beings. In faraway Australia, however, it was learned that if rabbits were on a diet deficient in glutathione, an
injection of an excess of the precursor of alloxan, namely, uric acid, also
would cause diabetes to appear.

There are two kinds of cells in the islands of Langerhans—the beta cells,
which are the more numerous and the ones which produce insulin, and the
alpha cells, which are less abundant and apparently secrete something which
raises the blood sugar and makes the diabetes worse. Quite recently it has
been found that just as alloxan will destroy the beta insulin-producing cells,
a mineral—cobalt—will destroy the alpha cells and thus abolish the action
of the alpha cells which makes the diabetes worse. The properties of alloxan
and cobalt are wonderful and almost past belief. Alloxan is so specific that it
is as though a bomb dropped from an airplane high up over a city with
800,000 blocks would invariably always select and destroy the same block!

What hours, days, months, and years must be spent to unravel the mystery of the marvelous action of these chemicals! Each diabetic should have a hand in furthering research. Think of what might be learned if each of the 1,500,000 diabetics in the country gave a dollar yearly for this purpose!

DOGS AND DIABETICS

The diabetic child does well because he leads a routine life, having regular hours for meals, exercise, and sleep. Note this, you older diabetics. You will do well to follow the example of a child, just as he in turn follows that of his dog and cleaves to him. In fact, I like every diabetic to own a dog, because a dog is a diabetic's thoughtful friend. A dog never says to a diabetic, "You are thin," never speaks about his diet, never tempts him to break it and to eat a little more, never refers to the delicacies he himself has eaten or the good bones he expects to eat; in fact, never implies by any sign or action that he knows his master has diabetes. A diabetic is never embarrassed by his dog. How often he wishes his friends were as considerate!

A dog is a diabetic's teacher. His dog shows the diabetic how to rest and sleep at odd moments, shows him how to exercise and play, indicates the value of sunshine, and sets him a good example by cleaning his paws every night. A dog is cheerful. The friends of a diabetic sometimes wish that he would take lessons from his dog.

From experiments on a dog Minkowski found out that diabetes originated in the pancreas. From experiments on a dog Allen learned that undereating helped and overeating harmed diabetes. From experiments on a dog Banting and Best discovered insulin, and from experiments upon a dog Young found that diabetes could be produced by injections of the pituitary gland, and Best showed that it could be prevented by the prompt administration of insulin.

Whenever I see a little boy named George, and his dog, Bob, and their devotion to each other, I am reminded of the million diabetics and future diabetics in the United States alive today, or who will be alive, enjoying better health and happiness, all because a few dogs, through the instrumentality of multitudes of scientific workers, have revolutionized the treatment of diabetes. Would you want to be a member of a society if it had for its object the prevention of a dog's saving the life of a child? Do you think this dog, Bob, would want to join such a society?

So deeply do I feel our indebtedness to animals for advances in medicine that in the foyer of the George F. Baker Clinic of the New England and Deaconess Hospital has been placed a plaque, suggested by the War Memorial Chapel in Edinburgh, with its memorials to men and women as well as to birds and beasts who also served and died.

DIABETES CONTROLLABLE

Diabetes is controllable, and that is the best news about the disease today. This is possible because of diet, exercise, and insulin, and a better understanding of the disease. No one need now die of diabetic coma which formerly was the chief cause of fatalities due to the disease itself. Tuberculosis, once the chief complication, also has almost disappeared, and the dreaded complications in the nerves, the blood vessels, and the eyes are preventable. Some doubt the latter statement, but my colleagues and I know it is true because we have the proof in faithful patients who have survived a quarter century of diabetes and are perfect. In contrast, we have seen thousands who illustrate the contrary. Years ago the Apostle Paul wrote, "The wages of sin is death," and it is just as inevitable if a diabetic breaks the rules of treatment that in time complications such as neuritis, premature hardening of the arteries, impaired vision, and even blindness will follow. The object of these pages, therefore, is to show how to control diabetes.

Education to replace ignorance about diabetes is the prime aim of all private and public endeavor.

DETECTION AND DIAGNOSIS OF DIABETES

No matter how good the remedies—diet, exercise, and insulin—are in the treatment of diabetes, they are useless unless one discovers who the diabetics are and sees that they are treated. This is the reason for the country-wide effort of the Detection Program—Diabetes Week—of the American Diabetes Association and the United States Public Health Service, namely, to find out who has the disease. Studies by the government in 1936 showed by house-to-house canvass that only one child under fifteen years of age in 2,500 had diabetes, but that among those adults above sixty-five years of age, one man in seventy and one woman in forty-five were reported to have it. Two thirds of the cases begin after forty years of age, but in my own special group, perhaps overweighted with children, there are as many cases with onset under ten years of age as among those we see between seventy and eighty years of age, and far more than after the age of eighty years. The median age of onset for men is 45.1 years, for women 50.1 years. Diabetes is decidedly more common in females than in males after the age of fifty, nearly twice as common, but so far as I have been able to discover it is no more common in single women than in men. Whether this is because married women weigh more—twenty more pounds, as I once found—or because of a more fundamental sex difference, I do not know. At any rate, after middle life diabetes is overwhelmingly more common in married women, and especially in all women who are overweight and the relatives of diabetics.

If you don't want diabetes, never get fat, and especially does this hold if you are a relative of a diabetic.

TESTING THE URINE FOR SUGAR

Every diabetic should learn how to test the urine for sugar. Then he knows whether his disease is controlled and, to a great extent, becomes the master of his diabetes. The urine on rising—the fasting urine—is the one most apt to be sugar free; the urine voided after a meal is the one most apt to contain sugar. If the fasting urine contains sugar, test another specimen half an hour later, because that urine may be sugar free. The reason for this is that the urine is constantly being secreted by the two kidneys day and night, and then passes through two tubes, called ureters, into the bladder. This has no compartments. Therefore, if a urine containing sugar was secreted at 2:00 A.M. by the kidneys, it would collect in the bladder, and even if no sugar was secreted by the kidneys at 7:00 A.M., when the bladder was emptied, the voided urine would contain sugar, because it would have been mixed with the 2:00 A.M. specimen.

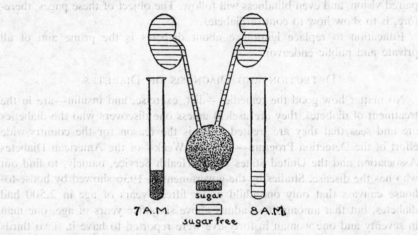

Fig. 45. Two Specimen Tests. If a separate specimen of urine is voided between 7 A.M. and breakfast at 8 A.M., a true idea of the presence or absence of sugar in the fasting state is obtained. This is very desirable for those patients taking both the regular and protamine insulin before breakfast. The 7 A.M. specimen represents the specimen which has been collecting for hours in the bladder; the 7:30 or 8 A.M. specimen represents urine recently secreted and is therefore a better index of the sugar in the blood.

The Benedict Test. The Benedict test is the test most generally employed for the detection of sugar in the urine. It requires a single solution and this keeps indefinitely. The test is sufficiently delicate to detect quantities as small as 0.08 or 1.10 per cent sugar, in which case a faint pea-green change in color takes place. This green color changes to a yellowish-green when the urine contains about 0.5 per cent sugar. When the solution loses the greenish tint entirely and becomes yellow or brown, the urine contains over 1 per cent sugar. Above this percentage the color of the solution gives very little aid in estimating the amount of sugar in the urine, although large amounts of sugar will produce an orange, brown, or red test.

The test is carried out as follows: Four (exactly 4) drops of urine are placed in a test tube and to this are added 2.5 cc. (an ordinary teaspoon holds about 5 cc.) of Benedict's solution. Eight drops of urine and 5 cc. of Benedict's solution are often employed, but the use of half quantities is just as satisfactory and more economical. The tube is shaken to mix the urine and solution, and then placed in water that is already bubbling boiling. In the presence of glucose (sugar), the entire body of the solution will be filled with a precipitate, which may be greenish, yellow, or red in color, according to whether the amount of sugar is slight or considerable. Particularly if 4 drops are used with 2.5 cc. of Benedict's solution, the test should be carried out in boiling water for five minutes rather than over a free flame, because of evaporation of the solution. If 5 cc. of Benedict's solution and 8 drops of urine are employed, as in the original test, the solution may be boiled over a free flame for two minutes, in which case a Pyrex test tube should be used. This latter method is liable to error because, unless one has a test-tube holder, the test tube gets too hot to hold with the fingers, and therefore the specimen may not be boiled for the whole length of time.

Tests of the urine for sugar should always be performed accurately.

THE BLOOD SUGAR

All of us have sugar in our blood. The kind of sugar is glucose. Glucose is grape sugar, and because a ray of light passing through a solution of it is turned to the right, it is said to be dextrorotatory and is called dextrose. The normal percentage varies between about 0.080 to 0.120 per cent fasting (often reported 80 and 120 milligrams) and does not exceed 0.160 after a meal. In diabetes the blood sugar is above normal after an ordinary meal and usually rises to 0.200 per cent, 0.500 per cent, or more. If the sugar in the blood is

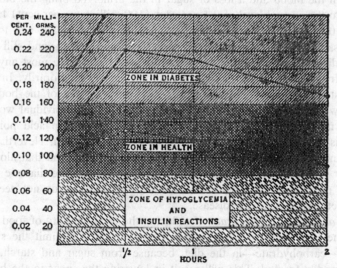

Fig. 46. Blood sugar zones, in health, in diabetes, during an insulin reaction. (Reproduced by permission of Lea & Febiger, from *Diabetic Manual*, 8th Ed., by Dr. Elliott P. Joslin)

above normal, it is termed *hyperglycemia;* if the blood sugar is below normal, it is termed *hypoglycemia.* The fasting blood sugar is usually elevated in diabetes, but may not be in the very early stages of the disease, particularly in children. The sugar in the blood corresponds to that in the urine only when compared with a specimen of urine which has been secreted by the kidneys and voided in the preceding few minutes—half an hour—the bladder having been previously evacuated.

DIAGNOSIS OF DIABETES

A diagnosis of diabetes is made when, in addition to sugar in the urine, the fasting blood sugar is 0.130 per cent, or 130 milligrams, or when after food the blood sugar is 0.170 per cent, 170 milligrams, or above. These values are border-line values, and one is very cautious about telling a patient he has diabetes unless they are later confirmed by the same or higher values.

Sugar in the urine which is unaccompanied by an increase of sugar in the blood is not diabetes. About 15 per cent of the patients coming to me with sugar in the urine do not have diabetes because the sugar in the blood is not above normal. Eventually about 10 per cent of such individuals become frank diabetics, and these are chiefly the ones with a diabetic heredity or who are overweight.

TREATMENT OF DIABETES
DIET

1. Reduce the Total Amount of Food. In diabetes there is an excess of sugar in the blood and a loss of sugar in the urine. To bring the blood sugar down to the normal level of 0.1 per cent (100 milligrams per cent) fasting, or below 0.17 per cent (170 milligrams per cent) after meals, and to prevent this loss of sugar in the urine, the earliest method known, and still the best, is the diet. Fasting, living entirely without food, will make most any diabetic sugar free, but naturally that can be employed only temporarily. In the very severest cases it would be dangerous, because even out of the body tissues sugar would be formed and lost in the urine, and the individual would burn up so much of his own body fat that he would develop acid poisoning— acidosis—which would result in diabetic coma and death. Nevertheless, the avoidance of overeating of any kind of food is helpful, and that alone in the mildest cases will prevent the diabetes growing worse. The diabetic therefore should never overeat, should never be fat, but today we do not need to fast a diabetic to control his disease.

2. Lower the Carbohydrate. If reducing the total quantity of food does not stop the loss of sugar in the urine, the next step is to limit the sugar and starch—carbohydrate—in the diet, because from sugar and starch, sugar is most readily formed. This will result in lowering the sugar in the blood and the escape of sugar in the urine. Today we need not omit all the carbohydrate, because one can take insulin to help utilize part of it. It is seldom necessary

DIETARY ESSENTIALS FOR DIABETICS

Table 4. Carbohydrate, Protein, Fat, and Calories in Common Foods

30 Grams 1 oz. Contain Approximately	Carb. C. Gram	Protein P. Gram	Fat F. Gram	Calories
Bread, 1 large slice	15	2.5	0	70
Oatmeal, large portion	20	5	2	118
Crackers, 2	10	1	0	44
Vegetables, 3% + 6% 4 large portions	20	6	0	104
Potato	6	1	0	28
Milk	1.5	1	1	19
Egg, 1	0	6	6	78
Meat, lean	0	7	5	73
Chicken, lean	0	8	3	59
Fish, fat-free	0	6	0	24
Cheese	0	8	10	122
Bacon	0	5	15	155
Cream, 20% light	1	1	6	62
Cream, 40% heavy	1	1	12	116
Butter	0	0	25	225

Vegetables and Fruits Arranged According to Content of Carbohydrate
Water, clear broths, coffee and tea, can be taken without allowance for food content

---

VEGETABLES, fresh or canned

*Reckon average carbohydrate, utilized,
3%; 6%; 20%*

3 per cent

Lettuce	Tomatoes
Cucumbers, raw	Radishes
Spinach	Water cress
Asparagus	Snap beans
Celery	Cauliflower
Mushrooms	Cabbage
Rhubarb	Egg plant
Sauerkraut	Broccoli
Endive, raw	Green peppers
Swiss chard	Kohlrabi
Beet greens	Kale
Dandelions	Summer squash

6 per cent	20 per cent
Turnip	Potatoes
Carrots	Shell beans
Okra	Baked beans
Pumpkin	Lima beans
Onions	Corn
Squash	Boiled rice
Brussels sprouts	Boiled macaroni
Beets	
Green peas	

FRUITS, fresh or canned
(water packed)

Food	Carb. 10	Grams 15
Grapefruit pulp	150	225
Strawberries	150	225
Watermelon	150	225
Cantaloupe	150	225
Blackberries	120	180
Orange pulp	100	150
Pears	90	135
Peaches	90	135
Apricots	80	120
Raspberries	80	120
Plums	80	120
Pineapple	70	105
Apple	70	105
Honeydew melon	70	105
Blueberries	70	105
Cherries	60	90
Banana	50	75
Prunes (cooked)	50	75
Ice cream	50	75

1 gm. carbohydrate,   4 calories
1 gm. protein,   4 calories
1 gm. fat,   9 calories

1 kilogram (kg.) = 2.2 lbs.
30 grams (g.) or cubic centimeters
(cc) = 1 oz. A patient "at rest" requires
25 calories per kg.

Table 5. Diabetic Diets in Grams

Diets	Total Diet				Carbohydrate (C)						Protein and Fat (PF)				
	Carbo-hy-drate	Pro-tein	Fat	Calo-ries	Vege-tables 3%-6%	Or-ange	Oat-meal	Po-tato	Bread	Milk	Egg	Meat	Bacon	20% Cream	Bu-tt
C1 PF1	137	60	61	1337	600	450	0	0	90	300	1	120	0	0	3
C2 PF2	149	65	74	1522	600	450	15	0	90	300	1	120	0	60	3
C3 PF3	167	78	86	1754	600	450	15	90	90	300	1	150	15	60	3
C4 PF4	184	89	103	2019	600	450	15	90	120	300	1	180	15	120	3
C5 PF5	199	101	116	2244	600	450	15	90	150	300	1	210	30	120	3
Acute Illness	160	52	52	1316	0	450	15	0	90	960	1	0	0	0	1

All above diets include 2–4 biscuits at bedtime

To add carbohydrate 15 grams, add bread 1 slice, potato 75 grams or 1 medium orange; to add 75 calories, add bread 1 slice, milk ½ glass, meat 1 oz. or 1 egg. One oz. bacon contains C.0 P.5 F.15 155 calories; one oz. butter 225 calories.

to reduce the carbohydrate below that contained in a slice of bread and a medium-sized orange at each meal, four portions of vegetables in the low 3 per cent and 6 per cent carbohydrate groups (Table 4), a portion of cereal, and oatmeal is the best because it contains the least carbohydrate, a glass of milk, and a few biscuits—4 saltines, 3 Uneedas, or 4 graham crackers. The balance of the diet would be made up of the usual quantity of protein—meat, fish, eggs, cheese—for the age, weight, and height of the individual, and finally of fat sufficient to maintain a normal weight or bring it to normal. Liquids are unrestricted, and as for minerals and vitamins, there are usually enough in the foods above mentioned.

The above diet can be increased or decreased according to age and size and activity, but there are few who would eat twice as much, and only rapidly growing boys and girls and very hard-working men three times as much carbohydrate.

COMPOSITION OF THE ABOVE DIET

What is the composition of the above diet? How much carbohydrate, protein, and fat does it contain?

Carbohydrate

The carbohydrate content in this diet is easily reckoned if one will remember that a slice of bread, if it weighed one ounce, or 30 grams by the metric system, would contain approximately one-half carbohydrate, one-half ounce, or 15 grams. A half ounce is equivalent to a tablespoonful of sugar, or 3 large lumps. A nickel weighs 5 grams.

The diet is easily learned by examination of tables 4 and 5.

Table 4 shows the vegetables which contain the least carbohydrate utilized by humans. Even four liberal portions of 3 per cent and 6 per cent vegetables contain only about 20 grams of carbohydrate, which is so little that few diabetics show sugar in the urine if they eat them alone without insulin. They are good for diabetics because they furnish bulk, contain many vitamins, and satisfy hunger. The vegetables in the 20 per cent carbohydrate group, like potatoes, contain much more carbohydrate, and about one third as much as bread. Many diabetics eat no potato when they take bread. Remember that sugar and starch are 100 per cent carbohydrate, bread 50 per cent, potatoes 20 per cent, fruit about 10 per cent, except bananas which are 20 per cent, and vegetables 3 to 6 per cent.

Vegetables in the 3 and 6 per cent carbohydrate groups were formerly listed as 5 and 10 per cent vegetables. They do contain these amounts, and animals eating them get 5 or 10 per cent value of carbohydrate from them, but human beings are not able to secure their full value. A cow gets nourishment from hay and grass, and even Nebuchadnezzar, when "he was driven from men, and did eat grass as oxen," acknowledged its good effect by saying "mine understanding returned unto me" (Daniel 4:33–34).

Diabetics like to eat. Therefore, give them bulky foods in which the percentage of sugar and starch, the so-called carbohydrate foods, is low. Such foods are the vegetables (the green vegetables, those which generally grow above the ground), termed 3 and 6 per cent vegetables. These bulky vegetables require a long time to be eaten, their use permits many minutes of happiness.

Diabetic vegetables, however, have other advantages in addition to the pleasure one derives while eating them. The sugar and starch in these low-carbohydrate vegetables take so long to get from the stomach into the blood that when the patient takes them, his blood is not suddenly swamped with sugar, which would be the case if he took pure carbohydrate such as sugar or cornstarch. I often tell my patients that the carbohydrate in vegetables *creeps* into the blood, the carbohydrate in potatoes and in cooked rice or macaroni *walks* right into the blood, whereas actual sugar in the diet *runs* into the blood, and if the blood is overloaded with sugar, it spills over and leaks out through the kidneys. Still another great advantage which comes to the diabetic who eats freely of green vegetables and fruits is due to the vitamins which they contain. Perhaps it is because of all these vitamins in vegetables and fruits that diabetic children have such good teeth.

Fruit is desirable, and most kinds contain between 10 and 20 per cent carbohydrate. The equivalent in grams of various fruits which contain 10 or 15 grams is shown in the table at the top of the fruit columns. A few fruits, like grapefruit and strawberries, can be taken in greater amounts than oranges to make up 10 or 15 grams carbohydrate. A medium-sized orange, peeled, contains 15 grams carbohydrate. An apple of similar size contains nearly half as much more. Diabetics must always be careful to compare an apple with its thin skin to an orange without its thick skin.

Fruit is the diabetic's best dessert.

Grapefruit is the safest fruit for a diabetic in that it contains only about 7 per cent carbohydrate. The sugar in half a medium-sized grapefruit is equivalent in weight to two nickels, or 10 grams. Oranges contain 10 per cent carbohydrate, and a small orange, peeled, weighs 100 grams and its sugar content is therefore equal to 10 grams, which is the same as in the half medium-sized grapefruit. A banana contains 20 per cent carbohydrate, and as the ordinary banana weighs about 100 grams, the carbohydrate in half a banana would be equivalent to that in a small orange or half a medium-sized grapefruit. Bananas vary so much in size that, as with potatoes, it is safer to weigh out the allowed portion. Potatoes and bananas, weight for weight, are alike in the percentage of carbohydrate, and it makes no difference whether they are cooked or not so far as the carbohydrate is concerned.

Protein

Tiny cells make up our bodies, and the essential component of these is protein. A horse likes his oats because there is more protein in the oats than in the straw. Protein we must have to replace old cells and to add new ones. Diabetics need protein just like the rest of us. Protein is found in concentrated form in meat, in fish, in eggs, and in its purest state in the white of an egg. The baby gets his protein in the curd or cheese of milk. The younger you are, the more protein you require, because not only have children worn-out cells to repair, but they need new cells to grow. Instinct teaches the baby to take three or four times as much protein for his weight as the old man. (Milk is an ideal food partly because it contains so much protein, and again because of its high content of calcium [lime] for the formation of bones.) Fortunately, diabetics can have as much protein as the ordinary individual and only seldom should have more.

Fat

Fat is the third component of the diet. This is to be found in a pure state in oil. Butter is 85 per cent fat, and cream is a transition from this percentage to the 3 per cent in milk as established by law. There is fat in meat and fish, and one should never forget that in nuts and cheese the percentages of fat are usually high. Oleomargarine can be reckoned as butter. A generation ago we doctors reduced the carbohydrate (sugar and starch) in the diet of our diabetic patients so low that we were compelled to raise the fat to furnish them enough nourishment to keep alive, and we overdid it. What happened? We satisfied their hunger, but we poisoned them with fat, because in the fat lurked danger. Soon we found out through the painstaking work done in many laboratories that if the proportion of fat to carbohydrate in any diet was unduly high, the patient's individual tolerance for fat was exceeded, acetone bodies accumulated in amounts greater than he could oxidize, which in turn caused acid poisoning and death from coma. For this reason today the fat in the diet of diabetics is watched quite as closely as the carbohydrate, and for this same reason we are testing the fat in the blood as well as the sugar to be sure it is not in excess.

As a rule, the diabetic is given as much sugar and starch (carbohydrate) as he can take without sugar appearing in the urine. If he cannot tolerate a considerable quantity—the 150 grams mentioned above in the form of bread 3 slices, oranges 3, 3 per cent and 6 per cent vegetables very freely, oatmeal one portion, milk 1 glass, biscuits 3—he is given insulin to help him get the benefit of it. He takes as much protein as the ordinary individual. As for the quantity of fat, he regulates that by what he needs to hold his weight, which seldom if ever should long remain above normal standards.

In the table on page 525 are recorded foods with varying percentages of carbohydrate, and, for certain commonly used foods, the quantities of carbohydrate, protein, and fat per 30 grams or one ounce. The values are approximate and not absolute.

A DIABETIC'S MENU

The average diet prescribed for a diabetic in the United States today, I suspect, is about as follows, and if it is not tolerated, the patient's doctor will probably give him insulin.

Breakfast:
> Half a grapefruit, a medium portion of oatmeal or a little less of any other cereal, one egg, a pat of butter, one slice of bread, coffee and cream.

Dinner (noon):
> A moderate portion of meat or fish, two liberal portions of 3 per cent vegetables or somewhat less of 6 per cent vegetables, a slice of bread or a medium-sized potato, a pat of butter, an orange or its equivalent.

Night:
> A similar meal to that at noon.

During the day:
> Half a pint of milk and ¼ pint medium rich cream.

With such a diet as a working basis, it is easy to add to it or detract from it according to the needs of the individual patient and to make definite the quantity of carbohydrate, protein, and fat. Such a diet probably contains carbohydrate 150 grams, protein 65 to 75 grams, and fat 80 grams. The food and caloric values are shown in the table on page 530.

If one wishes, such a diet can be reckoned in calories.

Food	Calories per Gram	Carbohydrate in Diet	Total Calories
Carbohydrate	4	150	600
Protein	4	70	280
Fat	9	80	720
			1600

The Diabetic Diet Is Simple

Food	Unit Portion	Grams in Each Portion				Total Daily Portions	Total Grams		
		Weight	C	P	F		C	P	F
Bread	1 slice	30	18	3		3	54	9	
Oatmeal	1 large	30, dry	20	5	2	1	20	5	2
Orange	1	150	15			3	45		
Vegetables, 3–6%	1 cup	150	5	2½		4	20	10	
Milk	¼ pt.	120	6	4	4	1	6	4	4
Cream, 20%	¼ pt.	120	4	4	24	1	4	4	24
Egg	1	60		6	6	1		6	6
Meat	1 small	60		16	10	2		32	20
Butter	1 square	10			8	3			25

Grand total grams (approximate)   C150   P70   F80
Calories per gram   x 4   x 4   x 9
Total Calories – 1600 = 600+ 280+ 720

Calories

Just as coal and gasoline furnish heat which can be reckoned in heat units, so the food we consume contains heat, and this can be estimated also in heat units, or calories. A calorie is a standard unit of heat and is equivalent to the quantity of heat necessary to raise one kilogram of water one degree centigrade, or approximately one pound of water one degree Fahrenheit.

All of us need calories—heat—to live. Babies and children need more heat than adults, because they are more active and must grow. A baby grows so fast that it requires about 100 calories for each kilogram—2.2 pounds; an adult requires about 30 calories with moderate activity, and an old man or woman less. Exercise greatly increases the need for calories and similarly rest in bed decreases it.

The caloric—heat—value of food varies with its composition, just as does the heat value of coal, whether it is of high or low grade. Pure carbohydrate and protein give off 4.1 calories for each gram burned; fat yields 9 calcries. Therefore, if we reckon up the grams of carbohydrate, protein, and fat in the diet, we can easily determine the calories. (See Tables 4 and 5.)

A person always eats, never truly fasts. He always requires heat—calories —and if he does not get calories from food, he eats up his own body: first, that part of it which is in the form of carbohydrate—glucose and glycogen, or animal starch; next, the fat; and, last of all, the protein which composes the various tissues.

A person needs from 100 to 25 calories per kilogram (2.2 pounds) body weight, according to whether he is a baby or an old man. The above diet would be about right for an adult who weighs 110 pounds, or 50 kilograms, because it would furnish a little over 30 calories per kilogram body weight.

Bouchardat, a hundred years ago, did not weigh diets, but he did almost better by teaching his patients to examine the urine. If, after eating a certain food, sugar showed, his patients knew that food contained too much carbohydrate—sugar or starch—for them. This is worth while doing today, and the oftener the urine is examined the better. Especially is this necessary if the diabetes is hard to control and it is difficult to keep the urine sugar free. One should never give up testing the urine. My patient with diabetes of over twenty-five years' duration, with three children born during her diabetes, omitted testing on a camping trip; her diabetes grew worse and she went into coma, and it took her more than six months to recover. Another patient, with a fabulous income, felt he could take no chances. He collected and submitted at least six specimens daily to his nurse. He never had diabetic coma or insulin reactions and lived over thirty-one years with diabetes, despite its having begun before the discovery of insulin. He could not afford a reaction, because it might have cost him his job as president, bank director, and trustee of many corporations.

EXERCISE IN THE TREATMENT OF A DIABETIC

The second steed in the diabetic's three-horse chariot of treatment is exercise. Years ago I learned its value from a diabetic patient who did unusually well. His favorable progress puzzled me, but after studying his case, it finally came over me that besides being a reliable patient and adhering to his diet, he did well because he exercised. He worked on a railroad, and railroad workmen are reliable, but apart from this I found out that his particular job was to drive an old-fashioned handcar and inspect the tracks over a stretch of many miles. Back and forth he bent his back to turn the crank of his handcar morning and afternoon in those days when one's motor was made of muscles, not steel, and in this way he could assimilate the carbohydrate which he ate. This man showed me the value of exercise in diabetes. About the same time I had a diabetic doctor, and he told me there was less sugar in his urine when he was camping and tramping and carrying his canoe in the depths of the woods in Maine than at home, where his diet was more strict and his exercise far less. Then I began to have all my patients exercise. Exercise does everything for a diabetic, but there are limitations. To drive this horse, Exercise, along with Diet and Insulin, requires judgment, and one must often lower the load for Exercise and increase it for Insulin. Exercise is good for the diabetic of mild or moderate severity, but for the severest diabetics before we had insulin, exercise did harm, and only recently a few patients told me they got along better if they stayed abed. Exercise to be advantageous requires insulin. The mild diabetic has enough insulin of his own available; the moderately severe diabetic produces some insulin; but the severe diabetic who manufactures practically none of his own must buy it and inject it, and then he can undertake as strenuous exercise as any healthy man or woman. In general, however, any patient who cannot exercise is handicapped. Such was the fate of the rare diabetic prior to the use of insulin who was crippled with rheumatism. One reliable patient tells me a game of golf is worth five units of insulin. Today doctors are careful to provide exercise in one form or another for their diabetics who must stay abed as a result of operations or for other reasons. Exercise should be utilized in the treatment of nearly every case of diabetes, but this steed must not be overdriven.

Exercise lowers the sugar in the blood just as does lack of food (fasting) and insulin. If one's diabetes is well controlled and exercise is greatly increased, while diet and insulin remain the same, the blood sugar may fall so low as to lead to an insulin reaction. The diabetic always should remember he is driving a three-horse team and he must think how to make Diet, Exercise, and Insulin pull together.

INSULIN IN TREATMENT OF DIABETES

The announcement of the discovery of insulin in Toronto in 1921 brought hope to the diabetic, and its general introduction in 1922 gave him life. The addition of protamine to it by Hagedorn of Denmark in 1936, and subsequently of zinc by Scott and Fisher in Canada, and more recently the new protamine insulin (NPH), devised also by Hagedorn, have led to his comfort and joy, because these improvements have reduced treatment from two, three, or four injections a day to once in twenty-four hours. It is one of the four

Table 6A. Average Duration of Life Subsequent to Onset of Diabetes Among 12,281 Deceased Ex-Patients in Each of the Important Eras of Treatment. By Age Group at Onset.

(Experience of Elliott P. Joslin, M.D., 1897–1951)

	Naunyn Era 1897– 5/31/14	Allen Era 6/1/14– 8/6/22	Banting Era 8/7/22– 12/31/29	Banting Era 1/1/30– 12/31/36	Hagedorn Era 1/1/37– 12/31/43	Chas. H. Best Era 1/1/44– 4/27/51
Age Groups at Onset	Dur. Yrs.	Dur. Yrs.	Dur. Yrs.	Dur. Yrs.	Dur. Yrs.	Dur. Yrs.
All ages	4.9*	6.1*	8.0*	10.3*	12.3*	14.3*
0–9	1.3	2.9	2.8	7.3	10.3	18.8
10–19	2.7	2.7	3.4	7.4	11.4	16.7
20–39	4.3	4.9	8.9	14.4	16.9	19.1
40–59	7.0	8.0	9.5	11.6	13.7	15.4
60 & over	4.4	6.4	5.5	7.0	8.6	9.5
Unknown	—	—	—	—	—	—

*Based on cases with known duration.
NOTE: Deaths reported through April 27, 1951.

Table 6B. Diabetes Mortality Among 656 Deceased Ex-Patients. Deaths Between January 1, 1950, and April 7, 1952
(Experience of Joslin Clinic)

Average Duration of Life Subsequent to Onset of Diabetes. By Age Groups at Onset

Age Groups at onset	Number of cases	Duration years
All Ages	656	15.2
0–9	27	21.2
10–19	52	19.3
20–39	102	21.1
40–59	314	15.5
60 & over	161	8.5

major medical discoveries thus far of the twentieth century. Even today none of us wholly realizes the good which insulin has done. *First of all, insulin enables a diabetic child to live, but, best of all, to grow and be happy.* Insulin protects the diabetic mother. Insulin allows the diabetic doctor, lawyer, teacher, laborer to resume his occupation and again to play an active part in the community. Years ago, before we had insulin or knew as much as we do now about diet, nearly one fifth of all diabetics died the very first year of their disease, and most of them were invalids. Today less than one in fifty die the first year, and this number is made up almost exclusively of old men and old women, with whom the date of onset of diabetes is uncertain, and of diabetics who have sustained medical or other accidents. Even if we do not grant to insulin the whole responsibility for the prolongation and protection of the lives of diabetics, it surely is responsible for 99 per cent of their health, because it affords them the opportunity to satisfy their longing for food and their desire to act as live men and live women and, if children, to rejoice in their play.

Insulin comes from a gland, the pancreas or the sweetbread, which lies behind the stomach in the upper abdomen. No one can live without insulin. Insulin regulates the percentage of sugar in the blood. If this percentage is too high, insulin removes the excess sugar and stores it as starch—glycogen—in the liver and muscles and skin, or helps in its change to fat for deposit throughout the body. Starch is an insoluble form of carbohydrate and thus is suitable for storage just as sugar is soluble and, if not used, is lost in the urine. For most of us our own pancreases suffice. The cells of the pancreas are so closely in touch with the demand and supply of insulin in the body that if there is ever a surplus or deficit of insulin in a normal person we consider it an anomaly. If we eat carbohydrate, the pancreas makes insulin to care for it, and the insulin factory is so delicately adjusted to the amount of sugar which should be in the blood that it does not allow this to vary as much as a teaspoonful, which, by the way, is the normal amount of sugar in the blood of the entire body in the fasting state. If 0.1 per cent, or 100 milligrams per cent—another scant spoonful—collects in it, sugar begins to appear in the urine. (The body contains about 5 quarts of blood or [5x32] 160 ounces [1 ounce = 30 cubic centimeters] or 160x30 = 4800 cubic centimeters or grams, and if multiplied by 0.1 per cent, we have 4.8 grams—and a spoonful is equal to 5.0 grams.) Sometimes normal individuals, who during violent exercise burn up most of their reserve starch (glycogen) and sugar in the body as a result of a Marathon run, a football game, or a four-mile boat race, suffer because exercise has done the work of insulin. Today trainers give to such athletes carbohydrate, tea with sugar, orange juice, etc., to offset the deficiency. Even a healthy child may go without a meal, and his pancreas may not stop manufacturing insulin soon enough, and as a result the blood sugar is reduced so low that he becomes unconscious. Recently four such cases were reported. The diabetic differs chiefly from the normal person in that his pancreas produces too little insulin, and to make up for the lack of insulin he must buy it. Few persons' intelligence is equal to their instinct, and so it is not strange that the diabetic occasionally gives himself an overdose of insulin. He is the one above all others who must learn what he needs, and no doctor can decide as well as the patient himself, provided he understands his diabetes and the workings of diet, exercise, and insulin. Few patients at first recognize the symptoms which demand an increase or decrease in the dose of insulin, but the diabetic of several years' duration does know these, and with the help of his physician he finally arrives at the proper amount which his system requires from day to day. The diabetic can test his urine one or more times daily and thus determine whether it contains sugar or is sugar free, and so whether he needs more or less insulin or no insulin. Unfortunately, as yet he cannot test the sugar in his blood, but I suspect that before long someone will discover a simple way to do that.

At one time it was the belief that a diabetic got worse the longer he lived, but today we know that this is not necessarily true. Diabetics can improve, and now it is a fact that the doctor must be as alert to detect his patient's getting better as he was formerly to note a downward course. Fortunately, every diabetic manufactures some insulin, even though the quantity is small, but we cannot tell yet how much a diabetic pancreas can be repaired, renewed, or how much it can grow when conditions are favorable. It is my impression that the belief is becoming general among doctors that the diabetic's pancreas is not so bad a pancreas after all, and that the reason a diabetic acquires his disease is not because his pancreas is wholly destroyed, but rather because in addition to the destroyed portion the remainder is not acting as it should. The possibility is still open that someone will discover a means by which the beginning destruction of the cells of the islands of Langerhans will be reversed and that the beta cells in the islands which make the insulin will again fill with granules and go to work, and I am hoping that in diabetes that discovery will be the next one. The few large alpha cells in the pancreas appear to make the diabetes worse. I wonder if one would be healthier without them. My idea is that there is greater hope for a new treatment of the diabetic along this line than for a form of insulin which can be given by mouth instead of under the skin.

I wrote the preceding paragraph some years ago, and the hope there expressed in part has been fulfilled. Haist, Campbell, and Best have demonstrated that the diabetes experimentally produced by injecting anterior pituitary extract into a dog can be prevented if insulin is simultaneously given. Lukens and Dohan have been able to cure this type of diabetes in the same way in a cat after it has gone on for as long as three months. These discoveries in one way or another will help diabetics because they will stimulate prompt and energetic treatment.

For patients who complain about taking insulin under the skin I have no sympathy. When I remember seeing a child six years old, or even as young as two and a half years, inject insulin into himself or herself and not whimper about it, it disgusts me to have an adult find fault. To buy insulin instead of making it one's self is a nuisance, but there are very few diabetic patients in the United States whose insulin need cost them more than twenty cents a day, because there are very, very few patients who require more than forty units of insulin a day.

Insulin can now be bought all over the world and has a fixed standard of strength in accordance with an International Standard adopted in 1935. The dose varies with each patient, but the total amount employed for the day ranges, as a rule, between ten and forty units, rising above this in the severer cases, and especially when the diabetic has a complication due to an infection or to diabetic coma. Under such circumstances a patient may require several hundred units of insulin in the twenty-four hours. An infection, whether general like influenza or local like a boil, always makes the diabetes worse, and in diabetic coma the insulin also acts less efficiently.

The cost of insulin should be kept as low as possible. One uses it to save life and not for fun. I hope the price can be kept low by wholesale methods and by allowing hospitals and clinics to sell it at a minimum profit. Everything should be done to encourage the purchase of insulin, so as to avoid giving it away, because that promotes wastage to an enormous degree.

The size of the dose, the number of units of insulin, not only varies with the severity of the disease, but with the amount of carbohydrate in the diet and also its relation to the fat as well. There is no absolute rule. Theoretically, one can reckon the total carbohydrate or glucose, sugar-forming material in the food, as follows:

Food	Per Cent Sugar-forming		
Carbohydrate	100 grams × 100% −	100	grams
Protein	100 grams × 58% =	58	grams
Fat	100 grams × 10% =	10	grams

However, this will not indicate how much insulin is required, because sometimes the carbohydrate from carbohydrate alone appears to be better utilized if the fat in the diet is relatively low.

Varieties of Insulin. The duration of the action of insulin varies with the type employed. Regular insulin, the first kind introduced by Banting's and Best's discovery, acts for six or seven hours and most powerfully at the end of one hour; crystalline insulin, the other quick-acting insulin (which is preferable because a purer drug, costing the same) acts an hour or two longer. Globin and NPH insulins are intermediate insulins and have a duration of action of about twenty and twenty-two hours respectively. Protamine zinc insulin, the long-acting insulin, acts up to twenty-eight and even forty-eight hours.

The immediate effect of regular or crystalline insulin is to lower the blood sugar rapidly for the first four or five hours after it is injected, while protamine zinc insulin acts slowly, and the blood sugar may not reach the lowest point for twelve hours. The intermediate globin and NPH insulins act most successfully in about eight hours, and so if injected before breakfast have the greatest effect in the late afternoon. Insulins fortunately do not accumulate in the body.

Table 7. Actions of Various Insulins

Name	Duration of Action in Hours	Peak of Action after Injection in Hours
Regular	6–7	1
Crystalline	6–7	1
Globin	20–22	8
NPH	20–22	8
Protamine	28–48	12–16

Sterilization

Equipment: 1. Saucepan   2. Strainer

1. Place syringe, plunger, and needle all disconnected in strainer. If no strainer used, place a cloth in bottom of pan.

2. Cover completely with cold water; heat to boiling and boil 5 minutes.

3. Lift strainer out of pan and pour out water. Place strainer back in pan.

4. Fill a clean dish or bottle with iso-propyl alcohol.

5. Pick up plunger by knob only and fit into cylinder. Handle needle by hub (thick end) and fasten to syringe by a twist to left or right to secure. Be sure nothing touches needle or plunger where they will touch insulin.

6. Place syringe with needle attached into covered dish or bottle containing alcohol to cool. (Steri-tubes to hold syringe and needle may be purchased.)

Entire equipment should be sterilized by boiling every week, or daily if iso-propyl alcohol unavailable.

Loading

1. Mix insulin by rotating bottle between hands. Clean rubber top of insulin bottle with alcohol.

2. Remove syringe from alcohol. Work plunger back and forth several times to expel any alcohol.

3. Draw air into syringe to equal insulin dose.

4. Cautiously but firmly push needle through center of rubber top. Push plunger down to expel air into bottle.

5. Invert the bottle. Pull down plunger to withdraw insulin. If air bubbles are present, holding syringe and needle point upward, expel insulin into bottle and slowly again withdraw dose. Remove needle from bottle.

Injection

Areas used: top and outsides of legs or arms. Abdomen. Never inject into same spot more often than once a month.

1. Clean skin with alcohol sponge where you plan injection.
2. Pinch up skin at site between thumb and forefinger. With syringe held at 45-degree angle to the skin, quickly insert needle its entire length. (The more quickly the needle is inserted, the less will be the pain.)
3. Force insulin from syringe. Cover area with alcohol sponge and remove needle.
4. Rinse out syringe with boiled water.
5. Replace syringe with needle in alcohol container.

Insulin, as already mentioned, acts by removing the sugar from the blood and storing it in the liver, the muscles, and the skin in the form of an insoluble carbohydrate, animal starch (glycogen), so that it can be utilized when required by the body. The sugar in the blood rises to its highest level from half an hour to an hour after meals, and to offset this insulin is usually administered one quarter to three quarters of an hour before a meal. This is necessary if regular or crystalline insulin is used. In fact, if insulin is given when the stomach is empty, it may lower the sugar in the blood so quickly that the symptoms of an overdose, the so-called insulin reaction, appear. Many patients can keep the urine free from sugar if they take one injection of protamine zinc insulin a day, but if they use the quick-acting but shorter-duration regular insulin they will require it twice, a few three times. Rarely is it necessary to give it four times.

When only the original regular insulin was available, I remember how frequently with children mothers would be obliged to waken with an alarm clock at 2:00 A.M. in order to inject the fourth dose into the child. During infections the patient may require insulin every three or four hours, in pregnancy three times daily, and in the treatment of a patient unconscious with diabetic coma it is often administered every thirty minutes until improvement begins to take place. Truly insulin is wonderful, and I know of nothing more dramatic in medicine than to watch an unconscious diabetic-coma patient come back to life with the use of insulin.

Protamine zinc insulin when given before breakfast day after day will act strongly enough to control the diabetes in about half of all cases for the entire twenty-four hours. In other words, it enables the patient to get the full benefit of (1) the food stored in the body as it changes from glycogen (animal starch) to sugar, or from protein, which yields 58 per cent sugar, and from fat, out of which 10 per cent can be formed, and (2) also takes care of the sugar which comes from the different foods at mealtimes. In the severer types of diabetes protamine zinc insulin is unequal to the task of utilizing the food which the patient eats rapidly enough. In such instances one supplements it with the quick-acting regular or, better, crystalline insulin plus protamine zinc insulin also before breakfast, and the effect of this quick insulin plus the slow protamine zinc insulin will protect the patient for the periods of meals.

When regular or crystalline insulin is given in the same syringe with protamine zinc insulin, a part of the regular or crystalline insulin changes to protamine zinc insulin because there is an excess of protamine in protamine zinc insulin. Fortunately, no such change takes place when the quick-acting insulins are added to NPH insulin and even to globin insulin, so that a single injection of insulin (both the rapid-acting and slow-acting being mixed in the same syringe) can be employed before breakfast.

During the course of infections or after operations, when patients eat irregularly, one usually depends upon an anchor dose of protamine zinc insulin once a day or a mixture of NPH insulin and regular or crystalline insulin, and also gives crystalline insulin every four to six hours as needed according to the following formula:

$$\frac{\text{Red}\quad\text{Orange}\quad\text{Yellow}\quad\text{Green}\quad\text{Blue}}{16 \qquad 12 \qquad 8 \qquad 4 \qquad 0}$$

The results of the Benedict tests are recorded in the numerator of the fractions, and the corresponding units of insulin to be given in the denominator.

Insulin is given by injection just under the skin. The patient should be systematic about this and not use the same spot of the skin for an injection

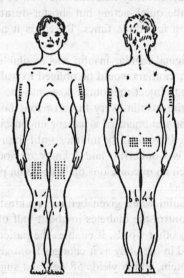

Fig. 47. These insulin maps show the regions of the body where insulin may best be injected.

oftener than once a month. A little planning will provide for this. If insulin is always injected in one place, lumps may appear, because the tissues are injured. As a result the insulin is incompletely absorbed, and the patient does not get his money's worth. And this is not the whole story, because in the injured tissue an infection may start. Abscesses from the injection of insulin, however, are extraordinarily rare and usually are due only to gross neglect.

The proper dose of insulin is not always easily determined because of the uncertainty as to when or how much the patient will eat or the amount of exercise that he has had or is to take. Obviously the trained patient who injects his own insulin can decide all this better than the doctor. Furthermore, sometimes people eat a meal but fail to digest it—and this especially occurs with children—or, if seasick, lose it, and so the insulin which may have been given with the expectation that the patient would eat has no food to work upon. If food remains in the stomach and so does not reach the blood, it is the same as if no food had been taken at all. For all these reasons it is not uncommon to see a patient who has had an overdose of insulin with a resulting "insulin reaction." Insulin is a drug, and symptoms will result from an overdose of any drug.

INSULIN ATROPHIES

In children and in women, rarely in men, insulin injections are sometimes followed by the disappearance of small portions of the fat layer of the skin. These make depressions in the surface of the body, and this hollowing out of the skin causes deformities. These are disagreeable but not dangerous. Eventually, if no insulin is injected in the neighborhood of such a fat-atrophied area, it will fill up. Treatment consists in using scrupulous care in the administration of insulin. Never inject near the same site twice in a month, use concentrated U-80 insulin, and employ sharp, perfect needles. One never needs to give up insulin on account of insulin atrophies. One can take advantage of the abdomen and lower back for injections.

When insulin was first discovered, its strength was weak and to get an effect it was necessary to inject several teaspoonfuls at a time. Gradually it has been made stronger and stronger, and so smaller quantities are necessary for an effect. At one time a syringeful—usually holding 1 cubic centimeter or one fourth of a teaspoonful—contained 10 units, but now insulin is usually dispensed in four times that strength, or 40 units in a cubic centimeter, known as U-40 insulin, although sometimes only twice as strong, as U-20 insulin, or eight times as strong, as U-80 insulin. At any rate, one unit is always the same no matter what the strength, even if as many as 500 units in one cubic centimeter. Sometimes syringes holding two cubic centimeters instead of one cubic centimeter are used. Obviously, one must always be very careful to note the strength of insulin to be injected as well as the type of syringe employed, so as to be sure of the number of units.

The one-cubic-centimeter syringes may be divided into ten parts, and then one tenth of one cubic centimeter would contain 1, 2, 4, or 8 units according to whether the strength of insulin was U-10, U-20, U-40, or U-80. Some syringes are marked for U-40 or U-80 insulin, and then one can read the desired number of units on the side indicated for the strength of insulin. U-10 insulin, now seldom available, comes in a bottle with a blue label, U-20 insulin in a bottle with a yellow label. U-40 insulin is sold in red-labeled bottles, and U-80 in green-labeled vials. NPH insulin comes in a bottle with four sides instead of in a round vial.

Be sure you know the kind of insulin you are supposed to use and the number of units. Show your insulin bottle and your syringe to your doctor to be sure you are making no mistake.

INSULIN REACTIONS

The symptoms which result from an overdose of insulin are much the same as those which occur in several other well-known states. If a dinner party is delayed by a latecomer, besides hunger and faintness even one's disposition may suffer, and those symptoms are characteristic of an insulin reaction. If one has been without food for many hours and even fasted, the percentage of sugar in the blood is lowered and may fall as low as after too much insulin or extreme exercise, and it is the low blood sugar which causes the reaction. I suspect that the old monks and anchorites, who wandered about the deserts and undertook long periods of fasting, and the Indian necromancers, with their weird and fantastic dances, often had experiences akin to those of persons who have an insulin reaction: Undoubtedly the sugar in their blood dropped; they became faint and feeble; their hands trembled; their minds were clouded and hallucinations appeared; they fell into trancelike states and could not be aroused. The common symptoms of an insulin reaction are weakness, faintness, and hunger. Patients often call these reactions the "shakes," because trembling occurs. Sweating, numbness, tingling of the lips, even unconsciousness, can come on quite rapidly, and if the dose of insulin has been extreme the patient may have a convulsion. Indeed, there are on record many instances where the diabetic has been supposed to have epilepsy when in reality he had nothing of the sort. An examination of the sugar in the blood will quickly show the true nature of the condition, because it will be far below normal. All diabetics are warned about these reactions, and all diabetics taking insulin should carry one or two lumps of sugar or other kinds of carbohydrate in their pockets. By eating carbohydrate, pure sugar, or sugar in fruit such as an orange, or starch as in bread or crackers, when they recognize the approach of a reaction, they can quickly raise the sugar in the blood and ward off untoward symptoms.

One of my patients, troubled with frequent reactions, took a saltine every hour when the clock struck. A saltine contains only 3 grams of carbohydrate, but this taken promptly might be enough carbohydrate to suffice. It is seldom that the body burns more than 10 grams per hour. If treatment with carbohydrate is delayed, larger doses are required; and if there is unconsciousness, very large doses of carbohydrate may be necessary and then one may need to give glucose intravenously. Usually when the sugar is taken, it acts rapidly. I have seen a child lying unconscious on the floor in an insulin reaction and three

Table 8. Differential Diagnosis Between Diabetic Coma and Insulin Reaction

	Diabetic Coma	Insulin Reaction	
Cause	Acid poisoning due to 1. Insufficient insulin 2. Overeating 3. Fever	Low blood sugar due to 1. Too much insulin. 2. Too little food or delay in eating after taking insulin. 3. Unusual exercise.	
Onset	Gradual over a period of hours or days.	After regular or crystalline insulin.	Sudden, usually in a few hours after taking.
		After protamine zinc globin or NPH insulin.	Slow, usually some hrs. after taking.
Signs and Symptoms	A feeling of serious illness, thirst, nausea, vomiting, deep and difficult breathing, pains in the abdomen, drowsiness, often fever.	After regular or crystalline insulin.	Hunger, tremor, sweating, nervousness.
		After protamine zinc globin or NPH insulin.	As above, though at times headache, nausea, drowsiness, malaise.
Prevention	Test urine reguarly. NEVER omit insulin except under doctor's orders when urine is repeatedly sugar free. If you feel ill 1. Send for a doctor. 2. Go to bed. 3. Drink a cupful of hot liquid hourly. 4. Keep warm. 5. Get nurse or friend to give care. 6. Take an enema.	Meals at regular hours. Those taking protamine zinc globin or NPH insulin should eat something between meals and on retiring. When driving a car, a diabetic should take carbohydrate 10 grams every two hours to prevent low blood sugar. Repeated reactions call for readjustment of the patient's daily routine with respect to insulin, diet and exercise.	
Treatment	Must be carried out by the physician, preferably in a hospital.	Give sugar immediately. Patients using protamine zinc globin or NPH insulin may need sugar more than once. Diabetics should always carry two lumps of sugar for use if an insulin reaction occurs. Adrenalin ½ cc. may be injected under the skin.	

The diabetic's best insurance against both coma and insulin reaction is to see the doctor as often as the latter thinks necessary and always every three or four months.

minutes after he was given a teaspoonful of syrup get up and chase his little railroad cars around the room. Obviously it is too dangerous for a locomotive engineer to take insulin unless it is given before his evening meal, so that twelve or more hours will intervene before he gets into his cab. An insulin reaction might come on quickly. Automobilists who take insulin invariably should eat 10 grams of carbohydrate (an orange, two lumps of sugar, or the equivalent of half a slice of bread or half a banana) if they drive a car more than two hours after a meal. A patient using insulin should carry his name, address, and directions for treatment of an insulin reaction, so that he can be protected if such a reaction comes on unawares and in strange surroundings. Non-diabetics can also advantageously bear in mind the dangers of being too hungry.

See other side

I AM DIABETIC

If I am found unconscious and if sugar, orange juice or sweetened fluids do not cause definite improvement in 15 minutes, call my doctor, or send me immediately to a hospital.

See other side

If I am found unconscious or behaving abnormally, my condition probably is the result of an overdose of insulin.

Name . . . .

Address . . . . Tel. . . . .

Physician's Name . . . .

Address . . . . Tel. . . . .

. . . .

Fig. 48. Identification Card.

Remember, one never attempts to raise money in a charity drive when the blood sugar is low but after the dinner when it is normal.

The reactions from protamine zinc insulin are quite different from those due to regular or crystalline insulin. Being a slow-acting insulin, they may not come on for eight or more hours after injection. Often if the PZI is taken before breakfast, these will develop during the following night or shortly before breakfast the next morning. If "quick-acting" regular or crystalline insulin is given at the same time as PZI before breakfast, or with NPH or globin insulin, the meal should follow within fifteen minutes, because the patient rises from bed with an already low blood sugar.

The symptoms due to a reaction caused by PZI differ materially from those caused by RI or CI. Lassitude, headache, nausea, and even vomiting are the most common, which in turn are followed by unconsciousness and convulsions. If a diabetic husband or wife wakes up "out of sorts," always assume it is due to a low blood sugar. At times the sequence from lassitude to unconsciousness is rapid, and rarely a state of reaction can develop during the night. It is for this reason many patients take about 10 grams of carbohydrate on retiring if their urine is sugar free. Occasionally they add protein and fat to promote a slow absorption. Such lunches might be (1) milk a small glass, 6 ounces, 180 cc. (carbohydrate 9, protein 6, fat 6 grams); (2) Uneedas 2 (carbohydrate 8, protein 1 gram) with cheese, one-half ounce, 15 grams (protein 4 grams, fat 6 grams); (3) peanuts 1 oz., 30 grams (carbohydrate 6 grams, protein 8 grams, fat 13 grams).

ORAL ANTIDIABETICS

One of the great discoveries of recent years is the substances which can be taken by mouth for the lowering of the sugar in the blood. Orinase, also called tolbutamide, is a product which lowers the blood sugar and decreases the amount of sugar found in the urine, also the frequency of urination and itching associated with diabetes. This drug is not used for diabetes in children or for cases in which the pancreas has suffered destruction or injury. It does however have great use particularly in cases in which diabetes occurs in middle age. Another similar product is known as DBI Oral Hypoglycemic. A third preparation, Diabinese, is recommended particularly for people with mild diabetes which is not well controlled by regulation of the diet. In each instance these products must be prescribed by the doctor in the amount necessary for the individual patient.

THE USEFULNESS OF DIABETES

It seems hardly conceivable that a disease should be useful, but really diabetes is a disease in which that is the case. We need our diabetics. The diabetic sets an example in cleanliness to his family, his friends, and, in fact, to all his neighbors. He is taught to be the cleanest citizen in the community, because if he keeps his skin in good condition, the chances for complications are slight, and in this way he avoids the carbuncles and boils and inflammations of the skin which years ago were a most annoying accompaniment of the disease. The diabetic is useful because he sets an example for temperance in eating, for control of body weight. He is an instructor in dietetics, and he diffuses through his family a practical knowledge of the properties and values of foods. He understands the meaning of a balanced diet. He knows that his 3 per cent vegetables, his fruit, his cream, his egg, his meat, and his cod-liver oil contain priceless vitamins. Diabetes is particularly useful because it is so evidently associated with overweight that it directs attention to the dangers of overweight in general, for these are by no means limited to diabetes. For years the insurance companies have pointed out that the expectation of life of the fat person is far less than that of the one of standard weight, because the fat person is more liable to diseases of the heart and the arteries. Lately they have shown that if a fat person loses weight and regains a normal value, his expectancy of life, which was shortened, will again rise.

Diabetes is useful because it brings before the public the advantage of cooperation between the physician and patient in the treatment of a chronic disease. The diabetic patient who does the best is the one who knows the most about the disease, and this soon becomes apparent to all onlookers. He thus demonstrates that it is desirable for the ordinary individual to know something about diseases, and particularly his own disease, so that he and his doctor can work in partnership. The diabetic is useful because today we know that diabetes is to a certain extent hereditary, and, having the disease, the patient must stop and think before he gets married. Not only must he consider whether he can take care of himself or herself, but he also must consider the health of his future partner before he gets engaged, because one diabetic should not marry another diabetic. In other words, the diabetic will spread the knowledge of eugenics, and when we remember the known one and a half million diabetics in this country and the two and a half millions now living who will acquire diabetes before they die, the necessity of thoughtfulness on the part of diabetics before they have children will be taught them and through them pass to the community as a whole. One can see how this idea of more care in contracting marriages will be spread. Almost any thoughtful father today demands a report of the physical examination and Wassermann reaction of the suitor of his daughter before he consents to her marriage.

For the doctor, the diabetic is a challenge because no group of patients is under his closer supervision, and therefore cancer should be detected earlier in them and more cures obtained, and tuberculosis always caught in its incipiency.

I feel that the diabetic who lives long lives usefully and that he deserves recognition. Unless he had used judgment in diet and treatment and care of his body, his duration of life would have been short. Therefore, I believe a diabetic who has lived longer with his disease than he was expected to live without it at the time it began should be given a medal in recognition of it. Such a practice has been followed, and for the encouragement of patients I can say that I know of more than two thousand diabetics who have earned such medals. Amelia Peabody, the designer, placed on the reverse side of the medal a child in a boat sailing toward the rising sun with this inscription, *"Explorers of Diabetes,"* because it is the child who is leading the way for improvement in the treatment of diabetics.

Quarter Century Victory Medal. A medal of greater distinction was created in 1947 by the Advisory Committee of the Diabetic Fund at the Boston Safe Deposit and Trust Company. It is awarded to that diabetic who after twenty-five years of known diabetes is perfect on physical examination; has eyes and blood vessels free from complications, as certified by a recognized ophthalmologist and a roentgenologist. Application for the Quarter Century Victory Medal should be sent to the Advisory Committee, Diabetic Fund, Boston Safe Deposit and Trust Company, Trustee, 100 Franklin Street, Boston, Massachusetts, or to Dr. Elliott P. Joslin, Chairman, Advisory Committee, 81 Bay State Road, Boston 15, Massachusetts.

If your physician or you think that you deserve a Quarter Century Victory Medal after your proved twenty-five years of diabetes, just get a complete examination by your family physician; if he thinks you will pass, second, secure an examination of the eyes by an eye specialist; if they are reported all right, then, third, secure X-rays of the blood vessels.

The letter of application should briefly summarize your history, with age and date of onset and course of diabetes, together with a statement of your physician about your physical condition. If he considers this perfect and that you are eligible, the report of the examination of the eyes by an eye specialist should accompany the doctor's report. In case you pass these tests by your family physician and the eye specialist, then X-rays should be taken to demonstrate whether there is calcification of the arteries. By experience we have found it necessary to have an X-ray examination of (1) the heart and aorta in the chest; (2) the abdominal aorta (film taken laterally to avoid the spine); (3) pelvic arteries; and (4) a lateral view of the lower legs, including the vessels about the ankles.

These medals are so rare and the discovery of such cases so important that eye and X-ray specialists, as well as the family physician, often will do the tests at minimum fees.

Already thirty-eight such diabetics have been granted medals. It is significant that the histories of these patients showed that they carefully followed treatment in their early years and that none was neglectful of treatment, although they may have controlled their disease in different ways. So far, no patient living on a free diet and careless of his diabetes has been able to pass the above tests.

A diabetic in the home after all may be an asset. To sum up, he knows about cleanliness, diet, the dangers of overweight, the use of a drug, the importance of heredity, and hence it is no wonder that often he lives long. He and his confrères constitute a great experimental laboratory for the benefit of the human race. I tell my diabetic children that each honest diabetic day they live is a great help to some diabetic old man or old woman, because from their young lives we learn how to treat those whose vitality and recuperative powers are less.

EMPLOYMENT OF DIABETICS

If a diabetic can secure employment which involves exercise, it is most advantageous, because exercise helps to utilize the diet and thus benefits the patient. If the diabetic must accept employment which does not involve exercise, then he must make up for it by taking exercise out of hours. I remember well those diabetics who progressed most satisfactorily while active in athletics in college, but who, after they graduated and took jobs which did not involve exercise, such as postgraduate work in the law school or in medicine, or in an office, found they did not do well unless they resumed exercise out of hours. These diabetics will not do as well as they might unless they arrange to secure exercise, even if it is only walking daily and a short period for calisthenics. Bouchardat was very insistent that his patients should exercise until they sweat. He said they should earn their bread by the sweat of their brows. He wanted them to use all the muscles of the body.

If a diabetic can work independently and be his own boss, that is often advantageous. Theoretically a diabetic who is a farmer should do especially well, because he can regulate his exercise according to his work and ask no questions of anyone.

Opportunities for employment of diabetics are many. Particularly was this true during the war when they were given positions which did not involve combat activities. Today I understand that more than one thousand types of positions in the United States Civil Service are open to diabetics. I know of no argument stronger than what has occurred in our own group. Formerly it was seldom that more than one diabetic doctor, nurse, technician, secretary, or camp counselor was employed by us, but this summer fourteen held such paid positions. (I hope a million diabetics will not apply for a job, because already we have quite a diabetic labor pool of our own.)

Employers in general are kind to diabetics. It is very important that any diabetic seeking or holding an appointment should do his or her work not only as well as but better than a non-diabetic so as to increase the opportunities for other diabetics to get a job. Diabetics may need to give up certain pleasurable activities, but if they can demonstrate their good health and their skill, then they will not need to fear for a position.

Certain occupations are unsuitable for diabetics. Recently the American Diabetes Association has suggested standards for the employment of diabetics, and below I record abstracts from the same.

1. A diabetic seeking employment should be required to present a note from his physician or the personnel manager, stating that he is a controlled diabetic and is examined at regular intervals.

2. Diabetics are capable of performing any type of work for which they are physically, mentally, and educationally equipped. Those diabetics who are taking large doses of insulin should not, however, be assigned work in which hypoglycemic attacks might result in injury to themselves and others.

3. An effort should be made to see that diabetics work the same hours on a steady shift; or, if they must work on a rotating schedule, that they avoid the "graveyard" shift from midnight to 8 A.M. This is the only concession in terms of hours that a well-controlled diabetic should ask.

5. Diabetics should carry cards or tags identifying their condition at all times, particularly when on the job.

6. The plant physician can save time for the company and also help the employee by performing blood sugar and urine examinations, whenever the patient's usual laboratory facilities are available only during working hours. Ordinarily, of course, this should be done only after consultation with the family physician.

7. A complete physical examination of each diabetic should be made regularly, at least once a year.

8. A plant physician is within his rights if he reassigns a diabetic employee to other work whenever the arising of new complications creates new risks for himself or for other employees.

9. The diabetic requiring insulin should be considered controlled if the fasting blood sugar is not below normal limits and not above 150 mg. per 100 cc. by Folin Wu method and the blood sugar three hours after a meal is not higher than 250 mg. per 100 cc. by the Folin Wu method and if the patient is under regular medical supervision. Although these or more nearly normal blood sugar levels are desirable, greater hyperglycemia alone, if not extreme or habitual, need not be considered a disqualification for employment in those cases where the patient's personal physician and the industrial physician both feel that other limits should be observed.

Naturally if diabetics have frequent reactions or develop diabetic coma, their chances for continuance in their occupations or for promotions are lessened. In a way this is fortunate, because it forces diabetics to study their diabetes thoroughly and to control it.

INSURANCE FOR DIABETICS

Until ten years ago practically no known diabetic was granted insurance. At that time the Manufacturers Life Insurance Company in Toronto undertook to insure diabetics. Gradually this company has increased the number insured and has broadened its policies and at lessened premiums. Its example has been followed generally, so that now approximately 75 per cent of all life insurance companies in the United States and Canada will accept diabetics on various terms.

The chief condition upon which insurance companies accept diabetics is proof that they are under medical supervision. Naturally all conditions which apply to non-diabetics apply to diabetics, but this one feature is apparently considered of more importance to the insurance company than detailed tests of sugar in the urine and blood. The longer diabetics live without complications and the better care they take of themselves, the more likely are they to receive insurance on favorable terms.

DIABETICS AND OLD AGE

Diabetes is predominantly a disease of older people. Two thirds of the cases begin above the age of forty years; the median age for its onset for males is 45.1 years and for females 50.1 years. About one half of our cases begin between forty and sixty years and one fourth between forty-five and fifty-four years. In my own series the onset is rare after seventy years, and extraordinarily rare after eighty years.

The patients live long, and the average age at death, which between 1898 and 1914 was forty-four years, is now about sixty-five years. The expectancy of life of a ten-year-old diabetic child is to pass his fiftieth birthday, even if no discoveries in treatment occur. Finally, medals have been given in one clinic alone to more than 1,000 patients who have lived longer with the disease than they were expected to live wthout it when it was first acquired. But despite all this it is regrettably true that up to the present time it has been the rule for diabetics to grow old too fast. This had long been suspected for the middle-aged diabetic, but it is in the children that the proof appeared. When the children lived only two or three years, of course this was rarely evident, but as improvements in diet came and children lived longer, the very same changes were noted in them which one sees in aging adults. Their arteries began to harden, and one could not only feel the hardening, but see the deposits of lime by X-ray examinations of the blood vessels of the legs. More important than the changes in the blood vessels of the legs were those in the arteries of the heart, and in comparatively young people it was found that clots in these vessels (coronary thrombosis) caused death just as in mature individuals. Sadder by far was another change of old age, which came on in the eyes, and diabetic children showed cataracts, hemorrhages, and exudates impairing the vision. I should hesitate even to record all this if it were not possible to add that in the last few years we know that in children this early aging has been deferred, and in some patients who have carefully followed treatment for even twenty-five years it has not appeared.

Old age has been deferred, because insulin permits the diabetic today to eat more nearly the diet of the normal individual. How can we help advancing the argument that if modern treatment has halted arteriosclerosis in diabetic children and is deferring it in the middle-aged diabetics, there must have been something in the disease itself or perhaps in its treatment by us years ago which was responsible for this arteriosclerosis? And is it not fascinating to seek for the greatest common divisor in the multitude of factors which caused this rapid growing old?

First of all, the evidence points to overeating. It appears to be not so much the particular character of the food, because all the foods break up into quite similar components which enter a common pool and are more or less interchangeable. For a long while the insurance companies have insisted that a man or woman above fifty years was not a good risk if he or she were fat, and although this has appeared to be due to the overweight alone, it is possible the additional fat tissue itself in the body has been the reason. At any rate, since our diabetic children have eaten less fat and have assimilated it better, and had it replaced with more carbohydrate food, which insulin has permitted, we have noticed less hardening of the arteries. At the moment excess in total calories rather than in those derived from fat appears to be the crucial factor.

In recent years the fat in the diet, particularly that known as cholesterol, has been thought to be of major importance in the development of hardening of the arteries. This fat is found in the walls of the blood vessels and is especially common in the blood of diabetics with arteriosclerosis. Nothing would appear easier than to exclude it from the diet and thus keep young. But it is not quite so simple. It happens that only 10 per cent of the cholesterol in the body comes from the diet, and the remaining 90 per cent is manufactured by the body itself. It would seem queer for the human body to produce so much cholesterol normally unless it was useful and surely harmless. One is on safer ground today to urge restriction of total calories rather than to urge extreme restriction of cholesterol. Cholesterol is most abundant in eggs. Up to now I have not excluded them, but I do believe at the present state of our knowledge it is wise to eat them in moderation.

Control of the diabetes by diet, exercise, and insulin is our best deterrent of degenerative disease of the blood vessels.

HEREDITY AND MARRIAGE OF DIABETICS

HEREDITY

Diabetes is an hereditary disease. I suppose about one in four of all the people in the United States has a diabetic relative and therefore harbors a tendency to diabetes. Among Jewish people it may be one in three. Proof that diabetes is hereditary is shown in various ways. When our diabetic children first come to us for treatment, the known heredity of these children is 20 per cent, but after the children have lived fifteen or twenty years, enough other of their relatives have developed the disease to show their diabetic heredity is over 50 per cent. Years ago Dr. White found that diabetes was seven times as frequent among the relatives of those of our diabetics whom she examined as among the non-relatives; and a few years ago in the United States Public Health Service studies in Florida, diabetes among the relatives of diabetics there investigated was five times as common. The most convincing argument that diabetes is hereditary is based upon twins. If the twins are similar, exactly alike (identical), one finds that if one of the twins comes down with the disease, it is not long before the other twin develops it. The non-diabetic twin of non-identical twins is no more liable to diabetes than the brother or sister of any diabetic.

Diabetes is considered to be *recessive* rather than *dominant;* it may skip a generation. As yet there are very few instances on record in which it has been shown to be present in four successive generations. Medicine must advance quite a good deal farther before we know what diseases our grandparents had or died of. My great-, great-, great-, great-, great-grandfather was hung for a witch on Gallows Hill in Salem in August, 1692, but was it not fortunate for me that his pregant wife was spared by the English Government so that she bore a girl baby?

In studying heredity among diabetics, one must remember that about one third of all diabetic patients begin to show diabetes under forty years of age, another third between forty and fifty-five years of age, and the remainder between fifty-five and one hundred years. These figures are only approximate.

It always takes two to make a diabetic, but if there is no heredity in one parent and none of the relatives of this non-diabetic parent has ever had the disease, then theoretically the children of such a marriage will never show it. Of course, with diabetes being so common that one in four in the United States has a relative with it and so carries a diabetic gene, there is always the possibility that it may have been in an ancestor without its being recognized. Consequently, if a diabetic marries a non-diabetic in whose family there is no known history of diabetes, theoretically it would be impossible for their children to have the disease. If they did develop it, it would be because, so far as we can tell now, some member of the non-diabetic parent's family had had it.

Realizing that heredity is so common in diabetes, how can one prevent the disease, and particularly how can the relatives of diabetics, who are more prone to it, avoid it? The best rules I know are that the relatives of a diabetic should never be overweight, always should work (exercise), and should avoid excesses of any kind of food, but particularly sweet foods. When one realizes that it is extraordinarily rare for diabetes to appear in middle life unless an individual has been overweight, one can see the reason for such advice.

MARRIAGE OF DIABETICS

As late as 1885, Bouchardat, the leading diabetes clinician in the world up to that time, said he had never seen a pregnant diabetic woman. Insulin has changed all this, and diabetic women now become pregnant as readily as non-diabetic women; and it is most exceptional for any pregnant diabetic woman today to lose her life on account of diabetes. On the other hand, even up to twelve years ago nearly half of the pregnancies of the diabetic mothers resulted unfavorably even with the use of insulin. Today results are far better, and it is reasonable to state that approximately 70 per cent will give birth to live children.

Pregnancies in very mild diabetics should result as favorably as in non-diabetics. In general, the outlook is good for live babies if the disease has gone on for less than ten years, whether the pregnancy is the first or a subsequent one. Danger begins when there are changes in the blood vessels, the kidneys, or the eyes. Consequently, no diabetic woman should become pregnant unless assured that her physical condition in these respects is good.

It is true that patients who have had diabetes fifteen, twenty, or twenty-five years can bear a healthy child, but until now it certainly has been extremely rare for a diabetic mother who had had the disease twenty years to have a successful outcome of her pregnancy. Dr. Priscilla White has had an unusual opportunity to follow such cases, and she has given me permission to state that between 1936 and August 27, 1952, she has had 625 viable pregnancies resulting in 520, 83 per cent, live births. Among these there have been 34 cases of diabetes of twenty years or more duration and 9 of twenty-five years or more.

Figure 84 is an exceptional picture in that the mother became pregnant twenty-five years after the diabetes began. This particular patient is a Quarter Century Victory Medal diabetic and therefore an unusually favorable case.

Two diabetics should not marry one another, because theoretically if they had a hundred children, all of their children would develop the disease. However, the outcome would not be quite so black as this. Actually only about forty-four of one hundred such children would ever develop diabetes, because only that number of children in either diabetic or non-diabetic families live to the period in life at which diabetes breaks out. The remainder would succumb to the ills to which all of us are exposed. Fifteen of the theoretical forty-four would be destined to develop diabetes before forty years of age, another fifteen to develop it between forty and fifty-five, and the remainder not until the age period of fifty-five to one hundred years. I have often thought that if a foreign ruler should issue a decree that diabetics in his country should not have children, my diabetics easily could conquer him, because two thirds of them would not develop the disease until after forty years of age, and therefore would make good soldiers, and the chances also are that a good many of those under forty also could serve in the army.

No one knows as yet the exact probability of the number of diabetic children in a family when the heredity is more remote than both parents having the disease, but of course it would be very much less.

DIABETIC GANGRENE

I enjoy writing about diabetic gangrene at this time because once, next to diabetic coma and heart disease, there was no cause of death of the diabetic more common, more harmful, or more distressing, and yet today this complication is disappearing. It is due to hardening and narrowing of the arteries in the lower extremities, and despite the diabetic of today dying twenty years older, at sixty-four instead of forty-four years of age, gangrene has dropped as a cause of death from 8 per cent to 1.1 per cent. This is proof that we are making headway even against those conditions which are due to arteriosclerosis— or growing old. This has been accomplished partly by better treatment of the diabetic, also by the use of sulfa drugs and antibiotics such as penicillin, which has lessened inflammation of the tissues that often preceded the gangrene, and by safer methods of anesthesia at operations upon the lower extremities, combined with greater experience and surgical skill employed in treatment. I do not think that it is due to medicines sometimes given to improve the circulation. Better treatment of the diabetes, along with education of the patient, prompt treatment of minor infections, and greater cleanliness of people generally have been the important factors.

The hardened arteries in the legs make the circulation and nutrition of the part poor. An injury to the skin, which would be of little or no account in a young or healthy person, in a diabetic heals slowly or not at all. Unless the skin is kept scrupulously clean, poisonous germs may get into superficial wounds, multiply, and spread, and very often a leg must be sacrificed to save a life. Old diabetics suffer especially from gangrene. This is not strange, because old people hear less well, see less clearly, and the skin is less sensitive than in the young. Thus they often cut themselves when they are caring for their feet and either don't see what they have done or don't feel it. In this way, trifling injuries progress, and the poor old man or woman may not realize for days or even weeks that a serious condition has developed. I have seen more than one patient who wore a shoe all day with a nail penetrating deep into the sole of the foot without experiencing pain. No wonder infections developed. It all goes on so gradually that when at last the patients go to a surgeon and he says a toe, a foot, a leg, must be amputated, it comes as a great shock. Approximately two thirds of our patients who undergo operations upon their lower extremities have never consulted us before. Every diabetic should care for his feet, or if he can't see well, get someone to do this for him. Chiropodists are a great help to diabetics. They know the dangers of neglected conditions in the feet of a diabetic and can recognize when the patient should see a surgeon.

CARE OF THE FEET

Injuries to the feet in the old must be avoided. New shoes should first be put on at night and worn for an hour or two. Shoe linings should not be broken; one should carefully avoid protruding nails in the shoe. The shoes should be large enough and long enough and flexible enough. The stockings should be whole, and if the feet are deformed with bunions, calluses, or corns, the shoes should be adjusted to overcome these difficulties. As the sensation is poor in the feet the diabetic should avoid exposure to their being burned or frozen. A woman from cold Canada came to the hospital, having burned her toes before an open fire; a woman from Cape Cod with its relatively mild climate entered, having frostbitten toes. A great many burn their feet with hot-water bottles and electric pads or even with hot water. We do not dare to trust the patients to use hot applications, because their skins are so lacking in sensation that they often do not feel pain. Never now do our surgeons allow our patients to soak their feet. Dry dressings are the rule!

The circulation in the legs of old people and of diabetics particularly should not be obstructed with round garters or by crossing the knees. It is a good plan to teach them to change the position of the legs often. Therefore we encourage patients to move about, and then to place their feet on a chair or stool or chaise longue, and sometimes go so far as to have them raise their legs for two minutes on an inclined board placed in the bed at an angle of forty-five degrees, then hang them down out of the bed for three minutes, then rest them in a horizontal position for five minutes, repeating this cycle six times an hour for even three hours a day. Repeatedly I have known this type of treatment recommended by Dr. Buerger to stop pains and help to heal an indolent ulcer on a toe. But it is far better to prevent the ulcer.

Diabetics cannot be too careful of their feet.

Nearly half of the diabetics who died in hospitals formerly died of gangrene; but today only one in a hundred of all our diabetics reach their end because of troubles with their legs.

Every diabetic should keep his feet as clean as his face. So few diabetics died with troubles of the face and so many with lesions of the feet that often I made it a practice to look at the feet of a diabetic, feel for his dorsalis pedis arteries, examine for athlete's foot—epidermophytosis—between the toes before glancing at his face.

Today amputations of an extremity above the knee are extremely rare because of the skill of the surgeons who can overcome gangrene and infections of the feet with local treatments or minor amputations.

Every old diabetic should show his feet to his doctor at each visit.

So serious have we found these complications in the feet that each year we increase preventive measures. Kind friends have been so impressed with the necessity of the prevention of all this nearly useless sadness and pain that they have provided in the hospital a beauty parlor for diabetic feet. Each diabetic receives special instructions in foot care. Monday mornings at eight o'clock sharp we have a combined medical and surgical conference and discuss lesions of the feet of diabetics then in the hospital. Similarly, I believe each hospital which treats diabetics should have a chiropodist on its staff.

INFECTIONS

Infections make a diabetic worse. Before the discovery and use of insulin and antibiotics the occurrence of an infection in a diabetic was a very serious matter, and a great number of patients succumbed to them. I remember one well-known physician who in the pre-insulin days predicted that pneumonia in a diabetic would invariably be fatal, but in these days of insulin we can combat infections successfully, although we recognize their gravity. During an infection it may be necessary to double, triple, or even quadruple the dose of insulin to hold the disease in control. Therefore, whenever possible, infections should be avoided and sources of infections should be removed. Abscessed teeth should be extracted; really infected tonsils should be taken out;

an infected gall bladder or appendix should be eliminated, and any pimple, boil, or run-a-round about a nail or callus on a hand or foot should receive prompt attention. Particularly is it desirable in children to remove an appendix if there is history of an attack of appendicitis, because the early symptoms and signs of diabetic coma can be easily confused with appendicitis.

When an infection is in progress in a diabetic it may be necessary to give the insulin every three or four hours; it is administered according to the results of the tests of the urine for sugar. Thus some doctors prescribe fifteen units for a red test with Benedict's solution, ten for a yellow test, five for a green test, and no insulin if the test is blue, showing no sugar. Mothers soon learn to vary the dosage of insulin which even so mild an infection as a common cold in a child may demand. Fortunately, when the infection subsides, the dose of insulin can be reduced to its former level. This makes us conclude that infections do not permanently injure the pancreas or indeed cause diabetes, but in some other way interfere with the diabetic state. By having all his lurking infections promptly treated, the diabetic may score a few points of health over the non-diabetic who is neglectful or careless about the same.

Remember an infection makes the diabetes worse.

Get rid of all infections.

DIABETIC COMA

Half a century ago sixty-four diabetics in each one hundred died of diabetic coma in my series of cases, but today a death from diabetic coma is as needless as a death from diphtheria. Only one in a hundred of all my diabetics, wherever in the world their lives end, now succumbs to it. All patients must learn how to escape it. Once I thought diabetic coma was the culmination of the disease, its final stage, and that it came on only in the severe diabetic, but now we know that it may occur in many of the milder cases and frequently in the very earliest stages, so that the diagnosis of the disease is first made when the patient is unconscious.

If you are a diabetic and want to dodge diabetic coma, or if you are a relative or a friend of a diabetic and wish to prevent it in your relative or friend, the rules are plain.

RULES TO AVOID AND PREVENT DIABETIC COMA

If you feel sick, take no chances, but call it diabetic coma and

1. Go to bed.
2. Call the doctor.
3. Never omit insulin if the urine contains sugar.
4. Take one cupful of a hot drink—water, coffee, tea, broth, gruel—every hour.
5. Get someone to care for you.
6. Move the bowels with an enema.
7. Keep warm.

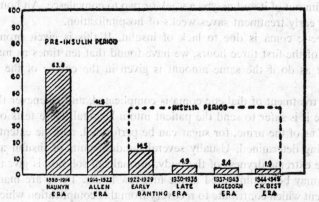

Fig. 49. Coma as a cause of death. Percentage of all deaths due to diabetic coma. Patients of all ages.
(Courtesy of the Metropolitan Life Insurance Company)

The symptoms of the onset of diabetic coma are notoriously obscure, and long ago I gave up trying to teach them. It comes on like a thief in the night. The patient usually feels "sick" and has discomfort or pain in the abdomen, nausea or vomiting; often he has given up insulin or broken his diet; he may have developed an infection and not realized that he required more insulin; he may have drawn too heavily on his own body fat because of extreme exercise or lack of food. Too much fat is bad for a diabetic, no matter whether it is his own body fat or some other kind of fat. Perhaps he has been seasick, or had diarrhea; perhaps he has goiter and thus, not getting enough food, he is living on his own body fat for nourishment to the exclusion of carbohydrate, which either he has not taken or has been unable to utilize because of want of insulin, either his own or that which he buys. He is weak, irritable, tired, nervous, and begins to have difficulty in breathing. All this comes on slowly and slyly: that is the reason for telling him if he feels sick to go to bed, get the doctor, and to call it the onset of diabetic coma until the doctor proves it otherwise. The cupful of hot liquid every hour will help to wash out of the body the fatty acids which cause the coma.

The onset of coma is slow, but its course is fast, and its outcome in death or recovery usually takes place in twenty-four hours, so that treatment must be prompt and active. Hence the patient needs a nurse or someone to care for him at once. As one patient put it, even get your mother-in-law, because it is touch and go. What is done in treatment the first two hours is worth more than what can be done the next twelve hours. The children know this. So do the well-trained hospital patients. When they get sick they telephone their doctors and start treatment immediately, and thus the coma is stopped before it gets a headway. If the patient becomes advanced so far in coma that he is nearly unconscious, then it means a day-and-night job for the doctor and the nurse to bring him out of it and maybe a week or two to convalesce. An hour of prevention or early treatment saves weeks of hospitalization.

Diabetic coma is due to lack of insulin. If this is given promptly in the course of the first three hours, we have found that ten times as many patients recover as do if the same amount is given in the course of the next twelve hours.

The treatment of diabetic coma is complicated, and whenever the diagnosis is made it is safer to send the patient into a hospital. Here tests of the blood, as well as of the urine, for sugar can be performed, and the extent of the acid poisoning determined. Usually several hundred units of insulin are required. For the extreme dryness of the body, normal salt solution is given and several quarts may be administered in the first few hours. There are many details of treatment which contribute to recovery from this complication which before the discovery of insulin was almost uniformly fatal.

The patient may be unconscious and yet not have diabetic coma, but be unconscious from other causes, and the danger is then imminent that he may be treated for the wrong condition. Accidentally he may have taken too much of a drug to produce sleep or relieve pain. He may have taken too much insulin. He may have had a stroke of apoplexy or some temporary nervous trouble which has made him unconscious. Children not uncommonly are unconscious at the beginning of various diseases, or even in health if long without food. Diabetic coma may be confused with a beginning appendicitis, and that is why it is so desirable to remove the appendix in a diabetic when there is a history of its being diseased, so that the question of appendicitis will not arise to confuse the picture if signs of acid poisoning, diabetic coma, appear.

The consequences of a wrong diagnosis between the unconsciousness of diabetic coma and an overdose of insulin (insulin shock) are tragic, and, I regret to say, in a few instances fatal. Therefore every diabetic should carry an identification card in his pocket, so that if by accident he should become unconscious from any cause, the strange doctor who first sees him will be given a hint of his condition. If a diabetic has symptoms of coma or does not recover from an insulin reaction within fifteen to thirty minutes, it is safer to send him to a hospital. An example of such a confusing situation is shown by the following incident. An old colored preacher whose kidneys were bad and blood pressure high in pipestem arteries became unconscious, and his wife thought he was having a stroke. At first, on reaching the hospital, this appeared to be the diagnosis, but a bright young house officer examined his blood and found the blood sugar to be below normal. He injected a little sugar into the vein and—a miracle—the colored preacher was brought back to life. If that young doctor had made a mistake and treated him for diabetic coma and injected insulin instead of sugar, in the place of a miracle there might have been a funeral. What happened was this: The pious old preacher took his insulin as usual before breakfast and then went into his garden. He worked hard, so hard, in fact, that his steed Exercise did all the work of his steed

Insulin. Insulin ran away with his blood sugar and sent it away below normal. The patient should have realized that the diabetic who takes unwonted exercise is entitled to an orange or a little additional carbohydrate in some other form. The extra carbohydrate would have protected him.

In diabetic coma the blood sugar is high and the urine contains sugar.

In an insulin reaction the blood sugar is low and the urine is either sugar free or a second test in thirty minutes will be sugar free.

Diabetic patients will never go into diabetic coma if they live on their diets, keep the urine sugar free, and are careful about their insulin. They must remember, however, that infections make a diabetic worse and so make changes necessary in the doses of insulin. Patients must not omit a regular dose of insulin without testing the urine within six hours to note its effect. A little experience will protect them.

If a diabetic patient can get into a hospital with a laboratory in which tests can be performed by night as well as by day, his chances for recovery from coma are good, and the younger he is the better the outlook for recovery. Of twenty-three children with diabetic coma recently treated in the New England Deaconess Hospital, none died, but we have had only one person as old as seventy-seven recover.

There are easy tests of the urine for the detection of acid poisoning by examining it for acetone and diacetic acid. Many doctors teach their patients how to make these tests. In general, I emphasize keeping the urine sugar free, and then coma does not appear; but one must remember that a patient voiding a urine which gives a green test with Benedict solution for sugar may in a few hours void a specimen which gives a red test. The tests for acetone and diacetic acid are recorded below.

The test for acetone is readily performed with Nitroprusside, which conveniently is put up in tablet form ("Acetest" manufactured by the Ames Company, Inc., Elkhart, Indiana).

The test for diacetic acid is also easily performed:

To 5 or 10 cc. of freshly voided urine carefully add a few drops of a 10 per cent aqueous solution of ferric chloride. A precipitate of ferric phosphate first forms, but upon the addition of a few more drops is dissolved. The depth of the Burgundy-red color obtained is an index to the quantity of diacetic acid present. The intensity of the reaction may be roughly recorded as 1, 2, 3, or 4+. If the color does not disappear on boiling, it is not a true test for diacetic acid, and is due to aspirin or some similar drug.

THE NERVOUS SYSTEM

It is seldom diabetics have imaginary ills or old-fashioned nervous prostration. In general, they accept their lot and plan to overcome any handicaps connected with it. On the other hand, they do have troubles with the nerves, but these occur almost exclusively as a result of the diabetes being uncontrolled.

I do not recall among the Quarter Century Victory Medal diabetics complaints of this nature.

NEURITIS

The nerves contain many fibers, both motor and sensory, and these may be involved individually. Thus occasionally there will be a paralysis of one of the motor nerves which controls the movement of the eyes, especially the Sixth nerve which supplies the external rectus muscle, and then one "sees double." Rarely, a nerve may be involved which supplies the muscles of the forehead and face, and the resulting condition suggests that of a patient who has had a shock, but it is distinctly different, being a peripheral paralysis and not a central paralysis which originates in the brain. In the lower extremities one may get a paralysis of the muscles, iliopsoas, which help one to rise from a chair, or of the peroneal muscle which when involved leads to a toe drop and a scuffling gait. All of these conditions are painless because only the motor fibers of the nerves are affected, and in time recovery occurs.

The sensory fibers may be involved without the motor fibers. Then pain may result along the course of a nerve and vary in extent or degree depending upon the severity of the attack. Instead of actual pain there may be sensory disturbances—numbness, prickling, pins-and-needles feeling—which are most annoying. They may be quite general or localized to a small area of the body. Occasionally the nerves of the digestive and urinary tracts are involved and symptoms related to these parts appear.

Neuritis is a most disturbing complication and may be serious, but one can reassure anyone who has it that eventually recovery will almost certainly ensue. It seldom occurs if the disease is controlled. Alcohol and tobacco in an attack must be avoided.

THE EYES

The eyes of diabetics temporarily may be affected when treatment begins, because of the lowering of the high sugar content of the blood to normal, thus changing the course of rays of light through the lens upon the retina at the back of the eye. This is a temporary condition and after a few weeks disappears. It is advisable, therefore, in the first few weeks of treatment for diabetics not to have new glasses fitted, because they would serve only temporarily, but to wait about a month until the eyes become adjusted to the return of the blood to normal.

Cataracts develop in diabetics as in non-diabetics, but it is not yet definitely proven whether they are more common in diabetics. Operations can be performed successfully even on very old persons.

Hemorrhages and exudates occur far too commonly in the eyes of diabetics. If these involve the macula in the retina, vision is seriously impaired. The best known way to avoid such conditions is to control the diabetes from the very beginning. Tobacco is harmful. Medicines may be of some value in preventing the hemorrhages.

DIABETIC CAMPS

Although the lot of diabetic children is steadily improving and they now enter into all the activities of a normal child, they carry heavy responsibilities. At each meal they are reminded of their disease; upon rising each morning they must have an insulin injection (only a few years ago it was two, three, or even four times a day); constantly their every act is watched, and they cannot help seeing the apprehension which their parents feel for them. Diabetic children need a respite, and for them the late Dr. Wendt of Detroit planned a diabetic camp. In the following year, 1926, Mrs. Devine at Ogunquit, Maine, opened her camp for diabetic children, and little by little these camps have sprung up in various parts of the country. Under the supervision of Dr. Priscilla White and Dr. Alexander Marble, some 200 diabetic girls go to the Clara Barton Birthplace Camp for girls in Oxford, Massachusetts, and 150 boys to the Elliott P. Joslin Camp for boys in nearby Charlton, Massachusetts. We know of at least eighteen other camps. We have found these camps to be most advantageous and strongly recommend their increase in number and size. A list of these camps can be obtained by writing to the American Diabetes Association, 11 West 42nd Street, New York 36, New York.

The change of food and surroundings, which a trip away from home involves, and the contact with many others who have the same disease, along with the pleasures of camp life, are splendid for the children. The revision of diets and dosage of insulin while under supervision which is as close as that in a hospital and yet not so obvious gives an excellent opportunity to improve treatment. But these camps soon disclosed another useful feature of almost equal value, and that was the vacation they provided for the children's parents and households. It is no joke to have the responsibility of a diabetic child day and night for years, and we soon learned that the mothers were quite as thankful for the freedom from care and the vacation they received as were the children themselves.

HOSPITAL TEACHING CLINIC

Bouchardat, that wonderful French diabetes clinician, taught us a hundred years ago that many a diabetic adult by attention to diet and exercise and good hygiene could attain his life's quota of years in comfort. The diabetic camps showed us that diabetic children could live joyfully and free from complications while under supervision. Ten years of life, even with moderate attention to diet and insulin, were available for almost every diabetic child even if dietetic rules were greatly relaxed. But soon it became evident that the second decade of diabetes in children as in adults was fraught with distressing and even fatal complications in the nerves, the blood vessels, the kidneys, and the eyes. At first it looked as if the children had been rescued from an early death in diabetic coma to suffer for months and years with impaired eyesight and then yield to weeks or months of invalidism ending in collapse of their arteries in brain, heart, or kidneys. For a short period the outlook appeared quite as hopeless as did the conquest of coma before insulin. But gradually our attitude has changed, for since that era we have had a patient here and there who, after fifteen, twenty, and even a quarter century of diabetes, appeared well. Little by little it dawned upon us, as these twenty-five-year exceptional diabetics were studied, that they were distinguished from other less fortunate diabetics by reason of their closer adherence to diet and insulin. Control of diabetes and not duration of the disease was the essential element for health.

The vital necessity to control the diabetes as soon as recognized has forced us to plan for the Hospital Teaching Clinic. To it young and old diabetics can be sent for instruction. All will be ambulatory because they are being assembled throughout the entire year, not for the treatment of complications but to learn how to avoid them. Complications demand a hospital, but a Teaching Clinic for diabetics can be built without operating rooms; and the ambulatory clientele can go to a cafeteria and thus save nursing expense, and they can do light housekeeping also—make their own beds, as in schools and colleges and in the Army—to reduce costs. Here diabetics can return for periods of instruction which will result in better control of the diabetes.

The Hospital Teaching Clinic I consider the most progressive idea in the management of the diabetic. Not only will he learn here inexpensively his own status, but along with it receive advice as to how to protect his family. Instructions will be afforded to his relatives and to all living in the neighborhood. Such a clinic will serve for continuous and inexpensive control of the patient and will also acquaint multitudes with the disease, and teach them how to detect it and its complications so that these can be attacked in their incipiency.

A million and more diabetics are now in our midst, and another sixty thousand will be diagnosed this year. Let us recognize the importance of this immigrant host which is springing up in every city and town in our country. Let us treat them rationally, appreciate all the good they do from their example in cleanliness and their temperance in diet and training in the advantage of close contact between doctor and patient and in the scientific progress of medicine. We must not forget their precocity and their wonderful leaders like Clemenceau, Edison, and Eastman, and strive to help them in their diabetic studies, knowing full well that in the end they are themselves an experimental laboratory and already the teachers of us all.

CHAPTER XXII

Blood Pressure

ARTHUR M. MASTER, M.D. and HARRY L. JAFFE, M.D.

MOST PEOPLE are extremely interested and anxious about the effects of high blood pressure and low blood pressure, and attribute various symptoms to these conditions. However, much of this anxiety and fear is unfounded. Only recently have the wide variations and limits of blood pressure among normal people begun to be realized. What formerly was considered either high or low blood pressure is often normal and without significance.

MECHANISM OF BLOOD PRESSURE

Blood pressure refers to the pressure within the arteries throughout the body, i.e., the blood vessels carrying the blood from the heart to the organs and tissues. The pressure in the arteries is produced by the beating of the heart. Each time the heart contracts (this part of the heart beat is called systole), the left side of the heart or left ventricle propels the blood within it into a large artery called the aorta. From this vessel the blood flows into its many branches which become smaller and smaller until they are exceedingly fine and connect with the veins through the capillaries. Because of the force with which the left ventricle ejects the blood into the aorta it flows with considerable speed, and a pulse wave is sent ahead through all the arteries. This pulsation is easily felt at the wrist, but may also be felt in the neck and feet and in other parts of the body. The arteries are elastic and flexible; in their walls are muscle fibers which contract and help send the blood along.

The pressure in the arteries is not the same throughout each heart beat; it is highest during the period of contraction, or systole, and lowest during the relaxation phase, or diastole. As a result, each person has an upper systolic pressure and a lower diastolic blood pressure, e.g., 124 over 82. Usually the diastolic pressure is about two thirds the systolic, but, as you grow older and the arteries tend to lose their elasticity and become rigid, the systolic pressure is apt to rise considerably whereas the diastolic increases only slightly. This type of change in the blood pressure is usually not at all serious.

Both the systolic and diastolic pressures are recorded. The instrument used to measure them is technically termed a sphygmomanometer. This name, derived from the Greek, literally means a measure of the pulses but is rarely used even by doctors. Most of them merely say blood-pressure machine. The device consists of two parts connected by a rubber tube. One part is a long cloth sleeve containing a rectangular rubber bag at one end. Two rubber tubes lead out from this bag through the cloth sleeve. One leads to a rubber bulb which inflates the rubber bag and has a valve which regulates the inflow and outflow of air. The second tube is long and is attached to the second part of the apparatus which consists of a glass tube containing a column of mercury. The glass tube is graduated in millimeters from 0 to 300.

When your doctor takes your blood pressure, he winds the cloth sleeve around your right or left arm. The pressure may differ by five to fifteen points on the two sides normally, but this does not matter. The doctor places his stethoscope in the crease of the elbow on the artery and squeezes the bulb. As he continues to do this, the pressure in the rubber bag on the arm increases, the mercury rises, and he hears the sound of the pulse through his stethoscope. He goes on inflating the bag until he is unable to hear the sound. Then he gradually releases his pressure upon the bulb until he hears the sound again. This is the systolic pressure; the exact figure is indicated by the height of the column of mercury. The doctor allows the bag to deflate gradually until the sound suddenly diminishes or cannot be heard at all. The level of the top of the mercury column is again noted and indicates the diastolic pressure.

NORMAL BLOOD PRESSURE

In the past normal people were supposed to have systolic pressure less than 150 mm. mercury and the diastolic under 90. These figures applied to all people over 40 regardless of their exact age, sex, or build. Therefore, if a man or woman of 55 or 65 had either a systolic pressure of 160 or a diastolic pressure of 95, he or she was considered to have high blood pressure or hypertension. As a result, these people were treated as if they were ill or potentially sick. As might be expected, this caused considerable emotional disturbances and even physical invalidism.

However, doctors observed that many of these people who were supposed to have high blood pressure remained in good health for many years. Therefore I began, in collaboration with Dublin and Marks, a new investigation into what blood pressure was normal at various ages. In order to find out, a large number of healthy people were required; the blood pressure readings were obtained in 74,000 men and women working in industry all over the country. They were 25 to 65 years old. The results were instructive, for we found that, after 40, at least half of the population had a systolic pressure of 150 or more or a diastolic pressure of 90 or more. Furthermore, the blood pressure gradually increases with age, and by 65 the majority of normal men have a systolic pressure up to 170 and normal women a pressure up to 175. At 65 many men and women have a diastolic pressure between 100 and 110. In fact, it seems that, at 65, even a systolic pressure up to 180 and a diastolic up to 110 may occasionally be normal. These facts are shown in the accompanying tables (1 and 2).

Table 1.—Normal Range and Limits of Hypertension

Systolic

	Normal Range		Hypertension Lower Limit	
Age	Male	Female	Male	Female
16	105–135	100–130	145	140
17	105–135	100–130	145	140
18	105–135	100–130	145	140
19	105–140	100–130	150	140
20–24	105–140	100–130	150	140
25–29	108–140	102–130	150	140
30–34	110–145	102–135	155	145
35–39	110–145	105–140	160	150
40–44	110–150	105–150	165	165
45–49	110–155	105–155	170	175
50–54	115–160	110–165	175	180
55–59	115–165	110–170	180	185
60–64	115–170	115–175	190	190

From the Bulletin of the New York Academy of Medicine, July 1951, vol. 27, pp. 452–65.

Table 2.—Normal Range and Limits of Hypertension

Diastolic

	Normal Range		Hypertension Lower Limit	
Age	Male	Female	Male	Female
16	60–86	60–85	90	90
17	60–86	60–85	90	90
18	60–86	60–85	90	90
19	60–88	60–85	95	90
20–24	62–88	60–85	95	90
25–29	65–90	60–86	96	92
30–34	68–92	60–88	98	95
35–39	68–92	65–90	100	98
40–44	70–94	65–92	100	100
45–49	70–96	65–96	104	105
50–54	70–98	70–100	106	108
55–59	70–98	70–100	108	108
60–64	70–100	70–100	110	110

From the Bulletin of the New York Academy of Medicine, July 1951, vol. 27, pp. 452–65.

In view of these results, it is necessary to change many of the notions about normal and high blood pressure which have been taken for granted in the past. People over 45 or 50 with a blood pressure of 170/90 or 160/100, for example, no longer need be upset and anxious, because at their age such a blood pressure is frequently normal and is not significant if the examination of the heart and blood vessels is free from abnormality. If such is the case, any symptoms the patient may have, e.g., headache, dizziness, throbbing in the head, should not be attributed to the blood pressure, and some other causes should be sought. In people over 65 even a systolic pressure of 180 to 190 or a diastolic between 100 and 110 may occasionally be within normal and therefore not serious. In such cases, particularly, periodic checkups are necessary.

In the past it has been accepted that high blood pressure either causes or leads to certain diseases, such as hardening or sclerosis of the coronary arteries (which supply blood to the heart muscle), enlargement of the heart, and heart failure. This assumption was based on the old figures of blood pressure. Now that the upper limits of normal have been raised, high blood pressure is probably in many instances much less of a villain than has been assumed.

Most people think of the blood pressure as being fixed and assume that the exact height of the pressure determines how they feel. Neither of these ideas is true. Many people, particularly those who are inclined to be nervous and apprehensive, have a variable or labile blood pressure. It may suddenly rise considerably in any situation of excitement, such as visiting a doctor, preparing for an examination, or experiencing pain. Because of this, the physician takes the blood pressure again if the first reading or two is high. If he wishes, the physician can obtain the "basal" blood pressure by placing the person being examined at rest or in bed for several hours or days and taking frequent blood pressure readings. In extreme cases the pressure may rise 40 or 50 mm. temporarily. As a rule, the systolic pressure rises more than the diastolic. One of our patients has a normal blood pressure of 124/74, but when she comes to the office, the first reading at times is up to 170 or 180 systolic and 110 to 120 diastolic. There is some difference of opinion among doctors concerning the importance of these transitory increases in blood pressure. Some doctors believe that such patients have a tendency to high blood pressure and probably will develop it later on. It has been our experience, however, that many of them retain a normal blood pressure over the years.

WHAT CAUSES HIGH BLOOD PRESSURE?

Several conditions increase the systolic pressure but not the diastolic. This type, which is called systolic hypertension, is not a true hypertension and is not significant. For example, we have already mentioned that, as many people grow older, their arteries become less elastic and their systolic pressure rises. However, in many of these the diastolic pressure rises only slightly or not at all. The blood pressure may be 200/80 but this need not be considered hypertension since the diastolic pressure is normal.

People with rheumatic heart disease of the type which prevents the aortic valve from closing properly, allowing the blood to flow back from the aorta to the heart with each heart beat, usually have a high systolic pressure but a low diastolic. In extreme cases pressures of 300 systolic and 10 or 20 diastolic are present. Similarly, when the thyroid gland functions excessively, a condition known as hyperthyroidism, a blood pressure of 180/60 is not uncommon but should not be labeled hypertension.

Among patients with diastolic or true hypertension, according to the newly established figures, the cause is known in only a small number and usually proves to be kidney disease, technically known as nephritis. This sometimes begins suddenly following a sore throat or scarlet fever and may develop insidiously over the years, resulting in high blood pressure. Examination of the urine shows significant abnormalities. In this connection there is a specific type of kidney disease which deserves special mention. When people have stones or repeated inflammation in one kidney, that organ may function poorly or not at all. As a result, a few of these patients develop high blood pressure. If the involved kidney is removed by operation, the pressure sometimes falls to normal. This type of hypertension is thus curable.

During pregnancy the blood pressure may suddenly become very high, should intoxication develop during the later months. The exact cause of this toxemia is not known, but the kidneys become involved. The frequency of this disease fortunately is diminishing because of better observation during pregnancy. If it does occur, it usually responds to the newer drugs now available in treating hypertension.

There are also ingenious experiments to show that kidney disease can cause high blood pressure. If a clamp is placed on the artery supplying blood to one kidney in a dog, the kidney gradually disintegrates and the animal's blood pressure may rise above 200 mm. However, it is generally considered unlikely that this is the way hypertension develops in human beings, except rarely.

Another known cause of hypertension is a tumor of the adrenal glands. There are two glands, each consisting of a small piece of tissue situated at the upper pole of each kidney. The inner portion of the adrenal gland secretes a substance called adrenalin which raises the blood pressure. When a tumor develops in an adrenal gland, it excretes an excessive amount of adrenalin at various times. As a result, the patient's blood pressure may suddenly rise to high levels, e.g., 220 or 240 mm., and the patient suddenly feels his heart pounding. He becomes dizzy and trembles and perspires profusely. Occasionally, the blood pressure is elevated continuously. When the tumor is removed surgically, the blood pressure becomes normal and the patient is cured.

In children and young adults with high blood pressure, the doctor looks for "narrowing" or a stricture of the aorta with which some children are born. This condition, called "coarctation of the aorta," is easily diagnosed because, while the blood pressure is elevated in the arms, it is low in the legs.

In over 90 per cent of patients with high blood pressure, a cause cannot be found. The condition is, therefore, called essential hypertension. Although the reason is unknown, in these people the smallest branches of their arteries throughout the body are narrowed or constricted. This increases the resistance in these tiny vessels, and the blood pressure must rise to keep the blood flowing through them.

A number of theories have been proposed concerning the cause of essential hypertension. The most popular view is that people who develop this disease are emotional and react more tensely and sensitively to the conditions of life. They meet most daily happenings, big and small, with anxiety and restraint. They tend to repress their conflicts. These inner tensions set up impulses in the brain which travel through a special part of the nervous system to all parts of the body, causing the arterioles to tighten. When this happens repeatedly day in and day out, these small vessels may become scarred and thickened. The resistance within them rises, and the blood pressure increases permanently.

Many situations in everyday life may cause emotional strain and anxiety in tense people. Among the commonest are financial difficulties, dissatisfaction with the job, failure to advance in work, jealousy, disagreement among members of a family, and physical disability or illness in a beloved one. Many people are full of fears about various things, many of which do not have any basis in fact.

Since anxiety and tension are almost universal, you may wonder why all people do not have hypertension. Quite likely there is another factor in people with hypertension, in addition to the specific type of nervous reaction already mentioned. This localizes the effect of this nervous sensitivity in the arterioles, resulting in hypertension, whereas other nervous people develop ulcer of the stomach, colitis (disease of the large bowel), or other diseases. This tendency to hypertension is more common in some families than in others. For example, we have observed a family in which the grandmother, her four daughters, and a grandson developed a high degree of diastolic hypertension at a relatively early age. As is not uncommon even in advanced hypertension, one of the sisters is alive at 77 and the others did not die until they were 69, 63, and 61, life spans not much different from the average. This is perhaps an unusual instance, but in a considerable number of families one not infrequently finds high blood pressure in one parent and one or two children. However, these members are usually a minority, and the majority do not develop high blood pressure. Hypertension is not hereditary, and the specific factor which predisposes certain families to develop it is not clear.

Observations have led some doctors to believe that there is a relation between high blood pressure and race and climate. Hypertension, according to some reports, rarely occurs in parts of China and the remainder of the Orient, and among people, particularly the natives, living in the heat of the tropics. These statements remain to be proven, and the results may not be comparable with those in the Western world because the life span of the people in the tropics may be much shorter. If hypertension is less common among tropical people, it is probably because of their type of diet, which is low in proteins, fats, and salt and because of their mode of life, which is slow and less tense than ours. When these people have lived among us, they develop hypertension pretty much as we do.

Overweight or obesity tends to increase the blood pressure and therefore favors the development of hypertension. Although it is an aggravating factor, it probably is not a direct cause, because many people with high blood pressure are of average weight or even thin. The popular conception of a person with hypertension is someone who is obese and emotional and has a florid complexion. Although this is often true, many such people have a normal blood pressure. However, obesity is significant and often serious when high blood pressure exists, and often merely reducing weight is sufficient to lower the blood pressure. Overweight increases the amount of work which the heart must perform, and loss of weight lessens the burden on the heart, allowing the blood pressure to fall. This was observed during wartime when malnutrition and starvation were common in many countries and the frequency of hypertension fell sharply.

Recently it has become evident that the endocrine glands play an important rôle in regulating the blood pressure and form a link in the development of hypertension in many cases. We have already mentioned how a tumor of the inner portion or medulla of one of these glands, the adrenal, causes bouts of high blood pressure or even constant hypertension. Similarly, high blood pressure may be caused by a tumor of the outer portion of the pituitary gland, another endocrine gland which is situated in the under surface of the brain above the nasal passages. The endocrine glands, which also include the thyroid, pancreas, and ovaries, secrete substances directly into the blood stream which are called hormones. The latter control many functions of the body such as growth, sexual development, menstruation, metabolism, and the distribution of salt and water in the body. Each gland secretes a specific hormone, but the functions of all the glands are interrelated, with the pituitary gland acting as the regulator of many functions.

One fact connecting the endocrine glands with hypertension is that many women develop high blood pressure during or after the menopause. At this period the activity of the endocrine glands undergoes a great change. In many of these women the blood pressure later falls.

The amount of salt in the body appears to be important in determining the blood pressure. We now know that the cortex of the adrenal gland plays a major role in salt metabolism. When this portion of the adrenal gland is destroyed by disease, as in Addison's disease, the sodium in the blood is decreased and the blood pressure may fall as low as 60 mm. Hg. When people with hypertension are given a diet low in salt, their blood pressure may fall to normal.

In the past a variety of other factors have been suggested as causes of hypertension. They include focal infections, such as diseased tonsils, abscessed teeth, or infected hemorrhoids; syphilis; gall bladder disease; constipation; alcohol; tobacco, and coffee. These conditions do not cause high blood pressure, but they may temporarily aggravate hypertension which already exists. For example, the pain of an abscessed tooth or of repeated gall bladder attacks may tend to elevate the blood pressure, and the removal of these sources of irritation often lowers the blood pressure. Also, excessive smoking or drinking of coffee or soft drinks containing caffeine may help to maintain high blood pressure. During the recent war it was not uncommon for officers to drink ten to twenty cups of coffee a day, and sometimes their blood pressure rose above normal. When they drank only two or three cups the hypertension disappeared. People with hypertension should follow their physician's advice concerning tobacco, alcohol, and coffee.

SYMPTOMS

It is a popular misconception that high blood pressure itself causes symptoms and that the severity of these depends upon the actual height of the pressure. It is quite common for a patient to come to a doctor's office because of a headache, dizziness, or noises in the head which he or she is certain indicates a jump in the blood pressure. Usually the doctor finds the blood pressure the same as in previous examinations. As a matter of fact, high blood pressure of itself often does not cause symptoms. Many people with a blood pressure, for example, of 200/110 mm. Hg., feel well. This is particularly true if they are unaware of their high blood pressure; on the other hand, the knowledge of having hypertension often produces a state of anxiety and tension which causes symptoms. For example, a man of 55 conducted a large business and had not visited a physician for some years. When the Red Cross called for donations of blood, he volunteered but was rejected because his blood pressure was found to be 180/100 mm. Hg. Almost immediately he began to feel tired and dizzy, and these symptoms persisted even though at times his blood pressure fell to 160/96. Examination of his heart and blood vessels was negative and, therefore, his symptoms were nervous.

Dr. Paul D. White has said that hypertension is the most important of all human illnesses. The reason for this statement is that it often leads to, or accelerates, hardening or sclerosis of the small arteries in various parts of the body. This does not always happen; many people with high blood pressure remain well for years without developing significant arteriosclerosis. Also, men and women differ in their tendency to develop arteriosclerosis. It occurs in men whether their blood pressure is normal or high, whereas in women it is usually found in those with hypertension. It is also apt to occur in both sexes when diabetes is present.

The commonest and most important organs affected by arteriosclerosis are the heart, brain, and kidneys. Recording the blood pressure is, therefore, only the beginning of the examination. The major part is the search for symptoms and signs of inadequate circulation to, or disease of, these organs.

When the arteries which supply blood to the heart, i.e., the coronary arteries, become hardened and narrowed, the person affected may experience two types of symptoms. The first consists of temporary heart pain (angina pectoris) when he walks or is excited, or a serious heart attack (coronary thrombosis). The second type includes shortness of breath, cough, and swelling of the ankles (congestive failure).

Hypertension often causes another change in the heart, i.e., enlargement. This happens because the heart must work against an increased pressure in the arteries and resistance in the arterioles. As a result, each muscle fiber in the heart increases in size, and the heart as a whole is enlarged. This is much like the large muscles in the arms which stevedores, boxers, and the like develop. At first the enlargement of the heart is not harmful, but beyond a certain size the heart becomes inefficient. At this stage sclerosis of the coronary arteries has usually developed, and both factors may produce heart pain or shortness of breath.

When the arteries in the brain are hardened, a change in personality and judgment may follow. The person may gradually become irritable and stubborn and his memory may be impaired. He may complain of weakness, headache, dizziness, noises in the head, and unsteadiness in walking, or he may suddenly have a stroke as a result of a hemorrhage or clot in one of the arteries. If it is severe, coma or stupor sets in; in less serious cases there is a paralysis of one or more parts of the body, usually the face and an arm and leg on one side (hemiplegia). Occasionally only the speech is interfered with. In most cases the paralysis recedes slowly.

When the kidney is damaged by arteriosclerosis, the person is apt to be weak and anemic and to vomit occasionally. His ankles and face may be swollen. The diagnosis is confirmed by making tests of the urine and blood.

Other evidence of hardening may be found in the arteries in the legs and in the pancreas. The latter causes diabetes. There is a special type of hypertension, called malignant, which occurs in younger people and progresses rapidly into severe diseases of the arterioles. In these cases treatment must be started at once.

To repeat, when hypertension is discovered, it is imperative that the patient have a complete examination to determine whether the heart, brain, or kidneys have been affected. If they have not, the patient may be assured that his condition is not serious.

TREATMENT

In caring for people with high blood pressure the doctor always looks for some condition which may be causing the hypertension. Some of these causes, such as a tumor of the adrenal gland, a single kidney damaged by chronic infection or stones, or narrowing (stricture) of the aorta with which some people are born, can be removed by operation and the hypertension permanently cured. At present there is no effective way to treat hypertension secondary to long-standing diseases of both kidneys or nephritis.

The vast majority of patients have primary or essential hypertension. Although its cause is not definitely known, we have already emphasized the importance of the nervous and psychological elements. It is essential to find out the patient's anxieties and fears. If his tensions can be released, his blood pressure may fall.

Since most people are filled with a dread of hypertension, the first step is to give them a true picture and clear understanding of the condition. The newly determined limits of normal blood pressure are of great importance; many people who are supposed to have hypertension may now be assured that their blood pressure is normal for their age. For example, a man, 65 years old, has had a blood pressure of 170/100 mm. Hg. for four or five years; he may now forget about his blood pressure instead of worrying about it and having it checked frequently. This habit of frequent taking of the blood pressure should be discouraged since the blood pressure normally varies a great deal from day to day, and even from hour to hour. Anyway, the exact level of the pressure is not significant. The remainder of the examination is far more important than the blood pressure reading.

Even if you have hypertension (according to recent figures), you should realize that many, if not most, such people remain well and lead normal lives; they run a benign course similar to people with normal blood pressure. Usually they need take only moderate precautions. We have observed people with blood pressures of 220/120, or even 250/140, remain well for fifteen to forty years! The wise person with hypertension is the one who accepts it calmly, makes whatever adjustments his physician advises, and then forgets about it except for an occasional examination.

It is often possible and valuable to modify the personality of hypertensive people. Many of them are full of drive and suppressed resentment; they have a tendency to flare up suddenly over unimportant matters. Pointing these facts out to them may alter their behavior and approach to life. They can learn to do things at a slower tempo and under less strain; in this way they can reduce the pressure of life. This approach is important also in younger persons who show occasional elevations in blood pressure and come of families predisposed to hypertension. If they can be taught to live with less intensity and more equanimity, it is likely that many of them can be prevented from developing hypertension later on, just as this approach can cause a drop in blood pressure in people with hypertension.

The person with ordinary degrees of hypertension should not consider himself an invalid and should go on working. People with hypertension perform their work as well as, or even better than, those with normal blood pressure. Naturally, people with hypertension should abide by the doctor's advice concerning hours and type of work, rest periods, and vacations. In many cases significant restrictions are unnecessary. Ordinary work is not harmful and often prevents anxiety.

The importance of avoiding or correcting overweight in people with hypertension cannot be overemphasized. The frequency of illness and death is directly proportional to the amount of overweight. When a reducing or low calorie diet is indicated, the doctor will prescribe one suitable for each patient. All reducing diets are low in fats and starches or carbohydrates and high in proteins; they include fruits, vegetables except potatoes, lean meats, fish and pot cheese; they avoid butter, sweet or sour cream, bread, cake and other desserts, dressing with oil, nuts, spaghetti, puddings, and custards.

SALT-FREE DIETS

In recent years another element in the diet of hypertensive patients has assumed the stellar role. When the salt in the diet is restricted, the blood pressure falls in many of these patients, often reaching normal levels. Many natural foods, e.g., milk, and most prepared foods, e.g., bread, contain a considerable amount of salt and are not permitted in a strict, low salt diet.

The diet which has the least salt content consists only of rice, fruit, and fruit juices. This "rice diet" contains a minimum of protein and fat as well as of salt. Tapioca may be used in addition to rice. Although this is an effective low salt diet, it is extremely unpalatable and difficult to follow beyond a short period. Also it is weakening and may have serious effects unless tests are made frequently. It is suitable, however, when the condition is serious and the person with hypertension is in a hospital.

The salt poor diets prescribed by most physicians are much more varied than the rice diet, but they are usually effective and quite palatable. Therefore, most patients will follow them for long periods. Here is a list of some of the common foods that contain considerable salt and should be avoided:

Bacon	Chili sauce	Popcorn
Beer	Corned beef	Potato chips
Beets	Crackers	Prepared flours
Bouillon cubes	Duck	Prepared desserts
Bran	Frankfurters	Pretzels
Cakes and cookies	Ham	Relishes
Canned fish	Kale	Salad dressings
Canned meats	Kidney	Salt butter
Canned soups	Malted milk	Salt pork
Canned tomato juice	Mayonnaise	Sardines
Canned vegetables	Meat soups	Sausage
Catsup	Mustard	Sea foods
Caviar	Nuts, salted	Smoked foods
Celery	Oleomargarine	Spinach
Celery salt	Olives	White bread
Chard	Pastries	Worcestershire sauce
Cheese	Pickles	

More and more foods are appearing on the market prepared without salt. These include bread and canned vegetables, soups, and meat.

No one should undertake a low salt diet except on the advice of a physician. He will decide what type of diet is required, if any at all, and will instruct the patient how to follow it. In addition, he must observe the effects of the diet from time to time.

There are several safe salt substitutes on the market which may be used to flavor the food. Much can also be accomplished with lemon, pepper, and other spices which are permitted in a low salt diet.

People on a low salt diet face another problem, for sodium, which is the important element in salt in combatting hypertension, is present in a number of articles used every day. These include many toothpastes; simple remedies for indigestion and heartburn, such as soda; laxatives and mild sedatives. It is important to read the list of ingredients printed on the cover of these items. In some communities the water contains an appreciable amount of sodium and special precautions are necessary.

RESINS TO REMOVE SALT

Recently the march of medical progress has led to the discovery of a resin substance which removes sodium from the intestines before it is absorbed into the blood stream. It is taken in powder form several times a day. It often increases the effectiveness of a low salt diet and, therefore, the diet may be less rigid. As in the case of diet, the effect of this substance must be watched by the physician.

OPERATIONS FOR HIGH BLOOD PRESSURE

Another method of treating high blood pressure is to perform an operation in which many of the "sympathetic" nerves are cut. These nerves run in a chain on each side of the spine and carry the impulses from the brain which cause the arterioles throughout the body to tighten. When these nerves are severed, this constriction is prevented and the blood pressure falls.

At first this operation, which is called sympathectomy, was popular because many patients felt better afterward. However, as time went on, it was found that the blood pressure often returned to its previous high level. Also the operation is a major procedure requiring an experienced surgeon and a lengthy stay in the hospital. However, the operation is sometimes successful and should be considered seriously when a patient has many symptoms which have not been relieved by a low salt diet and other measures.

DRUGS FOR HYPERTENSION

Recently several drugs have been developed which paralyze the sympathetic nerves, and it is hoped that they will accomplish the same result as the operation of sympathectomy. Among the most promising of these drugs are "Methium," "Apresoline" and "Hydergine." At times they seem to be more effective when combined. The required dosage of each must be determined for each patient, and they may have certain untoward effects. Another drug is veratrum. These drugs must be taken only under the direct supervision of a doctor.

Many other drugs have been used through the years on patients with high blood pressure. The majority of these are sedatives and tend to promote relaxation and allay anxiety. They include phenobarbital, chloral, and the bromides not containing sodium. These drugs are mild and helpful during periods of strain and emotional upset. They may also promote sleep, although a stronger sedative may be necessary. When these drugs are taken in the proper dosage under the supervision of a doctor, they are not harmful and often help keep the blood pressure at a lower level.

Other new drugs are derivatives of Rauwolfia or Reserpine, guanethidine, Diuril or chlorothiazide, Diupres, and other drugs which eliminate fluid.

In severe cases of hypertension a combination of several types of treatment (low salt diet, operation, and drugs) is more successful than any one alone.

The best approach to hypertension would seem to be a change in our way of living. We should strive to lessen the high tension and fast pace of modern life and live at a slower, more relaxed tempo. We should learn to be moderate in the way we work, play, and eat. (New drugs called tranquilizers include Reserpine, chlorpromazine, and Miltown or Equanil. These have been found helpful in lowering blood pressure.—Ed.)

LOW BLOOD PRESSURE OR HYPOTENSION

Many people believe that low blood pressure or hypotension is a common, even serious, condition capable of causing many symptoms. This notion is untrue! Low blood pressure in the true sense is uncommon and usually is the result of some condition, e.g., anemia; acute and chronic infections, such as grippe; disabling diseases like tuberculosis, rheumatism, and cancer, and malnutrition. For example, the blood pressure may fall considerably during a period of strict dieting in order to lose weight. As the patient recovers, his blood pressure rises.

What is ordinarily considered hypotension, e.g., a systolic pressure of 100, 110, or 120 mm. Hg., is, in fact, normal at any age. A significant number of normal women have a systolic pressure of 96 to 100 mm. While normal people with hypotension tend to be thin and narrow-chested, to feel weak, to tire easily, and to lack stamina, some are well developed and even athletic. Indeed, people with a low normal blood pressure have a greater life expectancy than the average. Their symptoms are not the result of their lowered blood pressure, but are part of their nervous, constitutional make-up.

We do not wish to give the impression that true hypotension, i.e., a systolic pressure under 96 mm. Hg., does not exist or that a low normal blood pressure may not be associated with some type of heart disease. As in the case of hypertension, it is essential to make a complete examination of the patient with a lowered blood pressure in order to determine whether or not it is significant.

The lowest blood pressures, e.g., 40 to 80 mm. Hg., are found in a rare disease causing destruction of the outer layers or cortex of an adrenal gland.

It is known as Addison's disease after the man who discovered it. It can be corrected by giving the patient salt and a drug (DOCA).

Following a heart attack or coronary thrombosis, a small number of patients maintain a blood pressure between 90 and 100 mm. for months or years. They usually feel quite well, and their heart function is quite satisfactory.

Narrowing of the aortic valve (aortic stenosis) is often associated with a blood pressure of 100 to 120 mm. Hg.

Thus far low blood pressure which is permanent or which lasts for days or weeks, e.g., following the grippe, has been considered. There are also several conditions in which the blood pressure or the heart rate suddenly falls, causing dizziness or fainting. This happens because the flow of blood to the brain is suddenly reduced, and that tissue is very sensitive to a lack of blood and oxygen.

This type of fainting in young people is usually nervous, but in others it occurs only when they stand up. Usually when people get up after having been sitting or lying down, the blood pressure rises. In certain people, however, it falls and they feel faint. This can usually be avoided by getting up gradually, by wearing an abdominal belt, or by a drug such as ephedrine.

These conditions with a sudden drop in blood pressure are not serious, but fainting may also be caused by heart disease and other illnesses. The correct diagnosis requires a through examination.

CHAPTER XXIII

Cancer

CHARLES S. CAMERON, M.D.

C ANCER IN THE PRACTICAL sense is not *a* disease, but rather a large family of diseases having in common the feature of uncontrolled, irregular cell growth, but differing widely in their manifestations, behavior, and response to treatment. This variation in the way cancer expresses itself, especially early in its course, makes its recognition more difficult than is the case with most other diseases. The process of growth is basically one of multiplication of cells—the units of which all living things are composed. Normal, controlled cell division in animal and human life is most active during the period between conception and birth when an entire new organism is being formed. It continues much less rapidly between birth and maturity, after which it slows down to a rate which produces new cells only to replace those which have worn out or have been damaged by disease and injury. For reasons yet unknown, cells occasionally begin to reproduce in the absence of any useful objective; when such purposeless cell division has gone on long enough to produce a mass of cells big enough to be seen or felt, a tumor or new-growth is said to have formed. There are two general kinds of tumor. A *benign* tumor is not very different from the tissue in which it originates and it is clearly separated from the surrounding tissue by a definite capsule. It usually grows slowly and remains in the same area. Such tumors do not endanger life as a rule, they are fairly easily removed and they do not tend to come back. Cancer is a *malignant* tumor. It differs from the tissue of origin in varying degrees. It sends rootlike branches into the normal adjacent structures, recurs unless every minute bit is removed or destroyed, and, sooner or later, tends to send fragments (metastases) off into distant parts of the body establishing new colonies, identical to the original cancer, which continue to grow. Such aggressive behavior obviously does endanger life. Cancers, in turn, fall into two groups, depending on whether they spring from connective tissue like bone and muscle (sarcoma) or from covering and lining tissue like skin and mucous membrane (carcinoma).

DISTRIBUTION

Cancer and related diseases are found throughout the world of living things. Tumorous growths affect plants, and cancer is familiar to all veterinarians. No race of man is free from it, although statistics from many parts of the world show decided differences in cancer death rates. Where high standards of health result in average long life, cancer is frequent, whereas in countries with poor living standards and high general death rates, people usually do not live long enough to get cancer which is mainly a disease of middle life and beyond. This explains in large measure why cancer has increased so strikingly in our own country in recent years; the proportion of older people in our population is steadily growing, and there are now over three times as many persons past the age of forty-five in the United States as there were in 1900. Control of typhoid fever, meningitis, diphtheria, tuberculosis, pneumonia, and other diseases is leaving little from which to die except heart disease and cancer!

CAUSATIVE FACTORS

While the basic cause of cancer remains unknown, a number of influences seem to favor its development. Among them may be mentioned long-continued exposure to strong sunlight, a factor in skin cancer in the light-complexioned. Cancer of the penis is unknown in males circumcised in infancy although it is seen in others. Cancer of the neck of the womb is commoner among women who have borne children and whose tears have gone unrepaired for years. In certain areas of the world absence of iodine in water and soil gives rise to numerous goiters in which cancer develops more often than it does in normal thyroid glands. Overexposure to the rays of radium and X-ray will result in cancer of the skin, as was the case with many doctors who used these agents before effective methods of protection were known. Several industrial operations formerly exposed workers to cancer-causing substances, but now that their danger is known proper safeguards assure adequate protection. There is no disease about which there are more misconceptions. Cancer is not caused by cooking with gas or by the use of aluminum pots. It is not due to white flour, chemical fertilizers, or hard liquor. In short, it is not a disease of civilization except insofar as civilization permits people to live on into ripe years.

DIAGNOSIS

The more advanced cancer is, the easier it is to identify and, conversely, the smaller or earlier it is, the more difficult diagnosis becomes, although that is when it is most important. The onset of cancer is quiet and gradual, in contrast with many diseases which appear suddenly, dramatically, and demand attention—diseases like appendicitis and pneumonia. Cancer, able to appear anywhere in the body, can manifest itself in a great variety of ways, but the commoner first expressions of the more frequent forms of cancer have been summarized as the Seven Danger Signals of cancer, and they have had an important part in alerting the public to the significance of certain signs and symptoms. They are:

1. Any sore that does not heal (cancer of the skin, lip, or mouth).
2. A lump or thickening in the breast or elsewhere.
3. Unusual bleeding or discharge (cancer of the uterus, rectum, lung, etc.).
4. Any change in a wart or mole.
5. Persistent indigestion (stomach) or difficulty in swallowing (esophagus).
6. Persistent hoarseness (larynx) or cough (lung).
7. Any change in normal bowel habits (rectum or intestine).

Doctors of experience can suspect the presence of many cancers early in their course after analysis of the patient's symptoms and can be reasonably certain of the nature of such tumors as can be seen or felt or visualized by X-ray. Nevertheless, the only completely reliable basis for diagnosing cancer is the biopsy—examination under the microscope of a small portion of the tumor. The procedure of removing a specimen of the tumor for such examination is simple when the tumor is easily accessible as in the skin or lip or neck of the womb (cervix). In other areas such as the rectum, more complicated instruments become necessary, and in such sites as the lung and bladder special skill is required to view and biopsy the lesion. Instruments like these make it possible not only to remove a fragment of the tumor, but to inspect its gross features—an important phase of diagnosis. When cancer arises in the breast, biopsy cannot usually be performed short of a surgical operation, and the same may be said of cancers in most internal organs. The presence of many such internal cancers (stomach, intestine, kidney) is established by X-ray examination, as is the case with cancer of the lung and tumors of the bone. Often X-ray appearance of such tumors offers strong evidence of their nature—strong enough to be used as the basis for treatment.

Recently careful study of individual cells from the surface of cancers has led to the diagnostic method known as the "smear test." The method has proven extremely valuable in determining the nature of tumors of the uterus and lung; it has been somewhat less widely used in studying conditions of the prostate, bladder, kidney, stomach, and large intestine. The smear method does not substitute for the biopsy; it does the scouting—turning up important evidence of cancer, but it remains for the biopsy to establish the final proof of it.

The diagnosis of cancer, then, begins in most cases with the patient himself who correctly interprets a danger signal—trivial though it seems—as a reason to see his doctor. There is no other disease which calls on patients themselves for so large a measure of responsibility for the outcome, because it is the patient himself who must be the first to seek diagnosis at a time when treatment can be successful.

TREATMENT

Effective treatment of cancer is of comparatively recent development. Surgery, as we understand it today, goes back only some seventy-five years, and surgical advances continue to be made as safer anesthesia, better drugs to prevent and combat infection, and wider understanding of nutritional needs make it possible to perform more extensive and hence more curative operations. Indeed, cancer patients are being operated on today, with prospects of cure, who ten years ago would have been classed as altogether hopeless and quite beyond the scope of any kind of treatment. Treatment of cancer by X-rays and radium began as recently as 1895, and much of the technical progress in the field of radiation treatment has grown out of research on atomic energy. X-rays generated by five and ten times the electrical power formerly used are now employed in treatment, and the rays from such machines are somewhat more penetrating and therefore more effective in attacking deep-seated cancers. Even stronger are the rays from the atom-smashing betatron. However, it is still too early to say whether such devices will actually cure more cancer.

While surgery, X-rays, and radium (and now radioactive cobalt used like radium) are the only established ways of curing cancer, other methods of treatment have lately come into use. These methods do not cure, but they do make the patient with advanced disease more comfortable and they often prolong life. Radioactive isotopes provide a means of introducing sources of growth-restraining radiations into the body and, to some degree, selectively into the organ in which cancer is growing (the target). Cancers of a few sex-linked organs, notably the prostate and breast, can be partially controlled in many cases by altering the circulating hormone pattern. This is done by castration (removal of ovaries or testicles) or by giving certain hormones derived from male and female sex glands. Chemical compounds which will restrain the growth of certain kinds of malignant tumors are now used (chemotherapy) in treating Hodgkin's disease which involves the lymph glands, and leukemia—the overproduction of white blood cells by the blood-forming tissues. As yet no such drug has been found which will do more than relieve symptoms for varying periods. However, even this can be of worth-while benefit, especially in acute leukemia which mostly affects young children and which up to now has been rapidly fatal. Today selected drugs (including ACTH and cortisone) will restore to apparent health up to two thirds of these young patients—always temporarily, but sometimes for over a year.

When cancer is treated is more important than how it is treated. Certainly there is no disease in which the factor of time is of more importance in determining the outcome. The differences in the results of treating cancer while it is limited to the organ in which it originated compared to the results once it has begun to spread elsewhere prove beyond doubt, that an early treatment of cancer is of the utmost importance.

QUACKS

The treatment of cancer, by whatever method, is always difficult and exacting, calling for the greatest possible experience and skill. Yet there are misguided or unscrupulous persons who belittle the efforts of honest doctors and who claim to have a treatment method far superior to any other. Their methods are usually secret, and the claims made for them are gaudy and assuring—such as no self-respecting doctor would dare to make. These cancer quacks sell their diets, pastes, powders, solutions, herbs, and what not to all comers—the hopelessly advanced patients who are grasping at straws and those with early, curable tumors who are trying to avoid the necessary surgical operation. Patients in the latter group lose whatever chance they had of really being cured when they do business with a quack. It must be remembered that it is as unlikely that a person with little understanding of cancer will discover a reliable treatment for it as it would have been for a plumber to have made the atomic bomb.

EARLY SIGNS AND SYMPTOMS

There can be no argument concerning the importance of the early diagnosis of cancer. And since the responsibility of the public in achieving early diagnosis is so great—a responsibility which cannot be delegated to anyone or any agency—all intelligent persons will accept it as their own by familiarizing themselves with the first signs and symptoms of cancer. Although these initial expressions of cancer are indistinguishable from many less serious, even trivial, conditions, a sensible man or woman will not assume that they are unimportant but will take immediate steps to make certain. The following brief description of cancer of various organs is limited to the commoner types and emphasizes those signs and symptoms which appear early and most frequently.

SKIN

Cancer of the skin is commonest of all but fortunately the most curable. It appears usually in the elderly, and those with light or "sandy" complexions seem to be especially prone to it in contrast to persons who tan readily. Negroes rarely have it. The first evidence of a skin cancer is a dry, scaly patch which persists in spite of the usual home remedy—salve of one sort or other. Such lesions are of slow growth, but they do gradually enlarge and involve deeper layers of the skin. As the growth proceeds the scaly surface grows thicker, forming a crust or scab beneath which the area is now found to be raw and moist—the first evidence of ulceration. As the tumor continues to grow its surface becomes fleshy—an open sore, which sometimes bleeds when irritated. It may project above the level of the skin around it or as is more common it may assume crater-like features, the depressed central ulcer being surrounded by an elevated, pearly rim. Skin cancers are apt to develop in warty brown to black lesions which are so common in aging persons, so that changes in such "senile warts" should receive attention. The exposed parts of the body—the face, neck, forearms, and hands—are the favored sites for cancer of the skin. Any sore which does not show signs of healing in a reasonable time, say three weeks, calls for investigation. The usual skin cancer is readily cured by surgical removal, X-ray, or radium. The small ones can even be treated by dessication—thorough destruction with the electric needle.

One kind of cancer usually originating in the skin, although not always, is the pigmented or black cancer called melanoma. Most of these begin in moles, particularly in dark moles, and there is some evidence that injury or repeated irritation of such moles may play a part in converting them to cancer. Melanoma begins most often as an enlargement of a pre-existing mole, and at the same time its color deepens; the lesion becomes raised, and ulceration with slight bleeding is apt to appear. Removal of pigmented lesions showing signs of such activity is immediately imperative. They should never be cauterized with the electric needle. Melanoma is a relatively rare tumor—a fact of much comfort, since the average person has twenty-one moles! Nevertheless, it is a wise health practice to have moles removed which are located where they are apt to be irritated.

Circumstances favoring the development of cancer of the skin are (1) fair complexion, with skin which sunburns repeatedly rather than tanning; (2) prolonged exposure to strong sunlight, and (3) overexposure to hot, dry wind with its drying effect on normal skin oils. Therefore, the only established preventive measure is avoidance of repeated and long-continued exposure to these influences, especially by those with fair skins. The skin cancers which result from exposure to arsenic, lubricating oils, and other substances involved in specific occupations are of little importance to the average person.

LIP AND MOUTH

The features of skin cancer previously described are often the same for cancer of the lip, which is nearly always on the lower lip. A scaly area appearing whitish in contrast to the vermilion lip surface, and which shows no tendency to heal but rather to enlarge slowly, suggests the possibility of cancer. The crust may grow thicker or may give way to a frank ulcer of varying depth, usually surrounded by a thickened elevated rim. Sometimes, however, as the lesion progresses the growth of cells piles up, layer upon layer, so that a mass of tissue protrudes well above the surface. The latter type is prone to have an irregular, pebbly or granular surface and has therefore been compared to a cauliflower. Cancer of the lip quite often develops in and is preceded by a condition of the membrane of the lip known as leukoplakia, which literally means white plaque. Leukoplakia has the appearance of a thin, white film or sometimes it resembles a bit of wet white tissue paper. It is not cancer—being merely a thickening of the layers of the lip's covering

—but in certain cases it becomes cancerous. Like cancer of the skin, lip cancer is treated by surgical removal or by X-rays or radium. Because it is a frequent forerunner of cancer, leukoplakia should also be treated promptly. Excessive exposure to strong sunlight is the chief causative factor in cancer of the lip, and, therefore, as in the case of the skin, protection of the lip from its direct rays is the sole accepted preventive.

Cancer of the mouth may involve the tongue, gum, floor of the mouth, inner surface of the cheek, or the palate (roof of the mouth). It may take the form of (1) an ulcer or "sore," (2) a raised, irregular, warty area, or (3) a lump or thickening. Such changes are frequently felt first by the tongue and should invite inspection in a mirror. Of course almost everyone has experienced sores in the mouth which after a few days or so disappear of themselves. The clue to the importance of any lesion in the mouth is its persistence beyond two weeks, and any such sore or lump which does not show a tendency to heal within that time should be seen without further delay by a doctor or dentist. Irregularities of the mucous surface of the mouth are sometimes caused by sharp, jagged teeth, especially broken teeth, or by poorly fitting bridges or plates. Although the cause of such lesions may appear clear to the patient, they should not be disregarded, and all such sources of irritation should be corrected. Leukoplakia occurs in the mouth, as on the lip, and it occurs more often in the mouths of heavy smokers. In fact, such white areas used to be called "smoker's patch." Since leukoplakia is so often precancerous, it must be taken seriously and eliminated. Sometimes it is enough to stop smoking, and in other cases vitamin therapy is indicated. But usually surgical treatment by excision or cauterization is necessary.

The factors widely regarded as tending to cause cancer of the mouth are (1) abuse of tobacco, (2) poor mouth hygiene, (3) sharp teeth or improperly fitting dentures, and (4) habitual ingestion of very hot food and liquid. These causes do not have as much proof as they ought to have in order to condemn them fairly, but their correction is so simple as to invite precaution even though proof of their rôle is lacking. Therefore, to reduce the likelihood of mouth cancer, if you must smoke keep it in moderation; keep your mouth clean by following your dentist's advice to brush the teeth twice daily; do not permit broken teeth or chafing dental appliances to go uncorrected; avoid insulting your mouth with food and drink which is too hot.

LARYNX

The cancers discussed so far can be seen and not heard, but the opposite is true for cancer of the voice box. It is not visible (to the patient), it cannot be felt with the tongue or finger, but it does give a sign of its presence which can be heard. That sign is hoarseness. Fortunately, in most cases this warning note is sounded early in the development of the growth. Hoarseness which develops without reasonable cause demands prompt examination of the larynx. Yet delay is the general rule; in fact, the average patient with cancer of the larynx waits three and a half months after hoarseness develops before consulting a doctor. To be sure, hoarseness is a common accompaniment of colds, and it is not unusual for it to hang on for a short time afterward. But any hoarseness—no matter from what apparent cause—which lasts for three weeks is cause for careful medical examination. The high rate of curability of early larynx cancer (nine out of ten cases confined to one chord are cured) makes early diagnosis of unquestioned lifesaving value. There are no generally accepted causes of this form of cancer, although it is claimed by some that it occurs somewhat more frequently among heavy smokers. Again, moderation in smoking appears to be the only available prophylaxis.

ESOPHAGUS

Cancer of the esophagus or gullet is fairly uncommon. The structure of the organ is such that diagnosis early in the disease is achieved all too rarely, and so it is among the more fatal forms of cancer. The chief symptom is difficulty in swallowing. At first this is slight, and food seems to hesitate for a moment on the way down, after which it progresses to the stomach. This sensation that food is sticking occurs in the beginning with bulky, dry foods such as bread and certain meats. Later the passage of all solid foods becomes delayed and eventually even liquids. Spasm of the irritated esophagus and actual obstruction by tumor are responsible for these signs. Treatment is by surgical removal in favorable cases and by deep X-ray treatment when the growth is more advanced. Recently X-rays generated at high voltage and the high energy particles emanating from the betatron have shown somewhat greater restraint of cancer of the esophagus and other deep-lying tumors, but it does not yet appear that actual cures can be obtained with them. There are no known causes of this variety of cancer which operate generally, although the somewhat higher than average rate in northern Scandinavian countries has been attributed to a diet deficient in vitamin B. This complex of vitamins appears necessary to maintain mucous membranes in a healthy condition, and when it is restricted or absent from the diet generative changes (including leukoplakia) may occur in these tissues.

STOMACH

Cancer of the stomach is, or was until recently, responsible for more deaths than any other form of cancer, one in every eight cancer deaths being charged to it. Two facts account for this high mortality—its frequency and the relatively small number of cases operated on in time to permit removal of all the disease. The delay before the diagnosis is made is appalling. Of all patients who develop cancer of the stomach, fewer than half are found to be suitable for operation—they are clearly too late. Of those who are operated on, fewer than half are found to have disease which can be removed. These are the patients of whom it is said, "They opened him and closed him right away."

Again, too late. Of the remaining few who have a chance and on whom a complete operation can be done, a few more will die before leaving the hospital. Finally a small group who could be operated on, whose tumors could be removed, and who survived the surgical procedure, are left. But they are not yet all cured, for within five years well over half of them will succumb to recurring cancer—to the hidden remnants of disease which eluded removal. All this adds up to the forlorn fact that of all patients who get cancer of the stomach, not more than 5 or 6 per cent are living free of the disease five years later. But this gloomy picture is not without its hopeful aspect, for much of the high mortality is due to the fact that these cancers are not usually diagnosed until late in their course, and some of this delay, perhaps a very important—even critical—part of it, should be susceptible of substantial reduction. The silent interval of cancer of the stomach—the period from its actual beginning to the appearance of signs and symptoms—may be as long as twenty months. Barring the discovery of a reliable, simple, and cheap diagnostic test, it does not seem likely that this portion of the delay period can be influenced. But after the development of digestive complaints, the average patient with cancer of the stomach waits another eight months before deciding to consult a doctor. This eight months, over which the patient and the patient alone has control, must be relied on for reducing the fateful interval between onset and treatment.

The bright side of the coin is that when cancer of the stomach is treated while the disease involves the stomach only (before lymph node spread has occurred), five-year cures in over 50 per cent are to be expected, and one large clinic has recently reported 64 per cent of such patients alive and well five years after operation. This is a heartening figure, especially when it is compared to the five-year results among the patients whose primary cancers were removed but where lymph node spread was present—only 12 per cent of whom lived beyond the five-year mark, and among the entire stomach cancer group, of which not more than one in twenty are living and well five years after they are stricken.

The opportunity to relieve this situation lies in the greatest possible reduction of the delay interval following the onset of stomach symptoms. Undoubtedly many lives could be saved if the average waiting time were to be cut to three or four weeks instead of the present seven or eight months. It is not easy to spot the symptoms of early cancer of the stomach because most of us have some mild stomach complaints from time to time and have come to accept them as the consequences of "something that didn't agree with me," or too much drinking, too much smoking, or overwork and what not. And most times we have been right. One has only to listen to the radio for a few hours or read a single magazine or newspaper to realize that "acid indigestion," "sour stomach," "heartburn," and "dyspepsia" must be widespread indeed to call for such numerous remedies as are advertised so intensively. So they are! The danger lies right here: the symptoms of simple indigestion or dyspepsia are no different from the early symptoms of cancer of the stomach. Perhaps the single term most expressive of the complaints of patients with stomach cancer is indigestion. True, this covers a multitude of conditions, and it is not a precise word—meaning different things to different people. On the other hand, its general coverage makes it useful to the public in describing the varied and subtle details of symptoms which may arise in the abdomen. "Indigestion," then, may be another way of describing (1) a vague sense of unease referable to the stomach, (2) a feeling of fullness or bloating, (3) mild nausea, (4) heartburn, (5) lessening of the normal healthy appetite, which often appears first as quick satiation—the feeling that one has eaten all he can after a few mouthfuls of food, (6) eructation of food, (7) excessive belching, and (8) pain. At the onset these symptoms are vague and they may be inconstant, coming and going with or without the usual medicine-cabinet remedies. How long then can one safely temporize? If a man or woman over forty years of age who has not had previous more or less chronic stomach trouble develops indigestion which lasts for two weeks, the possibility of serious organic disease is to be thought of, and even though such complaints will prove in most cases to have been due to something other than cancer, the wise man or woman will let the doctor determine the cause of the trouble.

There is another expression of cancer of the stomach which occurs often enough to be worth remembering. Shortness of breath from mild exertion, and fatigue from activity which formerly caused no tiring may be the first signs of this disease. They result from anemia which follows repeated small amounts of bleeding from the ulcerated portion of the stomach, and sometimes the quantity of blood lost is sufficient to produce obvious paleness. With older people who have had ulcers and "nervous stomachs" for years, the recognition of indigestion due to cancer is confused by the merging of their old complaints with the new. Of course, if chronic stomach symptoms change their character, become more intense or more frequent, suspicion should be aroused, but such changes are apt to be so gradual that a clear transition is rarely recognized.

Perhaps the best course for those past middle life with chronic stomach trouble and without it is to give the doctor a chance twice a year to re-evaluate the status of the digestive system. Let him be the judge of what tests if any need to be done. Let him share with you the responsibility of finding cancer early—which is another way of saying let him help you to live long and stay well.

INTESTINES

Cancer occurs less often in the small intestine than in the large, and when it affects the small bowel, its symptoms or warning signs are less definite and hence more difficult to interpret than is the case with tumors in the colon (large intestine). For this reason cancer of the small intestine has a less favorable outcome than that of the colon.

One of the earlier symptoms common to both is increased intestinal gas, that is, more than is usual, considering individual variations. Gas may be formed in such quantities as to cause discomfort varying from mild uneasiness to frank cramps. The content of the small bowel is liquid, so tumors here do not produce the signs of obstruction until they have almost closed off the intestinal passage. As greater obstruction is caused by the growing tumor, the symptoms of crampy pain often relieved by the passage of gas, and a change of bowel habits expressed by increasing constipation or diarrhea, become more insistent. Surgical removal of the tumor-bearing portion of the intestine is the one treatment, and when the growth is confined to the bowel the results are good.

The content of the large intestine is solid as compared to that of the small, and it becomes progressively more solid as it passes from the cecum at the beginning of the colon through the large bowel to the rectum. The solider the fecal mass is, the less obstruction is required to interfere with it and thereby produce symptoms. Therefore, as a general rule, the closer to the rectum a tumor of the colon is, the earlier symptoms will be produced and, theoretically at least, the more favorable the prospect for treatment in time. Cancers of the large intestine are associated usually with unusual quantities of gas, with varying degrees of abdominal discomfort or outright pain—usually not steady but appearing at first quite irregularly, later becoming more frequent and assuming the rhythm of cramps. This variety of cancer is apt to ulcerate early so that bleeding occurs in small amounts. This bleeding may be too slight to appear as blood in the stool (although chemical tests will reveal it) yet, continued week in and week out, it is often enough to cause a significant degree of anemia. The patient may look pale in the more severe cases; he may complain of fatigue, shortness of breath, or weakness; and in each case the blood count will confirm the existence of anemia. So consistently is anemia a feature of cancer of the colon that every patient having anemia without obvious cause should have careful X-ray studies of the intestine. When bleeding is sufficient to appear in the stool, the location of the tumor will determine how it appears. If the tumor is in the first portion of the colon —the part farthest from the rectum—the blood will be dark and will have become thoroughly mixed with the feces so that the stool will appear dark. The nearer the tumor is to the rectum or anus, the brighter the blood will be, and the more it will be separated from the stool itself, so that bleeding from cancer of the rectum located within six or eight inches of the anal opening will present as frank blood as seen in the toilet or on the tissue. A change in the bowel habits is apt to occur. Constipation, not previously troublesome, may develop; yet because of the irritation of the tumor and the production of larger quantities of mucus, diarrhea is also common; and often the two alternate.

Summarizing, the important early signs of cancer of the rectum and large intestine are (1) bleeding, seen in the stool or causing anemia or both, (2) a persistent change in the usual bowel habits—diarrhea or constipation or both, and (3) increased intestinal gas causing varying degrees of abdominal discomfort.

Surgical removal of the segment of the intestine involved by the cancer gives excellent results when the tumor is discovered and treated while it is confined to the bowel wall. Indeed, cures in 75 per cent of patients with cancer of the rectum treated while the disease was limited to the mucous lining have been reported.

With a single exception, causes of cancer of the rectum and large intestine have not been recognized. This exception is a precancerous condition known as polyposis, and it consists of the presence of small benign tumors called polyps which arise in and hang from the lining of the intestine or rectum. They may be solitary, but more often there are more than one, and occasionally there are many scattered along the length of the large bowel. Although not cancer, these polyps tend to become malignant as time goes on, and for this reason their removal or destruction is of great importance. Intestinal polyps tend to run in families; therefore it is a wise precaution for anyone who has had a parent or grandparent affected by cancer of the rectum or colon to seek a careful examination of his lower intestinal tract, including studies by X-ray.

BREAST

This is the cancer most feared by women, and for good reason, as it is the commonest major form of cancer among them. It is most likely to occur after the age of forty-five or fifty, although, as cancers go, it is not rare in the thirties. The first evidence of breast cancer is a lump in the breast, and this lump is usually painless. It may be present in any part of the breast, but the upper outer quarter is favored. As the mass of cancer grows larger, other signs appear. There may appear a suggestion of flattening of the normal convexity of the breast outline which later comes to look like obvious dimpling. The nipple may sink downward or "retract," and in time come to lie entirely beneath the adjacent skin level. Or, as the result of the pull exerted on the nipple by the tumor, the nipple may change its axis by tilting in the direction of the tumor. Later a portion of the skin covering the breast or much of it may grow tense, with the pores becoming prominent so that it resembles the skin of an orange. As the tumor grows to occupy more space, the breast may become larger, as would seem natural, but just as often it appears to shrivel, a paradox caused by the replacement of normally elastic tissue by the dense, hard tissue of cancer. Bleeding or other discharge from the nipple occurs when cancer develops in the larger ducts of the breast close to the nipple, but such abnormal nipple discharge is more often due to a benign tumor in a duct. But there is no way to know which it is—benign or malignant—short of surgical exploration, which is why operation is urged in all instances of bleeding nipple. Of course, benign tumors of the breast, which are very frequent, also present themselves as lumps so that the mere fact of a breast mass does not always mean cancer, and in women under fifty it usually does not. Again, examination by an experienced doctor will suggest the nature of the mass as a rule; but doctors with the greatest experience with breast tumors are the most ardent advocates of surgical removal of all true tumors arising therein, for microscopic examination is after all the most dependable and accurate of all diagnostic methods.

When the complete operation of removal is performed at a time when cancer is confined to the breast, the likelihood of cure is 80 to 90 per cent. When cancer has spread to the lymph glands in the armpit, as it is apt to do, there is still a worthwhile chance for cure, but it has dropped to 30 per cent or so. The administration of deep X-rays following surgery for breast cancer is widely employed in select cases.

The causes of breast cancer are unknown. A number of observers have recorded a lower rate of breast cancer among women who have borne children than those who have not, and a lower rate among women who have breast-fed their children than among those who have not. If any conclusion at all is justified on the basis of this evidence, it would be that the use of the breasts in fulfilment of their essential purpose is better than interruption of their normal function. The answer to the problem of breast cancer is to find and treat it before it has metastasized. This is not always possible, because some tumors spread to other parts of the body before they have grown large enough to be discovered. But the principle of "the earlier, the better" should nevertheless guide our approach to all cancer control, including the control of cancer of the breast.

Consider the fact that the average woman with this disease first consults a doctor at a time when the tumor measures roughly two inches across—about the size of a golf ball. This is a good-sized mass, and the question immediately arises, "Why do they wait so long?" The fact is that many of these women do not wait; rather, their oft-repeated story is, "I found this lump a few nights ago," and they usually add, "while I was taking a bath." In other words, they found the lump *accidentally*. Recently a number of doctors have wondered whether such women could not have found a lump many months before it grew to the size of a golf ball—when it would have been smaller, to be sure—if they had taken the trouble to deliberately feel for one. The answer is clearly yes. Experience has shown women can feel breast tumors as small as half an inch in diameter—indeed, can discover lumps so small that the doctor himself has difficulty identifying them. Six to twelve months are required for a breast cancer to grow from a size which can just be found to the size usually encountered at the time of surgery. Precious, wasted months—months of delay which could have been avoided! This delay can be avoided by any woman intelligent enough to adopt the practice of regularly methodically examining her own breasts once a month. The day following the end of each menstrual period should be checked as the proper time to perform the examination, but as the danger of breast cancer does not cease with the change of life, the practice should be continued on a monthly basis throughout life. An instructive film illustrating the proper technique of self-examination has been produced by the American Cancer Society and the National Cancer Institute and shown widely to audiences of women throughout the country. The essential steps in the examination, which need take no more than five minutes, are illustrated in Plates XXV-XXVI.

Any sensible woman, examining her own breasts regularly, will become thoroughly familiar with their structural features, and she can be relied on to recognize even very slight departures from this normal structure. Any such development must be brought to her doctor's attention at once. As has been said, not all breast cancers can be cured—even with early treatment—but it is possible that the general recognition of them while they are still very small would double the number of cures now being achieved. Everyone agrees to the value of brushing the teeth daily—and everyone does it. Yet judged by the standard of its lifesaving potential, monthly self-examination of the breasts is vastly more important.

UTERUS

Cancer of the womb is only slightly less frequent than cancer of the breast, and each year some 45,000 women develop it. It occurs about eight times more often in the cervix or neck of the womb than it does in the cavity or body of the uterus. In either case its cardinal warning sign is irregular bleeding from the vagina. When such abnormal bleeding appears during the active menstrual life, it may take the form of bleeding between the regular menstruations, or it may present as excessively heavy or prolonged monthly flow. Such irregularities are too often attributed to some minor cause—to a "cold" or irritation or to the beginning of the "change." When vaginal bleeding occurs after the change of life, its wholly unexpected appearance leaves little of excuse for failing to interpret it as an event calling for prompt investigation, for cancer is the most important, probably the most frequent, cause of bleeding at such a time. And yet even here mistakes are made; too many women are prone to interpret the unexpected flow as a "return of the monthly," and even to welcome it as an indication that they are not as old as they thought they were. It is during the menopause when bleeding is not according to schedule that the greatest confusion arises, and it may be difficult indeed to distinguish correctly the abnormal irregularity of bleeding due to a tumor from the normal irregularity attributable to the change of life.

While irregular bleeding is the foremost warning sign of uterine cancer, such bleeding need not consist of dark or bright red blood, though it often does. A vaginal discharge which develops in a woman of any age may be present in cancer, especially of the body of the womb, so that the cause of all discharges should be carefully sought. Vaginal discharge, while not uncommon and often due to benign conditions, is nevertheless always abnormal, and its cause should be determined and corrected. But when cancer is present in the uterus, the discharge is tinged with blood as a rule, and its color may vary from the faintest pink to the deep red of frank blood. Fortunately, women have the advantage of a method of protection against illness and death from cancer of the womb; the core of the control of this widespread disease lies in persuading *all* women to accept this protection. It consists of a thorough pelvic examination performed twice a year, even though there are no signs or complaints referable to the pelvis. It is not necessary for women to wait for abnormal bleeding to mark the presence of cancer—because such cancers can be found by meticulous search before they give rise to any signs whatever. In fact, it is now possible to identify cancer of the cervix before it can be seen by the eye of the examining doctor.

A pelvic examination is not difficult for the physician or unpleasant for the patient and takes but a few minutes to carry out. In the course of it the doctor will inspect all of the generative organs which can be seen—the vulva, the vaginal tube, and, most important, the cervix, that portion of the uterus which projects into the upper vagina. He will then examine the cervix with his fingers, and with his hands the pelvic organs which cannot be viewed—the body of the uterus, the ovaries, the tubes, and the adjacent supporting structures. He will possibly include a vaginal smear in his survey—a relatively new development which holds much promise for earlier diagnosis of malignant tumors of the uterus. By withdrawing a little secretion from the upper vagina and from the opening of the cervix and by staining the cells with special dyes, the nature of the cells present in the smear can be determined with a high degree of accuracy. Specifically, when cancer is present in the cervix, cancer cells can usually be seen in the smear; the reliability of the smear in cancer of the body of the uterus is slightly less than in cervix cancer. Of course, there is little difficulty in spotting cancer of the cervix when it is large enough to be seen and felt—that is, when it has been present long enough to be unmistakable. But when this stage is reached the outlook is often less favorable. The exciting feature of the smear method is that it can reveal or strongly suggest the presence of cancers so small that they cannot readily be seen or felt; and of course such cancers are early and highly curable. Smears are also of great value in identifying cancer in a cervix which is already so distorted by co-existing benign disease—tears, infection, and inflammation—that the malignant process is obscured.

The woman who is wise enough to play it safe, then, will do more than be alert for the danger signal of cancer of the uterus—abnormal bleeding or discharge; she will act before such signals have a chance to appear, by insisting upon a careful examination of her pelvis twice a year—no matter how strong and healthy she appears to be. The wisdom of this is obvious from a comparison of the curability of cancer of the uterus in very early, moderately advanced, and late stages of disease. Treatment of very early cancer of the uterus will cure 75 per cent or more. About 40 per cent of the moderately advanced cases, which is the condition in which most women with the disease are first seen by the doctor, can be cured. And of the late and extensive cases, fewer than 10 per cent can be saved. If you have to have cancer of the cervix (and don't say it can't happen to you), which group do you chose to be in? The choice is yours—and wholly yours.

Cancer of the cervix seems to be more frequent among women who have borne children than among those who have not, and one explanation for this is that childbearing often causes tears or lacerations which if unrepaired result in chronic inflammatory conditions which the doctors call cervicitis. Inflammation and chronic infections of this organ can and often do have other causes, but the cause is beside the point, which is that all such abnormal conditions can be eliminated; and since they appear to favor the development of cancer, they should be.

LUNG

Cancer of the lung is rapidly becoming one of the commonest types of malignant tumor. Fifty years ago it was almost unheard of; twenty years ago it was rare; but today it is second only to the stomach as a cause of death from cancer, and a few observers believe that it may now be the most frequent of all the major forms of cancer. No other kind of cancer has shown so striking an increase.

Lung cancer is chiefly a disease of the male sex, twenty men being affected for every woman. The most constant first symptom is cough. As is the case of other signs and symptoms which have been noted, correct interpretation of cough is made difficult by the fact that so many people have coughs more or less continuously. Chronic bronchitis, sinus trouble, the widespread "cold" with a cough that hangs on for weeks or months, and the "cigarette cough" are so familiar in most temperate climates that the cough, like the cry of "wolf" sounded too often, excites nobody. The fact remains that cough is one of the first expressions of lung cancer, and so it deserves more respect than it gets. A cough of long standing, even if it can be proved to be due to causes other than cancer or tuberculosis, deserves respect for another reason. The usual chronic cough which is not caused by a tumor is usually the result of inflamed, irritated, perhaps infected membranes of the bronchial tubes. Possibly this state of irritation is a predisposing factor in the origin of cancer, and therefore should be eliminated always. Besides, a cough is a personal inconvenience and a social nuisance. But since coughs are such frequent aftermaths of the simple cold, when does one make the decision that the time has come to make certain that it is not due to a more serious condition? The safest rule is to investigate the source of any cough—no matter how logically it can be explained on a trivial basis—which persists undiminished for *three* weeks. This rule holds for the cough that hangs on following a chest cold, and for the cough of chronic bronchitis which has been present for years (because a diagnosis of chronic bronchitis or anything else does not confer immunity from cancer).

The cough of lung cancer sooner or later becomes productive of phlegm or sputum, the character of which is extremely varied. It may be frothy and color-less or thick and containing pus, and so there are no features of the expectoration which can be said to be typical of cancer, with the single exception of blood. Blood in the sputum, even in very small amounts—as fine streaks, for instance—can never be regarded lightly, and its appearance, even once, should always be reported to a physician. Another sign which presents fairly often in lung cancer and at a relatively early stage is a faint wheezing sound which accompanies breathing. It is not necessarily constant. The patient himself is usually the first to notice this faint sound and he may do so only when he is quiet and undistracted by other sounds. Somewhat later in the course of the disease chest pain appears. If infection develops in the tumor or in the portion of the lung being interfered with by the tumor, fever and night sweats occur. Loss of weight and weakness are present eventually.

But as has proved true for some other forms of cancer previously discussed, the "early" signs or symptoms of lung cancer are not necessarily early in the tumor's growth and course. This explains in part why the curative operation of pneumonectomy, surgical removal of the infected lung, can be undertaken in less than a fourth of the entire lung cancer group; the disease is too far advanced in the rest. But there is a simple, inexpensive, painless, and reliable "test" which will reveal the presence of tumors of the lung *before* they are large enough to produce cough or other symptoms. This test consists of an X-ray picture of the chest. Such films can disclose small and unsuspected tumors both benign and cancerous in the lungs of presumably perfectly healthy persons, as the recent experiences with large-scale chest X-ray surveys have shown. And the early returns on patients whose lung cancers have been found through routine chest X-rays—persons, remember, who seem to be in good health and without any complaints—suggest that the treatment at such a stage of disease will cure as high as 75 per cent—or more than three times as many as can be cured once the symptoms have developed. This immensely important fact is all the proof that any sane man or woman should need as to the value of the routine chest X-ray twice a year beyond the age of fifty. (Lung cancer is extremely rare before then.) The first human being ever operated on successfully for cancer of the lung is living and carrying on an active medical practice nineteen years later, and since that historic operation was performed this has been a potentially curable disease. But only a fraction of this potential has been achieved up to now—and the reason is again—too late. The little time and cost of a chest film is a small premium indeed to pay for so large a measure of protection against needless, avoidable death.

Much has been heard in late years of virus pneumonia. It so happens that it seems to occur with surprising frequency in patients with cancer of the lung—and early in the course of the cancer at that. It is not uncommon for X-rays, taken in order to diagnose an acute infection of the lung—virus pneumonia, for example—to disclose an unsuspected lung cancer. But sometimes the area of pneumonia overlies or surrounds the cancer so as to hide it in the X-ray picture; therefore, it is highly important that X-rays of the chest be taken several weeks after recovery from virus pneumonia in order to be perfectly sure that evidence of infection as disclosed in the X-ray has disappeared as it should, and that no lurking cancer continues to cast its shadow.

A great many theories have been advanced to explain the remarkable increase in lung cancer in recent years. One which has received widest attention, especially in the past two or three years, is smoking. It is pointed out that the vast increase in cigarette consumption in our country parallels the increase in cancer of the lung. Several statistical studies have purported to show that heavy cigarette smoking is recorded in the histories of men with lung cancer more often than in the histories of control subjects of similar age but without lung cancer. More intensive investigation of this possibility is now under way. Until the question of smoking and cancer of the lung is answered, it would be best for all men and women to smoke in moderation, if they must smoke at all.

Inhalation of certain dusts or fumes generated in particular industrial operations is a proven hazard in respect of lung cancer causation, and other dusts and fumes are suspected. The fumes from anthracene oil, chromates, and nickel carbonyl are factors in cancer of the lung. However, most occupational dangers are recognized, and workers are protected by proper hygienic regulations.

BLADDER

Cancer of the bladder is given special mention here, not because it is especially frequent but because of the universal neglect of its early warning signs, which is largely responsible for the present poor results of treatment. Blood in the urine is the most important—in fact, the only—early signal of bladder cancer. It may first appear in several successive urinations, or it may appear but once. Usually there is a somewhat extended interval, amounting to weeks or months before it is seen again. During this period of freedom from bleeding, the alarm with which the patient reacted to the first shocking appearance of blood in his urine gives way to hopefulness that it won't happen again and, as time goes on, to varying degrees of assurance that it will not, but, soon or late —there it is again! The average patient—it is more often a man—delays six and one half months after he first passes bloody urine before telling his doctor about it. Blood in the urine does not always mean cancer, but cancer is the most important thing it can mean, and immediate investigation of the genital and urinary organs is called for. A single episode of bloody urine is enough to not wait for a second.

TESTICLE

Tumors of the testicle are rather rare—yet because they occur almost exclusively in young men in their twenties, with life before them, they are especially important to recognize. A life saved at this age means many more years of living than a life saved at fifty or sixty. There are but two signs calling attention to growths in the testicle: one is enlargement, so that one testis looks and feels bigger than its mate; the second is increase in density, so that the testicle in which the tumor is present feels heavier than its mate and this heaviness may be noted by the patient as a "dragging sensation." Most varieties of testicular tumors spread quickly, making the earliest possible treatment essential.

PROSTATE

Cancer of the prostate is probably the commonest cancer affecting men. It does not appear as the first cause of male cancer deaths simply because in many cases it is not diagnosed. This is understandable when it is realized that quite often the disease runs a slow, chronic course, and even when present may not be the primary cause of death and may not even give rise to symptoms. Yet prostatic cancer is responsible for some 10 per cent of cancer deaths in men, being third among the causes of such deaths. Cancer of the prostate may produce two quite different kinds of first symptoms. One kind, due to the enlargement of the prostate itself, consists of urinary difficulty of one sort or another. The other is pain in other parts of the body, for instance in the lower spine, resulting from spread of the disease to the bones of the skeleton. Thus symptoms may be local or general and, of course, both may be present together. The local symptoms—difficulty in urinating—often begin as a narrowing of the stream and a lessening of its force. Dribbling after urination becomes annoying. Later, as the prostate grows larger, it is necessary to force the urine out by contracting the abdominal muscles. Eventually complete obstruction may occur. If the tumor grows into the urinary passage or the base of the bladder, blood may appear in the urine. These signs are not necessarily proof of prostatic cancer, for they can also be caused by benign enlargement of that organ, termed hypertrophy, which is so common in elderly males. However, the possibility of cancer is so strong that immediate medical consultation should be sought at the first evidence of urinary irregularity. Certain cancers of the prostate remain relatively small within the prostate itself even while spreading by metastasis to other parts of the body—the bones usually. This explains why a man with no significant urinary symptoms may develop pains in the back or hip or neck and be found to have deposits of tumors scattered through the bones, as shown in X-ray pictures. As with all other kinds of cancer, cure is possible only when the disease is found to be localized, although, as will be seen, remarkable restraint of the growth, amounting sometimes to control, can often be achieved.

There is one way to discover cancer of the prostate at a time when it is localized and can be entirely removed; it is the periodic, twice yearly examination of the prostate of every man over fifty. This is a simple doctor's office procedure consisting of carefully feeling the prostate through the rectum. Actually examination of the rectum and prostate is performed at one and the same time. Even very small prostatic tumors can be felt in this way—still too small to cause any symptoms. The discovery of prostate cancer before it produces symptoms gives the patient an excellent chance of cure, and in view of the prevalence of this disease, no intelligent man can fail to concede the value of this form of life assurance—the regular examination of his supposedly normal prostate. Although surgical removal of the prostate while the disease is contained in that structure is the only means of effecting a cure, within the past few years it has become possible to greatly prolong the lives and relieve the discomfort of patients with widespread metastatic prostate cancer, and in some cases this growth restraint has amounted to a long-lasting arrest of the disease. This effect is achieved by castration or by the administration of female sex hormones or by both. Treated in this fashion, men with cancer of the prostate who a few years ago could expect to live no more than a year or a year and a half can now look forward to living twice that long, and, most important of all, in comparative comfort.

BONE

Malignant tumors of bone (bone sarcoma) are rather rare, but like tumors of the testicle their tendency to occur in young people from five to twenty years old makes them important. When the tumor arising in a bone grows large enough, it will appear as a swelling. Many bone tumors, especially malignant ones, are apt to develop at the ends of bones, near joints, and because of this motion of the joint may be interfered with fairly early—to a degree which causes slight disability or discomfort. Thus a tumor growing near the knee or hip may have the effect of limiting the normal movement of the adjacent joints so that a slight limp may be produced. Malignant tumors of bone constitute a notable exception to the generality that pain is not an early symptom of cancer. Pain is apt to occur early in bone sarcoma, and it tends to occur at night or to be worse at night. Swelling, mild dysfunction, and pain, then, are the signs of importance in bone tumors.

LYMPHOMAS

A large class of malignant tumorlike diseases differs from those which have been presented thus far in that they do not usually arise in one organ or site, but rather in entire systems or widely scattered parts of systems. Leukemia is a good example of diseases of this type, arising as it does in the blood-forming tissues of the body, notably the bone marrow, the spleen, and the lymph glands. Hodgkin's disease is another, originating in deposits of lymphoid tissue —the lymph glands. The lymphatic apparatus is also involved in lymphosarcoma, another of the generalized malignant tumors. The unique feature of diseases of this class is that they tend to be systematized or generalized from the beginning. There are exceptions to this, for occasionally lymphosarcoma appears as a localized lesion and has been treated successfully under such circumstances. However, Hodgkin's disease and usually lymphosarcoma are prone to involve multiple areas, with the lymph glands of the neck, armpit, groin, abdomen, and mid-chest (mediastinum) as the usual sites. At first the disease may seem to be restricted to the nodes of a single area, and thus be localized to some extent. The first evidence of either of these disorders is an enlarged or swollen lymph gland or several such. These initially large nodes are seen more often in the neck than anywhere else. Lymph node enlargement without obvious infection to account for it should be laid before the doctor, who may decide after reviewing all the evidence to remove the node in question in order to be certain of its nature.

Doctors of a few generations ago had a striking term for leukemia—"flowing cancer." It is thought of as a kind of cancer of the blood, and is fully discussed with blood diseases. While a tumor in the usual sense is not present, still the overproduction of white blood cells is a growth irregularity which is fundamentally similar to the cellular processes of cancer. In the case of leukemia the white cells are released into the volume of circulating blood. The number of white cells is sometimes very high (300,000 per cubic millimeter as compared with the normal 8,000), but sometimes the number is only moderately increased and occasionally it may be below normal. The age of the white blood cells, that is, their degree of maturity, is a more reliable basis for diagnosing and following the progress of leukemia than the actual number of blood cells. Leukemia may make itself known in a number of ways. The spleen or lymph nodes may enlarge and first call attention to illness. There may be an increased tendency to bleed, with troublesome oozing from gums or spontaneous small hemorrhages into the skin showing as small, perfectly flat, circular, rose-purple areas. A number of cases are diagnosed in consequence of persistent bleeding following the extraction of a tooth. Leukemia is usually associated with some degree of anemia; hence there may be pallor, fatigue, and shortness of breath. Most often the earliest symptoms are extremely vague, and patients will complain of little except not feeling up to par. Leukemia may be acute—running through its natural untreated course in a matter of weeks—or chronic, lasting for several years and showing alternating periods of activity and remission, the latter induced by treatment, or now and then occurring spontaneously. Patients with chronic leukemia can be kept quite comfortable and active, their lives perhaps prolonged, through judicious use of X-ray treatment and more recently, in selected cases, radioactive isotopes and a few chemical agents such as the nitrogen mustard compounds. Until three years ago there was no treatment which had any effect on acute leukemia, but through the administration of ACTH or cortisone and certain newly discovered chemical compounds called folic acid antagonists, it is now possible to induce significant regression of disease in up to two thirds of the young patients. (Acute leukemia is almost wholly a disease of children.) Hodgkin's disease and lymphosarcoma are usually managed for several years by carefully applied X-rays—and in later stages certain new drugs (nitrogen mustard compounds, triethylenemelamine, and others) prove useful in maintaining the patient in comfort.

CHILDHOOD

Cancer in children is rare, and yet it is an important cause of death in childhood, certainly more important than many of the usual childhood diseases. In fact, cancer causes more deaths between the ages of five and fourteen than any other disease. (Accidents lead the mortality table in this age group—accounting for one third of all deaths at this period of life.)

Cancers of all types occur in children, but sarcomas far outnumber carcinomas. Certain malignant tumors appear almost exclusively before the age of ten. In rare instances babies have been born with cancer. The organs and systems which are the usual sites of malignant tumors appearing in children are the eye; kidney; bones; lymph nodes; throat; nerve structures, including the brain, and soft peripheral parts such as muscle. All that has been said about the tendency of early cancer to imitate or resemble many benign and trivial conditions applies even more to young children, because the confusion is confounded by their inability to express themselves fully.

The commoner signs of the commoner malignant tumors of childhood are (1) a gray, greenish, or milky-white glint seen in the eye—in the presence of a tumor arising in the nerves of the posterior portion of the eye, (2) swelling seen or felt in the abdomen caused by tumor of the kidney or of the nerve tissues in the region of the kidney, (3) pain in an extremity worse at night, with or without associated swelling—suggesting bone tumor, (4) enlargement of the glands or bleeding tendencies, with or without small rose or violet discolorations in the skin, indicating the possibility of Hodgkin's disease, lymphosarcoma, or leukemia, (5) difficulty in swallowing or in breathing (causing audible breath sounds), pointing to tumors of the throat or chest, (6) persistent cough which steadily gets worse, caused by tumors within the chest, (7) stomach and intestinal symptoms not accounted for by infection or by inflammation within the alimentary tract, due to tumors of the nervous system (brain and sympathetic nerve structures), (8) continuing unexplained fever, (9) tiredness, lack of interest, decrease of appetite and loss of weight which persist beyond a reasonable period, say a week or ten days. The kinds of cancer which typically affect children seem to show unusually rapid growth. In general, treatment of them is not nearly so successful as the treatment of cancer in adults. Early recognition of the real causes of the complaints and abnormal signs in young patients offers the only hope of improving the results. It should be observed once more that cancer is rare in children, and no parent is justified in worrying about it nor in being oversolicitous in trying to interpret the early evidences of the usual childhood ills which can be quite perplexing. A reasonable rule would be to rely on the *duration* of any departure from normal. Because the great majority of children's affections are acute, developing quickly, running a relatively rapid course, and subsiding quickly, any mild evidence of illness or abnormality which lasts beyond ten days—even though it does not appear serious—should be presented to the doctor.

Many kinds of cancer have been omitted from this discussion. Most of the growths which have not been described are rare. Finally, for most of the tumors omitted, the factor of early diagnosis appears to be of less critical importance in determining the outcome than is the case for most of those which have been described. As examples of the tumors in this category, the following may be cited: (1) Tumors of the brain and spinal cord, whose signs—extremely diverse, depending upon the location of the lesion—include disturbances of sight (such as double vision), loss of balance, weakness, and paralysis of certain muscle groups and tremors. (2) Malignant tumors of muscles, tendons and the like, called soft part sarcomas. Here the sole sign which could possibly be of assistance in speeding the patient toward diagnosis is a swelling—that is the presence of a tumor mass. (3) Cancers arising in organs which are not removable or removable with great risk, such as the liver and pancreas. (4) Miscellaneous cancers such as those of the thyroid gland (a solitary lump in the neck or a goiter-like swelling), kidney, ovary, and so on.

RESEARCH

Many people believe that not very much is known about cancer and that not much progress is being made toward discovering its causes. On the contrary, probably more facts are known about cancer than about any other disease, although still not enough to provide effective means of control. Almost all that is known has come in the past fifty years, and still more encouraging is the fact that cancer research is now expanding rapidly—indeed, on the basis of cost, it has increased twelvefold in the past ten years and now amounts to about fifteen million dollars annually in the United States alone.

Research has disclosed evidence that for certain cancer in animals heredity is a factor. It has been possible by selective breeding to "bring out" cancer susceptibility in mice, for instance, so that almost every female will develop it, and conversely, the cancer tendency can be overcome by breeding so that resistant strains are established in which it never appears. Since heredity appears to be governed by the structure called genes, found in the nucleus of cells, much research attention is now directed at the gene and how it works. But the tendency to cancer in mice is evidently not wholly dependent on genes, because it has recently been shown that if the newborn offspring of cancer-susceptible parents are prevented from nursing at their own mother's breast and placed instead with foster nurses of a cancer-resistant breed, they will not get breast cancer as expected. Evidently breast milk is also a factor, and later studies suggest that it contains a virus which may be the cancer inciter. There is no clear evidence that such a factor influences human breast cancer, nor for any other kind of human cancer, although viruses are responsible for four kinds of cancer occurring in the rabbit, frog, and mouse. Genetic influences may also be modified by removing the ovaries of infant females of cancer-susceptible breeds; and cancer can be made to develop in the offspring of resistant strains by giving them large doses of female sex hormones. As noted previously, the course of cancer originating in certain organs controlled by sex hormones, as the prostate and breast, can usually be modified by altering the hormone pattern. This is done by castration and administering the proper hormone. The importance of hormones in cancer is also shown in the recent discovery that the make-up of hormones (as revealed in the way they are excreted in the urine) is different in cancer patients as compared to healthy persons. About 350 chemical compounds are known which will cause cancer under controlled conditions of the research laboratory, and efforts are under way to find out just how they convert the normal cell to a cancerous one, and whether any such chemicals can be "accidentally" formed by the body itself.

If, as has been said, life is a continuous series of chemical reactions, then so must cancer be. Up to now it has not been possible to analyze the chemistry of the body in minute detail, but recently developed machines and methods now are doing it. Radioactive isotopes enable the scientist to trace the fate of many substances within the body; microscopes of greater power than any used before and other physical equipment now permit determination of the chemical structure of the smallest parts of cells, and exploration of the complex changes which are the basis of life and growth and, very likely, cancer. Once these are understood, it is reasonable to expect that ways can be found to alter the chemistry of cancer, interrupting the chain of reactions leading to abnormal cell growth and setting the chemical balance to rights. Already under way is an intensive search for chemical compounds which will seek out cancer cells and destroy them, without harming normal tissues. Several such chemotherapy agents have been found which partially fulfil these requirements, not sufficiently, however, to destroy all the cancer cells in a given tumor. The most useful are derivatives of nitrogen mustard gas of wartime development, and the anti-folic compounds, which prevent the cells' use of folic acid, a vitamin which rapidly dividing cells need in large quantity.

Thus the general objectives of cancer research are to learn more about the causes of abnormal growth so that cancer may ultimately be prevented, and to find more effective methods of treating it, once it has occurred. From these brief references to research, it will be seen that cancer appears to be due to not just one cause, and it is quite possible that no one preventive or treatment method will prove effective for all tumors. As is always the way of science, each experiment undertaken opens up new paths to be explored, so that the opportunities for further research are increasing year by year. Sooner or later the great mass of information now being assembled will begin to assume meaning, and the outline of the picture we are seeking will gradually appear—not all of a sudden, but as the pieces of a jigsaw puzzle fall into place—bit by bit.

GOAL

Fortunately, it is not necessary to wait for research to forge the final answers to cancer in order to achieve a significantly larger measure of control over this disease than we now have. If present knowledge were to be fully put to use, if all cancer were to be treated within weeks instead of within months, as is the case generally, twice as many lives could be saved as are now being saved. The core of the problem of present-day cancer control is early treatment, and if it is to be achieved on a wide scale, the public must recognize that its responsibility is hardly less than that of the doctors. Your responsibility is twofold. First you must learn that you will be the first to receive the initial expressions of cancer and you must therefore prepare yourself for this possibility (a good possibility since cancer will affect one in every five now living) by learning its Seven Danger Signals. But it is now possible to forestall the appearance of certain of these danger signals and by the many months saved to increase greatly the chances of successful treatment. Methods are at hand for finding cancer in certain organs long before it would normally cause signs or symptoms, and these methods are simple, inexpensive, and applicable on a broad scale. Your second responsibility, then, is to take advantage of these cancer-detecting procedures by having a careful physical examination at regular intervals—no matter how fit you feel. Experience has proven that cancer may and does exist long before it calls attention to its presence—yet it can be found IF it is looked for. This is particularly true of cancer of the lung, womb, breast, and rectum, because of the ease with which these sites can be examined at proper intervals. The general physical examination including these organs and also an X-ray picture of the chest should be as routine for women over thirty-five and men over forty-five as the periodic visit to the dentist has become. It is likely to be a lot less painful, too.

The periodic health checkup has been advocated by doctors for years, but relatively few people have taken advantage of it. Its importance is increasing, however, because it offers the only means of coping with diseases which have now become our leading health problems owing to longer life. It is not possible to deal with cancer and high blood pressure and hardening of the arteries as the previous major health menaces have been dealt with. They are not controllable by vaccination or quarantine, by regulation of sewage disposal or water purification. There are no wonder drugs to combat them, no vitamins to build resistance against them. Instead, the responsibility for their control is squarely up to every man and woman, and it cannot be transferred to anyone else nor to any agency. Acceptance or rejection of this responsibility will largely determine how much farther the span of life can be lengthened—our life as a people and our lives as individuals.

CHAPTER XXIV

Occupation and Health

CAREY P. McCORD, M.D.
Revised by EDWARD E. DART, M.D.

INTRODUCTION: OCCUPATIONAL DISEASES

EVERY JOB ON WHICH *anyone works brings with it some degree of exposure to risk from contact with chemical substances, with electric power, with conditions of temperature, humidity or similar changes in the environment that may cause illness. The occupations are now recognized as of first importance as a factor in causing disability.*

The human body has in it certain factors for controlling its own temperature, but sometimes outside conditions become so severe that the body's own thermostatic function will not control. Cold constricts the blood vessels in the skin; heat expands them. Sudden changes of temperature, particularly from extreme heat to cold, result in discomfort and are believed to be associated with pains in the limbs and with catching cold. Excessive heat for long periods of time can produce changes in the body leading to unconsciousness and even to death.

In the article which follows, Dr. Carey P. McCord considers first the general conditions associated with occupational diseases and then classifies them according to the chief factor involved in bringing about the illness. For example, if anyone is exposed to extreme dry heat he can develop heat stroke. This is associated with fever, a rapid pulse, flushing of the skin, profuse sweating, and a fall in the blood pressure. Eventually, of course, exposure to extreme heat may so affect the organs and tissues of the body that anemia, inflammations of the skin, disturbances of the kidney, and breakdown of many of the other organs of the body may follow. There are innumerable occupations in which heat is a factor, particularly such occupations as those of blast-furnace and boiler-room workers, of workers in the chemical and cement industries, of cooks, laundry workers, tinners, and similar occupations.

Sudden changes in the temperature are particularly likely to occur to men in the ice industry, to butchers, to candy makers, cooks, drivers, electrotypers, fishermen, florists, miners, packing-house employees, soap makers, and similar occupations.

INDUSTRIAL SKIN DISEASES

Occupational skin diseases comprise about 75% of all occupational diseases. The number of substances used in various industries which may affect the worker is legion. Among florists there may be sensitivities to plants, as described under allergic diseases, or irritations of the skin from water, or poisoning from such substances as nicotine and arsenic used to destroy insect pests. Furriers may be poisoned by paraphenylendiamine, as described under diseases of the skin. Workers with chromium in electro-plating develop chrome ulcers. There are also inflammations of the skin from acids, alkalis, soaps, dyes, and drugs. The physician will usually inquire as to the occupation of his patient and as to any unusual substances used in that occupation.

Incidentally, all workers except those in a few especially hazardous trades are more likely to suffer from ailments unrelated to work than from occupational diseases that result directly from conditions in which the worker toils. Modern departments of industrial health in state and municipal health departments do much to control conditions of work.

DAMPNESS

Occasionally workers are employed in places which are exceedingly damp. This happens particularly in such occupations as those of the fisherman, leather preparers in the glove industry, laundry workers, packing-house employees, workers in the paper industry, pottery workers, sewer workers, and farmers. Most occupations in which dampness occurs are also associated with high and low temperatures and with high humidity.

There are, however, some conditions in which the wetness alone is the serious factor. Exposure to dampness is usually associated as a contributing factor with coughs and colds, in rheumatic disease, and in changes in the skin. Of course, the human being is not adapted to living in exceedingly damp areas; hence he should endeavor to avoid the dampness by wearing waterproof clothing, rubber boots, and similar protective coverings. Moreover, accumulation of water can frequently be prevented by digging channels or ditches to carry away the excess.

DUST AS A HAZARD

The most serious hazard today in many industries is dust. The dusts not only block the tissues, but in some cases act as an irritant, so that there are inflammation, swelling, and even destruction. Moreover, the dusts sometimes carry germs with them into the tissues, and once in the body the germs may set up inflammations.

Among the most dangerous of the dusts which affect mankind is silica. This produces a condition known as silicosis. X-ray pictures show the lungs full of nodules following the lodgment of the silica in the lymphatics. When the dis-

ease is well advanced, the lungs do not expand, and breathing is difficult, and there may be continuous coughing.

The dust from asbestos produces the same type of inflammation that silica produces, although apparently milder. In order to prevent silicosis, workers in any industry in which silica is much used should avoid inhalation, and the head of the industry can aid the worker with certain simple procedures. Water or oil may be used to wet the dust, thus preventing it from rising and filling the air. Exhaust systems can be applied to remove the dust at the point where it develops. Sometimes the work can be done in an enclosed chamber with the worker outside. Finally, where dust is exceedingly excessive, helmets may be worn by the workers to cover the head and neck, and they can get their air by breathing through pipes from a non-dusty area.

Workers in such an industry should have their lungs X-rayed regularly, and there should be a physician in the plant who is familiar with the changes that take place in the lungs under exposure. Whenever a worker in a dusty trade has a cough, a dryness of the nose and throat, pain on breathing and hoarseness, whenever he coughs or expectorates blood, and develops colds which simply refuse to clear up, he should begin to wonder whether or not the dust is affecting him unfavorably. There are hundreds of industries in which dust is a serious factor. In all of them it is a hazard, but when it is silica or asbestos dust, it is a menace to health and life.

INFECTIONS OF INDUSTRY

Certain industries are associated with the likelihood of special infections of the body. For example: workers with hides and animal hair are constantly exposed to infection with anthrax. This begins as a malignant pustule, an inflamed pimple or a boil, which becomes hard, has a purple center and a deep red zone around it. Gradually this breaks down and discharges a thick, bloody material, and eventually may even become gangrenous. The lymph glands in the neighborhood swell, and the veins become inflamed. Associated with this there may be a general weakness, including chilliness, loss of appetite, vomiting, and a high fever.

Anthrax is a dangerous disease, and workers with hides must do everything possible to prevent infection. Foreign skins or hair should never be carried on the unprotected shoulder. All hides and animal hair should be thoroughly sterilized. The workers should wash their hands frequently in antiseptic solutions, and those who sort hair should wear breathing devices to prevent inhalation.

As is pointed out elsewhere, the body may become infected from the tissue of infected rabbit with tularemia, from infected straw with actinomycosis, from a contaminated nail with tetanus, from infected milk with undulant fever, and so on, from various substances. Workers in mines and on farms who walk about barefooted may develop hook-worm infection.

Every cut, scratch, or abrasion sustained in any industry should be treated at once with suitable antiseptics, such as iodine, to prevent infection. Industries in which infections of the skin, such as boils, carbuncles, and abscesses, are most likely to develop are those of the butcher, the canner, feather workers, fertilizer makers, garbage workers, glue makers, hair workers, dairy workers, silk workers, soap makers, and veterinarians.

RADIANT ENERGY DISEASES

Among the most serious of the occupational diseases recently developed are those associated with the use of radium, the X-ray, and various radioactive substances. Exposure to X-rays and to the emanations from radium may produce serious burns and irritations of the skin which result in cancer. They also affect the blood and the blood-forming organs seriously, so that deficiencies of both the red and the white blood cells are exceedingly common.

Employees in watch factories who prepare the luminous dials have sustained generalized radium poisoning with disastrous results. Workers must learn to protect themselves against these hazards, first of all, by suitable screening against the rays through the wearing of aprons and gloves infiltrated with lead. Brushes for radium painting should never be pointed with the mouth or lips.

Another type of radiant energy which may produce damage to the human body is that associated with ultraviolet and infra-red rays. These are occupational hazards particularly in welding and cutting. The ultraviolet rays are invisible. They cause intense irritation of the eyes and a burning of the skin. Sunblindness and desert-blindness represent the type of injury that can be caused to the eye by ultraviolet rays. The infra-red rays are essentially heat rays and can cause all the damage that heat of intensity applied to the human body can cause in other ways.

Workers around ultraviolet or infra-red rays may protect themselves against these rays by wearing goggles, helmets, shields, and masks equipped with colored lenses especially designed to exclude dangerous rays. The rays cannot penetrate ordinary clothing, so that covering of the body with a sufficient thickness of clothing will prevent injury and damage to the skin.

Among the industries in which exposure to ultraviolet and infra-red rays are most common are blacksmiths, cutters who use oxyacetylene gas, furnace workers, glass blowers, iron and steel mill workers, and everyone working in the motion-picture industry. The welders who use the arc for cutting and welding steel are also constantly exposed to dangerous rays.

In the following article, Dr. Carey P. McCord has presented some of the general considerations associated with occupational diseases, and he presents a consideration of the one hundred and fifty most common hazards likely to be found in industry. Any worker associated with any of the poisons here listed should take steps to protect himself against exposure by inhalation, by contamination of the skin, and by other sources.

M. F.

OCCUPATION AND HEALTH

The outstanding characteristic of Americans is their zest for work. This willingness to work, along with great technical, economic, and social advances in our industrial world, have procured luxuries for all of us far beyond the dreams of kings of old—automobiles, good food, television sets, family-owned homes —to name but a few. The health to enjoy these good things has been enhanced by advances in medicine generally—the care of infants and the care of the aged; the new wonder drugs; new surgical techniques, including surgery of the heart; new procedures for diagnosis, and the improved organization of preventive medical programs in government and industry. Since nearly all adult men and many women spend forty or more hours per week at their jobs, occupational medicine has played no little part in this scheme of positive health promotion.

The industrial physician or medical department is the public health department for the worker at work. Safety programs to prevent accidents work effectively in industry. Carriers of workmen's compensation have found that excellent surgical care and the liberal use of specialists for sick workers is good for themselves as well. All large industries and most moderate-sized concerns have well-developed medical departments. There is also a rapidly increasing trend for small plants to procure good part-time medical consultation so that they, too, can participate in the positive benefit programs. Care for injured workers is by no means the only function of these medical departments and medical consultants. The pre-employment examinations prevailing in industry today are used not to prevent people from working, but rather to advise management of the type of work that a prospective employee can do without harm to himself or his fellow workers. For instance, a person with some disease of the heart might well do light work, whereas the work of a stevedore would soon disable him completely. Occupational medicine enables such men to work and earn, at the same time protecting health. Likewise by the pre-employment examination many people are for the first time made aware of some curable defect and encouraged to seek help from the personal physician of their own choice. However, people with communicable diseases may be prevented from exposing fellow employees until such time as they may safely mingle with them.

Nonetheless, the detection of disease or defects and personal health education do not complete the job of those charged with maintaining the health of the men and women who work. In the work environment there is sometimes encountered toxic vapor, fume, gas or dust, harmful radiation, undue alterations of temperature, excesses of humidity, noise or vibration, any of which may cause an occupational disease. An occupational disease is any abnormal state of the body or mind resulting from work. It differs from an accident in that some time must pass between the first exposure to the causative agent and the development of symptoms. A painter may be exposed over a period of days to the action of a paint solvent. This slowly irritates the skin, so that in the course of a week a rash appears on his hands or forearms. An employee in a battery-manufacturing plant where there is inadequate medical and engineering protection from exposure to lead may inhale lead dust for months and only gradually develop loss of appetite and weight, increasing constipation, and abdominal cramps. A miner may work for twenty or thirty years breathing silica dust before there is any evidence of silicosis as seen in X-ray films. These are occupational diseases.

Monumental research has been done by our universities, our government agencies, and above all by industry itself on the pathologic changes produced by exposure to these substances and on methods to control them in order to maintain healthful surroundings in which to work. The efficacy of these advancements in occupational medicine is attested by the rarity of occupational disease. In California in 1950 there were only 12,245 cases of occupational disease reported to the State Bureau of Adult Health. At the same time there were 136,814 lost-time industrial accidents.

Purely from an interest point of view, and to give some idea generally of the types of occupational disease which may occur, the reported cases are herewith broken down as to the organ affected and the principal groups of causative agents:

Infectious and parasitic disease		205
Diseases of the eye		1,726
Flash burns (from welding rays)	1,672	
Other	54	
Diseases of the ear		38
Diseases of the respiratory system		331
Diseases of the skin		6,615
Poison Oak	3,302	
Other	3,313	
Diseases of the bones and organs of movement		1,703
Strains & inflammation of the tendons	1,469	
Other	207	
Systemic poisonings by industrial chemicals		339
Poisoning by other substances, including venom (insect bites)		
& pharmaceuticals		620
Weather		273
Heat	246	
Other	27	
Burns (repeated exposure to chemicals)		234
Other specific causes		156
Not specified		5
Total		12,245

Much effort has been exerted to ascertain the effects of noise on people and to devise standards of noise tolerance. Also, with the advent of the atom bomb and the numerous radioactive substances that have been placed in common usage as a result of knowledge of nuclear physics, the increased control of radiant energy has become one of the greatest problems in the technical aspects of industrial medicine.

NOISE

Sound is that form of vibrational energy which produces the sensation of hearing. It is usually transmitted to the ear by air but may also travel through bone. Sound is propagated by vibratory disturbances. Whereas musical sound or tone is due to regularly recurring vibrations, a noise results when the impulses are irregular or confused. Both the loudness or intensity of the sound waves and their frequency play a part in the effect of a given noise on the ear. To be audible, vibrations must have a rate of at least 12 to 15 per second, and shrill, high-pitched tones may be heard with a rate of vibration of approximately 20,000 per second. High frequency sounds are more annoying and damaging than sounds of low frequency. The decibel is the usual unit of measure for sound. Some idea of the value of the decibel can be obtained from the following comparisons:

The tick of a watch at 3 feet may be measured as 10 to 30 decibels on the sound intensity or loudness scale; ordinary conversation as 40 to 60 decibels, and a pneumatic drill at 10 feet as 70 to 90 decibels. The threshold of feeling noise (in contrast to hearing it) occurs at 100 to 120 decibels, depending on the frequency. Since the bel, and accordingly the decibel, is determined on a base 10 logarithmic scale, 10 decibels is 10 times as loud, 20 decibels is 100 times as loud, and 30 decibels is 1,000 times as loud as 1 decibel.

Noise may produce effects ranging through mental inefficiency, nervousness, fatigue, indigestion, temporary deafness, and permanent injury to the ear. Deafness resulting from industrial noise may usually be distinguished from other types of deafness because occupational deafness occurs in certain frequency ranges peaking at 4,096 vibrations per second. Although there is no doubt that industrial deafness occurs, as illustrated by the old-time boiler maker, considerable duration of time, even with exposure to high noise levels, is necessary to produce permanent deafness. Opinion as to the exact levels at which noise may produce lasting detriment to the ear varies, but the majority of data indicates that some harmful effect may result from prolonged exposure to noise of intensities from 85 to 110 decibels. The incompleteness of data upon which to base standards of noise tolerance has been one of the deterrents to efforts aimed at controlling noise in industry.

Personal protection against noise and vibration is available. Airborne noise can be reduced by the insertion in the external ear of pliable materials such as wax, or foam rubber. Commercially produced ear plugs of various designs are available. Protection against bone-conducted noise and vibration requires the use of soft-soled shoes, felt or rubber mats, and chairs or platforms mounted on springs. However, these methods are employed only in situations where it is impracticable to control noise at its source.

The trend toward reducing industrial noise is apparent in the recent design of modern office machines such as the "noiseless typewriter." However, the same trend has developed in the field of manufacturing and processing equipment, and in many instances this has included alteration of production methods. Noise is reduced when welding replaces riveting, when hydraulic presses displace the old trip hammers, when V-belts replace growling gears, and when advanced foundry practice reduces or eliminates chipping and grinding of castings. The shock and noise created by metallic impact generally characteristic of metal fabrication may often be reduced at its source by damping materials such as rubber or the "hydro-pneumatic metal" of Chamberlain. The latter can be used as inserts in hammers, punches, dies, and as durable shock-absorbing mounts for heavy machinery. It was used successfully in World War II to prevent shock to delicate equipment on battleships and as shoe inserts to prevent fractured ankles when large bombs exploded under water in proximity to battleships.

Thus there are means of measuring noise, of determining its effect on organisms, and, to a certain extent, of reducing such harmful effects.

RADIANT ENERGY

The tremendous power of atomic energy for benefit or destruction was far from the minds of the German, William Roentgen, and the Frenchman, Antoine Becquerel, some fifty years ago when they respectively discovered the X-ray and what we call radioactivity. Becquerel found that uranium salts had developed a photographic film in the dark, and his pupils, Pierre and Marie Curie, went on to discover radium, the first known radioactive element always present in uranium.

Radioactivity, the giving off of charged particles, results from the breakdown of the element itself. As radium dissipates its energy it eventually turns into lead. Although this radiation from the atom is extremely harmful to human flesh and bone, no appreciable heat is felt and there is no way of immediately recognizing by the physical senses the dire effect of its penetration into the tissues, so that early there was no thought of the tremendous energy involved. What is this atom of which we speak so glibly? Everything is made up of invisibly small particles called atoms. However, small as they are, atoms are made up of even smaller particles known as electrons, protons, and neutrons. An atom consists of a nucleus (positively charged particles, the protons; and neutrons, without any charge) about which revolve the negatively charged electrons. The electrons are attracted to the nucleus, but their terrific speed of rotation exerts a centrifugal force that prevents their moving closer to it. It is the difference in the proportion of protons that makes one element different from another. Most elements are stable unless by bombarding with particles like those given off by radium or by slowed neutrons, a portion of the nucleus can be knocked off, producing a different element and giving off energy. This is the principle employed in the atom bomb.

The radiations produced in this manner consist primarily of three types of moving particles: alpha rays, beta rays, and gamma rays, which differ in their response to electric forces. Protons and neutrons may also be given off as energized particles. Similar to these are X-rays produced when a moving electrically charged particle strikes against a hard target. Such radiant energy produces undesirable effects in the human body whenever it is absorbed in excess of certain amounts to which the human organism has been accustomed in its natural surroundings. Injury results only when the radiation releases ions (electrically charged particles) within the cell structure, and the injury is proportional to the ionization produced. So far as the effect on the cell is concerned, it does not matter greatly whether these ions are produced indirectly by secondary emanations from X-rays or gamma rays or directly by the impact of primary particles such as beta and alpha rays.

The X-rays and gamma rays are penetrating radiations which, in contrast to other types of radiant energy, can pass entirely through any part of the body with only moderate diminution of their intensity. X-rays are used in the doctor's office to photograph bones and other parts of the body. In this instance the radiations are carefully controlled so that a single dose does not exceed the safe level.

Alpha particles have a very low penetrating power, and when originating outside the body produce no appreciable biologic effect. They are stopped by a few inches of air. Beta rays from radium and from many artificially produced radioactive substances have a much greater penetrating power and are able to traverse a fraction of an inch of animal tissue. Overexposure to beta rays will produce burns, most frequently of the hands.

Neutrons are known as slow or fast. They are without electric charge and do not cause ionization of tissue, but the fast neutron may collide with hydrogen atoms, imparting some of their energy to them and producing rapidly moving charged particles capable of harm.

Radiant energy may produce burns of the skin and cancer. Generalized radiation by penetrating rays causes nausea, vomiting, diarrhea, and anemia. Leukemia may result. Radium, if absorbed, is stored in the bones and affects both the blood-forming marrow and the bone itself. It is important to iterate that these symptoms are not immediately present. The senses give no warning of impending harm. Injury is only apparent after a latent period of several hours to one or two weeks or more. It may take many years for the results of repeated small exposures to radiant energy to become apparent. If the cells concerned in reproduction are injured, there is also the possibility of mutations (abnormalities) developing in subsequent generations.

Radiant energy may be encountered in an atomic explosion, in industrial X-ray processes to detect flaws in metal, in the work of medical technicians, in radium dial painting, and in the handling of radioactive isotopes, which are coming into more general usage.

Protection against the effect of radiation is twofold—medical and engineering. Pre-employment medical examinations are necessary to prevent exposure of persons already anemic. Periodic examinations of the blood to detect early changes, examination of the exhaled air for its radioactivity, and the wearing by workers of detecting devices or photographic film, are essential to protection. Shielding of processes by sufficient distance (remote control), adequate amounts of lead or other materials—in the case of fast neutrons, hydrogen barriers are used—and removal of contaminated air, are essential engineering controls.

In spite of the tremendous hazard from exposure to radiant energy with the development and application of atomic physics—once the problem was known —industrial medicine has done and continues to do an amazingly fine job in minimizing the harmful effects of radiation.

Toxic Substances That May Be Encountered in Industry

Acetanilid, which is well known as a dangerous drug in the treatment of headache, is extensively used in the manufacture of many chemicals, such as paranitranilin. It is commonly taken into the body under industrial conditions in the form of dusts. The action of acetanilid simulates that of aniline oil. An outstanding manifestation is a blue discoloration of the skin, notably of the lips, finger tips, and ears, which is due to the formation of methemoglobin in the blood.

Acetone (dimethyl ketone) is a much used industrial solvent, especially in the manufacture of munitions. It is representative of a long series of ketones, all of which possess about the same order of toxicity. While inhaled vapors may lead to some damage to the respiratory tract and other portions of the body, this takes place only when vapor concentrations are comparatively high. Acetone is much less toxic than such other agents as benzene or carbon tetrachloride. In contact with the skin, acetone is a defatting agent and thus favors the appearance of dermatitis.

Acetylene gas is in itself probably nontoxic, except that it may act as a simple asphyxiant; that is, it may displace oxygen in the air to an extent that life may not be supported. However, the use of acetylene as in torch welding may be associated with a number of other exposures. If acetylene welding be done on galvanized metal, zinc chills may arise from that metal used in the galvanizing. The same is true in torch work in brazing brass. Chemical rays from acetylene torch work may lead to injury to the eyes, producing such conditions as conjunctivitis or retinitis.

Ammonia gas causes profound local action on the skin, eyes, and respiratory tract. Four hundred parts of this substance per million of air constitute the threshold for immediate irritation of the throat. Prolonged exposure to one fourth of that amount is the maximum tolerable for prolonged periods. Although ammonia accidents may be severe and fatal, it is unlikely that ammonia as such enters the body.

Coatings, such as lacquers and varnishes, may contain *amyl alcohol* or related amyl compounds. Toxicity is not great, but it may lead to low-grade irritation of the eyes, nose, and throat.

Aniline oil is a much used chemical in a variety of industries, especially in the manufacture of chemicals. A large number of compounds derived from aniline exert a harmful action similar to that of aniline itself. Aniline is definitely toxic, producing both acute and chronic poisoning. It readily enters the body through the unbroken skin, leading to poisoning. Also poisoning may take place through inhalation or ingestion of the oil or its dusts or vapors. In severe acute poisoning there may be observed sudden prostration with blue coloration of lips, nose, and fingers, and unconsciousness with or without convulsions.

Both *arsenic* and its compounds are highly toxic. Arsenic is widely used in industry, and in addition is present in many industrial substances as impurities unknown to industrial workers. Unsuspected poisonings arise in scores of industries making no direct uses of this substance. It may enter the body in the form of gases, vapors, fluids, or dusts. Local action may be produced on exposed parts. In constitutional disease the principal systems or organs involved are: gastrointestinal tract, the kidneys, the liver, the nervous system, and the respiratory tract. The loss of hair and of nails, together with bronzing of the skin, are common features.

Asbestos, which is a complex calcium magnesium silicate, may from the breathing of its dust give rise to a lung disease known as asbestosis. This disease resembles silicosis, but in fact is not silicosis, which is only produced by silicon dioxide. Many years of dust exposure may be required to establish the disease. Once established, it is permanent. The X-ray picture of the lungs is fairly characteristic.

Asphalt is not a chemical entity but a tarry substance of inconstant make-up, found in nature or resulting from petroleum or coal distillation. Asphalt contains many toxic agents, notably skin irritants. Operations involving hot asphalt constitute greater practical dangers than the handling in cold form. Possible skin cancer may be caused by contact with asphalt.

Bakelite is the trade name for a synthetic resin produced from the interaction of phenol and formaldehyde. Several other trade names are associated with this product. In the manufacture of bakelite some exposures may be found in phenol, formaldehyde, various resin solvents, and "hex" (hexamethylenetetramine). The latter is a frequent source of dermatitis.

Benzene (benzol) differs from benzine. The former chiefly originates in coal-tar distillation but it is known that benzene or substances chemically closely akin to benzene may be obtained from some petroleums. Benzene is highly toxic. Concentrations above one hundred parts per million of air are to be regarded as harmful. Vapors enter the body along with respired air. High concentrations may lead to immediate action, characterized by convulsions, unconsciousness, and prompt death; but the greater number of cases are chronic and center about the results of destruction of several forms of blood elements.

Some persons are far more susceptible to the action of benzene than others. Chronic poisoning is characterized by damage to blood-forming organs, kidneys, liver, nervous system, and by increased susceptibility to ordinary infections. Hemorrhage into the skin, from the nose, mouth, and stomach, rectum, lungs, and genitalia, are prime manifestations. Benzene in contact with the skin may be absorbed and produce systemic poisoning, or local skin action may take place leading to a dermatitis.

Benzine is a nontechnical term applied to various derivatives of petroleum distillation, such as gasoline, naphtha, etc. The action of this chemical may be local on the skin, or systemic after the inhalation of vapors. This substance is more toxic than commonly believed, and may give rise either to "naphtha jags" (which is an acute disease resembling alcoholic intoxication), associated with respiratory tract irritation, or rarely to chronic forms characterized by profound changes in the nervous system, liver, and kidneys. Chronic benzine poisoning may simulate multiple paralysis.

Beryllium. There are many industrial processes in which beryllium may exist. It forms an alloy with several metals, most outstanding of which is beryllium copper, used in making springs and diaphragms for altimeters. Beryllium glass is used to filter out strong or reflected electrons in X-ray streams. Formerly the element was used extensively in the manufacture of fluorescent lamps and this was the chief source of poisoning. Although ulcers and nodules may be produced on the skin, the reaction in the lungs is of paramount importance. Beryllium causes weakness, shortness of breath, cough, nervousness, and loss of weight. Distinct changes in the lung, not unlike those found in tuberculosis, are produced.

Bichromates are extensively used in lithography, photography, blueprint work, the dye industry, etc. Their action is similar to that of chromates and chromic acid. Local action may be extensive and intractable. It may produce a dermatitis of unbroken skin, deep burrowing ulcers ("chrome holes"), perforation of the nasal septum, inflammation of the respiratory tract, and a condition akin to sensitization may be instituted by chromium, in which trivial exposures produce profound inflammation of large areas of the skin not in contact with the irritant. Damage from chromium is always slow in healing. Not all compounds of chromium are injurious. This depends upon differences in valency.

Bisulphide of carbon is much used in artificial silk manufacture and in the rubber industry. Its action is primarily exerted on the central nervous system, causing conditions resembling insanity. It may lead to blindness, paralyses of various groups of muscles, and in addition damage to the kidneys and the gastro-intestinal tract takes place. A rapid heart is the rule.

The manipulation of *brass* in cold form is not known to produce characteristic damage. Brass dust may induce a mechanical dermatitis, and the skin and hair may become green from the copper content of the brass. When, however, brass is in molten state, metal fume fever may arise, which primarily depends on the action of zinc rather than the copper or the brass. The disease produced is variously termed "zinc chills," "brass ague," "foundrymen's chills," etc. In addition, workers about molten brass may acquire lead or arsenic poisoning as the result of these metals being present as impurities in the brass.

Much stated in respect to the hazards of brass work applies to *bronze* workers. Especially, lead may appear in bronze, and lead poisoning is not a rarity.

Bronze powders is a term extensively applied to the divers metallic powders used in printing and decorating. All such bronze powders are capable of producing inflammation of the skin. Low-grade respiratory tract irritation is common. Some so-called bronze powders actually are colored aluminum powders. Fine aluminum powders are inflammable and explosions have occurred.

Butyl alcohol is a widely used ingredient in solvents. Its toxicity is believed to begin at about one hundred parts of the vapors per million of air. In addition to being a respiratory tract irritant, butyl alcohol may lead to damage to the kidneys, liver, lungs, and to the causation of anemia.

Various compounds of *cadmium* may enter the body through the lungs in the form of dusts or fumes, and to a lesser extent dusts may enter the stomach. Edema of the lungs may be produced, with or without pneumonia and related injuries. Some scar tissue may be produced. Cadmium likewise injures the liver, kidneys, and intestinal tract. Vomiting may take place, together with diarrhea. On a comparative basis, cadmium is more toxic than lead.

Wherever used, *carbolic acid* (phenol) is a potential source of severe injury. Harm may be either local, beginning with a slight burn and culminating in gangrene, or may be systemic, following skin absorption, inhalation, or accidental swallowing. Deleterious action is swift, and death may be produced within a few hours. Any portion of the body may be affected. Commonly the respiratory and intestinal tracts, the liver, the kidneys, and blood-forming elements are damaged.

Carbon dioxide is not toxic except as it displaces oxygen necessary in respired air. It is a simple asphyxiant. Deaths in industry from exposure to undue amounts of carbon dioxide are fairly frequent and commonly may be construed as accidents rather than occupational diseases. The presence of low quantities of carbon dioxide in the air constitutes no index of air vitiation. Instead, some carbon dioxide is essential as a stimulant to normal breathing.

Carbon monoxide is one of the most widespread and insidious hazards of industry. Carbon monoxide easily combines with the hemoglobin of the blood and inhibits the oxygen-carrying power of the blood. The commoner features of acute poisoning are headache, nausea, dizziness, visual disturbances, abdominal pain, discoloration of the skin, which may be pink, greenish or yellowish-red, followed by unconsciousness and convulsions in severer cases. This form of poisoning either in or apart from industry may be regarded as an accident rather than a disease. After severe poisoning with prolonged unconsciousness, various serious after-effects may arise of prolonged duration. Chronic carbon monoxide poisoning is at this time disputed. Prompt artificial respiration after removal from exposure is highly desirable when respiration has ceased.

The action of *carbon tetrachloride* is characteristic of a group of chlorinated hydrocarbons, including ethylene dichloride, trichlorethylene, and chloroform. The threshold of danger begins at about one hundred parts of the vapors per million of air. Poisoning may be acute, delayed, and possibly chronic. In acute poisoning the essential manifestations are headache, vomiting, diarrhea, abnormal pain, sense of moving masses in the abdomen, and irritation of the kidneys. The delayed poisoning may arise twenty-four to forty-eight hours after exposure. Delayed poisoning largely centers about destruction of liver tissues and damage from the subsequently produced guanidine. The damage from acute poisoning is believed to be readily repaired without significant aftereffects, but some physicians recognize the possibility of a chronic form of the disease. Exposure through inhalation is the usual mode of entry, but skin absorption is possible and local skin action has been observed. This material is widely used in industry such as in dry cleaning, metal degreasing, in fire extinguishers, etc.

In the manufacture and industrial use of *chloride of lime,* dusts and gases may lead to asthma, inflammation of the eyes, injury to the respiratory tract, and skin diseases. Harmful action is probably subsequent to liberated chlorine, although impurities may account for some damage.

Chlorine is an irrespirable gas, hazardous in small quantities, leading to prompt swelling (edema) of the lungs and air passages. The chronic form of intoxication, due to the intake of minute quantities over long periods of time, is characterized by severe bronchitis, persistent coughing, and pain in the chest.

Many of the widely used household *insecticides* consist of ground-up chrysanthemum buds used, as such, as a powder, or are extracted by such agents as ethylene dichloride, kerosene, etc. Both in the manufacture of these insecticides and in their use, extensive skin damage may be occasioned. In the powder form the offending agent may be pyrethrotoxic acid; in liquid forms, this combined with the solvent constitute damaging agents. In industry the disease state is more prevalent in summer months, due to the additional extracting action of perspiration. Allergic diseases from pyrethrum are more often in households than in industry.

Any toxicity connected with the industrial uses of *copper* is questionable, other than dermatitis and metal fume fever. Green perspiration and discoloration of hair may lead to an unwarranted degree of apprehension. The copper ion is no less toxic, if, in fact, it enters the body under any circumstance in quantities other than traces.

Creosote is an indefinite term covering various tarry substances from wood, coal, or petroleum. It contains many irritant constituents to the skin, eyes, and respiratory tract.

In the shaping of metal objects with lathes and similar machinery, coolants, cutting compounds and other *anti-friction agents* are in wide use. These agents may be oils or solutions of irritant salts, such as soda ash in emulsions. Irritation to the skin may be produced mechanically by the plugging up of the openings of the skin, sealing in effete materials, or by the direct action of the cutting compounds or their decomposition products. In addition, some harm may be created by bacteria from spitting into containers of these compounds.

Cyanides are extensively used in highly different industries, such as metal plating, case hardening, and insecticidal work. Action may be local, in the production of extensive ulceration, or systemic. The action is that of or is related to that of hydrocyanic acid. Cyanides are highly toxic industrial agents. Cyanides apart from causing skin disease act as internal asyhyxiants.

Dichloro-difluoromethane, used chiefly as a refrigerant, is a substance of low toxicity, acting solely or foremostly only as a simple asphyxiant, thus being dangerous only as it replaces oxygen in the respired air.

Dinitrobenzene is an intermediate in the manufacture of many chemicals, including dyes. It causes systemic disease, characterized by chocolate-colored blood, jaundice, marked loss of weight, labored breathing, mental sluggishness, impaired vision, and other changes. Its use by the obese to reduce weight is dangerous.

Ethyl benzene is a solvent for paraffins, resins, and lacquers. It causes dizziness, unsteady gait, trembling of extremities, slow, labored breathing, together with local irritation.

Ethylene dichloride is one of a series of chlorinated hydrocarbons with action similar to carbon tetrachloride. Its use is increasing in dry-cleaning plants, in the making of insecticides, in the disinfestation of grain elevators, etc.

Ethyl nitrate is a by-product in the manufacture of mercury fulminate. The latter is employed as detonator in gun cartridges. Exposure to fumes leads to low blood pressure, flushing of the skin, rapid heart, rapid respiration, excruciating headache, and abnormal temperature.

Formaldehyde is a gas, and when this gas is combined with water, formalin is produced. The liquid formalin exerts a destructive action on the skin. Formaldehyde vapors leave the solution. Systemic action is cumulative, leading to the degeneration of the liver and to nephritis. Severe damage may be done to the respiratory tract through irritation and subsequent edema.

Grain itch is a disease of the skin having many names, such as "prairie itch," "threshers' itch," "Texas mange," and "Ohio scratches." This disease is common around threshing operations and hay baling but may appear as a nonoccupational disease in bunkhouses where straw mattresses are utilized. This disease is due to an animal parasite, an itch mite technically termed *pediculoides ventricosus.*

Granite is a form of siliceous rock with a high content of free silica. It is a common source of silicosis, to which disease reference should be made.

Heat, or the absence of heat, is the source of a number of specific occupational conditions, such as thermic fever, sunstroke, heat exhaustion, chilblains, etc. Heat is not the source of characteristic occupational diseases, but of ill-

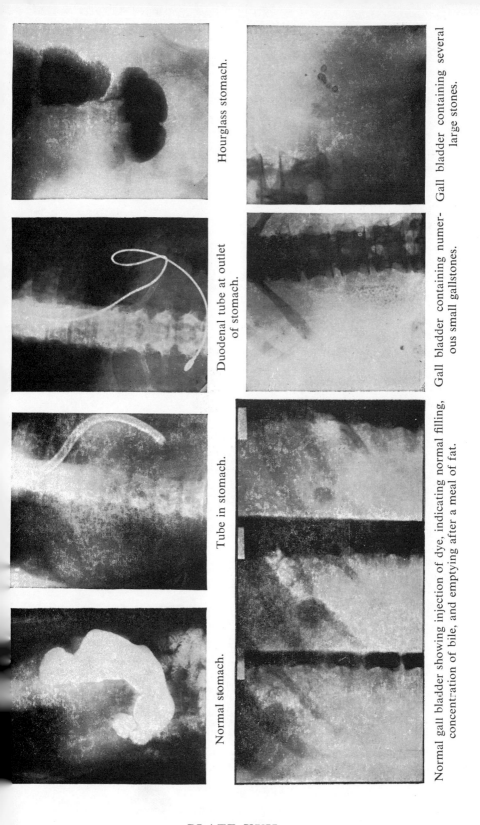

Hourglass stomach.

Gall bladder containing several large stones.

Duodenal tube at outlet of stomach.

Gall bladder containing numerous small gallstones.

Tube in stomach.

Normal stomach.

Normal gall bladder showing injection of dye, indicating normal filling, concentration of bile, and emptying after a meal of fat.

PLATE XVII

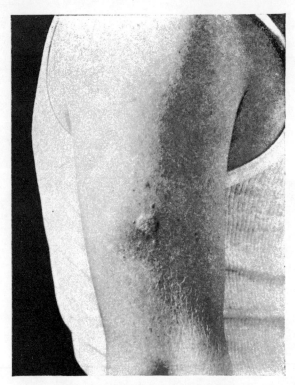

Positive skin test to ragweed pollen.

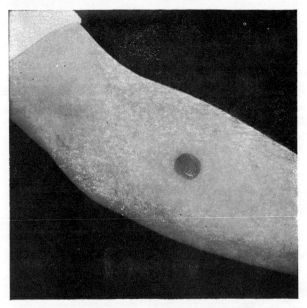

Positive patch test to streptomycin in physician who
became allergic to the drug after handling it.

PLATE XVIII

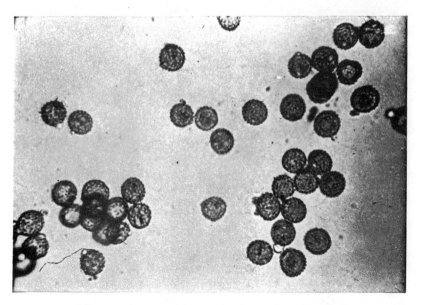

Microscopic appearance of ragweed pollen granules.

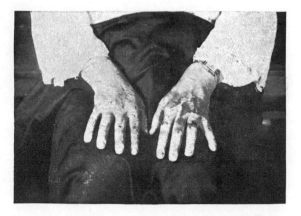

Contact dermatitis (occupational). Case 13. Patient, male, aged 49, a barber, had been troubled with a recurrent vesicular dermatitis of both hands for the past four years. This condition was associated with marked pruritus and was made worse by handling shampoos and face lotions. It was relieved over the week ends when the patient was not working. Patch tests corroborated the diagnosis of sensitivity to those substances.

PLATE XIX

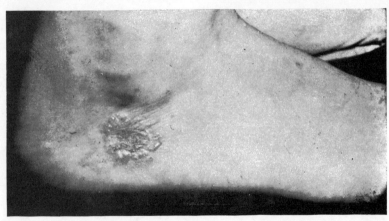

Contact dermatitis—poison ivy dermatitis. J. H., age 13. Patient states that she developed a vesicular dermatitis over her ankles following a walk through the park. She is definitely aware of the fact that she spreads this dermatitis to other parts of her body by contact of her fingers. She has had poison ivy every spring for the last few years. Patch test positive. Improved with treatment.
(Reproduced by permission of J. P. Lippincott Company, from *Essentials of Allergy* by Dr. Leo H. Criep)

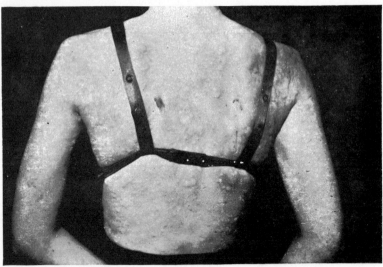

Urticaria and angioneurotic edema. Case 21. Patient gave a history of paroxysmal attacks of hives extending over a period of three years. These attacks were typical of urticaria and were accompanied by intense itching. The paroxysm causing her to seek treatment had continued for three weeks, involving practically all parts of her body. It came on about the time of final examination in school. The paroxysm was always worse during menstrual periods. The skin was very sensitive, so that even a mild stroking would produce welts (dermographia). There was a positive family history of allergy. The blood count showed an eosinophilia. There was evidence of skin sensitivity to many allergens.
(Reproduced by permission of J. P. Lippincott Company, from *Essentials of Allergy* by Dr. Leo H. Criep)

PLATE XX

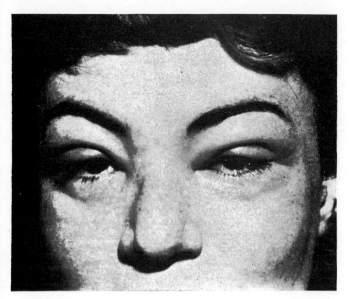

Giant hives of both eyes in young girl who presents marked
dermographism and hives.

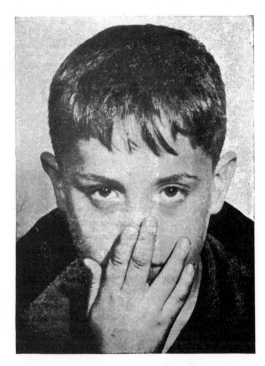

"Allergic salute" in nasal allergy.
(Reproduced by permission of
J. P. Lipppincott Company, from
Essentials of Allergy by Dr. Leo
H. Criep)

PLATE XXI

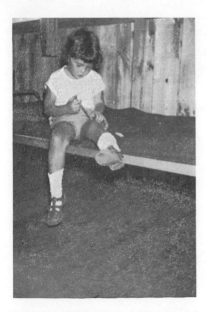

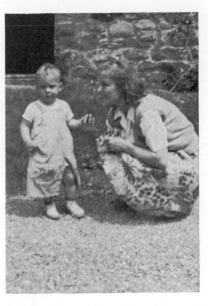

Self-subcutaneous administration of insulin by a child.

This healthy baby was born after the mother had h diabetes for twenty-five years and was a Quarter C tury Victory Medal case. She always tried to cont her diabetes.

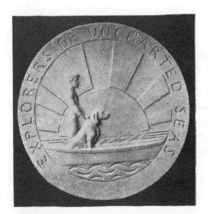

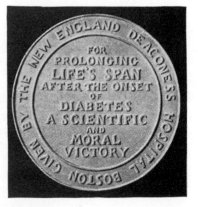

Expectation of Life Medal. To those individuals who have conquered diabetes by living longer with it than they were expected to live without it.

PLATE XXII

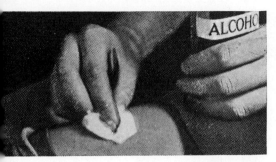

Cleaning the skin. The chosen spot on the skin is smartly rubbed with alcohol, *a different spot* each time: any convenient place on the body where a fold of skin can be picked up, but avoiding the *inner* surfaces of limbs.

Pinching up a fold of skin. A fold of skin is pinched up; the syringe is held by the barrel, *not* by the plunger. Some spots feel the prick more than others; feel around with the needle.

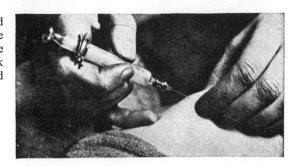

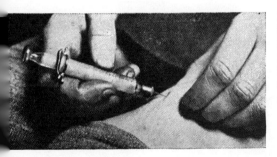

Inserting the needle. The needle is *suddenly* jabbed home, its point landing about midway between the tips of thumb and finger, well beneath the skin, yet not into the solid muscle. The needle goes *straight ahead,* so as not to bend or break it.

Injecting the insulin. *Then* the plunger is pushed in; some prefer slowly, some fast. After pulling the needle out, it is conventional to hold the alcoholic cotton on the spot for a few seconds, rubbing it in.

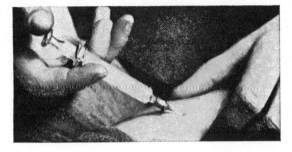

PLATE XXIII

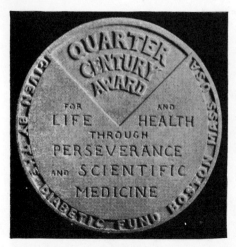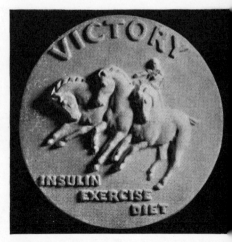

The Quarter Century Victory Medal for Health.

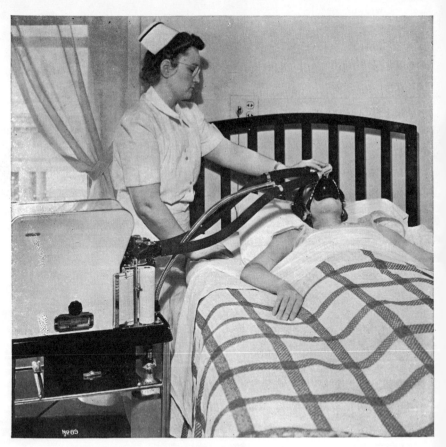

Basal metabolism test.

PLATE XXIV

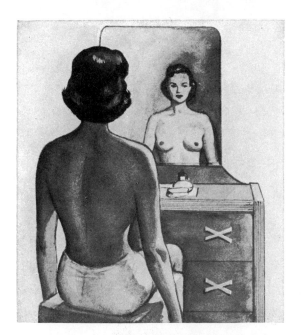

In first step of examining breasts, they are inspected carefully for changes in appearance — with special attention to puckering of skin, to size and contour of breasts and to nipple.

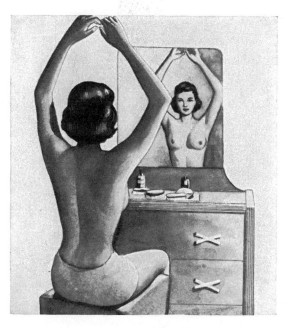

Step two is continuation of inspection with arms raised high. Again look for change.

PLATE XXV

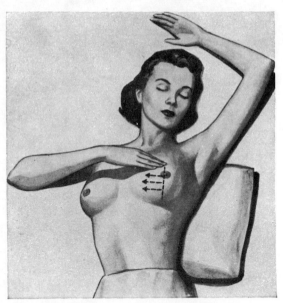

Step three is carried out lying down with a small pillow or folded towel under the shoulder of side being examined, and with arm of that side lying over head. Flat of fingers of opposite hand feel inner half of breast moving across and inward along imaginary lines — from above downward.

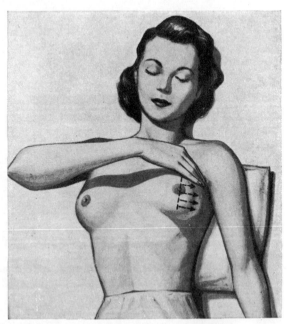

Step four, examination of outer half of breast, is carried out with arm brought to side, flat of fingers of opposite hand traversing breast from center line out, from above down.

PLATE XXVI

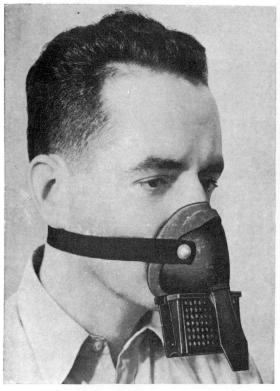

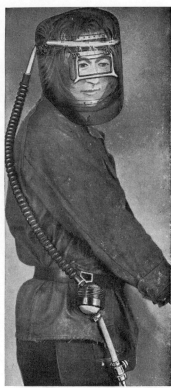

Respirator for protection against dust. Respirators in varying shapes, sizes, and weights are available for protection against all common types of harmful industrial dusts.

Some industrial operations call for and require helmets with hose line air supply. The above type is suitable for dangerous forms of welding.

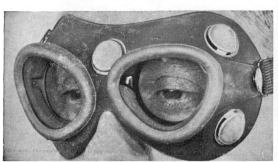

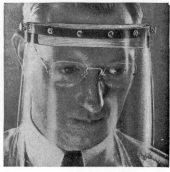

Numerous types of goggles are available for eye protection against dust, flying particles, harmful rays and vapors. Some types may be worn over spectacles.

In some industrial operations eye protection may be secured without the necessity of close-fitting goggles.

PLATE XXVII

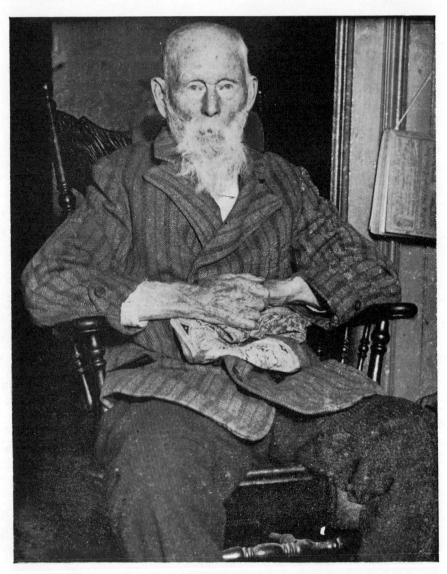

Skin of the aged.
(Courtesy of P & A Photos)

PLATE XXVIII

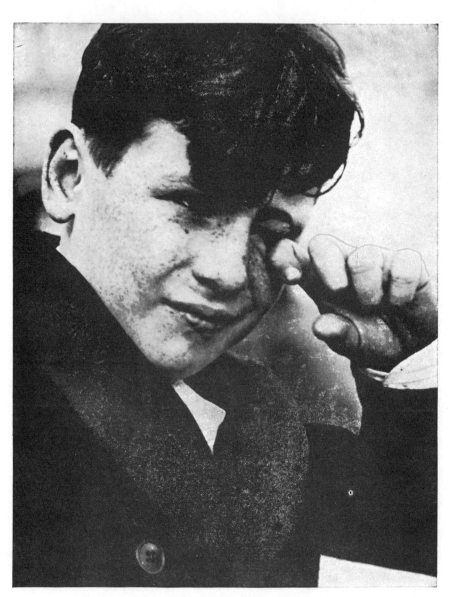

Wrong method of removing foreign body from eye.
(Courtesy by Ewing Galloway)

PLATE XXIX

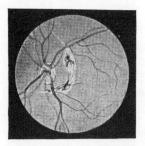

Rupture of the choroid.

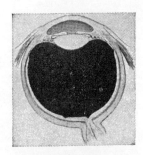

Intraocular hemorrhage with greatly increased tension. This may require enucleation on account of pain.

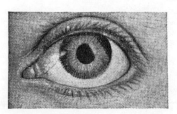

Rupture of iris and monocular diplopia. This is to be left alone. This requires very delicate operative measures. Under a conjunctival flap the cornea must be entered, the root of the iris grasped and a most delicate thread passed through it. This is anchored to the corneoscleral junction.

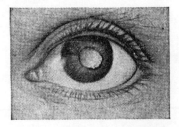

Traumatic cataract. Its management requires expert opinion based on considerable experience. An eye physician should be seen at once.

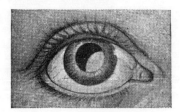

Dislocation of the lens. Often no treatment at all is necessary. If the eye becomes irritable or double vision results, an eye physician should be consulted. Treatment requires very delicate operative procedure.

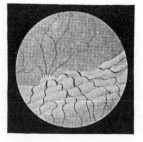

Detachment of the retina. This also requires very precise operative interference. New technic recently developed has improved the prognosis considerably.

PLATE XXX

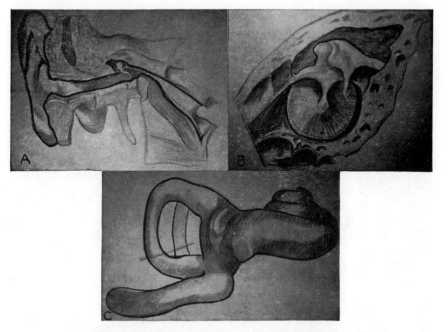

A. The outer ear, the middle ear and the Eustachian tube. The sound waves, caught by the shell-like outer ear, are carried through a canal to the drum in the middle ear, where the Eustachian tube equalizes pressure on the drum.

B. In the middle ear are located the drum and the ear bones, the entrance to the mastoid, and the Eustachian tube, which leads to the back of the nose. Closure of the Eustachian tube and infection of the middle ear are common causes of impaired hearing.

C. The inner ear is a spiral organ lined with different sized hairs like piano strings, for receiving the different pitches of sound. Connected with this organ (see diagram) are three small semi-circular canals by means of which we maintain our balance.

PLATE XXXI

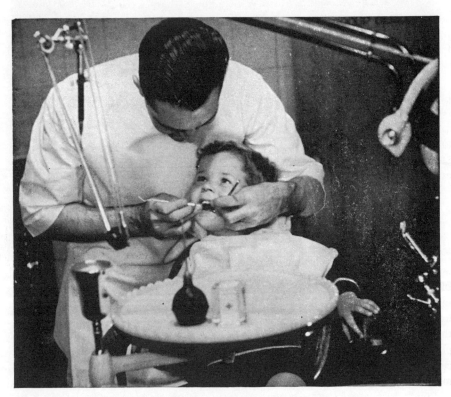

Every child should have his teeth cleaned regularly.

PLATE XXXII

defined systemic impairments productive of degenerative diseases and fatigue. The specified conditions, with the exception of chilblains, may, with propriety, be regarded as accidental injuries.

"Hex"—hexamethylenetetramine—is known in medicine as urotropin; it was formerly used in the curing of rubber. It is now used in molding plastic objects, such as in bakelite molding. It is a source of severe dermatitis, which occurs more frequently in summer.

Hydrogen is an explosive gas with a low degree of toxicity. It is a simple asphyxiant, causing the displacement of oxygen. It is also a slight irritant to the eyes and is found about plating vats, battery charging, etc.

Hydrogen sulphide, a highly toxic gas widely distributed in industries, such as tanneries, artificial silk mills, and oil fields, is a source of ulcerated eyes. The upper limit of tolerance for this gas is only 20 ppm of air. Its odor is characteristic and any general concentration that imparts odor may be regarded as dangerous.

Some complex compounds of *hydroquinone* eliminate all skin pigmentation after extended contact. The skin of the Negro may become albino-like white. No injury is known, the damage being cosmetic and usually temporary.

The manufacture of many *insecticidal* agents designed for use in households and elsewhere involves hazardous exposure. Among others, potentially dangerous agents are chrysanthemum buds, formalin, ethylene dichloride, hydrocyanic acid, etc.

Kerosene is a petroleum distillate with a higher boiling point than benzine. The toxic properties are the same as those for benzine, only less dangerous because of a higher boiling point.

Lead constitutes a foremost occupational disease danger, with potential exposure in no less than two hundred different industries. Practically all forms of lead are poisonous, although the less soluble compounds constitute less dangerous hazards. This substance may enter the body through inhalation of dust, ingestion of dust, or paste (such as lead in oil), the drinking of fluid, such as lead-bearing drinking water; some organic lead compounds are absorbed through the skin. Minute traces, such as 1.5 mg. daily, may produce lead poisoning as a result of cumulative properties. Some persons are far less susceptible than others to lead. The principal lesions are found in the neuromuscular system, circulatory system, gastro-intestinal tract, and brain.

Lime, chemically known as calcium oxide, may produce local burns of every degree of severity. These burns are deep, leading to tenacious eschars, which delay healing. Lime may contain impurities, including arsenic, that give rise to poisoning characteristic of these impurities.

Litharge is a form of lead oxide, much used in storage battery manufacture. The poison that may result from this substance is similar to that caused by other forms of lead.

Manganese is a metal associated in the ore form with zinc, lead, etc. Manganese enters the body primarily as a dust through inhalation and ingestion. After several months of exposure those who become affected gradually develop a deterioration of the central nervous system leading to permanent, irreparable paralysis. Patients develop masklike faces, become clumsy in all motions of the body, are unable to stop while in motion, and are permanently disabled. Manganese dust has been described as the cause of chemical pneumonia. This may be true in Europe, but is little known in the United States.

Meerschaum is a complex magnesium silicate. Mining and the shaping of articles from meerschaum lead to dusts that create a fibrosis of the lung tissues, similar to that from talc and possibly ashes too.

Mercury poisoning is one of the oldest occupational diseases, which has been well described by Ramazzini (1700), although he was not the first writer to discuss this subject. Both mercury and its compounds are the source of the poisoning. These intoxicants may enter the body through the skin, by inhalation, or by ingestion. No less than two hundred occupations provide exposure to mercury or its compounds or both. Outstanding manifestations are salivation, gastro-intestinal inflammation, urinary changes, skin ulceration, neuromuscular lesions, particularly tremors, and mental depression.

Mesothorium is a disintegration product of thorium, between thorium and radiothorium. This term, however, is applied to extensive series of similar bodies, such as thorium X, thoron, etc. Activity of commercial mesothorium is due to the presence of radium mesothorium I and its transformation products, alpha, beta, and gamma emanations.

Methyl alcohol, also designated by such terms as methanol, wood alcohol, Columbian spirits, wood naphtha, and wood spirits, may be made synthetically from the combination of carbon monoxide (or carbon dioxide) and hydrogen, under conditions of high pressure and temperature. The natural product is derived from wood distillation. Both the natural and the synthetic products are highly toxic. The threshold of toxicity is near the concentration of five hundred parts of vapor per million parts of air. Methyl alcohol may enter the body through the skin, by inhalation, and by ingestion. Characteristic lesions are optic atrophy, nephritis, toxic degeneration of the liver, gastro-intestinal, and pulmonary tract inflammation.

Methyl chloride is employed as a refrigerant and as such has been responsible for a number of cases of poisoning. Due to the fact that methyl chloride appears to decompose into wood alcohol in the body, the clinical manifestations are the same as those of methyl alcohol poisoning. Gross exposure leads to a primary intoxication, with death from narcosis. Known industrial accidents in hotels, apartment houses, etc., have been of the acute narcotic form. Death by methyl chloride from refrigerator leaks is well established.

Methyl violet is an aniline dye used in making indelible pencils. There is considerable variation in constituency of dyes termed methyl violet. This agent is especially toxic to the tissues of the eye. Necrosis of the cornea of the eye may readily be produced by flakes of indelible pencil lead material entering the eye. Puncture wounds from indelible pencils are healed with difficulty.

Mica is the name given various siliceous minerals, and dusts therefrom in any of its forms are siliceous. Silicatosis may be induced if the exposure to concentrated dust is prolonged. Mechanical injury of the skin from mica particles has long been recognized. Among other industrial uses, mica is employed in electrical insulation factories and in stove foundries.

Narcissus bulbs, which so closely resemble onions, contain a deadly alkaloid named narcissin. The eating of narcissus bulbs has caused deaths from the action of narcissin. Industrially, the only harm known to arise is a skin disease, which also is attributed to the narcissin.

The toxicity of *nickel* is often mentioned but rarely proved. Workers in nickel-plating departments truly develop divers intoxications, but in many instances these may be attributed to the adjuvants in plating departments rather than to nickel itself. The so-called nickel rash is a term covering practically all forms of dermatitis from whatever source arises around nickel-plating works. Nickel spectacle frames may cause a dermatitis on the wearer.

Nickel carbonyl is a clear, pale straw-colored liquid which boils at a temperature of 43° C. This salt is quite volatile and possesses toxic properties. In the milder forms of poisoning workers suffer from headache, giddiness, unsteady gait, nausea, and at times dyspnœa, which symptoms quickly disappear upon removal to fresh air. Severe poisoning is manifested by dyspnœa, which after a lapse of 12 to 36 hours is increased, accompanied by cyanosis, a rise in temperature with coughing, and with more or less bloodstained expectoration. The action of the heart is increased but otherwise normal. Delirium of varying types is generally present. Fatal termination of a case takes place usually from the fourth to the eleventh day of illness.

Nitrobenzene (oil of mirbane), an intermediate in the formation of aniline, may produce local skin burns, systemic disease from skin absorption, and intoxication by inhalation. Manifestations are weakness, loss of appetite, burning sensation of skin, abnormal sensation, anxiety state, reeling gait, stammering speech, abnormal reflexes, and convulsions. Later these may be followed by paralyses, amblyopia, brown-colored blood, methemoglobin, and in chronic cases yellow skin. Still later degeneration of red corpuscles and condition of hematoporphyrin are manifested. It is frequently fatal.

Nitrocellulose in its many forms is believed to be relatively harmless. Danger may arise from the many chemicals employed in its manufacture. It is possible that the coatings applied to nitrocellulose for special purposes, such as waterproofing, may be harmful.

Nitrogen oxides represent a series including the nitric, the dioxide, the teroxide, etc. High concentrations such as 100 ppm may cause pulmonary edema. These oxides may be produced in connection with arc welding and less so in torch welding. Nitrous oxide is the well known laughing gas anesthetic.

Nitroglycerin is responsible for "dynamite head," a condition well known to blasters. The characteristic picture of nitroglycerin action is an intolerable headache associated with a rapid pulse. The keeping of a small portion of dynamite, or other explosive, about the person, perpetuates the tolerance, which apparently is readily established. Enough nitroglycerin may adhere to the clothes of explosive workers to bring about nitroglycerin harm to other persons in their homes. When nitroglycerin explodes, toxicity from the resulting gas is not due to nitroglycerin but to products of combustion.

Nitrous chloride is a highly irritating and asphyxiating gas, possessing insidious delayed action leading to pulmonary edema and respiratory tract inflammation. This gas is highly explosive, notwithstanding which fact it is somewhat extensively used in industry.

Nitrous gases or oxides are frequently encountered in industry such as in arc or torch welding. Of the series, nitric oxide is probably the most toxic, but as such is seldom found. Nitrogen dioxide is the more stable form, but even this in the presence of moisture is changed over into nitrous and nitric acid. The threshold of danger begins at about 100 ppm, but many published standards are at lower levels, such as 40 or even 10 ppm.

Phosgene or carbonylchloride is used as a chemical warfare agent as well as in industry. Its harmful action is apparently limited to the lungs, respiratory tract, and the blood stream, with secondary cardiac impairment. Violent lung inflammation develops with edema, later followed by necrosis of the lung tissue. Death frequently occurs. Lesser exposure may lead to minor degrees of impairment, as mentioned above, which eventuate in emphysema, bronchitis, bronchiectasis, and dysfunction of the heart.

Phosphorus, because of its toxicity, is not employed to any great extent in the United States at the present time. It is utilized, however, in the manufacture of fireworks, in the making of phospho-bronze, and in the chemical industry. White or yellow phosphorus is severely toxic. Susceptibility to poisoning varies. Red phosphorus is essentially free from toxicity. Phosphorus primarily acts upon the bones, leading to necrosis and periostitis. The common site of this bone affection is the jaw, entry of the phosphorus being made by way of carious teeth. Soft tissues in the region of the bone become involved as a secondary process. Phosphorus necrosis is a continuous process and may result in deformity or death.

Extensive exposure to *phosphureted hydrogen* leads to prompt death without symptoms indicative of phosphorus poisoning. Symptoms are shortness of breath, marked gastro-intestinal irritation with vomiting and diarrhea, prostration, tremors, and finally active convulsions and death from respiratory failure. Long continued lesser exposure may lead to bone changes, nephritis, etc. Phosphureted hydrogen constitutes an insidious hazard in the manipulation of ferrosilicon, etc.

Recent advances in the field of insect control include the use of *organic phosphates,* examples of which are hexaethyl-tetraphosphate (HETP), tetraethyl-pyrophosphate (TEPP), which is the active toxic ingredient in HETP, and parathion, also known as Thiophos and Vapophos. These products are rapidly absorbed through the intact skin or by inhalation of their vapor or dust. Symptoms of poisoning are headache, nausea, vomiting, dizziness, abdominal cramps, and constriction of the pupils of the eye. Manifestations of severe poisoning are a feeling of tightness in the chest, diarrhea, difficulty in breathing, twitching of the muscles, convulsions, or loss of consciousness. Poisoning can be prevented by proper attention to safe methods of handling. Contacts of bare skin must be avoided, and natural rubber gloves must be worn. Material that gets on the skin should be quickly removed with large amounts of soap and water. Cleanliness of clothing and skin is necessary and repellent garments where drenching of the clothing is possible. Adequately designed respirators may be necessary.

Picric acid or trinitrophenol enters the body through skin absorption, by inhalation, and by ingestion of dusts. The commonest lesion is a dermatitis (picric itch). This may be brought about by use of picric acid and picrates. In addition to the dermatitis, there may be yellow pigmentation of the skin suggesting jaundice, gastro-intestinal disturbance with pain, degeneration of the blood, nephritis, and degeneration of the liver.

Putty commonly contains ground whiting and linseed oil, but rarely lead compounds. Colored putties may contain skin-irritating dyes.

Pyrene is a trade name for one brand of carbon tetrachloride. When decomposed by heating, pyrene may give rise to phosgene vapors.

Quinine compounds have been the cause of a dermatitis among pharmaceutical workers; also of edema of eyelids with conjunctivitis and itching. It is a low-grade respiratory irritant.

In the manufacture of rayon and other artificial silks, many harmful agents may be utilized as intermediates and adjuvants. The outstanding objectionable agent is *carbon bisulphide.*

Rotogravure ink has been associated with dermatitis. Paranitraniline red or a similar substance is probably the active agent leading to that type of dermatitis. Readers of freshly printed rotogravure newspapers may become affected.

Sandstone is a silica-bearing rock with a high free silica content. It is known as a source of silicosis.

Sealing wax of various brands may differ in composition. It may contain resinous materials from coal tar or petroleum or from vegetable matter. At times it is colored with arsenic. Turpentine and other harmful solvents have been employed.

Sewer gas may contain hydrogen sulphide, carbon monoxide, carbon dioxide, any of which may lead to disasters.

Shellac itself, which is an Indian resin, is probably nontoxic, but may be a skin sensitizer. The substances in which it is dissolved may be poisonous, and in the past have caused many scores of poisonings and some deaths. As a solvent, wood alcohol has been the source of blindness and death.

Free silica, in any of its many forms, when taken into the body through the respiratory tract, in sufficient quantity, slowly leads to a dusty lung disease known as silicosis. Silicosis is probably the result of chemical action of the siliceous materials. Cases may be produced within less than one year of exposure, but the usual case requires several years to develop. Patients may complain of difficulty in breathing, of pain in the chest, of coughing, but often the disease is symptomless until far advanced. No treatment is efficacious. Tuberculosis is a common concomitant. This disease is encountered among workers in granite and sandstone quarrying, in stone dressing, in mining, and in foundries among many other industries.

Silver, or its salts, as used in industry, significantly is harmful from just one standpoint, and that is that it produces black deposits within the skin, a condition known as argyrosis.

Sulphur dioxide is the commonest household refrigerant, with the exception of ice. It is also used extensively in a variety of industries or is the product of other materials. Twenty parts per million of air will produce some irritation; fifty parts per million is dangerous. Injury chiefly is limited to the respiratory tract and to reflex actions. Contrary to common belief, tolerance for sulphur-dioxide action is not established. Chronic bronchitis and other persistent manifestations are well known. It may also produce acidosis.

Talc is magnesium silicate. As such, it is capable of producing fibrosis of the lungs.

Tannic acid may attack the unbroken skin and may partially tan the skin. A dermatitis is universally present among hide handlers in the tanning yard using the tannic acid process. When the skin is broken, deep undermining ulcers may arise. In low percentages tannic acid solutions constitute a valuable medicament for the treatment of skin burns.

Tar is a general term applied to a variety of substances derived from wood, coal, or petroleum. Tar cancer is a rare affection among persons exposed. Skin diseases and irritation of the respiratory tract are common.

Tetraethyl lead is an organic lead compound utilized as an antiknock substance in motor vehicles. The opportunities for intoxication are largely limited to the manipulation of this substance in its manufacture. It is one of the few forms of lead entering the body through the skin. Apparently this form of lead has a special predilection for brain tissues, leading to encephalitis.

Thallium, a toxic metal, forms salts which are useful in the making of rat poisons, in the preparation of depilatories and other pharmaceuticals, in disinfectants, in dye manufacture, and in lead alloys. When taken into the body it causes loss of hair, optic atrophy, distorted color vision, lymphocytosis, etc. On skin contact, hair is destroyed and possibly through skin absorption the other actions mentioned may arise.

The *tin* industry is attended by some exposures in mining, smelting, and refining, but these are probably due to impurities, heat, etc., rather than to any toxic properties of tin itself under industrial conditions. At the present time scant proof of the toxicity of tin exists, but some compounds of tin may be injurious.

The *tobacco* industry affords a number of opportunities for injury. Tobacco workers may acquire nicotine poisoning, but rarely do due to the development of a tolerance for this substance as does the tobacco smoker. Tuberculosis and other respiratory disease rates are reported as high in this industry, but a direct causative connection is not established. Arsenic is a potential danger from its use as an insecticide during the growing period. In the curing of tobacco, carbon dioxide is given off which may lead to asphyxiation. Cyanides are sometimes used for tobacco disinfection. High temperatures and humidities characterize certain departments.

Toluene (toluol) is closely related to benzene. It is advocated as a substitute for benzol, owing to lesser capacity for intoxication. It is more active as a narcotic agent than benzene, but less frequently produces chronic intoxication. When poisoning occurs, the clinical picture is similar to that of benzene poisoning.

Trichlorethylene is a chlorinated hydrocarbon akin in action to carbon tetrachloride.

Pure gum spirits of *turpentine* is less dangerous than other types, such as wood or steam distilled or naphtha extracted turpentine. It may, however, produce irritation of the skin and mucous membranes, gastritis, salivation, genito-urinary manifestations, etc.

Vanadium is a metal of restricted industrial use. Its salts find use in photography and in the manufacture of steels. Toxicity has been attributed especially to the trioxid. The outstanding manifestations are marked irritation of the respiratory tract, eventuating in hemorrhage, rapid loss of weight, nephritis, optic atrophy, and general condition simulating nervous breakdown. This condition is so rare as to be open to question as to its existence.

White damp is a term used by miners for carbon monoxide in mines. Black damp is ordinarily carbon dioxide. Stink damp is usually hydrogen sulphide.

Xylene (xylol) is chemically related to benzene (benzol). It is more toxic than benzene in producing acute narcosis, and is less toxic in the production of chronic conditions. The clinical disease produced, although rarely, is similar to that of benzene poisoning.

Industrial *zinc* is probably nontoxic. Recently produced zinc oxide, as in the manufacture of brass or in galvanizing, may lead to zinc chills, also termed brass chills, brass workers' ague, etc. The condition is characterized by great thirst, marked chilling with or without elevated temperature, eventuating in deep sleep with profound physical depression. Zinc is not involved in any chronic form of poisoning.

Zinc chloride is much used in wood preservation as a fire repellent and fungicide. It is associated with the production of dermatitis. Zinc sulphate produces marked alimentary tract inflammation, culminating, in severe cases, in ulceration of the stomach or duodenum.

All of the above items are but examples of industry's injurious work materials. Several hundred additional items might have been listed.

CHAPTER XXV

The Skin
HOWARD T. BEHRMAN, M.D.

MANY PEOPLE think of the skin as a sort of envelope into which the rest of the body has been stuffed. This is far from true, as the skin is essentially one of the most important parts of the body and performs many functions which are necessary for both life and health. This complex and sensitive organ shows many different variations, depending upon age, sex, climate, and race; and, in addition, it shows considerable changes in different parts of the same person. For example, in some parts of the body such as the lips and the eyelids, the skin is soft, smooth, and exquisitely sensitive. On the hands and feet, as well as over the surfaces of the joints, the skin is tough and dry and sometimes even on the rough side. The skin is a useful part of the body. In its far-flung stretches, there are millions of minute factories at work producing oil, sweat, hair, and nails. So too, there are numerous waste-disposal stations where busy little cells and groups of cells are at work getting rid of waste products, bringing blood to the surface of the skin so that the temperature will be regulated, helping absorb or neutralize various substances from the surface, and trying to protect the skin from the ravages of various bacteria, chemicals, and all sorts of external irritants. In many ways the skin is a mirror of what is going on inside the body and will often show changes along its surface which indicate the presence of some internal illness. These illnesses vary from the minor ones, such as a sore throat beginning with a fever blister, all the way to the covering of the entire body by the ugly spots of smallpox. The skin plays a part of great importance as far as the human being is concerned, and the following paragraphs will show how these activities are specifically regulated.

STRUCTURE OF THE SKIN

The skin consists of two main divisions, an outer layer called the epidermis, or outer skin, and an inner layer called the corium or true skin. The corium is a sort of meshwork support for all the important little organs, blood vessels, and nerves which supply and nourish the skin. Underneath the skin itself is a third layer called the subcutaneous tissue, which also contains additional fat and fibrous supporting structures.

THE OUTER LAYER OF THE SKIN (EPIDERMIS)

The epidermis, or cuticle, is made up also of several layers. The main layers are the corneous or horny outer layer, and the mucous or deepest layer of the epidermis. The corneous or horny layer is the very top covering of the skin, and it is composed of practically lifeless cells which are being constantly shed from the surface as new cells from below move up and take their place. Its chief function is the protection of the skin. The deep or mucous layer is the most important layer of the epidermis because it is the living one and the one which produces new cells. It is composed of several layers of cells which are many-sided and joined to each other by tiny bridges of cell substance under which flow minute canals. As the cells in the deep mucous layer grow, and push those above them toward the surface, the top cells become flatter, dryer, and more shriveled in appearance. When they finally reach the surface, they are dried, horny, and wrinkled and are constantly shed from the surface as new cells from below take their place. The other two layers of the epidermis are called the clear layer and the granular layer. Their functions are relatively minor in importance.

The pigment cells, which are responsible for the color of the skin, are also produced in the mucous layer of the epidermis. These cells may vary from merely a few in number, or none at all, as in the albino, to the concentration of many cells heavily laden with pigment as in the darkly colored races. Pigment cells may also be found in the inner layer or corium of the skin. This is especially true in the colored races, in whom the pigment cells are more highly developed and the corium itself is deeply pigmented.

THE INNER LAYER OF THE SKIN (CORIUM)

The inner or connective tissue layer of the skin is its most important part. It is composed of parallel fibers forming a meshwork support for the blood vessels, nerves, oil and sweat glands, and hair which travel through it. As seen under the microscope, the line between the outer and inner layers of the skin is not a straight one because of the presence of little nipple-like prominences in the corium called papillae. These little structures dovetail into depressions on the under surface of the epidermis, thus serving to fasten the two layers together securely and increasing their flexibility. The papillae in general have two main functions, depending upon their origin. One type of papilla carries blood vessels and is responsible for the nutrition of the skin and all its minute parts. The other type of papilla carries various specialized types of nerves and is responsible for the feelings of touch, pressure, pain, and any of the many other sensations that originate in the skin. Even the sensation of tickling has a special type of nerve ending which notifies its owner that he should laugh. Estimates indicate that there are approximately five thousand of these specialized papillae to the square inch of skin surface. In addition to the papillae, the true skin is composed primarily of bundles of stringy fibers arranged in the form of an intricate mesh and forming sort of a crisscross network. This network runs directly into the third layer or sub-cutaneous tissue, and in many places is composed of a great deal of fat as it gets farther down in the skin. These layers form a comfortable cushion on which the skin rests and protects the delicate glands, vessels, and nerves from injury. In addition, it also gives the rounded appearance to the body which adds so much to beauty, provided it is not too rounded. Scattered through these layers are also found many little elastic fibers, which act like a layer of rubber bands in the skin. These fibers are primarily responsible for the elasticity of the skin, and if these fibers are numerous and healthy, the skin is likely to be smooth and have a good tone. If they are few in number, or shriveled because of age, the skin becomes saggy and wrinkled. Because of these fibers, the skin can accommodate itself to a moderate degree of stretch-ing, such as occurs during exercise, and still return to its original smooth con-dition. However, there are limits to which the skin can be stretched, and this is demonstrated during certain states such as pregnancy, when the elastic fibers often stretch to the breaking point, and subsequently return almost to normal, leaving the white lines often seen on the abdomen of women who have had children. It is also common these days to see these white lines in the skin of women who have undergone periods of rapid reducing. The skin which had been stretched to the extreme, as in the very obese, cannot accom-modate itself rapidly enough to the contraction of the fatty layer and hangs in apronlike folds. A similar process is in operation as we get older and the skin loses its elasticity, so that normal lines deepen and wrinkles become more apparent and noticeable.

Advancing age is inevitably associated with a certain degree of wrinkling of the skin. The only way really to escape wrinkles would be never to move a muscle in the face. Even such pleasant functions as eating and drinking re-quire the use of facial muscles, and the inevitable appearance of lines and wrinkles in the face. This brief survey of the anatomical reasons for wrin-kling and aging of the skin will not suffice to deter women from spending mil-lions of dollars a year in attempts to lessen or minimize the ravages of time.

SWEAT GLANDS

The sweat glands are corkscrew-shaped tubes beginning in the true skin and spiraling up to the cutaneous surface. Their openings in the skin surface are called pores, and literally millions of them are scattered over the surface of the skin, especially on the palms and soles. The larger sweat glands are found in the armpits and are primarily responsible for various types of body odor. The secretion of sweat is one of the most important functions performed by the skin.

SEBACEOUS OR OIL GLANDS

The sebaceous or oil glands are composed of a number of baggy pouches grouped together, along the sides of the hair shafts. They produce an oily, semifluid material of a whitish or yellow color, which is excreted directly along the upper part of the hair follicle onto the skin surface. This semisolid, greasy secretion lubricates the hairs and the skin surface, protecting it in part from all external agents and keeping it in a constant well-oiled state. As we grow older the oil glands function less and less adequately; for this reason the skin becomes dried with advancing age. Several million glandular oil factories are scattered over the body surface; the largest of these are found in the free margins of the eyelids, where they are called Meibomian glands. Beneath the sebaceous gland is a small involuntary muscle which is also associated with the hair follicle. During periods of stress or fear this muscle squeezes the gland and at the same time is responsible for the erection of the hair. Thus your hair can actually stand on end, as all of us who have had "goose flesh" at some time or other are well aware.

SKIN TEXTURE

The normal texture of the skin is smooth and fine, because the scales covering it are minute, oiled, and covered with delicate hair. The skin may be coarse, like that on many noses, because of large sebaceous ducts. Often faces that are scarred are referred to as having large pores. This is incorrect, as the scars are actually little pits unrelated to the pore openings. On the skin, as best seen on the palms and soles, there are many fine ridges arranged in patterns which are characteristic for each person and are often used for identification (fingerprints). On these ridges the sweat pores open. Coarser, less regular lines are caused by motion and stretching of the skin with eventual folding of the skin along these lines. Still larger lines are caused partly by motion and partly by the attachment of the skin to the underlying tissue about the joints and under the breasts. Dimples are caused by the attachment of the skin to the muscles of expression, thus drawing in the skin at this point when they contract. It almost seems a shame to break down the bare anatomical reasons for a dimple, but there you have it!

COLOR OF THE SKIN

The color of the skin depends upon the amount of pigment in the lower layer of the epidermis and by the color of the neighboring blood and the size of the surface blood vessels. Through the skin of the average blonde (if there is such a woman as an *average* blonde), the red color shows diffusely as through ground glass, with just enough effect of the pigment to make the color creamy. Brunettes have even more pigment, and other races than the white race have still more, until in the black race the red color of the blood is largely concealed. In many instances the skin may be quite light at the time of birth and become progressively darker with age. As is well known, the babies of the colored race are born with a comparatively light skin, and the pigmentation becomes progressively darker during the first few months of life, until the final skin color has been attained. In a few instances, when experiments have been performed with skin grafts, it has been found that a white man's skin grafted to the skin of a Negro will rapidly become dark and vice-versa.

The color of the skin may be temporarily affected by flushing or blushing of the skin surface. This momentary change in color is due to the opening of the small blood vessels near the surface and a flooding of the skin itself with blood. This may occur as a result of exposure to excessive heat or as a result of some local inflammatory change. However, the skin is so readily influenced by the emotions that even a mild degree of embarrassment will result in temporary redness of the face. Now you know what the humorists meant when they said that "your skin is showing." The skin reacts so vigorously to an emotion that we can see an immediate redness of the skin as a result of embarrassment, "goose flesh" as a result of fear, excessive sweating of the palms and under the arms prior to an interview with the boss or that quarrel with your in-laws, and so on down the line. The unusual person can develop a poker face. These examples illustrate how the skin readily mirrors not only the health and functions of the body but also of the mind.

NUTRITION OF THE SKIN

The skin feeds on the blood which seeps into its layers from the small blood vessels in the corium or true skin. These blood vessels also bring all nutritional necessities to the glands, the hair follicles, and the papillae. In the papillae the smallest blood vessels, which are called capillaries, exude a serum which passes into the little canals of the epidermis and circulates between the cells. As it circulates it gives up its nutritive substances and picks up the waste products, and flows down again to the papillae where it finds its way back to the blood vessels or lymph vessels, and is carried away. From this description of the structure of the skin it is obvious that food for the skin does not come from its outer surface. The skin receives its nourishment from the blood stream and from the essential ingredients of the blood stream. There is actually no such thing as a skin food because, like every other part of the body, the skin feeds on what is brought to it by the blood stream. Yet millions of dollars are spent yearly for nourishing creams, skin foods, and the like, under the mistaken impression that these preparations feed the skin and are responsible for its health and beauty. It would be almost as unintelligent to attempt to increase knowledge by rubbing the head with some learned treatise as it is to attempt to feed the skin from the outside.

THE FUNCTIONS OF THE SKIN

The skin has many uses and important functions. In general, these include the protection of the rest of the body from injury, to minimize the absorption of dangerous substances, to act as an organ of sensation and touch, to excrete waste products, and to regulate heat. Besides this, some of its nerve organs are connected with sexual gratification and other physiological stimuli.

The chief function of the skin is protection. A dry skin is a good insulator against all but high-voltage electrical currents. Insulation against body cold is aided by the contraction of the tiny muscles of the hair follicles, which lift the skin to form "goose flesh" and at the same time close off the surface pores and blood vessels, thus preventing the loss of the body's heat.

The prevention of evaporation of the body fluids is also of great importance. This provision against drying out made it possible, millions of years ago, for living beings to emerge from the sea and risk the drying effect of air, a bitter enemy of life.

Not less important than the loss of fluids from within is the prevention of the entrance of water and other harmful substances from without. The normal skin is almost entirely waterproof, but when its surface has been injured, water is readily absorbed. Usually, however, only small quantities of water filter through, and when this happens the cells of the outer layer "drink" it up and swell in the process. Have you ever weighed yourself before and after a long tub bath? The change in weight is due to the extra fluid absorbed by the cells in the top layer of the skin.

The skin can protect itself during long-continued slight exposure to mild acids but not to prolonged contact with a strong acid. Against alkalies the protection is only fair, for the alkalies soften the horn cells and, together with other chemicals of a fat-removing nature, they can reduce the resistance of the skin and favor penetration.

Radiation of heat is one of the chief functions of the skin, protecting it against the harmful effects of fever. In hot weather or during a fever the surface blood vessels become opened or dilated, thereby increasing the amount of blood exposed to the cooling air, and at the same time increasing the production of sweat which helps in the evaporation of heat. The production of sweat is also one of the important functions of the skin. Its value as an eliminant of waste products from within the body is slight, for only volatile bodies are eliminated in the perspiration. The odor of the sweat is the chief source of body odor, now popularized as "B.O.," about which so much is said by the advertising profession. The odor is due partly to these volatile substances from within and partly to the fatty acids in the skin. While sometimes unpleasant, giving the unfortunate possessor much mental distress, cases are also on record of a pleasant, violet-like odor of the sweat, but don't count on it! Recently there has been a great fanfare concerning the use of chlorophyll to lessen body odors. This harmless product does seem to cut down some mild odors but will not really lessen the obnoxious odor of large amounts of garlic and similar dietary indiscretions.

Under ordinary circumstances, absorption through the outer skin is slight even for greasy substances. By friction, fats may be forced into the hair follicles and absorbed, carrying other substances with them. The quantity of such absorbed substances is so small that while it may be valuable when strong medicines are applied to the skin, for the purpose of "skin food," it is too slight to be of consequence and must be redigested by the internal organs before the skin can use it. The popular idea that oils applied to the surface can feed the skin is a fallacy. Oils or creams thus applied only serve a useful purpose by keeping the skin supple, preventing scaling and cracking, and maintaining the resistance of abnormally dry skins, even though small portions of these creams or their ingredients may be absorbed.

The nerves of the skin protect the body against harm by warning us of the dangers of excessive heat or cold or sharpness. They also help us to become acquainted with the world about us, and provide one of our sources of pleasure in the feel of marble, fine woods, smooth skin, velvet, and the like.

By pigment formation the skin can protect the body successfully against exposure to ordinary sunlight and ultraviolet rays. The skin cannot protect itself from overexposure to X-rays and the rays of radium, and its efforts, though often manifested by pigmentation, are of no avail because these rays penetrate the pigmented skin as easily as they do the non-pigmented. And when it comes to the atomic bomb, the skin has no protective defenses whatsoever. If compensatory changes of evolution continue, we can conceive of centuries of exposure to atomic radiations resulting in a thick, bombproof skin if the human race has not been wiped out by some type of chain reaction.

Besides these more or less obvious functions of the skin, it has also the ability to clear its surface of germs within a short time. The mechanism of this action is not completely understood. Against some bacteria the skin is powerless; it cannot rid itself of them. Even against these germs the normal skin is an important first line of defense. Further, if germs do gain entrance to the skin, whether from without or through the blood stream, the normal skin can produce chemical substances which may inhibit their growth or wholly destroy them. Of course, some agents of infection are too strong to be controlled in this way, and the resistance of the skin is futile. These efforts of the skin to protect itself and the whole organism against infection often take the form of an inflammatory reaction in the skin. This skin reaction is the basis for many of the tests used to develop or determine resistance or immunity to tetanus, tuberculosis, diphtheria, scarlet fever, or other infectious diseases. Various skin tests have also been devised to detect allergic causes in asthma, hay fever, hives, and eczema. They are all of more or less value in diagnosis. Thus the skin has become a useful bureau of information, ready to report on the state of affairs in relation to protection against these diseases or on the presence of unusual sensitivities to organisms, chemicals, drugs, and the like, whenever requested to do so by the physician. Here again, we can understand why it is often referred to as the mirror of the body. In addition to its ability to protect against infection, the skin produces the vitamin (vitamin D) that protects against and cures rickets. This explains in part the beneficial effects of sun baths and ultraviolet light baths, particularly for infants.

Of course, there are still many functions connected with the skin about whose purpose we can only speculate. For example, we know that the secretion of the oil glands or sebum is of primary value in keeping the skin normally lubricated and also to supply a small amount of lubrication for the hairs. And yet recent work has shown that some of the secretions from these oil glands may become concentrated in certain abnormal conditions of the scalp and may actually result in the loss of hair, so that too much of some secretions may do harm rather than good. Another function of the oily secretion is to prevent the absorption of any toxic or poisonous material through the surface of the skin. Accordingly, if we wish to treat a certain area of skin with some drug or medication in a grease, it is important to wash the area thoroughly to remove its normal oily secretion and thus to get penetration of the specific drug contained in the externally applied grease.

Finally, one of the most unusual and important functions of the skin is to renew itself after it has been injured. The human being cannot quite compare with the lobster which can regrow a claw after it has lost one, but the skin certainly does show remarkable powers of regeneration. Very frequently extremely extensive areas of the skin will have been lost or injured, as in an accident or a severe burn. In many instances, these areas will completely regrow without leaving a trace of the original injury. However, if the injury has been extensive and deep, the normal skin will not regrow but the area will be replaced with a different type of tissue called scar tissue. Sometimes it is necessary to help the regrowth of this tissue by performing grafts with skin taken from other parts of the body. Modern science has made great strides in this direction and even now there are many ways in which ugly and disfiguring scars can be made almost insignificant in appearance.

NUTRITION

From a general point of view, proper diet is fundamental as far as the health of the skin is concerned. Faddist regimes and so-called health diets are not essential as far as the skin is concerned. A well-balanced diet, with proper attention to balanced meals and adequate vitamin and mineral intake is of fundamental importance. As shown in the chapter on diet, certain foods are required for health.

Special diets should be avoided unless you are allergic to some particular component of a diet. There are also certain diseases in which special diets are indicated, and the skin has its share of such disorders. In the last few years there has been much research concerning the fact that the skin is often the first indicator of a serious deficiency in the diet, and much has been written concerning the rôle of vitamins in the skin health.

In the following brief survey the vitamins are considered primarily from the point of view of their internal administration related to the skin and not from external application.

VITAMIN A

When vitamin A is missing from the diet, the effect on the entire system is pronounced. Some of these effects of vitamin A deficiency are lowered resistance to infection, poor appetite, disturbed digestion, eye disease called xerophthalmia, and loss of hair. The condition of the skin is also changed in deficient states. Generally, it becomes dry, rough, and darker than normal. Small spots, resembling goose flesh, appear on the arms and thighs, and gradually spread to involve the leg, abdomen, buttocks, and neck. Sometimes these tiny lumps resemble acne. Confirmation of the diagnosis of A deficiency may be obtained by various technical means, such as the biomicroscopic examination of the eyes under slit lamp illumination. Estimation of the vitamin A level in the blood is also helpful in diagnosis. The minimum daily requirements of vitamin A are approximately 4,000 U.S.P. units. The treatment dose ranges from 10,000 to 300,000 units daily. Large amounts of vitamin A should not be taken over long periods of time without medical supervision because an excess of this vitamin may give rise to toxic manifestations. Surprisingly enough, one of these symptoms may be loss of hair.

VITAMIN B COMPLEX

Slight deficiences of this vitamin lead to a decreased appetite, fatigue, and burning sensations of the hands and feet.

Vitamin B_2 or riboflavin is well distributed in our diet, and so deficiency states are not too common. A deficiency of it leads to itching and burning of the eyes, dimness of the vision, and a sensitivity to light. The skin shows characteristic changes as a result of a deficiency of riboflavin. These changes include scaling and redness of the lips, cracks at the angles of the mouth, and an oily scale on the nose and ears. These changes about the eye and mouth have been called "sharklike" in appearance. The tongue is usually bright and red and shiny. Recent studies have shown that the vitamin may be helpful in the treatment of psoriasis. The minimum daily requirement is 2 milligrams.

Vitamin P-P, or niacin or nicotinic acid, is still another member of the B complex. A deficiency of it leads to the disease known as pellagra. In medical parlance, this disease is known to produce the three D's—dermatitis (skin rash), diarrhea (intestinal upsets), and dementia (mental changes). The victim is usually nervous, restless, and easily fatigued, and complains of vague aches and pains. The skin changes are present on the exposed parts of the body (hands and face) and vaguely suggest sunburn. The minimum daily requirement is approximately 25 milligrams.

Vitamin B_6 or pyridoxine is considered necessary to the body because of its rôle in aiding in the use of certain essential fats in the food. This may be the reason for the lessened secretion of fat from the skin when pyridoxine is given to persons with oily and greasy faces. It may even help clear up the excessive oiliness and blackhead formation of a sufferer from acne or "pimples." Nothing is known of the minimal daily requirements of this vitamin. Therapeutically, as high as 50 to 100 milligrams daily have been used.

Pantothenic acid, another part of the B complex, is of interest in view of its alleged effects on hair. Also, a deficiency of it may be a factor in the development of gray hair. This effect may occur indirectly through its effects on the glands, as its exclusion from animal diet leads to the destruction of several of the glands of internal secretion. Workers in the field have not been able to demonstrate an exact relationship between the results in animals and in human beings. Accordingly, its value in the treatment of color changes of the hair is still questionable, as is discussed subsequently under the heading of gray hair. The daily requirements are not known, although 1,000 milligrams are tolerated therapeutically.

Inositol, a little known factor of the B complex, is a substance of extreme interest to scientists engaged in the study of hair growth. Experimental investigation has shown that inositol will cure baldness in mice. This dramatic change can sometimes be produced within as short a period as three days. This definite growth response has been checked by workers in different laboratories. The relationship of inositol to human baldness is still in the investigative stage, although it has so far proved of little value. Effects produced in laboratory animals cannot be applied directly to human beings. Perhaps the future will unveil this substance or some allied drug as the direct stimulant of hair growth.

Biotin, or vitamin H, is a term employed in the past to designate a number of different substances, but it is now considered a member of the B complex. Biotin concentrates prevent a scaly rash in chicks, but its importance to the human still remains to be clarified. It has recently been studied with reference to its preventive effects in minimizing the development of cancer.

Para-aminobenzoic acid, still another B-complex factor, has also received widespread publicity as a cure for gray hair. This publicity followed the announcement that this vitamin restored the black color to the hair of rats which had become gray on a diet deficient in the substance. This is another of those unfortunate examples of the ease with which a gullible public may be misled by results obtained in animals. Well-controlled studies on human beings have failed to substantiate the claims advanced for this substance. No drugs have been discovered, as yet, which will restore gray hairs to their natural color.

Choline is the last member of the vitamin B complex of any importance at the date of the present writing. It is related to growth, the metabolism of food, and the prevention of fatty livers in animals. It is still in the investigative stage.

VITAMIN C

Lack of this vitamin is the cause of scurvy. The value of foods containing it, as being anti-scorbutic, was recognized long before the vitamin principle was known. Whalers and other ships bound on long voyages kept supplies of lime juice and lemons and potatoes aboard as preventives of scurvy. The British sailor was called a "limey" for this reason. This disease manifests itself by bleeding gums, hemorrhage into various joints, swelling, and bloody diarrhea. The skin changes are of particular interest because they are easily seen and enable the doctor to make an early diagnosis. The changes consist of red spots around the hair follicles and openings of the sweat pores. This is most common on the legs and thighs or wherever pressure exposes the extreme weakness and fragility of the small blood vessels. Irritability, lack of stamina, and retardation of growth may be due to insufficient amounts of this substance, and there also results a susceptibility to infectious diseases. The minimal daily requirement is 600 U.S.P. units.

VITAMIN D

Vitamin D is abundant in the liver of fishes, chiefly the codfish. The discovery of this vitamin disclosed the secret of rickets. This disease is characterized by enlargement of the wrists, knees, and ankles, bowed legs, and other bony changes. It is closely tied with the absorption and use of the minerals, calcium and phosphorus. Accordingly, it is of importance in the growth and development of normal teeth. A very interesting fact here is that ultraviolet rays can produce the same effect on the bodily health and growth as vitamin D; and, as a matter of fact, children suffering from rickets improve miraculously under the ultraviolet-ray therapy, provided other necessary minerals and substances are present in the body. The minimal daily requirement is 400 to 1,200 U.S.P. units.

VITAMIN E

The wide distribution of vitamin E in natural foods has led to the belief that human deficiency of this vitamin is not likely. However, it has been found to play a rôle of importance as far as repair of the skin is concerned, and it is believed of increasing importance in the treatment of certain skin diseases where the corium or true skin is involved. It has also been found of some value in the healing of ulcers of the skin and certain long-standing disorders of the fibrous or connective tissue. The normal requirements of this vitamin are unknown. It is usually prescribed in the form of mixed tocopherols.

This brief discussion of the vitamins is merely intended to show that they are of importance as far as the health of the skin is concerned. It must always be remembered that vitamins are essential to health as accessory food factors and that they are not the *only* important factors from a dietary standpoint, despite the tremendous advertising campaigns which might lead us to believe otherwise. To maintain proper health of the body and the skin, proteins carbohydrates, and fats and a number of mineral salts are also necessary. Some of the minerals of particular importance as far as the skin is concerned are calcium, phosphorus, iron, sulfur, and other substances.

INTESTINAL FUNCTION

The health of the skin is definitely influenced by the functions of the intestinal tract. Failure to eliminate waste through the bowels and absorption of toxic substance from the bowels injures the proper sanitation and nutrition of the skin. For many years great stress has been laid upon the importance of inner cleanliness to skin health. Although this is true in great measure, it must be realized that the term "constipation" is a much overworked and little understood word. A slight degree of constipation is preferable to looseness, although healthy evacuation is more important. The irritative effect of cathartics on the bowels may favor the absorption of the so-called toxic agents they are intended to eliminate. Obviously, the routine administration of laxatives is to be deplored as it leads to looseness of the stools with consequent lack of muscular effect and tone, with resultant aggravation of the very condition which it is desired to cure. Today it is known that there is little absorption of poisonous toxins if the bowel contents are solid, but that unhealthy absorption of such contents may occur when they are rendered on the soft or even loose side, and that in this state bacterial decomposition is even greater. As far as the skin is concerned, the proper functioning of the intestines is important, and this should be regulated by diet and medical guidance, rather than by the constant use of cathartics. People who take mineral oil for constipation must recognize that mineral oil depletes the body's source of vitamin A, a vitamin, as we have already learned, of considerable importance as far as the skin is concerned. Where it is essential that the mineral oil be continued, the intake of vitamin A should be considerably increased.

THE ENDOCRINE GLANDS

The last decade has witnessed great strides in the direction of knowledge of the glandular secretions and their functions as far as the skin is concerned. These glands supply substances known as hormones which have profound effects on the skin and the structures within the skin.

THYROID

If hypothyroidism develops early in life, the individual remains small; the hair becomes dry, thin, and brittle. If an adult develops hypothyroidism, the condition is usually known as myxedema. The skin develops a peculiar swollen appearance, especially over the forehead, cheeks, nose, and lips. The skin is sallow or yellowish in color and dry, coarse, and cold to the touch. The nails are thin and brittle, and sweating is much diminished. The hair tends to fall out or is short, thin, and dry. It is often entirely absent on the chin, under the arms, and around the sex organs. The outer third of the eyebrows is frequently missing.

Overactivity of the gland leads to hyperthyroidism or excessive secretion of thyroxine. This produces an increased metabolism, loss of weight (body fuel is burned up too rapidly), and a rapid pulse. In addition, excessive sweating, shortness of breath, and nervous symptoms are usually present. The latter include trembling of the hands and fingers, restlessness, fidgety motions, mental irritability, and troubled sleep. The eyes occasionally protrude and the heart may become enlarged. The skin becomes hot and flushed. The hair is usually thin and silky. The nails are frequently lined and ridged. Treatment consists of the proper use of iodine, and surgical removal. Milder cases respond to sedation and drug therapy, especially to new drugs of the thiouracil group.

PARATHYROID

These glands are small bean-shaped masses located in pairs above and below the thyroid. A deficiency of the secretion from these glands gives rise to a condition known as tetany. In this disease the nerves become irritable. The nails are ridged and brittle and the teeth show defects of the enamel. The skin may develop a peculiar hardness known as scleroderma. In animals the hair frequently falls out, and this occasionally occurs in humans.

ADRENAL

The cortex, or outer part of the adrenal glands, has a direct relationship to the skin and to hair growth. A deficiency of the secretion of the cortex produces a condition known as Addison's disease. In this disease the victim shows extreme fatigue following a slight exertion. A peculiar pigmentation often develops which first attracts the patient's friends. The degree of color ranges from a bright yellow to a bronze-brown or tan, so white persons are often mistaken for mulattoes. The pigmentation may be difficult to distinguish from "sun tan," for, in both, the color is deeper on exposed parts. The patient gradually loses weight, the blood pressure drops, and diarrhea occurs. If treatment is not instituted, death may result. Primarily, it is in conditions due to hyperfunction (overactivity) of the adrenal cortex that we see effects on the hair structures. Overactivity of this gland gives rise to a peculiar chain of symptoms. In affected people there is an increase in hair over the entire body. This hair growth may be very heavy. The eyebrows are usually bushy and thick. The skin becomes thick and the sweat glands large. It is the overfunction of this gland in children which produces the so-called "infant Hercules." These children are much taller than their age, of broad stature, great muscular development, and especially well-developed sex organs. A boy of five may require daily shaving and have the hairy chest and mature sexual organs of an adult. A girl of five may have well-developed breasts, hair around the genital region, and may even menstruate. An adult woman may show the secondary sex characteristics of a man (growth of a beard, deep voice, and flat chest). The new wonder drug, cortisone, is produced by the adrenal cortex. It has been found helpful in the treatment of certain skin diseases. It must be taken with great caution because of certain side effects. As far as the skin is concerned, these side effects include the development of acne and the growth of facial hair.

PITUITARY

In those people who suffer from an oversecretion of the anterior pituitary growth factor, in addition to their tremendous increase in size, the skin becomes dry and yellowish in color. The entire body usually shows an increased growth of hair. In individuals who show an oversecretion of the pituitary sex hormone, a peculiar group of symptoms may develop. These symptoms also appear when ACTH (one of the pituitary hormones) or cortisone is administered in the treatment of disease. These symptoms include a rapidly progressing weight increase of the face, neck, and abdomen (buffalo type). In addition, these individuals develop high blood pressure and peculiar purplish lines on the abdomen. An extreme degree of hairiness is present. In conditions due to an undersecretion of this pituitary sex hormone, the individuals are known as Fröhlich types. Pickwick's "fat boy" is an example of this disorder. The victims are fat around the face, breasts, abdomen, and hips. The skin is delicate, soft, and cool. Dryness, falling hair, and nail changes are rare. The genitals remain undeveloped and infantile. Even when maturity is reached, the men have a distinctly feminine appearance and manner. The face remains hairless, fat deposits occur about the hips, and the voice remains high-pitched.

The posterior lobe of the pituitary has various effects on the blood pressure, lungs, intestines, and kidneys, but it bears no known relationship to skin changes or hair growth.

MALE SEX GLANDS

The testes are the primary sex glands of man. They produce secretions which are responsible for the male appearance and development. They also produce the sperm cells, which are responsible for the propagation of the race following fertilization of the eggs produced by the female organs of reproduction. The secretion produced by the testes include the androgens or male sex hormones. These hormones are extremely potent, and a study of their behavior effects in animals is amusing; female canaries given male hormones sing like males, and hens crow; the social order of chickens can be manipulated, because birds receiving the hormone become very domineering and quarrelsome. A deficiency of this hormone in humans leads to retention of a high-pitched voice, reduction of hair growth, particularly around the sex organs and the chin, a slim figure, and poorly developed sex organs. The extreme form of this deficiency is evident in castrated individuals or eunuchs. It is extremely interesting to note that these people rarely if ever lose the hair from their head. Whether this fact is due to a deficiency of androgen or to other secretions contained in the testes, or through remote effects on other organs, is discussed in detail under the heading of hair growth. An excessive amount of male hormones is also considered to play a causative role in the development of acne or "pimples," and this fact must be considered when treating resistant or severe cases of this disease.

FEMALE SEX ORGANS

The ovaries are two in number and are located on each side of the lower abdomen. The ovaries usually produce one egg each month. Fertilization of the egg leads to pregnancy. The ovarian hormones are responsible for the characteristics of the female and influence the development of the breasts, uterus, and accessory female organs of reproduction. At the time of puberty these secretions lead to slight alterations in the voice, the enlargement of the breasts, and the acquisition of feminine characteristics. They also influence the development of hair under the arms and around the genitals. The average woman goes through several periods of glandular change. The first of these occurs at puberty, then at sexual maturity, and finally following the menopause or change of life. During the first cycle, an irregularity of the secretions may lead to acne of the face, chest, and back, and an increased hair growth on the face. The hair may also be affected at the time of the menopause when there is frequently an increased fall of hair from the scalp and a thinning of the individual hairs. Due to lessened activity of the oil glands, dryness of the skin may also accompany the menopause. Pregnancy may also be followed by a diffuse loss of hair, which is usually due to a temporary lack of hormones almost in the nature of a "miniature menopause." With proper treatment, this hair loss may be restored. Pregnancy may also be accompanied by an increased growth of facial hair. Certain tumors of the ovary and the adrenal cortex are frequently accompanied by masculine changes in the affected women, as shown by an increased growth of hair over the entire body but especially on the face, under the arms, and around the genitals. This is due to an excessive production of male hormones similar chemically to cortisone and ACTH, and the same changes may also be produced by these drugs.

ALLERGY (HYPERSENSITIVITY)

Many skin conditions are produced or aggravated by a peculiar idiosyncrasy to a food, a drug, or some external application. Many people show an unusual susceptibility in their reactions to various foods and develop annoying rashes on their skins if they eat these foods. The most common offenders are eggs, strawberries, fish, chocolate, and related substances. In the majority of cases these foods produce a skin reaction known as "hives" or urticaria, which shows itself as itchy, raised "bumps" frequently shifting to involve different parts of the body. This is not always the case, as there are various other forms of skin reactions to foods and drugs. Sometimes it is possible to determine the offending agent by performing so-called skin or allergy tests. The suspected agent is either injected into the skin or scratched into the surface of the skin, and the sensitivity of the individual is determined by the development of an irritative patch of skin around the tested site. These tests are not infallible, and in many instances the allergic manifestation can only be brought out by swallowing the food or actually taking the drug, rather than by the performance of skin tests. The doctor must always be on the lookout for these drug eruptions as there are many old and new drugs which are capable of producing such reactions. In the early days of penicillin therapy this wonder drug was considered completely harmless, but as time went on numerous people were found to be sensitive to penicillin in various forms. Many of the newer drugs which are constantly being discovered are heralded in the beginning as completely harmless and incapable of doing damage. As their usage continues for long periods of time, many side effects and complications are observed to develop, and the skin is often the first to show these complications.

Nervous Tension and Emotional Disorders

Many eruptions on the skin are related to nervous tension, emotional upsets, and the like. We have all become familiar with the term "psychosomatic" and recognize the fact that it means the interplay of body functions with emotional or psychic factors. At present many diseases are called psychosomatic or "nervous" which are not entitled to the use of this term. Before dismissing a skin complaint as being due to nerves or emotions, it is advisable to obtain the opinion of your doctor first. The great strides that are being made in medicine are still due to the early recognition of disease rather than dismissing it on the basis of some emotional upset. Nevertheless, relaxation and rest are helpful in the treatment of many disorders of the skin, and understanding and insight into your own emotional background is also of great benefit. We have advanced too far in the treatment of ulcers, heart disease, and similar illnesses from the standpoint of their origin along the lines of emotional difficulties ever to dismiss the subject lightly in the matter of long-standing and resistant skin conditions. Our modern daily life provides many factors of tension and strain. The nerves especially suffer from the tension under which we live, and the skin is indirectly affected by it. Where skin disturbances are associated with an accompanying emotional disturbance, the physician can be of great help in assisting the patient to express his fears and worries, and to bring them out in the open for a frank discussion and understanding of their nature. It is amazing how much benefit can be observed in some chronic skin conditions following a reassuring discussion and a helpful adjustment in a life situation.

THE CARE OF THE NORMAL SKIN

It is of importance to understand how to take care of the skin and how to apply external preparations to keep it healthy and free from disease. The measures discussed in the following paragraphs are those accepted as adequate for maintaining a healthy skin.

BATHING

Local care is, of course, of great importance to the skin. Besides the removal of grease and dirt, bathing, particularly if the bath is ended with a cold shower, has a beneficial effect on the circulation. This is accentuated by the rubbing necessary to drying, especially because of the feeling of vigor consequent on the cold shower. Frequency of bathing is an individual problem. Some find frequent bathing enervating, while on others it has the opposite effect. Some people cannot get a good reaction to cold baths and therefore should not take them. Often such persons react better to a mild application of cool water and can train themselves to the cold shower by gradual increase in the duration and decrease in the temperature of the bath. People with dry skins should not bathe frequently because constant washing removes their own meager supply of oil and merely degreases and defats a skin which desperately requires all of its own available oil supply.

The use of soap in the bath is to be regulated according to the kind of bath and the kind of skin that is being bathed, and according to the season of the year. In the summertime we perspire so profusely that soap can be used more freely by most of us. In fact, we usually start to produce more sweat and oil immediately following the bath, and there is no danger of depriving the skin of the oil necessary to its welfare. In winter, however, the skin secretes less sweat and oil, the cold air is dry, and so is the warm, overdried air of our steam-heated dwellings. Frequent bathing only serves to aggravate the dryness of the skin. The skin resents it by becoming flaky and itchy, especially after a bath. This can be corrected by limiting the use of soap during the winter months to the armpits and groin and to the parts that get the dirtiest, the hands and feet.

Some women and a few men find that their abnormally dry skins will not tolerate soap on the face at any season. The skin becomes scaly and itches and, if the irritation is carried farther, becomes red in patches, the condition known as chapping. For such people cold cream is a justifiable substitute for soap. More refreshing, however, is oatmeal water, made by boiling oatmeal for five minutes in a bag made of several layers of gauze. A handful of oatmeal should suffice in a gallon of water. It removes dirt better than plain water, taking the place of soap to a considerable degree, and can be used on some irritable skins with impunity. The introduction of sulfonated oils as soap substitutes for cleansing the skin has given us another method, valuable for those whose skins are sensitive to soap. The best of these oils are acid in reaction, as is the surface of the normal skin, and they cleanse without forming suds and without drying the skin. Those with greasy skins, however, must recognize that these methods are not for them; but that their skins are best cared for by vigorous washing with hot water and soap, followed by a cold shower.

For long periods of immersion in water, as in the use of a tub bath containing some medication intended to soothe the skin, the water temperature is best kept lukewarm. Ordinarily, both hot and cold baths are stimulating, and the greatest effect of this kind is obtained from a hot bath followed by a cold shower, which stimulates the circulation, preventing chilling and increasing resistance against infection. Rubbing the skin with the hands or the washcloth while in the water and vigorous rubbing while drying assist in obtaining this effect. The duration of the bath should be short, unless a soothing effect is desired. We are all aware of the relaxing and soothing effects of a warm bath at night. On the other hand, a short cold shower in the morning is stimulating and helps wake one up in preparation for a day of activity. Sweat baths, among which the Turkish bath is the most popular, are not essential and are, in fact, enervating. If benefit can be derived from them, they should be taken with the approval of the physician. The same rule applies to medicated baths, mud baths, and sulphur baths, for under some circumstances they may prove to be too much of a strain and should, therefore, not be taken indiscriminately. Certain types of skin conditions are made worse by excessive sweating, and this type of bathing is absolutely contraindicated in the presence of these disorders.

Open-air bathing is one of the most popular of the sports of today and of past ages, and deservedly so. At the beginning of the season care should be used to avoid too long exposure to the sun, and the same warning applies to those who go to the southern beaches during the winter. The skin, long protected from light, cannot stand much of it at first. Severe sunburn damages rather than benefits and should be avoided. This applies particularly to people with blue eyes and light complexions, inasmuch as constant exposure of such skins to strong sunlight may eventually lead to extreme dryness, warty growths, and even cancer of the skin.

SOAP

The surroundings of our present-day life, with constant exposure to the smoke and dirt of the cities, make frequent washing and the use of a good soap a necessity rather than a luxury.

As the result of the application of modern scientific research, there have been tremendous advances and changes in the formulation of soaps. A good soap must cleanse the skin thoroughly without irritation and without removing all of the skin oils. It should not be harsh nor excessively alkaline. It should preferably produce a thick creamy lather in both soft and hard water, without leaving an insoluble scum in the water. The manufacturing chemist has set his sights on the production of such a preparation, and there are several excellent soaps on the market. When fats are boiled with a solution of an alkali, they are split into glycerin and fatty acids and the latter unite with the alkali to form soap. The glycerin is a valuable by-product. Potassium hydrate forms soft soap, of which the green soap used in the hospital is the familiar example. Sodium hydrate forms hard soaps such as ordinary laundry or toilet soap. The solution of these in water is viscid, that is, it has the power of holding together, illustrated by the formation of bubbles, which are globules of air separated from the rest of the air by a film of soap. This viscid character of soapsuds enables it to emulsify the grease on the skin, carrying with it the dirt, and they both then dissolve in the water and are carried away.

In the making of soap there is always a part of the alkali not combined with the fatty acids, and this is the "free alkali" so often mentioned in connection with toilet soap. It makes the soap strong, loosening the dirt and grease so that it can better be removed. For rough work considerable free alkali is needed; but for the average skins it is desirable that the free alkali should be reduced to the minimum. Strong soap removes more fat from the skin than is good for its health and leaves it red and irritated, an easy victim to skin eruptions and infection. In good toilet soap the free alkali should not exceed ¼ of 1 per cent. For dry and delicate skins superfatted soap is made by removing as much as possible of the free alkali and adding wool fat. This does not become rancid and leaves a film upon the skin to replace that removed in washing. These superfatted soaps are only a little less efficient as cleansers than the regular soaps and are particularly recommended for infants and for older persons with dry skins.

Green soap is strong; that is, it contains a considerable amount of free alkali. The surgeon prefers it because of this fact, in order to get his hands and arms as free from germs as possible. Not uncommonly, however, he suffers from its irritating quality. Pure green soap is not green but yellow. At present most hospitals have discontinued green soap because of its harsh reactions on the skin after long periods of use. Some of the newer antiseptics, such as hexachlorophene, are even more germicidal in action, and may be incorporated in a mild soap mixture, thereby minimizing the dangers of skin irritation.

Hard water soaps are often only ordinary soaps with an excess of coconut oil. This oil enables them to form suds more readily with water containing too much calcium. Coconut oil is an ingredient of most soaps and is not harmful as long as the amount is small; but in excess it may be irritating to delicate skins.

There are now available various types of water softener. When these substances are added to hard water, they prevent the combination of calcium and soap, thus softening the water and enabling it to form soapsuds more readily. The solution of such a salt in hard water prevents the deposit on the skin of a scum which holds and protects bacteria. Thus the water softener aids in ridding the surface of the skin of infectious agents. Sodium hexametaphosphate is one of the best softening agents.

Soap is not only cleansing in its action, but actually kills most of the ordinary germs. Unfortunately, two, the typhoid bacillus and that cause of most of the boils and other skin infections, the ubiquitous staphylococcus, are able to resist it. It seems better to maintain the normal germ-killing efficiency of the skin by proper care rather than to attempt direct action upon the bacteria with antiseptics combined in soap.

The best soaps usually contain approximately 20 to 30 per cent of water. The best type of soap is a comparatively neutral form containing no more than ¼ to 1 per cent of free alkali. Transparent soaps contain more water, 25 to 35 per cent. Floating soaps also contain large amounts of water, although their brilliancy is due to the air stirred into them during their manufacture. Superfatted soaps are milder and less irritating due to the fact that the alkali has been neutralized by the addition of lanolin. A good soap need not be expensive, as the well-known brands put out by the leading manufacturers are usually priced within a reasonable range. For the average skin they are adequate. The highly perfumed soaps made up in expensive packages and given misleading names are not superior to the average inexpensive toilet soap. As a matter of fact, they are frequently less effective from the standpoint of cleansing and minimal irritation. Choose a soap adapted to your need and made by a leading manufacturer, and it should be adequate for the average skin.

POWDERS

Dusting powders and face powders are soothing, cooling, and drying, as well as protective and decorative. Each tiny particle of powder acts to increase the available surface for the evaporation of insensible perspiration, thus cooling and drying the skin. It also protects against the irritation of cold air or sunshine and the rubbing of clothing. The requirements for a good powder are that it be fine and non-irritating. Talcum is the best known and most widely used powder. It is of light weight, very fine texture, and adheres well to the skin. Zinc stearate is heavier and also a good adherent. The starches, potato, wheat, or corn, are useful but absorb moisture and swell, making them less desirable where moisture is present in any quantity. Boric acid in small amounts is often added to dusting powders for its action in deterring the growth of germs. Stout people and babies are the chief beneficiaries of dusting powders. Without them, they are apt to suffer from irritation in the folds of the skin (armpits, groin, buttocks), known as intertrigo. In applying powder to the infant, great care should be taken to have it in one of the patent containers made to prevent the possibility of the baby getting the open end of the container into its mouth, for severe consequences have been caused by the baby's shaking an antiseptic powder (boric acid) into its mouth and inhaling it. For this reason I prefer a bland type of baby powder with a minimum of added antiseptic ingredients. Where the skin folds are irritated (as in the diaper region), a powder of a more adherent nature with water-repellent powers, due to its content of cod liver oil (Desitin powder), is often of value.

Since powders are widely used on account of the smooth and cooling feeling which they give to the skin, they must be correctly formulated in order to exert this cooling effect. Although a good powder could be made from talc alone, it would not have good absorbing properties, and for that reason various metallic salts are usually added. In addition, when powders are used as aids to the complexion, they must have additional chemicals added in order to cover defects of the skin and to lessen the shine of the oil secretion. Unfortunately, the trend in recent years has been to mask completely the shine due to the secretions of the sweat and sebaceous glands, and the resultant powder gives a smooth, masklike appearance to the face. Aside from the appearance, the use of these heavy powders (cake make-up, foundations) results in the undesirable side effect of blocking the skin secretions for a period of time. The constant use of heavy foundations and cake make-up, without adequate cleansing of the skin, often results in the appearance of blackheads and other minor complexion difficulties, much to the distress of the wearer. If a woman must use a foundation, she should apply it infrequently and cleanse her skin thoroughly following its use.

LOTIONS

Most lotions are actually water solutions containing powder. The usual preparation often requires thorough shaking prior to its use. The lotion is then spread on the skin and allowed to dry. The evaporation of the fluid leads to a cooling off of the skin, and the residual coat of powder which it leaves on the skin continues its action and so soothes both normal and inflamed skin. The well-known calamine lotion is just such a mixture. Part of its effectiveness is due to the fact that it is extremely bland and cannot irritate or aggravate an already inflamed skin. If most home remedies applied to the skin were of a similar bland and harmless nature, the doctor would see fewer cases of aggravated and irritated skin disorders.

COLD CREAM

The oil in the skin is an important ingredient. It keeps the horny layer of the skin soft, flexible, and watertight and forms a thin protective film on its surface. When oil is deficient the skin becomes rough, dry, and scaly, often inflamed, and much more liable to infection. The owner of such a skin is notified of this condition by a feeling of stiffness or even itching or pain. In common words, the skin is chapped. This happens most often in the winter, when cold dry winds are prevalent. To counteract it, oil may be supplied to the skin in the form of cold cream, supplementing nature. Creams are oils that contain water. When applied to the skin, the water evaporates and the cream absorbs water from the skin. If there is inflammation present, this results in a cooling of the skin, whence the name, cold cream. To avoid the overly frequent removal of oil by ordinary washing with soap and water, cold cream is rubbed on the skin and wiped off, removing much of the dirt with it. This does not compare, of course, with the cleansing attained by the use of soap, but is fairly efficient. Cleanliness may be next to godliness, but is not an unmixed blessing for those with dry skins. It can be overdone, or, rather, it can be done in the wrong way. In those with greasy skins, however, cream is harmful if it takes the place of hot water and soap cleansing. Cream adds to the grease already too plentiful in the skin, and in cases of blackheads and acne increases the tendency to form pus pimples.

Many different fats are available for anointing the skin; but cold cream, ointment of rose water, a perfumed emulsion of fat and water, is deservedly the most popular. There are many formulas for it; but all have about the same effect upon the skin. Light, soft creams are called cleansing creams and are sometimes advertised as "skin foods," which of course is a misnomer and a false claim, for the skin is fed only through the stomach, as the rest of the body is fed. Other preparations advertised as greaseless cold creams and recommended as cleansing creams are not creams at all but soaps made with sodium carbonate. Of course, they cleanse better than real cold cream, but they also defeat the purpose of creams, for they take oil out of the skin instead of adding to it. Some cold creams become rancid in time. This can be delayed by adding a small amount of boric acid, 5 or 10 per cent, to the cream. Many of the commercial cold creams are now made with petrolatum (mineral oil) in place of animal fats. Petrolatum is not a fat, but a derivative of petroleum which has many of the properties of fats but does not become rancid.

Creams are best used at bedtime following thorough washing of the skin with soap and water. From the point of view of their true value, the chief use of creams is to cleanse and protect the skin as well as to supply a small amount of oil and fat when the skin is on the dry side. In recent years there has been a great deal of discussion concerning the value of hormones in creams as an aid in minimizing the aging process. Up to the present time there has been no specific proof that hormones in creams will halt or lessen the process of wrinkle formation and maintain or produce a constant state of rejuvenation. If you are actually deficient in sex hormones, they should be administered in adequate dosage by your physician. It is very difficult for the average person to read between the lines of a skillful advertisement proclaiming an easy method for obtaining glamour and facial beauty. Experts in the field can do no more than advise caution and intelligence in reading highly publicized reports concerning a new easy road to perpetual youth and a beautiful complexion.

ANTISEPTICS

For application to small wounds, tincture of iodine is probably the most widely known antiseptic. It should be painted on, one coat only. More than this does not add to the good effect and increases the danger of irritation. The bottle must be kept tightly stoppered, preferably with a rubber stopper, for if the tincture is exposed to the air it evaporates and becomes so strong that even one application may cause a severe reaction. After iodine has been applied, no preparation of mercury should be used on the same area for several days for fear of an unpleasant skin irritation. The stain of iodine can be removed by alcohol, and it is usually advisable to follow an iodine application with an alcohol application.

Boric acid in saturated solution is a deservedly popular household remedy. Though it does not kill germs, it limits their growth and is soothing rather than irritating to inflamed skin. It should be made by filling a clean (boiled or scalded) fruit jar or large bottle one fourth full of the boric acid crystals, then adding boiled water to fill the jar. When this has cooled, it is a saturated solution, and what is needed can be poured off. By keeping crystals at the bottom, water above, a saturated solution is always ready for use. These bottles must be carefully labeled and kept in a safe place out of the reach of a child, as the solution is poisonous if swallowed. For infections, the boric acid solution should be heated and applied on a large dressing covered to retain heat as long as possible. For most acute skin irritations, however, it is best applied cool on a thin compress, allowing for evaporation. The compress should be kept thoroughly saturated if it is to be effective.

The solution of hydrogen peroxide is a useful household remedy. It does not kill germs, except those that cannot grow in the presence of oxygen. These occur in the mouth and other cavities of the body. More often, peroxide is used for cleansing wounds. It attacks and destroys pus and blood, and at the same time gets into small crevices where it forms oxygen gas and loosens dirt so that it can be wiped or washed away. It should not be applied too frequently as it may delay the healing of a wound. Care must be taken not to put peroxide into a cavity from which it cannot easily escape, for under these circumstances the gas may form under pressure and cause great pain and actual damage to the tissues.

Carbolic acid, often used in the household, is a dangerous chemical. It does not dissolve well in water, and when the attempt is made to make such a solution, concentrated carbolic acid often comes into contact with the skin and burns it. It should be used only under the direction of the doctor.

Within the past few years many new drugs and chemicals have been discovered. These agents have the common effect of killing or at least inhibiting many of the organisms which are present on the surface of the skin. A partial list of their names would have to include the sulfa drugs, penicillin, bacitracin, streptomycin, terramycin, aureomycin, chloromycetin, and many others. Although these drugs are effective from the standpoint of sterilizing the surface of the skin, they should be taken only under the supervision of a physician because of their capability of producing undesirable toxic or allergic reactions. Also their use in a skin cream for a minor infection may result in the development of an allergy to the drug, thereby preventing its use at some later date, for a more serious internal infection.

WET DRESSINGS

Wet dressings are helpful in the treatment of minor skin disorders, and some of them have already been described under the heading of antiseptics. Sometimes the application of a wet solution to an inflamed area of skin will accomplish a remarkable degree of healing and soothing action within a short period of time. In most instances it is important to apply the wet dressing every few hours for at least twenty to thirty minutes. Wet dressings are one of the most effective ways of removing crusts and dried secretions from the surface of the skin and in maintaining some drainage from infected areas. They serve as very effective local applications of heat, and may also be used to prevent rapid changes in the temperature of the skin surface. They are very useful in the treatment of skin eruptions with extensive blister formation, in that they tend to open these blistered sites and bring the effective medication in the wet dressing to the irritated area. The most widely used and effective wet dressings are a weak salt solution, Burow's solution (usually used in solutions containing ten to twenty times as much water); potassium permanganate solution in a weak form (approximately 1 part of potassium permanganate to 5,000 parts of water), a 2 to 5 per cent boric acid solution, and a magnesium sulfate or Epsom salt solution containing approximately ½ to 1 tablespoon of the salt to a quart of water. There are two main types of wet dressing, and it must be realized that their effects are considerably different. The open type of wet dressing, in which the solution is merely soaked in several layers of cotton or gauze and applied to the skin, is used when cooling is desired and maceration of the underlying skin is not advisable (poison ivy, burns). The so-called closed type of wet dressing, in which the layers of gauze or cotton are covered with oiled silk or cellophane, is used where local heat and maceration of the top layer of the skin are desired (boils, carbuncles). It is important that the dressing be kept sopping wet by constantly changing the entire thickness of gauze or cotton, or applying a completely new and fresh application. The hands and feet can also be treated by merely soaking the affected part in a basin containing the solution.

MASSAGE

Massage, including rubbing and kneading, is a well-established means of maintaining circulation in those prevented by disease from exercising, and of restoring circulation to parts of the body in which it is deficient. The face, however, seldom lacks exercise. Our days are full of facial exercise. At mealtimes we chew our food thoroughly (let us hope), and between meals we talk and allow the play of our emotions to find expression on the face. The rubbing in of cold cream is not necessary, for it exerts all its benefit on being applied gently. Massage is refreshing, however, and if followed by a good washing, as it always should be, does no harm in most cases. In any active inflammatory condition of the skin massage is harmful. In acne it is of doubtful benefit, and the grease that always accompanies its application is harmful. In any real infection, such as boils, it is dangerous, particularly on the face.

STEAMING

Steaming the face or other involved parts of the skin (back, chest) is a valuable measure in greasy skins containing blackheads. It causes increased perspiration and acts more vigorously than washing with hot water. It should not be carried to the point of causing the face to get very red and should always be followed by a cold application to restore tone to the vessels. Like the hot bath, if used too frequently, it may cause drying or even chapping of the skin.

SUN BATHS AND ARTIFICIAL SUBSTITUTES

The use of arc lights and quartz mercury vapor lamps in the home is being popularized. There is no doubt of the beneficial action of these rays and of the sun's rays under proper conditions and control. Light baths of any type should be given cautiously, allowing the skin to become accustomed to the light and to respond with pigmentation, instead of being burned. People with blue eyes and fair skins should exercise particular care to protect the skin from the harmful effects of light. The overly frequent exposure of the normal skin to ultraviolet rays for the purpose of a temporary cosmetic effect is not without the possibility of ultimate harm to the skin. There are some abnormalities and diseases of the skin, as well as some internal conditions, in which light is actually harmful.

On the water or snow the reflected rays may greatly increase the degree of the skin's exposure to ultraviolet irradiation. Hats are no protection against these rays, which contain the ultraviolet rays that are most active in producing irritation. Particularly at high altitudes, their penetration is great, and the effect of sunlight much greater than its visual intensity indicates. At low altitudes these rays are largely absorbed by the atmosphere, and comparatively few of them reach us. People who are strongly sensitive to the sun may now protect themselves by the use of creams and lotions containing physical or chemical sun screens. One of the best chemical sun screens is para-aminobenzoic acid and its derivatives, and it has been incorporated in several preparations now commercially available.

CARE OF THE SKIN AT VARIOUS PERIODS OF LIFE
INFANCY

The skin of an infant requires gentle treatment. Soap should be of the mildest superfatted kind, and even this should be employed only when absolutely necessary. It is preferable to clean an infant's skin with a bland oil containing small amounts of one of the newer and less irritating surface antiseptics such as hexachlorophene. After the bath a bland powder should be used, care being taken that the baby cannot get the opportunity to shake the powder into its mouth and lungs. The folds of the body should receive more powder than the rest of the skin. The clothing should be soft, carefully rinsed after washing, and not too heavy. Many infants are kept too warm and suffer from heat rash, which may, as a result of scratching, become infected and eventuate in more serious skin disease. Infants frequently develop chafing of the skin in the diaper region due to prolonged contact with urine and feces. This area may be protected by the application of soothing creams of a slightly water-repellent nature due to their cod liver oil content (Desitin ointment).

CHILDHOOD

The same rules apply as in infancy, except that the young child and the older small boy or tomboy girl require for their hands (and too often for other parts of the body) more soap and water. The mother should not, however, let her love of cleanliness carry her too far with the scrubbing process, for it is better that the child be a little less than perfectly clean rather than hampered in its exercise. Precautions against overcleanliness can be safely left to the defensive power of the child in most cases. Both boys and girls, if they have blond skin that freckles, should be urged to wear hats in the sun and to protect the skin before going outdoors. Modern sunburn protection includes the use of preparations containing para-aminobenzoic acid and derivatives, as well as salol, menthyl and benzyl salicylates, and other agents. The average sunburn is effectively soothed by applications of cold, weak boric acid solutions and a mild lotion such as calamine containing 1 per cent of phenol. The fair-skinned youngster should be taught in childhood that severe sunburn is dangerous and should be taught how to protect the skin from the sun's rays.

ADOLESCENCE

The chief change seen in the skin at puberty is the greasiness which appears in so many skins at this time, often accompanied by blackheads and pimples. The measures to be described later under the heading of acne must be instituted at once, and include frequent washing with hot water and soap and the insistence on good habits of hygiene.

MIDDLE LIFE

This is the active, strenuous time, when health is most often neglected for the sake of work or even sometimes for the sake of play. Loss of sleep, irregular meals, worry, all have their effect upon the health of the skin, as well as on the rest of the body. Worry, hurry, and impatience hasten the onset of age, which is often announced too early by the condition of the skin. The use of cold cream upon the female skin becomes more generally justifiable because of lessening oil production and decreasing glandular activity.

Age brings lessened nutrition to all parts, including the skin, and the latter loses both elasticity and oil to become wrinkled and rough. The skin loses its resistance and tolerance to the sun and various chemicals such as soap. Oil should be applied artificially, soap used sparingly, and the skin protected as much as possible. If hormones are necessary, they should be used only under the guidance of a physician.

INFLAMMATIONS OF THE SKIN

ECZEMA

Years ago almost any skin disease involving a patch of red, scaling, itching, and weeping skin was attributed to eczema; no one really knew what produced the symptoms. Accordingly, at some stage in development more than half of all skin diseases were called "eczema."

Eczema is a common inflammation of the skin. Its symptoms are: redness, itching, small blisters, and the discharge from the skin of a fluid that stiffens linen and tends to dry into scales and crusts. Incidentally, eczema is *not* catching.

This sounds specific enough—but, unfortunately, many other skin diseases have exactly the same symptoms. Actually, a skin disease is called eczema when it has all the features just mentioned, and is apparently caused by some unknown agent, either inside or outside the body.

For example, a man visited his physician and complained of an eruption of this type on the outside of his thigh. Without modern scientific investigation, it was classified as eczema of an unknown origin. Later, when the eruption had spread to the hands, face, and neck, the patient became seriously worried. Again he consulted a physician, this time a specialist in diseases of the skin. The second doctor made a detailed investigation. It revealed that the patient always carried a box of matches of foreign manufacture in his trouser pocket. The box rested against his thigh at the spot where the trouble began. The doctor found that the sulphur and phosphorus mixture on the striking side of the box and also on the match heads had an irritating effect on this particular patient's skin.

This man's reaction to these chemicals was so violent that he would have become a hospital case, with an entire body rash, had the cause not been discovered and the matches removed from his pocket.

Another instance, also an actual case, concerned a woman who asked her physician about an itching, red rash on her hands and forearms, a type of irritation that many chemicals and substances produce. This woman did not normally come in contact with strong chemicals, soaps, or other irritants. She was the sort of woman who used her hands for holding cocktails, waving people out of her way, and playing Mah-Jongg (before the days of Canasta). After questioning, the doctor discovered that a friend had given her a beautiful set of Mah-Jongg tiles, made in Japan. It was finally discovered that these Japanese tiles were covered with a lacquer made from a distant relation of poison ivy! The Japanese Mah-Jongg sets sold well, and, as a result, many women developed skin rashes from playing with the "poison ivy" tiles.

Neither the woman nor the man mentioned here had eczema. If the cause of their skin eruptions had not been discovered or determined, it would have been diagnosed as eczema, for want of a better explanation.

There is a lesson to be learned from these illustrations. It is of the greatest importance for patients to provide their doctors with all details of their daily lives when consulting them about skin condition.

There are other examples of specific skin diseases.

Among these are those fellow Americans who would develop a rash on Sunday nights, after a relaxing, restful day spent with pipe, slippers, and the Sunday papers. This rash improved during the week and flared up again on Sunday night.

"Aha, my friend," exclaims Sherlock Holmes the dermatologist, "you're rather fond of the rotogravure sections."

"Yes—so what?" replies our fellow American.

Well, you've guessed it! The rotogravure sections of the Sunday papers were the clue to the mystery of the Sunday-night rash. The ink from which they were printed frequently contained a red dye, which is an irritant to some people's skin. The irritation took several hours to develop—if it did not, it might have been a Sunday-afternoon rash. The rotogravure sections have disappeared from the Sunday papers, although an occasional person may be found sensitive to ordinary newsprint.

From the foregoing examples, there are irritants that affect certain people and not others. Likewise, there are certain substances that affect only certain parts of the body. For example, the scalp, face, and neck may react to a hair dye, a cold wave lotion, or to a perfume; the forehead to hat bands, especially those recently cleaned; the ears and nose to plastic or metal eyeglass frames; and the eyelids and neck to nail polish. The latter may sound strange—but the damage is done by contact with the fingernails.

Underwear shorts may affect the thighs or abdomen. Plastic watch straps may inflame the wrists. Even, forgive me, nylon stockings might affect the legs! I can hear the American housewife say: "Just give me the nylons; I'll take my chances."

And, she is right. Ill effects from wearing nylons are infrequent. Yet the few women who are susceptible can develop an annoying and itching eruption from wearing these stockings.

There are innumerable other instances where diagnoses could not be made until after long and detailed investigations. A baffling case was that of an attractive young woman on whose lips a severe itching and burning broke out. Many tests were made, with lipsticks, cosmetics, foods, and other substances.

Yet these and other precedures produced no effect. At long last the cause of the irritation was tracked down—her fiancé's mustache wax!

We seem to be concerned not with what eczema is, but with what it is not. This is necessary. The importance of the cases described is that there are some diseases classified as eczema that are due to specific agents. These agents can only be discovered by means of painstaking examinations.

The number of cases classified as eczema has been shrinking steadily. It will continue to do so as our methods and means for ferreting out hitherto unknown causes improve.

For our purposes, eczema can now be defined more exactly. It is a skin eruption in which there are certain complex internal factors more important than the local existing cause. In other words, though there may be a local existing cause, such as a matchbox, Mah-Jongg tile, or mustache wax—the removal of this cause, while essential, may not affect the cure. What is more, a skin irritation due to some such simple cause may develop into an eczema. Even though you track down and remove the primary cause, the irritation process goes on as eczema.

Again heredity comes into the picture. Some people are apt to develop eczema because of family tendencies. Blondes and redheads usually have sensitive skins that are irritated by sun, wind, and other agents. Other people are susceptible to eczema because of an infection in the teeth, tonsils, or sinuses. People with dry or oily skins may be predisposed to skin eruptions. People with dry skins are easily irritated by soap and, in general, lack sufficient resistance to skin infections. There are people whose sweat glands do not function well. Consequently, they don't perspire enough to remove irritants from the skin or cool the body.

Poor nutrition may also cause eczema. Lack of vitamins may lower skin resistance to the disease. Lack of vitamin A can cause a type of eczema complicated by pus formation. Lack of vitamin B can cause scaling of the nose and lips. Deficiency of various elements of the vitamin B family can cause a peculiar eruption on the arms and legs.

Various internal parts of the body influence the skin in the development of eczema. Among these are poorly functioning glands, such as the thyroid and others; and upset stomachs, livers, and kidneys. Often a good doctor tracks down some unsuspected disease elsewhere in the body following an eczema clue.

These conditions, and others, can predispose a man or woman to eczema. In other words, they are indirect causes. There are also causes directly responsible for it. Some people are hypersensitive, or allergic, to drugs or proprietary remedies which may do others good. If the hypersensitive individual takes these drugs, it may easily produce a skin disorder, or predispose him to it.

If you have a skin eruption, it may be possible that a supposedly harmless laxative, tonic, or blood purifier in your medicine chest is either the cause or part of the cause of your trouble. Perhaps you get a rash in the spring or fall of the year. You probably attribute it either to the weather or astrology. It's more likely to be caused by the insect spray or moth destroyer you use during these seasons.

Of course, there are many more factors which bear on this disease than can be briefly mentioned. Nerves also enter the picture. A period of emotional tension can produce inflammation of the skin. Does this sound far-fetched? If so, reflect on what happens when you are embarrassed—your face gets red. What happens when you're nervous or excited?—you break out in little pimples, known as "goose flesh." So—you see—mere thoughts and emotions do produce definite skin changes. When these thoughts and emotions take firm hold, they can also play an important rôle in the production of skin eruptions.

The patient, on being convinced that he has eczema, next wants to know the answer to the question that doctors hear many times a day, "All right, what can you do for me?"

The answer is—a great deal. One of the first jobs is to determine the cause and to eliminate it.

Another decision the doctor must make is whether the condition is acute or chronic. If it is acute, the itching must be relieved and the inflammation reduced as soon as possible. Normally, the patient will be given wet dressings and soothing lotions at this stage. The doctor will urge him to avoid such irritants as soap and water. If there are any predisposing factors—such as the matchbox, Mah-Jongg tiles, hair dyes, or hat bands—and also specific worries or digestive troubles—these must be eliminated or modified. Proper diet is important; so is proper intestinal functioning.

In chronic or long-standing eczema, the skin becomes thick and leathery. The irreverent medical student calls it "pigskin" or "elephant's hide." When this stage is reached, the cure becomes a long and difficult task. It is important for the doctor to study the patient minutely, to eliminate all potential irritants. Each person presents an individual problem. The doctor must decide what investigation and laboratory tests to make and he must analyze and interpret the results. Careful attention should be given to the patient's diet. The rate at which the patient's body absorbs sugar from his food must be checked. Functioning of the glands should be tested, and a search made for specific infections.

In addition to his chronic eczema, if the patient has some mild skin eruption elsewhere, such as "athlete's foot," this should be treated at the same time. If not treated, it may aggravate the eczema.

A word of warning—if a local remedy is prescribed—the greatest care must be exercised in applying it. To apply it skillfully is often as important as to choose the right remedy. It is also essential to carefully follow instructions. Strong remedies require careful judgment, and you may be sure your physician has assessed your requirements.

In some cases of obstinate eruptions X-ray treatment, administered by an expert, may produce a cure when other methods have failed.

Eczema, then, occupies a unique position in the field of dermatology. It is not only the wastebasket for all unexplained eruptions with characteristic symptoms, but it is also the keystone of skin diseases. The specialist in this subject deals with the commonest and most distressing skin disorder. If he knows how to treat this disease, you may be certain that he is able to treat most skin disorders.

DRUG RASHES

Within the past few years rashes on the skin due to drugs taken for some reason or other have become one of the most important causes of skin disease. Every doctor who prescribes a drug is well aware of the many problems which arise both on the skin and elsewhere on the body, as a result of the same drugs which may do so much good internally. Although the physician may be well aware of the pitfalls and disadvantages of these drugs, the patient usually is not. This is especially unfortunate in view of the fact that many drugs may be bought in the neighborhood drugstore without the necessity of a prescription. Accordingly, the occasional person may be taking some proprietary remedy which is doing him more harm than good. As far as the skin is concerned, while many of the drugs embodied in these various remedies are harmless, many others produce skin eruptions varying from an occasional attack of hives to an extremely serious rash involving almost the entire body. At the present time it is probable that the two most important causes of drug eruptions are the sulfa drugs and penicillin. Even a drug as simple as the salicylates (most popular member of which is aspirin) may be the cause of a troublesome itch or recurrent eruption, often baffling to both the patient and to his doctor.

This brief paragraph cannot be regarded as adequate in view of the vast importance of the rôle played in chronic eruptions of the skin by one or several drugs. It may, however, serve to impress upon the reader that he must seek the services of a physician for advice concerning any chronic skin disorder and, of even greater importance, as to the necessity of continuing some highly vaunted home remedy or drug mixture. Many people, on being asked whether they take a drug, state that they do not. On further questioning, it develops that the remedy they have been taking over a period of years for constipation or for their liver, or whenever they have a headache, is just the drug that is producing the trouble with their skin. Even that so-called "harmless" hang-over remedy may be the cause of their troublesome rash, and that special cure of Grandma's may not only irritate the skin, but affect various other parts of the body even including the blood cells and certain vital structures. Don't take any of those home remedies unless you know exactly what is in them and the mixture has been approved by your physician.

DERMATITIS FROM EXTERNAL IRRITANTS

The common example of this type of rash is the inflammation caused by poison ivy, poison oak, or sumac. The plants, chemicals, fabrics, and other substances that may cause this form of dermatitis are as numerous as those causing eczema, and in fact the two are closely related, so that it is at times impossible to say definitely where one leaves off and the other begins. Children should be taught to recognize the appearance of poison ivy so that they may avoid it in their excursions to study nature. It has glossy foliage, arranged three leaflets on a stem. In the fall among the first to change color, the leaves turn a beautiful red, and are often collected for this reason by uninformed enthusiasts. A good working adage is: "Leaves of three, let it be!"

If contact with the plant has been unavoidable, the next procedure should be to wash thoroughly with soapsuds and hot water, followed by rinsing with strong grain alcohol. If the dermatitis has hardly begun, this may lessen the severity of the attack; but when it has become well established, this treatment comes too late and will irritate the skin and result in a more severe skin reaction. It should be employed preferably within a two-hour period following exposure to the plants.

Among house plants the primrose is a common cause of dermatitis. Tincture of iodine that has been allowed to become strong by evaporation, or the too enthusiastic application of the fresh preparation, often is responsible for it. One coat of a fresh preparation is all that is necessary, and more will not have any better effect but may have a bad one. In bygone days the mustard plaster also was a common cause, but today it is scarcely used. However, there are many new household cleansers, chemicals, and cosmetics which may result in skin irritation.

Severe cases of dermatitis may be caused by contact with certain chemicals. The conditions are just about the same as those caused by poison ivy. Paraphenylenediamine and mercury are among the most important of these chemicals, as they are contained in many hair dyes and toilet preparations. New York City has an amendment to the Sanitary Code prohibiting the sale and distribution of preparations containing these chemicals, except with certain precautions.

Paraphenylenediamine is a coal-tar derivative and a strong poison. It is commonly used in hair dyes and has recently become a source of common exposure due to the sudden popularity of home hair dyes. The scalp may react shortly after the hair is dyed, with severe itching, followed by swelling and blistering of the scalp and surrounding skin. On the other hand, the reaction to a hair dye may not appear for several days, depending on whether the reaction is due to irritation alone or to an allergy to the dye.

Mercury is another chemical often used in liniments, ointments, and lotions. Most freckle removers contain mercury. While it is a valuable agent for many purposes, it is sometimes an acute irritant, and it should not be used except when specifically prescribed by a physician.

Another frequent source of inflammation of the face and neck is traced to dye used on furs, a dye similar to that in hair dyes. The inflammation is usually severe, prolonged, and recurrent. Another form of dermatitis on the forehead is caused by the action of sweat on the dye and other chemicals contained in cheap sweatbands in hats. Mouth washes, lipsticks, and toothpaste may cause a dermatitis around the mouth, face, and neck. Many cosmetics and cosmetic applicators (rubber sponges) may also be the cause of unpleasant and uncomfortable facial rashes.

For these forms of dermatitis the treatment consists in the detection and removal of the source of irritation, whatever that may be. The doctor must really do some detective work in order to ferret out the cause of some of the more obscure skin eruptions. After the cause has been eliminated, soothing remedies are all the treatment that may be required.

CHAPPING

Chapping is one of the simplest forms of inflammation of the skin. It is seen commonly in the wintertime, on the tender skin of children and on the hands of housewives who do not protect their skin from constant contact with soap, detergents, and other household chemicals. The combination of a cold, dry, wintry climate and a dried-out, steam-heated room conspire with hot water and soap to remove the oil from the skin, causing red, dry, scaly areas. Ordinarily such areas, when spared the irritation of soap and lubricated with some oil, will promptly return to normal. This same combination of overdried and steam-heated rooms together with the winter season not only dries out the skin but the mucous membranes of the nose and throat. Do you have a very dry and rough skin during the winter together with frequent colds and sore throats? If so, get hold of a monkey wrench and fix the radiators so that no one can heat your rooms to that blood-drying level where your skin, nose, and throat literally pant for a little atmospheric moisture. Or at least keep a pan filled with water on the floor so that the hot air can pick up some of the fluid. The Eskimos hardly ever catch cold, and their skins are in excellent condition—and all this without steam-heated igloos.

Some people have a distinct tendency toward chapping. Usually their oil and sweat glands do not function adequately. Accordingly, it is important for them to wash as infrequently as possible, and to minimize their contact with harsh, strong soaps. They are far better off using bland oils, either mineral or vegetable in nature, for cleansing purposes, and lubricating their skins whenever possible with a soothing cold cream. Some of the new lotions and emulsions containing ingredients whose purpose it is to increase the oil content of the surfaces of the skin are also very helpful.

CHAFING

This occurs commonly in babies and obese adults. It is caused by the rubbing together of parts moistened by sweat, offering an excellent opportunity for infection to take place. The parts should be kept scrupulously clean and well powdered. If this does not suffice, a flat bag made of gauze may be filled with talcum powder and suspended between the opposing surfaces to prevent rubbing. Of value also are various lotions and pastes which absorb some of the excessive secretions and excretions from these sites (i.e., Lassar's, Desitin). In women with heavy thighs, chafing between the legs may be minimized by wearing a light, porous pantie specially designed to lessen friction in this region. If these simple measures are not successful, it is advisable to consult a physician because some form of infection may have been superimposed on the simple chafe.

SUNBURN

Sunburn is an inflammatory reaction of the skin to the rays of light, not to heat rays. It occurs on snow fields as well as in the hottest climates. The redness does not appear at once, but several hours after exposure to light. If given an opportunity, most skins can produce enough pigment to protect themselves against any ordinary exposure to the sun; but when they receive a large dose of light without any preparatory hardening, they react with an acute inflammation. Some skins do not produce pigment in all parts but only in small scattered patches—the well-known freckle. And the albino has a skin that apparently cannot produce pigment at all; sunburn in the albino can be a very serious malady.

People vary in their reaction to the sun's rays. Blondes, as is well known, are apt to grow very red, to burn instead of tan. Brunettes frequently do not redden at all but merely take on a tan color, due to increased pigmentation in the skin. If the exposure to the sun is prolonged or if the redness (erythema) has lasted for some time, the skin becomes dry, harsh, and what is called "dead." The top layers scale or peel off. Very sensitive skins, or those exposed to intense sunlight, may become severely inflamed. There is much swelling, blistering, oozing, and disfiguring. The eyelids, mouth, and nose swell greatly. Some persons react so severely to sunburn that after a short exposure which is only sufficient to cause a slight burn in the average person, they are generally upset and nauseated. Stronger exposures lead to more violent reactions with fever, chills, and severe surface burns.

Brunettes as a rule do not suffer from these reactions nearly so acutely as do blondes. The normally high percentage of pigmentation in brunette skins is what protects them. Pigmentation is the skin's chief protection from the sun's rays. The pigment-containing cells are called chromatophores, literally meaning "color-loving cells." Blondes have fewer chromatophores than brunettes. The colored races, naturally, have the greatest number of chromatophores, and therefore have greater resistance to the sun's rays.

Prevention against sunburn is worth many pounds of cure to those who react. Large, wide-brimmed hats should be worn. Parasols and the large type of beach umbrella are of great help, especially at the seashore, where the strongest rays are felt. Applications of oils, lotions, and creams keep the rays from penetrating the skin to some extent. Para-aminobenzoic acid in various liquid or solid forms is a very efficient protection against sunburn, as is red veterinary petrolatum (a very effective but messy preparation). Salol (5 to 10 per cent) in a vanishing cream base is also pleasant and efficient. Other new drugs are effective and not unpleasant for application, but when trying a new sunburn cream, use it carefully for the first few times. It may not protect sufficiently, or the very chemical designed to protect your skin may do just the reverse if you are allergic to it.

When the first signs of sunburn appear, a cold cream should be applied. If there is swelling, a wet dressing of a slightly astringent and cooling solution, such as 5 per cent of Burow's solution, boric acid, or witch hazel, should be applied, followed by a powdery liquid such as calamine lotion. These reduce the heat, cool the skin, and help absorb the water in the skin.

The action of cold creams is excellent. They cool, soothe, and protect the skin, and counteract the drying effect of the sun. They do not make hair grow on the face, as some people would have us believe. (If cold cream did that, it would do as much for the scalp, and every bald-headed man in the country would be frantically massaging his scalp with his wife's newest and most expensive cold cream.)

Exposure to strong sunlight occasionally results in a very severe burn, usually of a first- or second-degree character, but never third degree. The so-called first-degree burns are really comparatively mild and produce only a redness of the skin. Second-degree burns occur simultaneously with the first-degree type, and in addition to redness, there are many blisters scattered over the burned area. The second-degree burns do not destroy the complete thickness of the skin, so that the remaining tissue can spontaneously regenerate the burned areas. It is only in third-degree burns, which practically never occur from sunburn, which cause complete destruction of the entire skin, and are far and away the most serious in that the burned victim is seriously ill and requires various types of plastic operation in order to correct the permanent damage to the tissues. First- and second-degree burns occur not only from some sun exposure, but primarily as a direct effect of exposure to heat. This heat may be due to exposure to fire, hot liquids, steam, and flash burns. Although we worry to a certain extent about the dangers of atomic bombs, the real medical problem of exposure to the atomic bomb is not the atomic radiation but the direct effect of heat.

Although the principal measures involved in the treatment of burns are primarily medical problems, their main features are the relief of pain, the prevention of shock and infection, and the actual treatment of the burned areas. With sunburn, the ordinary first-aid measures are adequate, such as the use of a simple mineral oil ointment containing a mild cooling agent such as menthol in a very weak concentration, in order to help relieve the pain. If not available, the application of a heavy paste made of water and sodium bicarbonate is also a useful first-aid measure. The more severe burns resulting from the direct effect of heat rather than sunburn should only be treated by a physician. While waiting, however, the victim may be made more comfortable by the application of a cool wet dressing, minimizing contact with the hands so that infection is not apt to occur. These extensive second- and third-degree burns are best covered with a clean, freshly ironed towel or sterile dressing moistened with a weak bicarbonate of soda solution until the doctor arrives. The newest method of treatment includes the surgical removal of all blisters and dead tissue, preferably in a sterile operating room. Subsequently, the burned area is washed with an antiseptic soap and sterile water, but in a very mild fashion, in order not to remove any of the still living tissue. The soap is then removed by rinsing with a sterile salt solution. There are many variations in the treatment of severe burns, depending upon the training of the physician. At the present time the most popular methods include the use of pressure dressings over a simple mineral oil application to the wound itself. Although many authorities feel that the ointment should contain some antiseptic or antibiotic, it would seem as though the best results have been secured by using the antibiotic internally, rather than locally. Another strange thing that has been found out is that it is preferable to leave the dressings in place for several days rather than to change them frequently. The reason for this is that there is less chance of infection developing, and the tissues seem to heal better when they are not disturbed.

Certain people are extremely sensitive to sunlight and should never expose themselves unnecessarily. Still others, particularly those suffering from a skin disease known as lupus erythematosus, should avoid sunlight as they would a plague. One strong exposure might initiate a fatal flare-up of the disease. People with a tendency toward skin cancer must also avoid the sun.

FROSTBITE

The skin may become irritated as a result of exposure to extreme cold. Usually it is most evident on prominent parts, such as the cheekbones, tip of the nose, ears, and chin. This is frostbite or chilblain, and it usually begins with a painful whiteness of the frozen part. Subsequently, the skin becomes cold, dark red, and painful. It may then lose all sensation. If the exposure is prolonged, the extremities may turn a black color, and in extreme cases the skin becomes gangrenous or dead.

The recent war has resulted in a considerable knowledge concerning the treatment of frostbite. These measures were learned, unfortunately, by the observation of aviators whose hands were frozen at high altitudes, and also from poor "G.I. Joe," who developed trench foot due to exposure of the feet to cold and wet for days at a time. Formerly we were all aware of the age-old custom of massaging the skin with snow, but this has long since been thrown out. In fact, massage of these almost brittle areas of the skin may actually lead to gangrene. The present methods of treatment of frostbite include gradual increase in the skin temperature by putting the patient first in a cool room and allowing the frozen part to thaw out slowly. It is of the utmost importance that the frozen tissue be thawed out slowly, because any rapid increase in the skin temperature will result in death of the skin cells and gangrene of the tissue. Gradually the frostbitten victim is warmed up with hot stimulating drinks, and if the freezing is extensive, transfusions of blood or plasma are usually necessary. Very little is done with the skin itself, other than keeping it extremely clean. The trend has been to give all the necessary antiseptics and antibiotics internally rather than locally, and this procedure has resulted in fewer cases of lost fingers and toes.

EXCESSIVE AND ABNORMAL FUNCTIONING OF THE SKIN OR OF ITS OIL AND SWEAT GLANDS

EXCESSIVE SWEATING

Excessive sweating may prove annoying, and the pads worn in the armpits and the various chemical applications to this area are not fully satisfactory remedies. Many chemicals act as deodorants when externally applied, and some are also anti-perspirants. The most effective anti-perspirant preparations are the aluminum salts, although some people may be allergic to these chemicals and they must be tried out with caution. As a deodorant, plain bicarbonate of soda as a dusting powder is effective. In recent years some of the newer internally acting drugs such as banthine have been successfully used for the control of excessive sweating, but only under medical supervision because of their effects on other parts of the body.

BODY ODOR

Body odor is usually synonymous with the odor of the sweat. Certain perfumers advise the use of perfume suited to the body odor of the client, but that sounds rather unpleasant. Foul-odored sweat is a great affliction, fortunately not common. Some of the newer soaps and deodorants are effective in the control of unpleasant body odors. Many of these preparations contain hexachlorophene and other effective antiseptics. Chlorophyll enjoys great popularity, not entirely deserved.

PRICKLY HEAT

Heat rash (prickly heat) is an acute inflammatory disorder due, obviously, to an inability of the skin to adapt itself to an increase in temperature. It occurs more often in infants than in older persons, and is most prevalent during periods of heat and humidity.

The eruption consists of tiny elevations ranging in size from a pinpoint to a pinhead and usually containing a clear fluid. Actually, these tiny elevations are present over the pore openings and are due to the fact that the sweat secretions have been blocked by a surface inflammation of the skin. The surrounding skin is usually of a pinkish shade. The prickles may remain separate, but not infrequently they join with one another and form large patches of irritation, as in eczema. If these areas are not properly treated, secondary infection may result with pus formation and rapid spread.

Prickly heat is best prevented by the avoidance of too heavy clothing and frequent use of bath and dusting powder. Do not dress babies and children too warmly during the summer months. Bathe them frequently, and make certain that they drink enough water and other fluids. After the eruption is present, it will frequently yield promptly to cooling measures such as weak, cold applications followed by the use of a bland dusting powder or calamine lotion. The skin should not be cleansed with soap, which is very apt to irritate the condition. For the purposes of cleansing, mineral or vegetable oils may be employed in alternation with the local applications of powder and soothing lotions. If these simple local procedures fail to improve the condition, a physician should be consulted, as such eruptions afford an excellent invasion center for infections of the skin.

EXCESSIVE OILING

Excessive oiliness of the skin is one of the commonest causes of large pores and a generally poor complexion. It is most common around the age of puberty or adolescence, and this may be considered due to the increased activity of the sex glands during this period of life. The oiliness of the skin occurs about equally in both sexes, although it is presumed to be due to the secretion of male, rather than female, sex hormones. It is usually referred to medically as seborrhea, and is characterized by the presence of an excessive amount of oily secretion on the face and the scalp, and occasionally elsewhere on the body. This greasy secretion appears as oily droplets oozing through the pores of the skin and often on the scalp. The result is a greasy layer of oil droplets which can be wiped off the surfaces of the skin with a handkerchief at frequent intervals. In time the pore openings become blocked with oily secretion which can be squeezed out in the form of little wormlike bodies. In addition, these oily droplets serve as sort of a catch-basket for all the dirt floating in the air, and so the surface of these oil droplets or the secretion in the pores themselves is often of a blackish color and is referred to as "blackhead." The black color is not actually dependent on dirt, as certain chemical changes are responsible for the blackish color. The scalp is always affected, and the free oily material results in a glistening and shining appearance of the scalp. In women with long hair the secretion may be so extreme as to mat the locks together in a sort of gluelike paste. Although in former years this was believed to be responsible in great measure for early baldness, the relative importance of oil secretions in producing baldness is still an unsolved problem.

Although the glands of internal secretion are primarily responsible for the excessive greasiness and oiliness of the skin, other predisposing causes include any internal change which lowers the vitality and general nutrition. Seborrhea may appear following any one of a number of infections and is often associated with constipation, lack of fresh air and exercise, and poor diet. When sebor-rhea has persisted for a long time, it may be responsible for the formation of crusts and scales on the scalp and around the ears and nose. This may even go on to a more severe form of the disorder, often referred to as seborrheic dermatitis.

In the average case of seborrhea frequent washing with soap and water and the use of a mild astringent may be all that is required. However, in the usual instance it is important to take care of both the external and internal factors if an effective cure is desired. Ordinary common-sense hygienic measures are indicated. Sunlight, nutritious food, and plenty of fresh air and exercise are important. An adequate intake of vitamins, especially of members of the B-complex family, is especially indicated. The latter vitamins contain substances which have been shown to lessen the greasiness and scaling of the skin both in animals and human beings. Vitamin B_{12} has been reputed of particular benefit in this disorder. For the direct treatment of the skin, frequent use of soap and water on the face and frequent shampooing of the scalp are highly recom-mended. Bland soaps or soap substitutes such as sulfonated oils are of value in many instances, especially if the skin is sensitive and easily irritated. One thing that is definitely contraindicated is the use of massage by the beautician and barber, both of the face and scalp. Massage of the face is not only valueless in this condition, but will often increase the local irritation and accentuate the blocking and oil secretion of the skin. In addition to frequent washing of the skin, the use of a mild astringent at frequent intervals is effective.

Where the condition is more of a rash, rather than merely excessive oil secre-tion, various drugs have been employed and recommended, and these include sulfur, resorcin, salicylic acid, and similar agents. They are usually made up in the form of pomades of various types, although lotions are better adapted to some skins. Repeated application and patient care of the face and scalp are necessary to secure complete relief in the case of a disease as essentially chronic as seborrhea. These conditions require the services of a physician, as the local and internal measures require close watch and frequent change.

EXCESSIVE DRYNESS

This condition is the exact opposite of seborrhea, in that there is an in-adequacy of the secretions of the oil glands. As a result, the skin is not satis-factorily lubricated, and this may occur as a natural phenomenon or as a result of constant bathing of the skin, or as a result of immersing the body in strongly alkaline solutions in the course of various occupations. Dryness of the skin frequently occurs in the wintertime in cold climates, and is often ag-gravated by the lack of humidity in heated rooms. It is often associated with other disturbances of the skin, and is not infrequently a forerunner of eczema. In extreme instances the skin is not only dry but becomes cracked, chapped, and split. Dryness of the skin is more typical of the older age groups, but it must be realized that various internal factors may also produce this state. For example, when the thyroid gland does not function adequately, the skin often becomes extremely dry and scaly.

If the dryness is merely due to various external causes, the condition can usually be simply remedied by the use of oils such as lanolin, almond oil, mineral oil, and other agents. The skin should be bathed as infrequently as possible, and soaps confined primarily to the skin under the arms and in the groin. Even the face should be cleaned with oils rather than soaps, and a protective layer of cold cream should be left on the skin overnight. Other effective solutions for the face include glycerin in rose water and the occasional local application of the white of an egg rubbed gently into the skin. If the condition does not respond to simple applications of creams and oily lotions, a search for some internally causative factor, such as a hormone deficiency, may often be rewarding.

ITCHING

The skin is the source of many peculiar sensations, including smarting, burning, prickling, tingling, creeping, and crawling. However, one of the most common sensations in the skin is itching. As a result of this sensation, we are provoked into rubbing and scratching the affected area in an attempt to relieve the undesirable sensation or to change it almost preferably to one of pain. When the itching is severe, self-control can seldom be mustered even by persons of unusually strong will power. These unhappy efforts of the sufferer to relieve himself result in the formation of bumps and infection as a result of the entrance of bacteria through self-inflicted wounds. Often the irritation is far more acute at night than during the day, and sleep becomes a thing of the past.

The causes of itching are many. In some instances it may be as simple as contact with a new soap, shaving lotion, hair tonic, or the like. In other instances it may be due to infection with some germ or parasite. Occasionally it may be a symptom of a severe underlying disease such as diabetes. Obviously, then, the only intelligent approach to the treatment of itching is to find out what has caused the symptom. To a trained observer, this may prove to be a simple problem, although, on the other hand, it may require an extremely careful medical and laboratory investigation.

The occurrence of itching is divided about equally among men and women, and, while no age level is exempt, there is a tendency for it to be more frequent after forty. Adults with dry skins often develop itching during the winter, especially if they bathe frequently and use more than their share of soap. It may also make its appearance during the menopause and result in itching of either one portion of the body or the entire body surface.

If the itching is due to a specific cause, removal of the offending substance will result in prompt and speedy relief. This relief will be increased by the use of cold wet dressings and soothing lotions. Within recent years new antihistaminic drugs have been found extremely effective in controlling sensations of itching, whatever their cause. Of course, these drugs should be taken only under the supervision of a physician. Unfortunately, the tendency at present is to employ them as a cure-all for all known skin diseases, but, as might be expected, they will not perform miracles. Not infrequently dietary measures are also of value in itchy states, and the elimination of tea, coffee, and alcohol may be of considerable benefit.

Itching of the skin may also be due to an associated nervous disorder, and the treatment of a difficult emotional situation may sometimes result in relief from that extremely uncomfortable and maddening itch. Where an itching condition has persisted for any period of time, do not attempt to treat the condition yourself but consult your physician.

INFECTIONS OF THE SKIN

BACTERIAL INFECTIONS

Impetigo is the commonest of all skin infections and one of the easiest to cure. It is most frequently seen in children and is caused by pus germs, the streptococcus and staphylococcus. In the newborn baby, it can be serious because the baby has no immunity to the infection and it is fatal in approximately 25 per cent of all cases. For this reason children are not permitted to visit the maternity floor of the hospital. The disease is highly communicable and spreads rapidly from child to child. It can usually be recognized by the appearance of honey-colored crusts which look as though they were stuck on the skin. Impetigo prefers to attack children, and the face is the favorite site. The scalp is not uncommonly involved, especially in children with head lice.

The treatment of impetigo is based primarily on the use of antiseptics and general cleansing with soap and water. If the crusts do not come off easily, the application of a wet dressing or a soap poultice will serve to take them off in short order. Following removal of the crusts, the application of any one of several antiseptic ointments, such as those containing ammoniated mercury, or some of the newer antibiotic agents is extremely effective. Where the condition is widespread and serious, it may be necessary to employ some of the newer antibiotics, such as penicillin or terramycin, by mouth or by injection.

Folliculitis is similar in nature to impetigo, but the infection is in the hair follicle rather than on the surface of the skin. In other words, the infecting germs, either the staphylococcus or streptococcus, penetrate the deeper parts of the skin, usually through the mouth of the hair follicle or pore opening. Within a short time the skin surrounding the hair follicle becomes inflamed, sensitive, and tender and discharges pus. As with impetigo, the infection spreads rapidly from one hair follicle to another, most commonly on the beard or in the scalp. The infection sometimes is transmitted from unclean instruments or unsanitary procedures in the barber shop, and is more common in people with diseases such as diabetes. Even if true diabetes is not present, persons whose blood sugar or skin sugar content is high show a particular tendency toward the development of pus infections of the skin such as folliculitis, boils, and carbuncles. Recurrent attacks of these conditions are often successfully treated by a low sugar and starch diet in combination with proper hygiene and anti-septic agents.

Boils. When the same pus-forming bacteria that produce impetigo and fol-liculitis dig farther in and attack the deeper parts of the follicles and the oil glands, a deep, round, inflamed mass develops. The result is a boil.

Boils are common enough to be considered slightly amusing by everyone except their victims. They are painful, hard, red lumps like marbles surround-ing each hair follicle. Some tend to soften and form a soft, pus-discharging core. That is, the center around the follicle discharges the pus and the rim re-mains hard and bright red. When the center has softened sufficiently, it may be removed. A pus-discharging ulcer is then left, which empties itself and heals, often leaving a scar.

Boils are quite frequently the accompaniment of constitutional disorders. Almost invariably they indicate a run-down condition, if not a serious disease. Diabetes is often accompanied by boils. Frequent boils should send the patient to a physician for a general examination and treatment.

When the rim or wall of a boil is soft—because of a poor general resistance —the infection is not well confined and tends to spread and invade the blood. Abscesses may develop in other parts of the body, such as around the kidneys, and general blood infections may result. Sometimes these infections are fatal. Boils with firm borders are, therefore, more easily cured and less dangerous.

In certain occupations in which the skin is likely to be injured or exposed to dirt, tar, petroleum, or other chemicals, there is a constant danger of con-tracting boils. Bromides and iodides taken internally may produce boils and folliculitis. Both boils and folliculitis may affect any part of the face and neck. Folliculitis, of course, is more likely to occur on the bearded parts of the face. It is more chronic and obstinate, but boils are more painful.

A boil on the upper lip or in the nose is especially to be watched. It is ex-tremely dangerous and may cause death. This is because the blood circulation of the upper lip is extensive, and also is upward to the brain. Poisons draining from the lip, therefore, may cause meningitis and abscesses of the brain.

Carbuncles. There is a widespread confusion of ideas about boils and car-buncles. A great many people rather naturally think they are the same thing. They are distinctly different, but the difference is more in degree than in kind.

A carbuncle is larger, deeper, more destructive, and vastly more serious than a boil. It is an infection by a pus-forming germ, like the boil; but it is always accompanied by the symptoms of a severe and acute illness.

A carbuncle is a hard, rounded, inflammatory mass, extending down through the corium into the subcutaneous tissues. It goes deeper than the boil, which seldom extends below the upper part of the corium. A boil affects only one hair follicle. A carbuncle affects several, through which pus is discharged from the inflamed center.

With carbuncles may be fever, chills, loss of weight, and general discomfort.

In addition, there may be symptoms of a metabolic disease, such as diabetes. Because of this, a main feature of the treatment of carbuncles is the employment of every measure that will build up the body and help it to fight the disease.

THE TREATMENT OF PUS-PRODUCING INFECTIONS
(FOLLICULITIS, BOILS, CARBUNCLES)

In the treatment of folliculitis, boils, and carbuncles, the doctor finds out if any constitutional disease is present and corrects it. Even if no such disease is discovered, it is advisable to clean out the bowels, remove sweets and indigestible foods from the diet, and take any measures necessary to bring the system's powers of resistance up to par. Plenty of fresh air and sunlight and a great deal of water, outside and inside, are highly desirable. Irritation, dirt, and harmful chemicals should be avoided, of course.

The physician may decide to rely on immunization in order to stimulate the defensive forces of the body. Either the so-called stock vaccines, or a vaccine made from germs in the pus given off by the patient may be used. It is necessary to regulate the dosage carefully, or there will be severe reactions. In recent years the sulfa drugs, penicillin, aureomycin, and other potent remedies of modern science have been remarkably effective in curing episodes of these diseases. They are usually not effective in the chronic and recurrent types, although small doses carefully supervised over a period of time may prove effective.

There are two main fallacies about the treatment of folliculitis and boils. One is that the face must not be shaved, and the other is that boils must always be cut. Actually, the face should be shaved daily. The reason for keeping hair off the face is that infection is minimized and the local applications can penetrate more readily. Boils usually need not be cut. Cutting breaks down the rim, or defensive wall that the body builds around the infection, and this opens up the blood and lymph vessels and so permits the spread of the infection. It is rarely necessary to cut boils, as a matter of fact; but when it is done, the most thorough asepsis and antisepsis must be enforced.

The main aim of treatment, indeed, should be the enforcement of cleanliness and personal hygiene and the administration of measures that will reduce and remove the infection. The boils and the skin around them should be washed several times a day with soap and water. Following the washings, alcohol and water or antiseptic solutions should be lightly dabbed on and then antiseptic dressings applied. Avoid irritating and infecting the skin around the boils.

When the boils are tense and tender, a wet dressing of a 5 per cent Burow's solution or a 5 per cent sodium propionate solution—not a compress—relieves the pain and encourages the softening and evacuation of pus. It is a mistake to put heavy bandages, oilskin, or gutta-percha over the gauze to form a compress. The dense texture of these materials causes a retention of the heat and the pus discharge, and nurtures the growth of the germs. In early cases wet applications are aided by X-ray treatments. Ultraviolet rays also are useful in improving some local infections. Of even greater value are a whole score of new drugs, including the sulfa drugs, penicillin, bacitracin, aureomycin, and terramycin. These drugs may be used either locally or internally, depending on the severity of the infection.

The same sort of treatment is employed for carbuncles, but here surgery may be necessary if wet dressings, the antibiotics, and X-ray therapy are not effective.

As may readily be imagined, these pus infections are not trivial. The best way to treat them is not to have them. And the best way to achieve that happy state is to keep the general constitution up to its highest tone, and to make a habit of strict cleanliness and an intelligent, balanced diet.

Spirochetes—Syphilis

Syphilis is no longer considered as a disease to be discussed in whispers by both younger and older generations. This is an era in which prudery has little, if any, place. We are more concerned in measures and effects that will improve the public health and which must be known by those who wish to protect themselves. We must understand the early and beginning symptoms of a disease such as syphilis, so that any suspicious symptom may be promptly investigated. At present the ease and speed of eradication of the disease depend chiefly on the early diagnosis of the condition. A disease such as syphilis does not merely affect one part of the body, but can spread to affect almost any organ or tissue in the system. Furthermore, if the initial symptoms are disregarded, the germs which cause the disease quietly dig into the internal organs and produce serious damage which cannot be remedied if it has been persistent for many years. In this chapter the purpose for describing and discussing this disease is not so that it can be treated at home. The average person is no better equipped to take care of syphilis than is the quack who preys on frightened and uninformed youngsters without a real knowledge of the proper treatment and fundamentals of medical care. If you develop any symptoms such as those mentioned under this disease, discuss them with your family physician and not with your friends or a so-called sex disease expert who may not even be a qualified physician.

The cause of syphilis is a tiny corkscrew-like germ which swims around in the fluid discharging from a syphilitic sore. It is an organism called a spirochete, and in fresh syphilitic sores the fluid literally swarms with these corkscrew-shaped organisms. This germ is rather delicate and is usually promptly destroyed outside of the body. For this reason, syphilis is usually transmitted only by direct contact with a person who is infected with the disease. Although syphilis may also be acquired and transmitted in other ways, these transmissions are quite uncommon and the disease is truthfully called a venereal disease. The germ usually requires the presence of an open wound or slightly irritated mucous membrane such as the mouth, rectum, or outer male and female genital organs, to enter the body. Although syphilis may be transmitted through the sputum, after kissing, this method of transmission is slight in comparison to sexual intercourse as the primary means of infecting another person with syphilis.

Syphilis is usually divided by the physician into three stages. During the first stage the infection usually appears as a small sore on the genital organs. This sore usually appears within two weeks following sexual intercourse. Any sore which develops on the genital region at this period of time should be examined by your physician. He can usually perform a test known as a dark field examination, which will promptly disclose the presence of spirochetes if the sore is due to syphilis. If it is not, you are better off being told that such is the case, rather than waiting to see what happens. At this stage the germ has only started to get into the blood stream and so the Wassermann test does not become positive until a later date. If this primary stage is disregarded, the sore usually heals in a few weeks and the glands in the groin, which are swollen at the time of this primary sore or chancre, usually go down. The germ is now being transported around the body, and the unfortunate victim is passing into the second stage. If the second stage is mild, the infected person may not know that he has syphilis for many years, when it will either be disclosed by the performance of a routine blood test, or by symptoms of a serious nature.

In the secondary stage of syphilis, which appears within six weeks or so, the chief symptoms are an extensive rash, a peculiar loss of hair, and often what seems to be an ordinary cold or sore throat accompanied by slight fever and achy or "grippy" symptoms. One of the unfortunate features of the disease is that the secondary stage may be mild, and the patient may feel that he merely has a slight cold. The rash may be mild enough to be overlooked, and he may be completely unaware of the fact that his entire system is going through a mighty battle in order to build up resistance against the germs which have spread to every part of the body by way of the blood stream. Another unfortunate feature of the disease is that lack of awareness of this stage means that the victim can easily transmit it. During this secondary period the saliva and all other body secretions are loaded with the organisms, and it is very easily transmitted. To get back to the rash, it may be stated that it looks like measles and is usually present on the body rather than on the face. The hair fall is of a peculiar type in that it usually consists of either a diffuse thinning of the entire scalp, or of the appearance of small bald patches. These bald patches are so characteristic, in that they look mangy or moth-eaten, that it is described in medical textbooks as the typical moth-eaten appearance of the scalp in secondary syphilis. During this stage the blood shows a strongly positive Wassermann test and the diagnosis can readily be established.

After several weeks or months the secondary stage passes, and the symptoms gradually disappear. If laboratory tests have not been performed on the blood and spinal fluid, the disease may pass unnoticed until the person passes into the final or tertiary stage of syphilis. This stage may not appear for many years and it is due to the destruction of various internal tissues and organs by the spirochete which eats away insidiously at these tissues over the years. This stage persists until the end of the patient's life and may even remain undiscovered if the symptoms are not sufficiently pronounced to bring the patient to the doctor. In the ignorant and uninformed this occasionally is the case. The average person with the tertiary stage of syphilis has usually had such mild primary and secondary stages that he was never aware of the presence of the disease. At some stage in his life either a routine blood test or a general examination brings to light the presence of the disease. The symptoms of the tertiary stage may consist of extensive sores on the skin, or changes involving any portion of the body, including the eyes, ears, nerves, blood vessels and heart, the liver, and the brain. These changes are usually so extensive and severe as to shorten the life span.

The symptoms described present the picture of a serious and unpleasant disease. The disease will only be eradicated in time by early diagnosis and prompt examination following any suspicious exposure. Don't let fear keep you away from the physician! He is sworn to secrecy and will protect your privacy as well as your health. Fortunately, public health authorities have made tremendous strides in wiping out the sources of infection among prostitutes and other groups which are responsible for the constant transmission of the disease. Only with lessened secrecy and more intelligent knowledge and information concerning the disease, will it eventually disappear. Modern treatment methods are such that the disease can be completely cured and its transmission prevented if an early diagnosis is made. Even the late and severe stages of the disease can be dramatically helped by prompt and adequate therapeutic measures. The old methods of treatment with arsenic, bismuth, and other heavy metals have to a great measure been displaced by the newer drugs, especially penicillin. Whereas formerly it was necessary to treat patients over a period of years, the disease is now practically completely eradicated in weeks with massive doses of penicillin, as well as some of the other drugs. The advances of science will eventually force the disappearance of this dread disease, but this will only come about with intelligent understanding and co-operation on the part of the general public.

VIRUS INFECTIONS

FEVER BLISTERS (HERPES SIMPLEX)

Small groups of blisters break out on the face when we catch cold or get too much sun. They usually appear around the mouth or nose as tender and tense small blisters which rapidly become crusted and sore. Herpes are due to a virus and are actually an infection, difficult to transmit. Some people seem to be peculiarly susceptible to them and get herpes regularly whenever they get a cold or sore throat. Others get herpes whenever they are exposed to too much sun or wind. The blisters seem to have a favorite site for recurrence so that some people always develop them around the mouth, yet others only get them around the nose or elsewhere on the body. They also occur in association with certain severe infections or high fevers, for example, pneumonia. They also occur at the time of menstruation, but this may often be due to some drug taken for the relief of menstrual cramps.

Herpes usually dry up and disappear within one week to ten days. The healing process may be accelerated by the use of drying lotions and powders. In the initial stage spirits of camphor or tincture of benzoin may make the tender area less sensitive and hasten the drying of the blisters. Of value also is plain zinc oxide ointment containing a fraction of a per cent of menthol. When herpes simplex recur constantly in the same spot, this may be prevented by a few X-ray treatments to the affected area. Other people who develop recurrent fever blisters may be immunized against them more or less permanently by four to eight smallpox vaccinations at intervals of two weeks. It seems as though the smallpox vaccination immunizes against the herpes virus as well as against the smallpox virus.

SHINGLES (HERPES ZOSTER)

Shingles is also a virus infection like herpes simplex, but is more severe in its effects. The name *zoster* is derived from the Greek and means girdle. It got that name because the virus infects part of a nerve and the eruption appears all along the course of the nerve, thereby girdling or encircling the body. Only one side of the body is involved, and so the rash appears as a group of blisters traveling from back to front along one side of the body. Because the nerve is infected, this eruption causes severe neuralgia and the pain may be very distressing. In fact, the pain often lasts long after the rash is gone, and the poor sufferer complains far more because of the neuralgia than because of the rash.

If shingles is treated early with antibiotics such as aureomycin or terramycin, the infection may disappear quickly. In other instances, if the pain is not great, the whole process may be treated satisfactorily with drying powders, lotions, and salves. The neuralgia may be so severe that drugs like codeine and others may be necessary. The occasional severe attack may even require blocking or destruction of the sensitive and irritated nerve. Fortunately, dangerous complications of shingles are rare, and the disease hardly ever recurs.

PARASITES

VEGETABLE PARASITES (RINGWORM)

This old name of ringworm was given to the disease because of a misconception of the cause of the ring shape of the patches on the skin. It is a complete misnomer, because the disease, in most of its manifestations, is not in the shape of rings. Of course, worms have no part in producing the disease. It is due to many different cousins of the common molds which attack bread left in an open moist place. This has been known for many years by the medical profession. Only lately have the doctors realized how important and widespread these infections are.

On the feet this disease is carried between the toes of a large percentage of those who consider themselves perfectly healthy. The wonder is not that it breaks out in other parts now and then; but that this happens so seldom. So far as is now known, it is spread chiefly by walking on moist, infected floors of bathrooms, gymnasiums, and golf clubs, and in evidence of this fact is the more modern name "athlete's foot."

The treatment of these infections is often difficult and taxes the ingenuity of the physician. The hair and nail infections are most difficult of all forms to treat, and the latter is one of the important sources for the spread of the infection. Fortunately, many new remedies are now available both for control and treatment of the ringworm. The majority of these effective agents are derived from non-irritating, fatty acids first discovered in human sweat. These acids may be incorporated in liquids, powders, and ointments. Cleanliness of the feet and frequent powdering, particularly care to keep the clefts between the toes clean and dry, is of great importance in preventing infection. Women have less ringworm than the men, probably because of better care of their feet. There is little doubt that a great difference of susceptibility to these organisms exists, and those afflicted may not be lax in regard to cleanliness but only unfortunate in their susceptibility.

Treatment of most cases of ringworm should be kept up for a long time after cure has apparently been obtained. The organisms lurk among the skin cells and await an opportunity, perhaps in the form of simple moisture, to multiply rapidly and cause another outbreak.

Everyone has a pet remedy for his own case of ringworm, but the same remedy may wreak havoc on someone else's skin. If your athlete's foot or jockey itch does not get better from simple hygienic measures, don't use your friend's remedy but seek professional advice. Some of the newer drugs such as the undecylenates, propionates, salicylanilides, and many others may actually cure that "old faithful" ringworm of yours, so don't give up hope!

ANIMAL PARASITES

1. *Lice*—The three forms of lice which feed on man obtain their nourishment from blood sucked from the hair follicles. In procuring this food they inject a poison into the skin, which causes intense itching. Among ordinary folks the best known of this disgusting family of parasites is the head louse, pediculus capitis. The children of the family too frequently bring home samples of the parasite in the hair. Its eggs, called nits, are tiny white pear-shaped bodies glued to the hair. The parent louse has a semitranslucent gray body and is not easily distinguished through the hair. Scratch marks and bloody crusts, sometimes pustules and matting of the hair are seen.

Thorough soaking of the hair and scalp with a mixture of equal parts of kerosene and sweet oil is an old method of eradicating the lice. A cap is formed of cloths soaked in the mixture and left upon the head overnight. The next morning a thorough shampoo is given, and after this hot vinegar applied to loosen the nits, which then are removed with a fine comb. Modern methods of cure are much more effective. They include the use of DDT, HCH, and similar chemicals in the form of ointments or lotions applied for comparatively short periods of time. When large groups of children are infected, powder sprays of DDT have been very effective. They kill the parasites with speed and efficiency.

The body louse lives in the clothing and only moves to the skin at mealtime. It attaches its eggs to the fibers of the underwear. To obtain blood it marches over to the skin. This explains why the bloody crusts and itchy pimples which are typical signs of this disease are found most plentiful on parts like the waist and shoulders, where the clothing rests closely upon the skin. The derelict and the hobo, as well as those who neglect cleanliness of body and clothing, harbor body lice though it must be recognized that some people are much more attractive to the louse than are others. Body lice carry typhus, a dangerous disease fortunately rare in the United States, but a great problem when our troops entered Italy during the last war. A mild form of typhus is associated with rats, possibly carried by their fleas.

"Crabs" are caused by the pubic or "crab" louse, and this nasty parasite is found clinging to the pubic hairs with its head down close to the skin. At times the parasite travels to the armpits, the chests of hairy men, or even to the eyebrows and eyelashes. Although formerly a great nuisance and difficult to eradicate, the parasites are now destroyed with ease due to the use of DDT and similar chemicals in a form suitable for application to the pubic region. What a transition from the weeks of constant observation and the shamefaced isolation endured by the victims of "crabs" in former years!

2. *The Itch* (*Scabies*)—The itch mite, a member of the spider family, is small. The male mite is smaller than the female. Living on the surface of the skin, his only purpose in life seems to be the propagation of his kind because the female often destroys him after impregnation. She then burrows into and along the upper part of the skin, depositing her eggs as she goes, producing a small canal about one fourth of an inch long. As the eggs hatch the canal loses its roof and appears as a dark, wavy silk thread, seen most easily between the fingers. Itching is more severe at night, because the female itch mite is a night worker.

The diagnosis of scabies is often difficult. A doctor should always be consulted. Much damage can be done by unsupervised home treatment of this disease and the other conditions frequently confused with it, whereas proper medical treatment employing benzyl benzoate, DDT, and sulfur may promptly eradicate the mites.

3. *Insect Bites*—Many insects use man as their source of food supply. Mosquitoes, flies, bedbugs, and fleas are some of the many insects which disturb our travels and trips to the country. They all produce somewhat similar reactions in the skin, depending upon the individual. Some people are completely immune to their bites, but the usual reaction consists of a tiny red

spot at the site of the bite, followed by itching and a small, whitish swelling or bump. There are even reports of people so sensitive to these bites that fever, chills, and severe constitutional reactions may result from them.

The first problem is one of prevention and this may be accomplished by extermination of the particular pest. DDT sprays and various new insect repellents are effective with precautions taken to avoid overexposure to these chemicals by the humans rather than the insects. Thorough housecleaning and removal of dust and rubbish may also be necessary.

Treatment consists merely of soothing lotions and tinctures. Calamine lotion with 1 per cent phenol is still a useful remedy. The more severe reactions respond well to the antihistaminic drugs.

Skin Growths
corns

Corns are caused by pressure, as everyone knows, usually that of improperly shaped shoes. The world is slowly becoming more sensible in its dress, but tight-fitting shoes are still much in favor, and corns still flourish. The only effectual treatment is protection from pressure. Removing the central horny plug with a knife, or softening with a salicylic acid preparation, followed by soaking in hot water and scraping out the plug is good treatment, but is of no lasting benefit unless the pressure is removed. Sometimes a soft felt pad may take the pressure off the callus or corn and cause it to disappear. Anything that does not yield to such treatment over a period of a few weeks is probably a wart and requires treatment for that condition.

warts

Because they are at first tiny, flat, skin-colored elevations that are inconspicuous, warts are often neglected until they have had an opportunity to show their ability to grow and spread. The original wart may remain single and stationary for a time, but a month or so later a new wart may appear near this spot. This property is called autoinoculability; that is, we can infect ourselves again and again. In this way whole crops of warts are raised, like dandelions, where they are least desired. It is plain, therefore, that warts should not be picked with the teeth or fingernails or pared with the pocketknife. The virus that causes warts belongs to the interesting group of "filtrable viruses," whose ability to pass through the finest porcelain filter has given them the name.

Ordinarily warts are painless; but sometimes on the fingers, and commonly on the soles of the feet, they are tender, causing exquisite pain during walking, dancing, or as a support for someone else's feet.

Ever since prehistoric time warts have been treated successfully by suggestion. Tom Sawyer's method and many others like it which are still used by boys all over the world are survivors of the ancient practice of the witch or voodoo doctor. The modern child is often too sophisticated, even at an early age, to have any faith in such practices, and other methods must be used. The only objection to the faith cures is their encouragement of false beliefs and gullibility, which is even worse than warts. Warts respond to treatment with various chemicals, X-rays or radium, and the "electric needle." Some of the newer "wart" remedies include extremely potent chemicals such as tri-chloracetic acid and mixtures of podophyllin. Because warts are sometimes difficult to cure even with the most modern methods, the treatment is best left to the physician. A popular home treatment is the use of nitric acid. This is mentioned only to be condemned, for it often results in unsightly scars or even keloids.

Seborrheic warts are the brown to black-topped elevations that occur on the trunk, less often on the face or scalp, of people in middle life or later. They are of no consequence except for the fact that they are sometimes hard to distinguish from senile keratoses, which are important lesions in that they may be the forerunners of skin cancer.

SEBACEOUS CYSTS (WENS)

Sebaceous cysts or "wens" usually occur on the face, back, or scalp. However, they may appear on any part of the body surface in which there are oil glands. They are a result of a blocking of the mouth of the oil gland or hair follicle with an accumulation of oily or cheesy material under the skin. The skin around this cheesy secretion develops an actual cheese bag or pocket in order to contain this material. This bag or cyst continues to grow larger until it is a large lump in the surface of the skin. Sometimes a small black pore communicates with the interior of the cyst, and some of its cheesy contents can be squeezed out through this opening. Often several cysts of different sizes are scattered about this surface of the body. They should be removed because of the possibility of infection, and in a small percentage of cases of cancer.

These cysts may be cut out surgically, but they should not be opened unless a complete removal is planned. However, the resulting scar may be small if one of the newer techniques for removal is employed. By one of these methods, an electric needle is inserted into the cyst and its contents are actually "cooked." Subsequently the cooked cheesy material expels itself with the wall of the sac. Other methods include injection of the cyst with penicillin and other drugs and a gradual expression of its contents. When performed with painstaking care, this method may result in removal of the cyst with practically no scar formation.

MOLES

Moles are birthmarks, even though, as often happens, they do not appear until adult life. The ordinary skin-colored or brown mole, whether covered with hair or not, seldom becomes dangerous except when exposed to chronic irritation. When located so that the clothing rubs upon them, or so that they are frequently cut in shaving or possibly irritated in some other way, they should be removed thoroughly by the physician. Any mole that starts to grow rapidly, bleed easily, or show any type of unusual change, should be examined promptly by a physician and as promptly removed if the doctor considers it necessary.

Blue moles, much less common than the brown kind, but not rare, are in a class by themselves. They may last throughout life without change. Consult your physician about them if there is any question as to change in the mole.

KELOIDS (OVERGROWN SCARS)

Keloids are benign tumors (tumors that practically never become malignant) which grow in scars. At times there is no history of a preceding scar; but it may have been so slight that it was not noticed. Some people have the peculiar tendency to form keloids in their scars, or these tumors may occur in some of their scars and not in others. They should not be cut out because of their ability to return promptly, thereby resulting in a larger tumor than before the operation, unless treated at the same time with radium or X-rays which have a very beneficial effect on them. The careful application of solid carbon dioxide ("dry ice") by the physician has also been found of value in the treatment of keloids.

XANTHOMA (YELLOW SPOTS)

Xanthoma is the name given to the yellow tumors caused by the deposits of fat in the skin. Some of us seem to have an inability to dispose of fats in the normal way, and the skin serves as an exit station. The only form of this disease seen frequently involves the skin around the eyelids, most often the inner part of the lower lid, in the form of small yellowish elevations. They can be removed by the physician with the production of very slight scarring. They may return if the internal condition that causes them is still operative, though seldom sufficiently so to cause other symptoms.

VASCULAR BIRTHMARKS

Vascular birthmarks may be flat "port-wine marks," slightly elevated, flat-topped "strawberry marks," or egglike swellings composed of groups of veins in a grapelike mass. The large swellings are easily compressed, but return immediately to their original shape, and tend to become bluish and still larger when the baby cries. Often the skin over such a mark is the site of one of the flat kinds already mentioned. All these growths should be treated during infancy, when the skin is able to renew itself most readily and the resulting scars are smaller. Furthermore, although some of these bloody tumors may disappear, many of them grow larger rather than smaller.

The vascular tumors respond well to proper methods of treatment. The flat or port-wine stain may be improved by abrasive scraping with an electric drill. The strawberry mark can be removed by the electric needle, "dry ice," or by injection with a strong solution (sclerosing solution). The deep or cavernous type of bloody tumor may be removed by the two latter methods or by means of contact X-ray therapy or radium applications.

KERATOSES

Keratoses are of two kinds. The soft or seborrheic variety are brownish, velvety plaques which appear during middle age. They are of no significance and can easily be removed from the skin. They are commonly seen on the face and back.

The hard or senile keratosis is more serious in nature. It is a rough, scaly spot often found on the face and backs of the hands. People who are exposed to a great deal of sun and wind over a period of years often develop these spots. Farmers and sailors are particularly apt to develop these spots because of their constant exposure to the elements. These small scaly or warty growths must be removed because they may turn into cancers of the skin. Removal may be accomplished by cutting or burning them off. The only important fact is to make certain the removal is a complete one. People who develop senile keratoses should protect themselves from the sun and wind, following the removal of these growths.

CANCER OF THE SKIN

Cancer of the skin offers the doctor one peculiar advantage over cancer in other parts of the body in that it can be seen at its beginning and treated early. Inability to do this is the chief reason why cancer elsewhere cannot be cured as readily. Any unusual growth on or in the skin should be shown to the physician at once, without taking the great risk of home treatment or delaying treatment until ulceration occurs. The idea that cancer always causes pain is another very harmful one, for skin cancer seldom causes pain until it is in the last stage, when it is too late to save the patient's life. Home treatment is worse than simple delay, for it is like trying to put out a fire by pouring on gasoline. If anything will insure the change from a harmless to a malignant growth, or encourage one that is already malignant, the usually irritating home treatment will do so.

Scaly spots, warts, or growths on the lips and the hands should have attention early, for cancer occurring on these parts is apt to be more malignant than upon the face. The great strides made in the treatment of malignancy are due to the early recognition and removal of suspicious growths. Any "mole," "wart," or similar spot on the skin should be examined by your doctor promptly if it becomes sensitive, enlarges in size, bleeds readily, forms a crust, or ulcerates. Make certain that the wart or lump on your skin is harmless by having it examined rather than by waiting for trouble!

MISCELLANEOUS SKIN CONDITIONS
ACNE VULGARIS

Acne vulgaris is a disease of the oil glands of the skin. At puberty, along with other changes in the body, these glands develop and frequently take on excessive activity, causing the skin to become greasy and plugs to form in the pores. These plugs of grease undergo a chemical change and show as black points on the skin, commonly called blackheads, and by the doctors, comedones. These plugs cause some irritation, as do all foreign bodies in the skin (wood, glass), and nature tries to eliminate them by the formation of pus. When the pustule breaks, the comedo is forced out with the pus. Unfortunately, if the pus remains too long in the deeper lesions before being freed, the pressure and dissolving action of the pus destroys the tissue about it. This loss must be replaced by scar tissue, leaving a permanent disfigurement. If scarring does not follow the pustule, the process may be repeated many times in the same follicle. Acne tends to clear up as the patient grows older, but the risk of scarring is too great and the distress of the young person at the disfigurement too acute to justify neglect of treatment. Don't neglect the early treatment of acne if you wish to have your child develop as few holes or pits in the skin as possible. And remember, at this impressionable age the seeds of an inferiority complex are easily sown. The physician, opening the pustules with a tiny knife, is not causing scars, as many think. He is preventing them by releasing the pus before it has time to destroy tissue.

Since acne occurs usually in greasy skins, acne is benefited by the free use of hot water and soap. Children affected with the disease should not be accused of causing it by reluctance to use these measures. No amount of scrubbing can cure a real case of acne. Neither is acne a sign of sexual irregularity, as some ignorant persons insinuate. The unfortunates afflicted with the disease are embarrassed enough because of their facial blemishes without the added cruelty of such insinuations.

In mild cases pustules may be few and comedones many, forming small yellowish elevations with a yellow, brown, or black point in the center. When the horny layer of the skin forms completely over the surface, the end of the fatty plug cannot become dirty but remains as a white pearl-like body called milium, or whitehead. These remain without much increase in size until removed and do not recur as promptly as the blackheads.

Acne is not always confined to the face, but also involves the chest, upper back, and outer sides of the arms. In persons of low resistance it becomes a disfiguring, distressing, and indeed serious disease. Cold cream or other greasy applications should not be used, for the skin already has too much fat. Massage is apt to do harm because of the cream employed. Patent medicines called "blood purifiers" are apt to make acne worse, because many of them contain iodides. The acne patient does not need this type of "blood purifier."

Removal of blackheads is beneficial, as can easily be understood when the method of formation of pus pimples is considered. It should be done with care, however, not to injure the skin by too much force. Many nervous patients increase their disfigurement by too enthusiastic attempts to remove blackheads by squeezing without preliminary loosening. The face should first be washed thoroughly with hot water and soap, hot towels applied for about ten minutes and then the skin sponged with alcohol. If necessary a needle, sterilized by flaming, or a blackhead remover, a small instrument with a hole about 1/16 of an inch in diameter in one end, may be used to help remove the blackheads. After the blackheads have thus been removed, the application of hot towels should be repeated, followed by a short application of cold water and drying with a towel. This second application of heat lessens the inflammatory reaction to the pressure. Deep pustules, the kind that are most apt to cause scars, should be opened by the physician.

Care of the health is important in all children, but particularly in those who have acne. Fresh air, good food, proper exercise, and plenty of sleep are essential to good health. Strict dieting seldom cures acne and may do harm if not properly supervised. Many youngsters with this disease need restraint, however, in the matter of eating and drinking, and should be particularly warned against the bad effect of sweet carbonated drinks, nuts, greasy foods, excessive condiments, chocolate candy and ice cream. Irregularity in the eating and sleeping schedule is also harmful. Constipation should be avoided by the generous use of vegetables and fruits and by the formation of regular habits of bowel evacuation.

This somewhat lengthy discourse on acne is not intended to convey the idea that acne can be cured by home treatment. Only the mildest cases can be handled without the help of the physician. Under medical supervision, the proper use of some of the newer drugs (both internally and externally) may result in rapid improvement of the condition.

Cleanliness is essential. Soap and water are fundamental, and the face should be vigorously washed several times daily. A good astringent should be rubbed into the skin after each washing. At night salves containing chemicals such as sulfur and resorcin are left on overnight to soften the blackheads and peel off the top layer of affected skin. In addition, your doctor applies various chemicals such as a carbon-dioxide slush and various peeling pastes to accelerate the cure. Ultraviolet light performs a similar aid in treatment. Although X-ray was formerly used in the treatment of many cases of acne, it is seldom used now except in the resistant and stubborn cases of acne. However, modern science has found out that certain hormones and chemicals such as the antibotics may be helpful in the treatment of acne. Even the pits and scars produced by the disease can be removed by the newer techniques of facial planing and drilling. Don't neglect your child's skin, because acne is a disease that can and should be controlled from its onset.

ROSACEA

Rosacea, or acne rosacea, is the disease that reddens the nose and cheeks, and in extreme cases causes enlargement of the end of the nose, popularly called "whiskey nose" or "grog blossom." This title is not justified, for many sufferers from this disease are strict abstainers from alcoholic drinks. The trouble is caused by a nervous reflex flushing of the sensitive blood vessels of these areas on the face as a response to internal changes or abnormal local conditions in the mouth or nose. Anything which tends to cause flushing or heating of the face should be avoided. The patient can do much to restrain its development by the avoidance of hot foods or drinks, spicy or peppery foods, and particularly alcoholic beverages. Alcohol irritates the stomach and sets up the reflex already mentioned, at the same time that it acts directly to dilate the peripheral blood vessels. After frequent dilatations, the vessels become paralyzed and remain as disfiguring red or bluish lines. The consequent slowing of the circulation is probably the chief reason for the enlargement of the end of the nose. This can be improved by treatment with proper diet and astringent, local measures including powdered carbon-dioxide "slush."

For direct treatment of the skin, the main thing is merely washing the face frequently. But it should be washed with soap and cold water, or rubbed with ice. This is a marvelous tonic; it peps up the muscles and blood vessels and keeps them small and contracted. It is difficult to resist the temptation to break into eulogy of water. No cosmetic ever devised can compare with plain cold water as a tonic, cleanser, and beautifier combined. The only drawback to water is its cheapness. If it could be obtained only in tiny, ornate flasks at ten dollars an ounce, it would sweep a vast amount of perfumed trash off the toilet table!

There are, however, certain preparations which help cold water in fighting rosacea. They are all astringent in nature. Rose water and boric acid solutions and emulsions containing sulphur are especially valuable. The best sulphur lotions, such as lotio alba, tend to prevent grease formation, and as they evaporate cool the skin, contract the blood vessels, and leave the sulphur powder on the skin.

Where there is irritation in addition to the redness, the skin should be soothed with wet dressings of boric acid (2 per cent), or zinc oxide lotions, such as calamine lotion, before the sulphur is employed. In using these preparations, some of the mixture should be poured into a saucer and applied with a piece of clean flannel cloth. The best time to apply any such preparation is at night, so that it can remain on the face until morning, when it should be washed off with cold water and soap. After this, a fine powder or a thin, invisible lotion may be dabbed on.

Vinegar, witch hazel, and weak alum in solutions of less than 5 per cent are good, mild astringents. Too strong a reaction of the skin is harmful; but drugs such as resorcin, ichthyol, and camphor are sometimes used successfully.

There is a general delusion that massage of the face is necessary in treating rosacea. Barbers are apt to prescribe it, as well as operators in beauty parlors. The fact is that massage of a diseased face is injurious. It irritates an inflamed skin and spreads infection. When the skin is unhealthy, it is very easy for it to contract infection from the masseur's fingers.

Electrolysis can do much to reduce telangiectasias—the enlarged blood vessels which show as purplish streaks. The operation is the same as that for the destruction of the follicles in hypertrichosis, or superfluous hair. The electric needle is inserted along the course of the vessel and the current allowed to flow until the vessel is destroyed. The application of the electric cautery will also destroy the unsightly vessels, if done skillfully. After such treatment, cold applications and astringents are applied.

These same methods of treatment are employed for cases where the nose is tremendously enlarged or has a hanging growth; but the quickest and best method is removal of this growth by surgical operation. The growth is cut away surgically; if the bleeding is profuse, it is easily stopped by pressure and ice. Operations by this technic usually produce excellent results. X-ray or caustics prevent the regrowth of tissue after the operation, and caustics are used to destroy the follicles which have produced the excess growth.

Rosacea is no longer a difficult problem. With proper diet and internal measures, plus effective external applications, the victim may again regain a normal complexion. It requires self-control and patience on his part, and both proper diagnosis and therapy on the part of his physician.

HIVES

Hives or urticaria affect many people. You may get it the first time you eat strawberries or peaches. Or you may spend an uncomfortable night after that delicious lobster. Or that last injection of penicillin which cured your boil shows up again one week later in the form of little swellings or wheals all over your body. The hive itself is a small whitish or pinkish bump which can appear anywhere on the body. It means that you are allergic to something or other, and if you are lucky you can quickly blame the strawberries, the lobster, or the penicillin. Alas, not all hive sufferers can find the cause of their symptoms so quickly, and a long, tedious search may be necessary if the hives keep on appearing over a prolonged period of time.

Usually the wheal is what is called evanescent. It comes and goes. It may last only for a second, or it may remain twenty-four hours. It sometimes appears so suddenly that it can actually be seen swelling. The wheals vary in size from that of a pea to a patch big enough to cover the whole face. Usually round or oval, they are sometimes irregular or ring-shaped, or they may develop like a map or become scalloped in shape.

There is usually itching, and sometimes burning or tingling or creeping sensations in the skin. Frequently the itching is intense. Another condition occurring with the hives is dermographism. This phenomenon consists in the appearance upon irritation of elevated white spots bounded by pink borders, which take the outline of the irritation that causes them. The irritation may be only slight pressure, or it may be pinching or scratching. In medical schools it is demonstrated to the students by stroking the patient's skin, or writing on it with a finger. The elevations appear whenever the finger touches the skin.

The wheal is produced by practically anything which affects the blood vessels of the skin. It is supposed to be due to a combined action of the nervous system acting on the blood vessels. The blood vessels are first closed in the central zone which results in the white area of the wheal. Those on the border are open to make the pink area.

Although hives may be produced by almost any kind of external or internal irritation, the more serious types are associated with constitutional and emotional disorders. Even when external causes are apparently the only ones, there is almost surely some disturbance or defect in the vasomotor system—the mechanism which controls the blood vessels and their nerves.

The internal disorders which produce hives fall into special groups. There are those due to allergy or to a sensitivity to proteins; those due to the taking of such drugs as quinine, aspirin, cathartics, or any other drug for which the individual has an idiosyncrasy; disturbances of the metabolism; disturbances of the blood; and nervous disorders. Still another group is due to intestinal disorders. Another group is due to the reaction from eating certain foods. Children especially suffer from this type of hives.

An attack of hives is usually of short duration. Twenty-four hours at most should cover the appearance and disappearance of the wheal. There are, however, short attacks which recur for several weeks. Other cases last for a long time. The itching is intense in the prolonged cases.

The great point is to discover the cause. In acute cases a simple diet is usually ordered and a thorough cleansing of the bowels. Large amounts of water should be imbibed—alkaline water is especially good—and a brief diet consisting mainly of skimmed milk, wheat-free cereal, lamb, and toast is advisable.

Chronic cases require a general examination and the care of a physician. Tests should be performed to determine sensitivity to various foods, pollens, and other possible causes of allergic reactions. Laboratory tests may be necessary, before the constitutional cause can be determined.

Certain drugs are of benefit in treating the hives. These include the new and potent antihistamine drugs, which work wonders in recent and acute attacks of hives. These so-called anti-allergic drugs are less effective in the chronic types.

Adrenalin, one of the most powerful of all drugs, is also valuable in acute cases. It has the special effect of causing the blood vessels to contract, thus diminishing the formation of the wheal. Frequently adrenalin causes the immediate disappearance of the wheals and itching. Ephedrine is also given. But all these drugs are to be taken only on a physician's orders. They may injure the eyes, heart, or nervous system, and may cause peculiar eruptions.

PSORIASIS

Psoriasis is a strange and capricious skin condition, characterized by the appearance of bright red, coin-shaped patches on the skin, especially on the knees and elbows. These bright red patches are often covered with delicate silvery-white scales. When these scales are scraped off the skin, a bright red surface with tiny bleeding spots is characteristic of the disease. Although this disease is not serious in that it does not affect the general health, it can be very annoying in that its constant appearance and reappearance, with spread to involve many different parts of the body, can be a source of great unhappiness. No one knows why this disease occurs. Strangely enough, the condition doesn't seem to bear any relationship whatsoever to various forms of internal or external illness and often affects people who are otherwise in the best of health. It is not infectious or communicable. In a small number of cases the condition may be associated with some form of arthritis.

One of the features of psoriasis has been that patients with the condition usually improve following exposure to sunshine. An old adage used to be that psoriasis does well with grease and water, soap and sunshine. This would mean, of course, the use of some drug in an ointment, following removal of the crusts by soap and water. The average patient with the condition requires a little more than the preceding if he really wants to know how to take care of the condition. Unfortunately, the permanent relief of a severe case of psoriasis cannot be promised as there is no remedy which will produce a permanent cure of the disease. However, the sufferers from this disease often find that common sense and the help of a physician who has had special experience in the treatment of this condition can get him through the severe episodes more rapidly and will often lessen the violence of a flare-up in the condition. The local measures which have been found to be of the greatest value include preparations containing tar, ammoniated mercury, salicylic acid, and chrysarobin. These are strong drugs and capable of doing a considerable amount of damage unless closely supervised by the physician. This is particularly so because the concentrations of the drugs to be employed are usually high if they are to be effective. Continued diligent treatment will often bring about the disappearance of large patches of the disease. Specialists in diseases of the skin have also found that, in certain instances, the use of various drugs taken by mouth will be helpful in improving or controlling the condition. Again, intelligent co-operation between the patient and his doctor is of great value. At the present stage of our medical knowledge, the patient with psoriasis must learn how to live with the disease rather than constantly to fight it. This knowledge can be gained from a combination of expert medical therapy and guidance, plus an intelligent approach to the problem.

Locally, wet dressings and tub baths containing starch or oatmeal may be comforting. The wet applications are more comfortable when cold. On the skin itself lotions or powders containing camphor, phenol, or menthol often afford considerable relief. The antihistaminic drugs (Benadryl, Pyribenzamine) in a cream or lotion form are also effective in relieving itching, but must be carefully watched as they may produce local irritation. In severe cases both cortisone and ACTH have been found to be useful, preferably for a short period of treatment.

LUPUS ERYTHEMATOSUS

This condition is an example of one of the skin diseases which can affect both the skin and the internal organs. The internal form is far more serious and may even occur in the absence of a rash on the skin. However, in the usual case it is associated with a reddish eruption involving the nose and the cheeks in what has been described as a "butterfly pattern." This form occurs most frequently in younger women and is related to overexposure to sunshine. In other words, there is a probability that a strong sunburn in a person who has had a preceding infection, or is predisposed to this disease, may be the aggravating or precipitating factor which touches off the whole process. The subsequent occurrence of changes in the heart, kidneys, and other internal organs would indicate the serious and often fatal nature of the condition. Although the disease has been treated with some success with cortisone and ACTH, these drugs usually serve merely to arrest or lessen the condition rather than result in a complete cure.

The external form is of a somewhat different type in that the victims are not necessarily sick. It also bears some relationship to preceding excessive exposure to sunshine, and is most often present on the nose and cheeks as a red butterfly-type of rash. In addition to the red rash on the face, the scalp is often involved and the skin may show patches of crusts, scars, and bald areas in the scalp. This disease is a serious one, and no attempt should be made to treat it at home. It requires the services of a skilled physician and the use of various internally acting drugs, such as bismuth, gold, arsenic, and others which may be potentially dangerous when taken without constant supervision.

PEMPHIGUS

This is an extremely serious disease involving the skin. Its cause is unknown, although recent research would seem to indicate that it may be in part an infection and in part some disturbance in the general metabolism. It usually begins around the nose or mouth as a series of blisters or crusts, which get better or worse and never seem to heal completely. In time practically the entire body becomes covered with small and large blisters. These blisters may join together to form large areas of raw weeping skin. The unfortunate victim literally leaks his life fluid through these open surfaces of the skin. In the majority of instances the disease is fatal within a period of six months to several years. Within the past few years, the occasional patient may be helped considerably with cortisone and ACTH, although the results may merely be a prolongation of life, rather than an actual cure.

SCLERODERMA

This disease is also a serious skin problem. The sufferer develops the condition gradually after having complained of previous circulatory changes in the skin. The hands and feet are cold and bluish in the beginning and eventually become hard, tight, and ulcerate easily. In time both arms and legs may become stony hard and firm to the touch, and the process may even involve the entire body. Not much is known about its cause except that the fibrous tissue and small blood vessels in the true skin have been severely damaged by an unknown toxin. Treatment is not too satisfactory, although some patients have been helped by warm climates, measures designed to improve the circulation of the skin surface, and some of the newer drugs such as sodium paba, cortisone, and ACTH. None of these measures have proved constantly satisfactory or curative.

DISORDERS OF PIGMENTATION

FRECKLES AND TANNING

These changes in the skin are brought about by exposure to sunlight. The natural reaction of the skin to light and some other forms of irritation is the formation of pigment, tanning. Some skins, notably those lacking in pigment, are not able to produce pigment as readily as the darker ones and often produce it only in spots. Freckles, therefore, are the indication of a weakness of the skin in this important function. Such skins should not be needlessly exposed to light, for they cannot protect themselves or the owner from its sometimes harmful effects, which do not appear at once, but may come to notice much later as senile freckles, liable to change to rough, scaly spots and end in cancer of the skin. These are larger and fewer than the ordinary freckles of youth and are more persistent. Such a skin should be protected as much as is possible from direct sunlight; though, of course, this is locking the barn long after the horse has been stolen, for such a skin should have been protected since early childhood. After the damage has occurred, its progress may be delayed somewhat by the daily application of a good cold cream. Treatment of senile freckles is usually not necessary unless they are disfiguring or show some tendency to become rough and horny. They should then be eradicated. The freckles of youth are best treated by preventive measures, as already stated. The mild applications suggested for chloasma may be tried if the freckles are disfiguring; but time and protection from light are the most successful measures.

CHLOASMA

Chloasma is the unequal browning of the skin of the face that occurs in women more often than in men and, like all increases of pigment, in dark-complexioned persons oftener than in blondes. Its popular name is "liver spots"; but the liver cannot be held responsible. (Apparently a hormone from the pituitary called the MSH or melanocyte stimulating hormone is respon-sible.—Ed.) The treatment often unsatisfactory, consists in trying to remove the surface layers of the skin by means of an inflammatory reaction produced by irritants. These, when strong enough to be effective, are hard to control and often cause too great an inflammation with most unpleasant consequences to the patient. Peroxide solution, made active by the addition, at the time of using, of about 20 per cent of ammonia water, may be beneficial to some; this is questionable, however, and care should be used to stop the application be-fore too great an irritation has been produced. All such remedies act by causing scaling, and this is seldom deep enough to affect the pigment without causing an unpleasant inflammatory reaction. In some instances careful electro-surgical removal of the pigmented patch may be successful. (A new ointment called Benoquin has been reported useful.—Ed.)

VITILIGO

This disease is almost the opposite of freckling. White spots suddenly appear on the skin, usually around the face or on the backs of the hands. In time they get larger in size, and new white areas appear elsewhere on the body surface. These white spots are due to a loss of the pigment cells in the affected areas, but no one knows why they occur. They may be due to deficiencies in the glands of internal secretion, metabolic alterations, or vari-ous unknown factors. They sometimes appear at the same time as alopecia areata (see p. 703), and may be due to similar emotional problems.

The spots become more conspicuous if the surrounding skin gets sunburned —so stay out of the sun. The whitish areas may be effectively concealed by Covermark. A new Egyptian chemical, derived from an herb, has been found of value in some instances. (This product is now marketed under the name of Oxsoralen. It must be prescribed by a physician.—Ed.)

BERLOCK DERMATITIS

This relatively common disorder appears as flat, dark brown spots, usually in a necklace or droplike appearance. It is more common in women and is due to the action of sunlight on skin previously covered with a sun oil, lotion, or perfume containing an essential perfume oil (bergamot). The usual sites are the sides of the neck, face, arms, and armpits, but any part of the body may be involved. The eruption is often produced by dripping or running down of the fluid on the skin, and this gives it the droplike appearance. It is due to light sensitivity, and the brown spots can appear with redness, inflammation, and even blistering. Treatment should consist at first of soothing creams and later of bleaching lotions. Cosmetics or other substances containing the essential causative oils must be avoided if recurrences are to be prevented.

THE HAIR
ORIGIN AND STRUCTURE

The hair is formed by a dipping down of part of the epidermis, which forms a pouch, at the bottom of which is a papilla, like that of the epidermis; but this one is a specialist among papillae in that it is able to build hair. From this a cylindrical body of skin cells forces its way up through the pouch, called the follicle, which is now long and narrow. Soon after they leave the parent papilla the cells of this cylindrical body become horny like those of the surface of the skin, and form a spine that extends beyond the surface for a distance. After the cells turn to horn they are no longer alive but form only a mechanical projection. As the hair grows by the formation of new cells in the papilla, the part above pushes out until it has attained its destined length. It then ceases to grow, unless cut off, and after a period of rest falls out, leaving the papilla in the skin to form a new hair. As already mentioned, the sebaceous duct joins the hair follicle near its upper end, filling the follicle with oil which is forced into the body of the hair. Below the gland the erector muscle of the hair joins the outer part of the follicle. During periods of excitement this muscle raises the hair from its normal slanting position to an erect one. Contraction of this muscle also helps to force out the contents of the sebaceous gland, and, during excitement or when the body is chilled, puckers the skin into the condition we call "goose flesh."

Most of the hair on our bodies is only a remnant of the hairy covering of our ancient ancestors. It is fine and consists of two layers, the cuticle, a layer of tiny flat scales surrounding the hair, overlapping one another like shingles on a roof, and the cortex which consists of long strands of spindle-shaped horn cells with tiny spaces between them, presumably for oil. These fine hairs are called lanugo hairs, from the word for wool. Coarser hairs, like those of the scalp, contain in addition to the two layers mentioned a third, a fine pithlike center filled with a few larger cells. The cortex contains the pigment of the hair in the form of granules and also as a fluid within the cells.

The average area of the adult scalp approximates 120 square inches. It is the site of a profuse growth of hairs varying in thickness, length, straightness, and color, depending upon the individual's racial characteristics and sex. As in the skin, the oil or sebaceous glands are located along the hair shaft and secrete an oily fluid which appears to supply a protective oily coating to the scalp and gives it a gloss. As has been stated previously, the secretion of the sebaceous material is stimulated especially by the male sex hormones and is most marked at the time of puberty. As the person grows older, there is less and less secretion, until in old age both the skin and the scalp are dry. One of the constituents of the sebum, or the oil secretion of the sebaceous glands, is a chemical known as squalene. Recent work has shown that this chemical in adequate concentration acts as a depilatory on animal skin. This has led to the interesting theory that as male sex hormones are essential for the development of ordinary baldness, and the male hormones are the most powerful known stimulants of the secretion of oil, this sebaceous material may be related to and, in fact, may be a fundamental cause of baldness.

The entire body, with the exception of the palms and soles and a few small areas, is entirely covered with hair. The greatest percentage of this hair is a soft, delicate type of hair which is referred to as lanugo or fuzz and easily escapes notice by the naked eye. It has been estimated by a painstaking count that there are approximately 1,000 hairs of all types per square inch of scalp. Since the average surface area of the scalp encompasses approximately 120 square inches, it requires 120,000 hairs to cover it. The finer the hair, the more numerous are the shafts present in a given area; blond hairs are usually finest, and average 140,000, and black hairs average 110,000 per scalp. It is possibly distressing to the average redhead to learn that she has the fewest hairs on her scalp, namely, approximately 90,000. When hair is allowed to grow its full length, it will measure between 22 and 27 inches and sometimes grow as long as 36 inches, but this is indeed rare. As is well known, the hair does not live forever but is shed and regrown constantly. The life span of a single hair averages from 6 months to several years, and in the instance of extremely long hair the age can be figured from the length of the hair. The rate of hair growth approximates between ¾ and 1 inch per month, so that a hair 24 inches in length may be considered to be about 2 years in age.

Another feature of the hair that is not generally recognized is the fact that hair varies in form from a straight hair to variations of curves, with the resultant kinky hair in the Negro, as contrasted with the straight or wavy hair of the white race. Hair is extremely elastic and can be stretched very considerably. If it were not for this fact, it would be impossible to wave the hair, and this is the basis of most of the so-called "permanent" waves.

EXCESSIVE SWEATING

Excessive sweating of the scalp is not uncommon and often gives rise to unpleasant odors which are increased by infrequent washing and the use of various perfumed types of hair tonic. The condition is easily remedied by proper local hygiene and frequent washing of the scalp.

GRAYING

The color of the hair is due in part to hereditary and racial factors. Its appearance to the observer is actually due to the presence of tiny pigment granules scattered throughout the shaft of the hair. These granules make their appearance at the base of the hair under the scalp and do not change once they are scattered through the hair shaft itself. In other words, once the pigmentation has formed, it cannot be changed because of internal reasons, but only through external applications such as dyes. In other words, hair does not turn white overnight, but the pigmented hair shafts are shed and are replaced in time by new hairs which do not have these tiny pigmentation specks. Few persons have hairs of an identical color over their entire scalp, and detailed examination under various lights shows that many shades of hair occur on one head. Blonds, in particular, sometimes reveal hundreds of varying shades on a single normal scalp. Graying of the hair is still somewhat of a mystery, and the exact chemical mechanism which takes place in the hair bulb just before the hair loses its pigment and becomes white is unknown. Premature graying may begin in childhood, and by the age of twenty-five or thirty the scalp has a sort of salt-and-pepper look, and by forty or forty-five the patient is completely gray. Contrasted with this comparatively rapid type of graying, normal grayness begins at thirty-five or thereabouts, with a few non-pigmented hairs around the temples and a gradual slow whitening over a period of many years. There was a great deal of publicity given to a report that gray hair might be prevented by certain substances in the vitamin field. These substances were members of the vitamin B complex family, and are known as para-aminobenzoic acid and pantothenic acid. Unfortunately, subsequent studies have not confirmed this report, and sufferers from grayness cannot expect to be cured with vitamins. At the present time the only method of changing hair color is to resort to a dye. Although comparatively harmless dyes are available, they do not impart a satisfactory color to the hair. The stronger dyes are not entirely harmless, and the decision to proceed with hair dyeing should not be undertaken lightly.

ENDOCRINES AND HAIR GROWTH

The glands of internal secretion, which play such an important rôle in the physical and emotional well-being of the human race, also influence the scalp and the hair. The problem of relationship of hair growth to endocrine secretion is a very involved one, and the problem is often to recognize which gland is the primary factor and which the secondary, as far as the hair and its growth are concerned.

The sex glands are of the greatest importance with reference to the growth of hair. The female hormones have a very specific effect on oil secretion and on the growth of hair. An excess of female hormones, either of natural origin or due to some form of administration, results in a decreased activity of the oil glands, a shrinking of the hair follicles, and a lessened formation of skin cells. Accordingly, the administration of female sex hormones is often followed by the appearance of smooth, delicate skin, dryer and fluffier hair, the lessening of dandruff, and the softening of the beard. If the woman taking female hormones is afflicted with acne, there is usually a decreased amount of blackhead formation and even the disappearance of acne pimples. Although the statement is often encountered in the medical literature that the female hormones increase or stimulate the growth of scalp hair, this cannot be stated with absolute certainty, although the weight of evidence is in its favor. On the other hand, the male sex hormones, which are primarily responsible for the growth and development of the male organs, also have a specific effect on the hair follicle and the skin surface. They are probably the greatest single factor responsible for the production of the oil secretion, and they are also responsible for excessive growth of the skin around the hair follicles, and finally, they are of primary importance in the production of ordinary male baldness. The most interesting feature of these sex gland secretions is that while the male hormones encourage the growth of body hair, they discourage the growth of scalp hair. On the other hand, female hormones encourage the growth of scalp hair and discourage the growth of body hair. Men who have been castrated before puberty, and whose sex glands have remained infantile accordingly, have scanty body hair, of a female type, and very sparse beards but thick luxuriant hair on their scalps. Such persons do not become bald. However, if these eunuchs are treated with large doses of male sex hormones, they will become bald if their family or racial background is one of ordinary baldness. Although these scientific facts are well known, these secretions cannot be used in the treatment of ordinary baldness because they have other effects which might be of a serious nature for the person concerned. However, when hair is lost following pregnancy or during the period of menopause, this loss of hair can be checked and frequently regrown by the appropriate use of the female sex hormones.

The adrenal gland also produces hormones which affect hair growth. For example, the new wonder drugs cortisone and ACTH often increase facial hair while they are being given for the treatment of some other condition. In some instances, they even produce a mild degree of acne. These unfortunate side effects are usually temporary in nature and should be disregarded where the use of these drugs is necessary for the treatment of a serious disease. When the outer layer of the adrenal gland is overly active early in life, the person is frequently affected so that he appears far more advanced and older than his actual age. These "Young Hercules" often have an early growth of hair on their face and body, long before the time of puberty. When this gland becomes overactive in woman, the person begins to take on masculine features and there is often a considerable increase in body and facial hair.

The pituitary gland, especially one of its parts, also secretes hormones which affect the growth and development of hair. There is a disease which is due to a tumor of this gland and was first described by the famous brain surgeon, Harvey Cushing. It is known as Cushing's Syndrome and it affects women primarily. The women suffering from this tumor show certain color changes in the skin which look as though the skin has been bruised and stretched. In addition, these women develop a heavy beard. In other instances of disturbances of the pituitary gland there is an undersecretion of the pituitary hormones, and the individuals are known as Fröhlich types. These youngsters often have soft white skin and fat hips. They become so feminized as to even develop breasts. The face often remains free of hair, although the scalp growth is usually a good one.

As we have already learned, in connection with the skin, the thyroid gland regulates the metabolism and affects body growth. Where the thyroid gland is overactive, scalp hair is usually abundant but fine in quality and given to early grayness. In those instances where the thyroid gland does not supply an adequate amount of hormones, the skin is usually dry and puffy, and hair growth is scanty.

From the preceding brief description, it is evident that hair growth and glandular function are very closely related. At the present stage of our knowledge, no one glandular secretion can be said to be directly responsible for the growth or absence of hair. Each secretion is dependent in part on a secretion present in another gland which may either accelerate it or neutralize it, and that is why no specific gland can be definitely stated to be responsible for the sole production of hair.

NUTRITION

The relationship of diet to hair growth is of great importance, but is still a matter for speculation and future research. A few facts are available to us. The secretion of the sebaceous glands may be changed by either an excessive intake of fat or by an intake of special kinds of fat. For example, we know that certain types of fats are necessary for proper nutrition in rats, because a diet extremely low in this type of fat results in severe dandruff, scaliness, and baldness of the rats. If they are continued on this diet long enough, they will die at an early age. We also know that certain proteins are necessary for skin and hair growth. The reason for this is that these proteins contain a substance known as cystine which is found in far greater quantities in the skin and hair than in any other organ in the body. We know, too, that vitamin deficiency may affect the scalp.

If the system is deficient in vitamin A, the hair loses its sheen and luster and then becomes dry and eventually falls out. Surprisingly enough, almost similar features will occur in rare instances where too much vitamin A has been supplied to the body. In other words, don't take too much or too little of any of these substances without your doctor's approval. Other vitamins have some effect on the secretion of the oil glands as well as hair growth, and these have been mentioned elsewhere.

CARE OF THE NORMAL SCALP

The care of the normal scalp and its hair is the day-to-day attention which we give our scalp and hair to maintain its health and to increase its beauty. This definition would therefore not only include the usual brushing, combing, and cleaning, but also the cutting and waving, and the application of lotions and similar preparations which have been developed to satisfy the hair fashions of the day. There are so many nonsensical theories and superstitions which have been raised about the values of the many things done to the scalp and hair that the truth and validity for their application will be briefly presented.

BRUSHING

The implement chosen to brush the hair is just as important as the manner in which the brushing is to be performed. The one characteristic which these brushes should have without fail is the ability to undergo frequent cleaning without injury. The bristles should be well spaced to allow washing to free accumulations of dirt at their base, and should be set in frames able to withstand soap and water. Lacquered or polished wood is not satisfactory because repeated immersion causes the varnish to disappear, leaving the porous grain to absorb foreign matter. Metal frames are preferable though unattractive, but best of all are the ones more recently manufactured of pastel-colored plastics which seem capable of taking all kinds of physical punishment. Brushes should be washed in soapsuds and water regularly, whether they show signs of dirt or not. Natural bristles, when immersed too frequently, may become soft and too yielding to have any value as a medium for brushing the hair. Nylon bristles are more resistant. They may be wiped dry immediately after washing, while natural bristles must be allowed to dry in the sun or near, but not too near, artificial heat. It is unnecessary to use boiling water for antisepsis of one's own brush when the scalp is a normal, healthy one and the brush has been used by one person only. When frequenting a beauty shop, however, one should insist upon the use of a sterilized brush which is brought into the booth wrapped in a sterile container. Since one prevalent theory is based on the premise that dandruff may be transmitted by a germ, insistence upon sterile implements is merely a normal precaution, and reputable shops have long made this a practice.

Brushing should be performed regularly night and morning, not because a hundred brush strokes each time were thought by our grandmothers to evoke luxuriant heads of hair, but because it aids combing by unknotting tousled hair in a gentler fashion than the comb, and because it temporarily affects the circulation of the scalp.

The hair should be divided into strands and brushing should begin near the bottom of each strand, which is held firmly between the thumb and forefinger. When a two- or three-inch sector at the end of the strand seems to have been freed from all snarls, the hair should be grasped several inches higher and brushed down as before. This process should continue until finally the brush is allowed to begin at the scalp and sweep down the entire strand of hair to its end without encountering any tangles. Careful treatment of this nature excludes the breaking and tearing out of individual hairs by too hasty and too violent tugging. Such procedures are, of course, for long hair. Short hair may be brushed directly from the scalp. The value of brushing is the exercise which it gives the scalp by pulling at it, no matter how gently. Recent observations claim to show that exercise which involves bending or keeping the head in a position lower than that of the rest of the body is just as effective in producing a temporary improvement in scalp circulation as brushing was thought to be. For this reason lying for periods of time with the feet well above the level of the head causes a temporary increase in the blood supply both to the scalp and to the face.

Although brushing of the normal scalp is of some value, it must be modified in diseased states involving the hair. Where the hair is weakened and its attachment is less than normal, frequent and vigorous brushing may increase hair fall and result in further damage to the sick hair. Under such conditions gentle massage of the scalp and the discontinuance of daily, vigorous brushing are advised.

COMBING

Combs are employed not only for unsnarling tangled hair but also for the parting of the hair and its arrangement. No matter of what material the comb is made—whether ivory, shell, metal, or plastic—the teeth should be evenly spaced and separated sufficiently to make thorough cleaning between the teeth not too arduous a task. It is important to see that the teeth have rounded, blunt ends to avoid accidental scratching of the scalp, since we now know that many diseases of the scalp would not have been transmitted without an initial scratch or irritation which simplified the development of inflammation and infection.

Since combs are used even more frequently than brushes, both men and women carrying them about in pockets and pocketbooks, it is most important that their cleanliness be maintained and that no borrowing whatsoever be tolerated. As with brushes, soap and water are adequate cleaners. A small nailbrush may be used to clean between the teeth to be certain that all grease, dandruff scales, and city dust and grime have been removed. Sterilization may be assured by using weak solutions of alcohol or ammonia.

CUTTING

The only reason for cutting the hair is to add to one's comfort and to keep up one's appearance. The old-fashioned notion that frequent cutting of the hair and even shaving the scalp would augment its thickness has long since been completely discarded. The source of this fallacy must have been the gardener's successes at "cutting back" rosebushes and other shrubs to make them grow more successfully. The hair of the head which the naked eye discerns is fully developed, so no shaving or cutting can possibly affect the rate of its growth or influence its thickness. Painstaking research has proved the scientific fact that no part of the hair shaft above the surface of the scalp is capable of independent growth. All growth develops within the hair sheath.

SINGEING

When the ends of otherwise healthy hairs split, there is no cause for concern. If this is objectionable, it is only necessary to cut the hair shaft above the section which has already shown signs of separating. There is no scientific value whatsoever in singeing the hair. It is true that the flame eliminates the split end, but it also chars the hair shaft and tends to dry it higher up. Microscopic examination reveals the charring of the inner layers of the hair far above the point where the cuticle has been singed.

The unscientific notion that singeing is preferable to cutting was originally based on the erroneous belief that the entire hair is constantly nourished by a life-giving fluid which flows through a hollow canal in the hair shaft. These pseudoscientists thought that cutting would open an end of the canal and through this orifice the nourishing fluid would be lost, with resultant death of hair. Singeing, they believed, would weld the end into a closed point which would act as a stopper to the vial of nutritive elixir. Since, as stated above, the hair shaft with which we are dealing is to all intents and purposes a matured appendage beyond the scalp surface and not an animated one, this whole theory is nothing but primitive folklore.

SHAMPOOING

Shampooing was originally intended for the purpose of cleansing the hair and scalp, and this should still be its primary objective. However, when one reads the advertisements for a constantly growing list of new shampoos, and those "brought up to date," one reads not of their detergent and grease-dissolving value, but of their ability to leave the hair with a lustrous sheen. In other words, instead of just cleansing the hair shaft of all foreign matter, the advertisements brag that the shampoo adds to the glory of milady's tresses. Actually, the new synthetic detergents now being used in shampoos are such efficient cleansing agents that they actually remove the natural oils in the hair too completely. The proper treatment is to cleanse the hair and scalp first, and then, after the shampoo is completed, to add to the hair an appropriate oil to put the hair back into condition with regard to manageability and luster.

The question always arises as to how often the hair should be washed, particularly hair which is characterized as "dry." As a general rule, once every five days is ample when the hair is not excessively oily, although the more often it is washed, the better it is for the hair and the scalp. Some believe that once every ten days is sufficient for the greasy head, and once every two weeks for the dry. If dried properly, and subsequently treated according to the type of scalp, it is believed that the hair may be washed with impunity as many times as one has the energy to do so. Proper drying does not mean rubbing the wet hair briskly with a towel. Experimentation has shown that the tensile strength of hair when wet is considerably lessened, so, rather than risk breaking the hair, it should be exposed to heat, preferably that of the sun, although a warm current of air propelled by the fan of a hand dryer is also adequate. The inquisitional dryers which completely cover the head must be carefully regulated, since overheating will injure the hair by excessive drying, rendering it brittle, with the danger of damage when exposed to brush and comb.

The ideal shampoo should cleanse the scalp without either irritating the skin or causing excessive reduction of its natural oil. A shampoo with too alkaline a reaction or one with too great a detergency will dry the hair and make it brittle, instead of leaving it soft and lustrous. Since shampoos are designed specifically to remove all foreign matter, they should not themselves produce, either alone or in combination with water, any scum or gritty material remaining on the hair shaft. And lastly, for purely psychologic reasons, when combined with water they should evoke an instantaneous creamy lather.

All shampoos except those characterized as "dry" depend upon the addition of water. Hard water should be avoided for shampoos, or, if no soft water is available, it should be treated until it becomes soft. So-called "hard water" is water with a sufficiently high mineral salt content to interfere seriously with the lathering of soap. Usually hard water can be softened by simply boiling the water; but if chlorides and sulfates of magnesium and calcium are components, boiling is no help and the water will remain "permanently hard." When this type of water is used during a shampoo, the soap leaves a deposit on the hair shaft, thereby dulling the hair, and the scalp becomes irritated by the action of the harsh residue.

When soft water is totally unavailable, the permanent type of hard water may be softened at home by distillation. A Permutit system for home use has also been made available, but the simplest expedient is to add a 1 per cent solution of Calgon, a sodium hexametaphosphate. To test whether the water supply is soft or hard, one needs only to shake up the same amount of soap solution in two test tubes, one filled with the questionable water and the other with distilled, and compare the subsequent lathering. For the water to be sufficiently soft to use in shampooing, the lather should persist for a mimimum of two minutes after agitation.

The best sources of soft water are rain, which is usually pure but may become contaminated passing through smog or being collected in unclean receptacles, and distilled water, which is the condensation of steam arising from boiling water. Water from subsurface springs becomes purified as it wells through the soil, which acts as a filter, and water from artesian wells may have varying degrees of hardness, and, whereas it is pure, treatment may be required to soften it.

The perfect shampoo should clean the scalp without producing irritation or causing excessive reduction of its natural oil. There are three types of shampoos in most popular use, and these are the soap shampoos, the dry shampoos, and the soapless shampoos. The most popular types are the soap shampoos in liquid form, and these are composed primarily of oils such as coconut oil, which have been made into a soap and then diluted in water or in a mixture of water and alcohol. The "dry" shampoos are so-called not because they are not liquid, but because they do not contain water. They are actually dry cleaners for the hair and should only be used for special reasons and indications. The soapless shampoos are a type of detergent and are very efficient cleaners. In fact, the main disadvantage of shampoos made of such substances is that they are so efficient that they actually clean the hair too well, and remove from it the last trace of oil. To get around this difficulty, it is often necessary to add substances such as egg yolk or various other oils in order to decrease this cleansing action. In some instances these soapless shampoos can be used on an irritated scalp where an ordinary shampoo might prove to be very irritating.

HAIR LOTIONS

So many nonsensical and fantastic claims have been made by manufacturers of hair lotions that there is a tendency among intelligent persons to deride their use altogether. Actually, a good antiseptic conditioning and stimulating lotion is useful in the scalp. The use of such a lotion, together with ordinary scalp hygiene, may help to keep the hair and scalp as bacteria-free as possible, as well as improve the appearance of the hair. None of the advertised lotions is capable of growing hair, for the simple reason that there is as yet no known preparation which will effect such a miracle. When applied with enthusiastic friction, they help to free the hair mechanically from dandruff, and to make the scalp less liable to bacterial infection. Persons with oily scalps may use a lotion frequently, but those with dry scalps should be careful not to increase the dryness of their scalps.

WAVING LOTIONS

For the past few years we have heard more and more about permanent waving of the hair. Unfortunately, there is no such thing as a truly permanent wave, inasmuch as only the hair which projects from the surface of the scalp can be waved. As soon as this hair grows out, the new hair will be of the same uncurled state as it was previously, according to the shape of the hair follicle under the surface of the scalp. Artificial waving has been practiced on the scalp since the earliest recorded times. There have been many methods of waving hair, varying from the simple metal and leather curlers up to the present vogue for the cold wave lotion. Although some of these lotions were considered unsafe unless used by extremely skilled operators, the passage of time has showed that intelligent application according to the directions listed in the merchandised product render the applications a safe and effective way of waving the hair.

The reverse of the permanent waving process is called the hair straightening process. Actually, it is the same procedure done in reverse, and it is very popular not only among the colored race, whose characteristic hair kinkiness is well known, but among all persons with extremely curly hair. Inasmuch as these chemical solutions are all comparatively strong, it is recommended that proper attention be paid to directions and that their use be limited to the periods of time recommended by the manufacturer.

HAIR DYES

There are four main types of hair dyes. In the first group, the dye is a vegetable color such as henna, and is of a comparatively safe type. Unfortunately, the process is painstaking, the color is not very attractive, and the results comparatively unsatisfactory. A rinse is also a hair dye, but the word is apparently more acceptable to the public than the word "dye." Nevertheless, any substances which change the color of the hair are hair dyes and not rinses. Blond hair is usually kept in its state of natural beauty by removing the dark pigment from the hair rather than by the use of a hair dye. The bleaching agent usually employed is a peroxide and ammonia mixture, although too large an amount of ammonia will impart an undesirable reddish shade to the hair. So-called platinum blond hair results from excessive bleaching and will occur if the peroxide and ammonia solution is kept in longer contact with the hair than usual. Although the average bleaching preparation is relatively safe to use, continued bleaching will result in dryness and brittleness of the hair, with resistance to permanent waving, and a generally unattractive and unflattering appearance.

Another form of dye is the metallic group, containing silver, copper, or lead. These dyes are only successful when frequent applications are made, and the desired color emerges after a series of treatments which progressively darken the hair. They are not too desirable from a standpoint of attractiveness and nuisance of application.

Far and away the most popular hair dyes are the synthetic types, containing a substance known as paraphenylenediamine, and its derivatives. The para dyes are effective in that they produce a desirable shade of hair color. Unfortunately, they have to be applied at frequent intervals and are comparatively expensive. In addition, a certain number of people become sensitive or allergic to these hair dyes, and may develop uncomfortable and annoying skin reactions. There has been a recent trend toward the use of home hair-dyeing preparations, and although this type of dyeing may be carried out with some degree of safety, it is probable that the future will result in the development of more and more cases of sensitivity to these preparations. In most cities the local boards of health insist on the performance of various tests for the application of these hair dyes, and the reading of these tests should be performed by a person with some degree of training. It is difficult to see how the incidence of reactions to these dyes can fail to increase when there is even an apparent difficulty in the performance of dyeing procedures by a skilled professional operator, let alone the inexperienced home amateur.

IRRITATION OF THE SCALP

The term "contact dermatitis" is used to describe an acute inflammation of the scalp due to the application of some chemical or other agent. Just as we have seen with the skin itself, the scalp may be considerably irritated following contact with chemicals such as shampoos, hair lotions, and hair dyes. The subsequent inflammation results in redness and itching of the scalp. In severe cases there is often an appearance of blisters and crusts throughout the scalp. Usually the entire cycle of the dermatitis is completed within a few days to a few weeks, but if the offending substance has not been discovered, a chronic eruption may result. The dermatitis of the scalp is dependent primarily on the strength of the offending agent, the condition of the scalp, and the presence of an allergic state due to a preceding contact with the same substance. If the person has already become allergic to the chemical as a result of a previous exposure, the reaction occurs quickly. The fine balance between the scalp's capacity to withstand exposure to a new substance may be upset by a variety of factors. Scalp resistance may be lowered by frequent washings with strong soaps, by excessive secretion of the oil and sweat glands, and by overexposure to sunlight. The presence of an associated local disease such as dandruff, or extreme dryness of the scalp, may also play a rôle.

The diagnosis of the scalp condition is sometimes made easy by a history of an itching and burning sensation following the application of some new preparation to the hair. An acute eruption spreading down the neck and about the ears should often make the doctor suspicious of hair dyes or some recent chemical agent applied to the scalp. The tendency is for most people to deny that they use hair dyes, and some of them honestly believe that they never have because of clever advertising and promotion which allow the dye to masquerade under the name of "hair rinse" or "color restorer." However, dyes are not the only offenders. There are many other substances which will not only cause a reaction when brought in contact with the scalp, but may produce a dermatitis after a week or so. According to the Food and Drug Administration, the government agency which controls and supervises all types of cosmetic applications, the para dyes sooner or later produce skin eruptions in four out of every hundred people if they continue to come in contact with them.

Other substances which have been known to produce acute or chronic irritation of the scalp include perfumes, hair lotions, hair lacquers, hair straighteners, waving lotions, and even the ordinary skin enemies such as poison ivy and other plants. Dermatitis of the scalp and near-by skin has also resulted following contact with hat bands, rubber caps, and hat dyes.

The treatment of dermatitis of the scalp is similar in nature to the treatment of skin disorders of this type in general. The first step consists in the detection and elimination of the suspicious chemical. Sometimes it may be a simple matter to discover the cause, and then again it may be extremely difficult and even impossible. After the suspicious agent has been detected, it may merely be necessary to stop using the preparation. Where the exposure has been going on for a long time, it is also important to shampoo the suspected preparation out of the scalp or, in extreme cases, even shaving the head. The local inflammation should then be treated with mild wet dressings, such as weak boric acid or salt solution, as well as with bland and soothing ointments and lotions. Ointments containing weak dilutions of Burow's solution and mild vegetable oils are inexpensive and effective. They should be made up in a greaseless type of base so as not to mat the hair together. If the scalp is extremely irritated, some of the newer drugs which have been found of value in the treatment of itching may be necessary. This, of course, is a matter for the physician to decide, although in general it may be stated that the anti-histaminic drugs are often of great value, and in the extreme case both cortisone and ACTH have been found very useful drugs for the acutely uncomfortable stage of the eruption.

ORDINARY BALDNESS

The common or so-called garden variety of baldness is referred to medically as male pattern alopecia. Alopecia means baldness, and male pattern means of the typical form common to men. It is responsible for more than 95 per cent of all the cases of baldness. The loss of hair occurs with far greater frequency in men than in women, although women occasionally become bald also. In the usual case the loss of hair first manifests itself by a thinning of hair along the side margins between the scalp and forehead, and a slight moving back of the hairline over the temples. In time the hairline gradually moves itself back, and a small bald patch makes its appearance in the middle of the back of the scalp. With advancing age, the bald patches in these two areas gradually enlarge, and in extreme cases of baldness eventually meet, so that no hair is left except for a little fringe around the scalp. At this stage the victim's friends state that he has a "nice head of skin." The rate of hair loss is more or less an individual matter. In the early stages of beginning baldness hundreds of hairs may be shed in one day. After a period of time, these decrease to approximately fifty to a hundred. Because of these slowed-up periods of hair fall, advanced baldness is seldom noticed in a man before he is thirty years old. During these periods exempt from profuse hair fall there is the usual slight growth of new hair, but these are never of sufficient nature to compensate for the preceding loss. Furthermore, these newer hairs are usually of a fine and delicate type, being produced by a half-dead papilla. Their appearance is often glibly prophesied by the quack hair grower, and their actual appearance is attended by great fanfare and mutual congratulatory exchanges. Unfortunately, they rarely turn into a normal healthy type of hair. Beware of the quack who promises to grow a new head of hair for you!

Numerous theories have been advanced in an attempt to explain ordinary male baldness. According to studies performed by competent scientists, especially Dr. James Hamilton, the essential reason for the development of common baldness is an inherited racial tendency. We know that members of certain races inherit tendencies either to retain hair or to show certain definite types of baldness. Just think of different racial groups that you are familiar with, and you will realize that each group has a somewhat similar pattern of hair growth and hair loss. Another factor of importance in the production of ordinary baldness is the hormone secretions, particularly that provided by the secretions of the male and female sex glands. We know that baldness does not appear in men who for any one of several reasons did not mature sexually. Baldness can be produced in these men if they are later treated with male sex hormones, but only if their pedigrees show their families to be susceptible to baldness. And don't let the bald men use this fact as proof of their virility because it just is not so. The third reason for ordinary baldness is the simple process of getting older. Advancing age is always accompanied by an increase in the number of bald people and the extent of the usual typical baldness. These three factors—namely, an inherited racial tendency, the male sex hormones, and the aging factors—act singly and in unison to increase the tendency toward baldness. Although typical male baldness is limited to men, women may also lose their hair in similar fashion although this occurs far less frequently and is never as extensive as the advanced cases observed among older men. Other causes which have been blamed for baldness may play a small rôle, and some of these include tightness of the scalp, and the presence or absence of dandruff and seborrhea. In all probability, the association of dandruff, excessive oily secretions, and other local diseases may not be of primary importance in the loss of hair, but they are certainly aggravating factors and may increase the extent and rapidity of hair fall. Inasmuch as baldness develops far more rapidly in the presence of circulating male sex hormones, and inasmuch as male sex hormones are the most powerful known stimulants of oil secretion, there is probably a relationship between the two which accounts in certain measure for the occurrence of baldness with greater frequency in the male sex.

At the present stage of our knowledge, there is no 100 per cent effective remedy for ordinary baldness, either from the standpoint of prevention or cure.

Nevertheless, general massage of the scalp rarely does any harm, and the local application of remedies of value in the treatment of dandruff and similar states may lessen the degree and extent of the baldness. It can be stated with almost complete certainty that the many so-called "scalp institutes" and "hair growers," whose advertisements fill the daily newspapers, have never been able to prevent or treat ordinary baldness with success. If you are losing your hair and you are worried about it, consult your family physician or a skin specialist if you wish to know what, if anything, can be done for the condition.

OTHER TYPES OF BALDNESS

Although ordinary male baldness accounts for by far the greatest number of hairless scalps, the remaining examples of baldness may occur for any one of many reasons. First of all, a certain amount of baldness may occur in association with various types of scalp or skin disease, varying from the loss of hair in small patches to complete baldness involving all the hairy areas of the body. A diffuse shedding of the scalp hair often occurs following the ordinary childhood diseases if they have been associated with high fever for any period of time. This type of hair fall may occur after scarlet fever or measles and is usually temporary in nature, as the hair starts to grow in within a few weeks to a few months following the shedding. In addition to the childhood diseases, various toxic conditions, especially if associated with a high fever, may also produce a temporary or permanent loss of hair, and this has been noticed in diseases such as typhoid fever and influenza. The loss of hair is quite general over the scalp but seldom complete, that is, only a thinning of the hair occurs rather than complete baldness. These scalp changes may also occur in chronically ill people who are suffering from tuberculosis and other wasting diseases. Infections such as syphilis often produce loss of hair during certain stages of the disease. In syphilis the hair loss is fairly typical in that the hair falls out in small bald patches, giving the scalp a somewhat typical mangy or moth-eaten look. In most instances, with proper treatment, these types of baldness are followed by complete restoration of the hair.

THE SEBORRHEIC DISORDERS AND DANDRUFF

The most common malady to involve the scalp is dandruff. In this condition the scalp often becomes covered with loose dry scales or with fine branny flakes which result in a process of constant peeling of the scalp due to a flaking off of the outer layers of the skin. The scales are gray or white and fall off the scalp when they are disturbed by combing, brushing, or scatching. Much to the annoyance of the individual, they then appear in large quantities along their hairs and as "snow" on their shoulders. The scalp often feels itchy and even slightly irritated. Inasmuch as the oil secretions cannot flow freely in this condition, the hairs become dull and unruly. In the average person dandruff appears in early childhood and may persist as such for many years. However, in the majority of people the scales in time become greasier, yellowish, and more numerous. At this stage, the underlying scalp is apt to be more irritated and there are occasional crusted areas in the scalp which may even extend down the forehead. In other cases the scalp becomes excessively oily, and the face, especially around the sides of the nose, may show a similar extremely excessive oily condition. This profuse secretion of oil bathes the hair and the scalp and contributes to the glossy, greasy appearance of the latter. At times the secretion is so pronounced that drops of oil form and have to be wiped off. This is usually referred to as "oily seborrhea." These conditions are related in part to certain germs, to changes in glandular secretion, and to various general factors such as poor nutrition, chronic intestinal disturbances, and various unknown mechanisms.

The treatment should be managed by the physician, but the patient must expect to co-operate fully if he wishes to achieve a result. The main features of the treatment consist in the frequent shampooing of the scalp, and the constant use of ointments and lotions applied with massage, without neglecting the massage of daily brushing. There are various other methods which should be employed by the physician in his office, but the chief points in treatment are the patience and persistence of the individual with the scalp condition. The state of the general health has much to do with the recurrence of the different types of seborrheic conditions. Over-fatigue, worry, emotional disturbances, and loss of sleep are some of the causes of lowered resistance which may play a rôle in the continuance of these disturbances. It should also be mentioned that there are several new preparations which have been found very effective in the external treatment of these conditions. One of these new drugs is a chemical known as selenium which should be employed only under the supervision of a physician, as its toxic properties have not yet been fully studied.

The very oily forms of seborrhea require even more skillful treatment. If local measures are going to be effective, the scalp must first be freed of its fatty covering by bathing it in softening solutions such as olive and almond oil, with a small amount of glycerin. Even when the oily secretions are unusually large and crusted, soap and water will free the scales and cleanse the oily surface of the scalp. After this cleansing operation has been completed, alkaline rinses may be used to lessen the oiliness, and this would include mixtures of borax and ammonia carefully diluted to proportions harmless to the scalp itself. It is important to use an oily application immediately after such a mixture in order to prevent possible irritation of the scalp, and vegetable or mineral oil are usually effective for this purpose. Here again, measures which will improve the general health are very important. In many instances it has been found that people working indoors are most apt to suffer from these oily forms of seborrhea and they are often helped by fresh air and exercise in addition to the local measures. Of course, a well-balanced diet and the elimination of any local infection are also of value.

SEBORRHEIC DERMATITIS

This disease usually follows the preceding local scalp disturbances such as dandruff and the oily forms of seborrhea. It is a more severe form, and usually shows, in addition to the features of the conditions mentioned, a considerable degree of greasy scaling, crusting, and redness involving both small and large areas throughout the scalp. In some instances the condition becomes so extensive and severe that it may spread to involve the face, ears, and many other parts of the body. In such instances it becomes a serious and difficult skin disease to treat and requires the services of a skilled dermatologist.

The ordinary forms of seborrheic dermatitis are considered due to the same causative mechanism that produces dandruff and the oily forms of seborrhea. The excessive flow of oil on the surface of the scalp depends in turn upon the production of excessive amounts of male hormones by the gland of internal secretion. The question as to whether or not the process is also related to bacterial infection is still undecided. There has also been considerable research to show that poor nutrition plays a rôle, as do certain hereditary factors, chronic intestinal conditions, inadequate personal hygiene, and various emotional disturbances.

The treatment of the chronic type of seborrheic eczema or dermatitis is difficult. It may be helped by proper diet and the administration of vitamin B complex, combined with crude liver extract. Vitamin B_{12} has also been found of value in this disease. No matter what therapeutic measures are advised, it is necessary for all the victims of this condition to follow an intelligent daily routine with regular periods for rest and sleep, frequent bathing, the use of soap substitutes if soap proves to be an irritant, a diet high in protein and low in fats and carbohydrates, and the elimination of alcohol. In the acute stages of the condition it is often necessary to resort to wet dressings in order to lessen the inflammation. After the condition improves, a soothing ointment or lotion is of value. In the scalp the most useful preparations contain chemicals such as sulfur, salicylic acid, and resorcin. If infection is present, it is often necessary to add some of the new antibiotics, such as penicillin or terramycin, to the therapeutic measures. This, of course, is only done under the supervision of a physician, as it is recognized that any of these preparations are capable of acting as irritants to the skin and scalp, and they must be watched with great care. (A newly discovered product is Selsun and this is now recommended by doctors as a specific method of controlling seborrhea and dandruff.—Ed.) I routinely advise a low fat and low carbohydrate, high protein type of diet, with the elimination of alcohol and excessively hot foods and drinks. In the heavy and red-faced individual, it is often necessary to make sure that the mundane pleasures of steam cabinets, Turkish baths, and daily massage are not indulged in. These simple measures are important in combination with actual medical treatment of specific value in individual instances.

INFECTIONS OF THE SCALP

The same bacterial infections that involve the skin may also appear on the scalp. Impetigo, boils, and carbuncles occasionally occur in the scalp and are similar in appearance to the condition when it involves the skin. In impetigo the scalp shows typical honey-colored crusts scattered throughout the hair, often in children having head lice. Boils start as an infection in the hair follicle, with swelling and discharge of pus. In neglected cases they may spread throughout the entire scalp. This is especially true when the boil starts in the back of the neck, and rubbing and friction from the collar cause it to spread. These conditions all respond promptly to local measures with wet dressings, antiseptics, and antibiotics, such as penicillin, terramycin, aureomycin, and chloromycetin. It is of the utmost importance to exercise proper local hygiene if a recurrence is to be prevented. Such measures include frequent washing and shampooing of the scalp and adjoining skin, the wearing of clean, soft collars, and a proper diet, including the avoidance of excessive sweets, starches, fatty and greasy foods.

Ringworm of the scalp is a far more serious condition and is due to the attack of the hair and scalp by a fungus. This organism primarily occurs in children before the age of puberty. It is characterized by the appearance of scaly, bald patches, sometimes covered with brittle and broken hair stubs, and in certain cases with small pustules. Any bald patch in a child's scalp should be considered as a possible ringworm infection until the doctor rubs it out. The disease is highly communicable and may be spread from animals to humans, or, depending upon the type of ringworm, from children to other children. In the epidemic that occurred during the last war it was found that the backs of theater seats and barber shops were often a source of contagion. Insist that your barber clean his instruments before cutting your child's hair, and you may save yourself a serious problem. Also, if your youngster loves to go to the movies and rest his head on the back of the seat, tell him to put his handkerchief on the seat or bring along a little paper towel that he can put on the seat before sitting back and relaxing.

The most common type of ringworm of the scalp is a so-called "gray patch" or human type. In this variety the diseased area is usually round and bald except for a few hairs which have been broken off above the surface of the scalp. It may be impossible to see any bald areas in the scalp, the only sign of infection being the presence of a few scaly or crusted scabs in the scalp. In these instances a doctor should be consulted so that the child can be examined under a special light known as a Wood's filter. Under this very helpful light, the infected areas show up as bright green fluorescent hairs which are immediately both typical and diagnostic. This little gadget has been of great help in screening the scalps of hundreds of school children and in preventing the spread of epidemics of the disease. It is also of value in diagnosing other forms of ringworm, although certain unusual types of the disease do not cause the hair to fluoresce under the light.

The second type of ringworm most commonly encountered is that which is transmitted not only from child to child, but by domestic animals such as dogs or cats. It differs from the simple gray patch type of ringworm because there is a certain amount of inflammation and pus formation present. These are the two most common types of ringworm, although there are many other less common forms observed in different parts of the world. The doctor has a rule that any child showing scaly or bald patches on the scalp must be considered as having a ringworm infection until the Wood's filter and the examination of the hair shows it to be otherwise. In addition to the Wood's light as a means of diagnosis, it is also of importance to the doctor to examine the hairs directly under the microscope and, in suspicious cases, to attempt to grow the organism from the hair by planting the hair in some type of culture medium.

The treatment of ringworm of the scalp depends upon the type of fungus producing the disease. When the organism is of the so-called animal type, which results in infection of the scalp, the use of local remedies such as sulfur, ammoniated mercury, and some of the newer chemicals, combined with frequent shampooing, is usually effective. The reason for this is that the infection around the hair loosens the hair and causes it to be shed from the surface of the scalp. Unfortunately, in the other types of ringworm, where no infection is present, the infected hair is held tightly in the scalp and any attempts to pull it out only result in breaking the hair and the continuance of the infection in the hair under the surface of the scalp. Where this type of infection fails to respond to local measures after a suitable period of time, it is often necessary to treat it by means of X-ray therapy. The X-rays are usually administered at a single session and in a dose sufficient to cause complete falling out of the hair within a few weeks. This procedure requires great training and technical skill on the part of the doctor, and should only be administered by an expert. After the hair has fallen out, regrowth begins after several weeks and the new hairs show no signs of the infection where the X-ray treatment has been properly performed.

HEAD LICE

The head is frequently infected in young children by the head louse referred to medically as pediculosis capitis. The head louse is a small animal approximately 2 mm. long, of a gray color and with black spots around the margins of its body. It inhabits the scalp, especially in children of both sexes and of questionable cleanliness. These lice set up severe itching of the scalp, due to the fact that they feed on and bite the scalp surface. As a result of itching, the child scratches the scalp and often produces a secondary infection. This infection may be so severe that the occasional child develops large glands of the neck due to drainage from the infected areas. Where the social environment is one of absolute neglect, an occasional child may be found to have the head covered with a hairy mess teeming with lice and covered with hundreds of eggs (nits). This combination, plus secondary infection and crusts, leads to a nauseating odor and the accumulation of pus and infected debris on the scalp. Fortunately, these conditions are rare at the present time, although an occasional refugee or neglected child may be seen with such an extreme degree of lousiness. The eggs look like tiny white or grayish grains stuck to the hairs, near the surface of the scalp. In many instances the duration of the infection can be determined by the distance from the egg to the hair shaft, inasmuch as the egg is deposited at the scalp margin and grows out with the hair shaft. In other words, if the egg is approximately one inch from the scalp, the infection would be approximately one month old, inasmuch as hair grows at the rate of approximately one-half inch every two weeks.

There are many local remedies which bring about a speedy and rapid cure of pediculosis capitis. First, it is necessary to remove all sources of the infection and to observe the normal rules of cleanliness if a recurrence is to be prevented. This means that hats, combs, and brushes which have been recently in contact with the scalp should be cleaned very thoroughly or thrown out. The present methods of treatment include the use of DDT in various powders or ointment forms, as well as other newer killers of animal parasites, including benzyl benzoate, Eurax, and Gamergent.

It is also of importance to loosen the eggs with scalp rinses of vinegar or similar substances, and then slide the eggs off the hair shaft with tweezers.

ALOPECIA AREATA

Alopecia areata is a fairly common disease of the hair, occurring more often in children than in adults but not uncommonly in the latter. Often without warning, a bunch of hair may be found upon the pillow in the morning, or a small completely bald patch suddenly noticed in the scalp. There may be only one small spot, but frequently others appear and join to form large, queerly shaped areas. In rare cases this hair loss progresses until all the hair upon the body has disappeared. Such cases are difficult to cure, but to the ordinary case with a limited amount of baldness of the scalp a much more cheerful outlook can be given, for they usually clear up after some months of treatment. In the bald patches the hair may grow in blond at first, even in dark-haired persons; but this usually changes to the normal color later. In those of middle age the hair may come in white and remain so. The afflicted one need not be frightened if the first growth of hair falls out, for continuation of treatment is usually successful in causing a permanent growth. The cause of the disease is not known, but bears a definite relationship to various psychosomatic factors. Within the past year resistant cases of this disease have been successfully treated with cortisone, but this treatment is still in an experimental stage and must be carefully supervised. It is most effective in recent rather than in old cases of alopecia areata. A more permanent cure depends upon a thorough understanding of the physical and mental causes of the disease.

SUPERFLUOUS HAIR

Undesired hair on a lady's face is a greater trial even than the lack of it upon the head of her husband. This common form of irregular hair distribution often begins in early adult life and causes great mental distress. The mild form appears as lengthening and darkening of the ends of the mustache or groups of long hairs on the sides of the chin; but in severe cases the beard is complete and fairly thick. Efforts to relieve this condition have been made since time immemorial, and the old methods are still in use: the razor, the depilatory, and the resin-wax method. Shaving and the use of an epilating paste are alike in removing only that portion of the hair which projects from the follicle. After their use the hair grows out stiff. The resin-wax method pulls out the whole hair, and it grows again only after a considerable time and then as a young hair, pointed at the end.

When X-rays were first studied, it was thought that they might be the long-desired means of wholesale removal of hair; but it was soon found that it could not be done by this method without great danger of injury to the skin. That such injury might not make itself known for months or years after the treatment did not make it any less serious. All reputable dermatologists have agreed that this method is unsafe. Only the electric needle is left to give lasting relief to the sufferers from this deformity. It is slow and tedious; but safe, certain, and not very painful.

If fine hairs become dark-colored, they can be made less conspicuous by bleaching with peroxide solution, to four parts of which one part of ammonia water is added just before applying it on a cotton pledget. This should not be used often enough to irritate the skin.

THE NAILS

The nails are horny plates designed for protection of the ends of the fingers and toes and also for weapons of defense and offense. These latter uses have to some extent gone out of style, although some women are unaware of that fact. These plates are produced by the epidermal cells much as are the hairs. Normally they are smooth, curved from side to side, and very slightly curved in the long axis. At the base is a light-colored oval area where the active growth of the nail is going on, and over it, next the fold of skin under which the nail grows, is a special membrane, popularly referred to as the "cuticle." As the nail grows, the free end wears off in those doing rough work, or in those who have itching skin disease and keep their nails worn short and highly polished from constant scratching. Nervous individuals often keep their nails short by biting. When protected from friction and injury, the nail may grow several inches long, a good sign of inactivity and the so-called "leisure class."

HYGIENE OF THE NAILS

They should be kept cut fairly short. Fashion decrees at times that they should be trimmed so that they are pointed. This does them no harm. Neither does the polishing, if it is done in a way to avoid infection, nor the various colored nail polishes in popular vogue. Careful pushing back of the cuticle is also harmless if gently done with a smooth, clean instrument, preferably of wood. The manicurist should have some knowledge of cleanliness and should sterilize her instruments by boiling after each use. The polishing pad has gone out of style, and the present-day use of a liquid polish is much more sanitary. After trimming off hangnails, the little tags of skin that become loosened along the sides of the nails, the spot should be touched with an antiseptic. Do not bite or pick hangnails, for these methods favor infection, especially an infected swelling called paronychia or "run-around." Cleansing of the nails should be done after thorough washing, that the dirt under the free edge may be well loosened. A sharp instrument should not be used for this, because it will roughen the inner side of the free portion, dirt will adhere more tightly, and more scraping will be necessary to dislodge it. If the skin of the hands is dry, the nail folds should receive special attention in applying cold cream, for deformities of the nail may result from lack of oil. Dry and brittle nails are common complaints. The causes of nails of this type are not completely known, although in specific instances the reasons are definite. For example, a certain type of nail polish was only applied to the nails after a so-called "base-coat" had been applied first. Many women were allergic to this particular base-coat and their nails became dry, brittle, and deformed. In some cases the reaction was so severe that they lost their nails. Fortunately, the cause was detected and the base-coat taken off the market. In other instances dry and brittle nails may be due to a vitamin deficiency (especially vitamin A), a mineral deficiency (especially calcium), a protein deficiency (especially cystine), or a glandular deficiency (especially thyroid). Don't attempt to be your own doctor, but get professional advice if you are worried about your nail condition. It may be as simple as stopping your nail polish or avoiding soap and water to the best of your ability!

Transverse grooves appear in the nails commonly after illness, sometimes after so trivial a disorder as seasickness, and gradually disappear by growing out to the free end. Any disturbance to the nutrition of the nail may cause this deformity. Even overenthusiastic care of the nails—such as pushing down the cuticle too roughly, cutting it, or injuries received in other ways—may lead to nail deformities. The same is true of other deformities of the nails—longitudinal ridges, pitting, splitting—and often it is impossible to find the cause of these irregularities of growth because they are so slight that the nail changes are the only evidence. Loosening of the nails at the sides may occur in the absence of any other sign of disease; but is usually only temporary. Spoon-shaped nails and other abnormal changes may be hereditary, with accompanying hair and tooth deficiencies, or may result from malnutrition or anemia.

White spots on the nails, "gift spots," may be caused by general disease or local injury. They are the result of imperfect formation of the horny plate as the nail grows and usually disappear in time.

Thickening of the nails may be caused by nutritional disorder, skin disease, or more frequently by ringworm infection of the nail. It occurs most often on the nail of the big toe, and if not due to infection may be kept in check by paring and scraping. Ringworm of the nails is important because, owing to the fact that it is unobtrusive in its manifestations, it is often not noticed, and if treated is very difficult to cure. Therefore, it is likely to remain as a focus of the disease from which infection is spread to other parts. The most successful treatment entails weekly removal of the nail surface by means of an electric drill and the subsequent painting with a fungus-killing chemical such as ammoniacal silver nitrate. These severe nail changes are not hopeless, but take time and skill if a cure is to be obtained.

Ingrowing toenails are caused by improper nail cutting, tight shoes, or local injury. They can be cured, before they become severely inflamed, by carefully cutting out the ingrowing part at the sides of the free border of the nail and preventing regrowth in this direction by padding with wool. This procedure should be performed with the utmost attention to cleanliness in order to minimize infection. Once infection has occurred, wet dressings and some of the newer antiseptics result in rapid cure under medical supervision.

ACKNOWLEDGMENTS

Acknowledgment is hereby given to the following articles and books which were used as a source of material and actual text matter in the preceding chapter.

1. *The Modern Home Medical Adviser* edited by Dr. Morris Fishbein. Chapter 25—The Skin—by Dr. Arthur W. Stillians.

2. *Your Skin and Its Care* by Dr. Howard T. Behrman and Dr. Oscar L. Levin. Emerson Books, Inc., New York, 1951.

3. *Your Hair and Its Care* by Dr. Oscar L. Levin and Dr. Howard T. Behrman. Emerson Books, Inc., New York, 1947.

4. *The Scalp in Health and Disease* by Dr. Howard T. Behrman. C. V. Mosby Co., St. Louis, 1952.

5. "Eczema" by Dr. Howard T. Behrman was reprinted in part from *Hygeia Magazine* (Today's Health), American Medical Association.

CHAPTER XXVI

The Eye
MORRIS FISHBEIN, M.D.

DISEASES OF THE EYE

THE EYES are used constantly almost from the moment of birth to the time of death, except for the hours spent in sleeping. Good eyesight is necessary to an enjoyable existence, and the handicap of blindness one of the most serious that can affect a human being. Although the human eye is one of the finest instruments of which mankind has any knowledge, even a normal eye has certain defects. The visual field of a human being is not nearly as great as that of many other species of living organisms. A bird or a fly has a much wider range of vision than does the human being.

The mechanism of vision is complicated and difficult to understand, except by those who have some knowledge of the construction of the eye. The chief factors involved in seeing are the optic nerve and the center in the brain for vision; the retina, which is the portion of the eye that acts to convey things seen through the optic nerve; the lens, which is the focusing tissue; the muscles, which control the lens; the iris, which makes the pupil and which controls the amount of light entering the eye, and, of course, the associated fluid material, which is necessary to the proper working of the mechanism.

The eye is one of the most adaptable of organs. The distinctness of vision varies with different parts of the retina. For example, as one goes from a bright light into darkness, the vision is, at first, very bad, but after some minutes improves rapidly. The retina has the power to adapt itself to correspond with variations in the intensity of illumination. The various parts of the retina vary in this manner.

PREVENTION OF BLINDNESS

About seven million children in the United States are failing to secure proper care of their eyes because their parents and teachers fail to realize that they do not see well. Children are not likely to complain because they do not

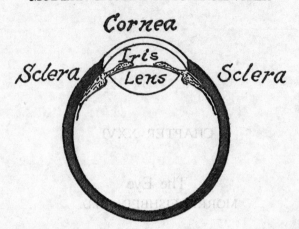

Fig. 50. Cross-section of eye. Clear cornea. Colored iris with hole showing the pupil. Lens and scera or white of the eye.

recognize that they are not seeing well. They do not know what they ought to be able to see. Here are some warning signs of possible visual defects.

The child rubs its eyes frequently, frowns, or tries to brush away blurring.

The child shuts or covers one eye, or tilts the head sidewise or forward trying to see better.

The child has difficulty in reading. Thousands of children have difficulty in reading ordinary print but can easily make out larger print now recommended in sight-saving classes.

The child blinks more than other children and becomes irritable when asked to do close work like stringing beads.

The child stumbles or trips over small objects.

When reading or drawing or painting the eyes must be close to the material used.

The child is sensitive to light and avoids it.

The eyes and eye-lids are reddened, swollen and perhaps have crusts.

The child has frequent infections with styes.

The eyes are inflamed and watery.

Any of these symptoms means that the child should have an examination after which proper care and the provision of suitable glasses may save eyesight and permit the child an even break with other children.

CROSSED EYES

When people say "crossed eyes" they usually mean that the two eyes do not track together. What people call "crossed eyes" doctors call strabismus or squint. With the craze for system which is the soul of science the different varieties have been classified in various ways. Eyes that turn inward are "crossed eyes." When the eyes turn outward they are "wall eyes." When the eyes turn upward they are "vertical eyes."

Near or far vision, blows on the head, defective development of the muscles of the eyes and the effects of a number of diseases may result in malpositions of the eyes such as have been mentioned. When the eyes are unable to focus on the same object at the same time the brain sees two images. The images do not fuse together. When trying to get them together the child turns his head or partly shuts the eyes or tries the use of one eye at a time.

The National Society for the Prevention of Blindness notes that the longer a child is cross-eyed the more difficult it is to improve the vision. Treatment should be started preferably before the age of four. Some forms of treatment can be started before one year of age. Even cross-eyed children up to nine years of age can occasionally get back normal sight if they receive correct treatment. Exercises may help; sometimes glasses help; often an operation is necessary.

The eyes of very young babies may seem to float. A tendency to close one eye, to tilt the head or to rub one eye means that a doctor's attention is necessary.

SPOTS OR SPECKS IN VISION

Because of the nature of the construction of the eye, several visual disturbances occur which do not represent actual defects but are the result of the construction. As you look up at the blue sky or as you look suddenly at a white ceiling, you may notice a number of minute specks that move in front of the eye. These specks are the blood corpuscles moving in the smallest blood vessels of the retina. As will be shown later, such specks constantly seen may be a sign of changes in the fluid material of the eye. If the heartbeat is increased by exercise, the corpuscles will move faster, and the specks, which represent the corpuscles, move faster.

SEEING COLORED LIGHTS

Bright lights seen at night, as for example street lamps, may appear to be surrounded by areas of color or colored rings, blue inside and red on the outside. These are due to the tissue of the lens and of the cornea, which is the membrane over the eye. These tissues are ordinarily not seen.

BLACK EYE

One of the most common disturbances of the eye is injury caused by a blow of some type. Indeed, these injuries are so common that they have become common material for the cartoonist. Anyone who shows up at the office with a black eye is sure to be the victim of several presumably comical remarks as to marital conflicts. Actually, it may merely be the result of running into an open door. Anyway, that's your alibi if you stick to it. The immediate effect of a blow on the eye with a blunt instrument may not be serious, but the later effects may be extremely serious. It is, therefore, best to treat every severe blow of the eye as a serious condition until sufficient time has passed to indicate the extent of the damage. Sometimes there is merely bleeding of the small vessels in the white of the eye. An X-ray picture may show that the bones of the skull which surround the eye have been broken.

It is safe, whenever one has had a blow on the eye, to go to bed immediately and to put an ice-bag on the eye and to have competent medical attention as soon as possible.

PENETRATING INJURY

Much more serious than a blow with a blunt instrument is the penetrating injury, such as may be brought about by a sharp probe, or by flying particles of glass, steel, or similar material. If any of the fluid material of the eye has escaped through the injury, the condition is especially serious. Fortunately, the X-ray is now of great aid in indicating whether or not a substance has actually penetrated the eyeball.

The removal of the foreign substance from the eyeball is a most difficult process, and one of which only trained physicians are capable. The use of a magnet is sometimes helpful. There are many substances which are not attracted by a magnet and which may cause great harm if they remain in the eye. Sooner or later destruction of the tissue occurs around the foreign substance. Sometimes there is infection, and not infrequently complete loss of vision.

Flying particles of hot steel are usually free from infection. However, even when germs are not carried into the eye with the foreign substance, they may be brought to the eye by the blood and localize in the spot which has been damaged by the irritation.

SYMPATHETIC OPHTHALMIA

Most serious in connection with any penetrating injury of the eye is the serious inflammation of the other eye, known as sympathetic ophthalmia. This occurs some fourteen days after the injury to the first eye, most frequently in from four to six weeks, but may occur many months or even years later. The appearance of the eye first injured helps the physician to determine the possible onset of such an inflammation in the other eye. In the majority of cases, proper preventive measures are taken immediately. If the first eye is severely damaged and inflammation is serious, it is customary to remove the injured eye promptly before any signs of inflammation have appeared in the second eye. In some instances cortisone has been helpful.

No one knows yet just why sympathetic ophthalmia occurs. It is such a serious condition, however, as it means loss of both eyes rather than of one, that the physician must give the benefit of the doubt to the patient. If the vision of the eye first injured is destroyed, if the eye is soft, if it is painful, and if the condition seems to be progressive, the physician may feel that to remove the eye immediately is safest for the patient.

CARE OF EYE IN INDUSTRY

Another fairly common type of injury to the eye is the burn by caustics of one type or another, such as lime or acids. In industry, it is well to follow certain rules for all workmen who happen to suffer injuries to the eye:

1. Under no circumstances should an untrained or inexperienced employee attempt to remove any foreign body from the eye.

2. Immediately after an accident, the eye may be bathed with suitable mild aseptic or sterilized solutions, preferably a weak solution of boric acid made with sterilized water.

3. The eye should be covered with a sterile bandage moistened with this solution.

4. The person whose eye is involved should be sent immediately to the physician who is in charge of such cases. If the factory or workshop does not have a first-aid department, arrangements should be made with some near-by hospital or medical institution to give prompt attention to such cases. This will mean the avoidance of a great deal of unnecessary blindness and furthermore a much shorter period of disability than is otherwise the case.

FOREIGN BODIES IN EYE

This brings up the question of removing foreign bodies from the surface of the eye. There are hundreds of superstitions as to how this is best done. They concern sneezing, rubbing the other eye, and similar methods. It is much safer to rub the other eye than to rub the one in which the foreign body has lodged. In most instances, rubbing tends to push the foreign substance farther into the eye.

People who understand how to remove foreign bodies are exceedingly careful to make certain that their own hands are clean and that every instrument or other material used in the process is clean or sterilized. The eye itself must be handled with the utmost delicacy. The person first looks upward so that the lower lid of the eye may be pulled down and carefully studied. He then looks downward while the upper lid is turned back. It is impossible to turn the upper lid back safely while the person is looking up or moving the eyeball constantly. With practice, skill can be developed in turning back the upper lid. This is then carefully studied. If the foreign substance is not seen, the physician then looks at the surface of the eyeball, changing the light so as to catch the reflection of any foreign substance which may be imbedded in the cornea.

Of course, the competent physician has means of anesthetizing the surface of the eye and of avoiding injury to it in the removal of foreign substances. He is careful not to introduce infection, and to follow up the removal by later inspection to make sure that no untoward results are occurring. Secondary infections may bring about ulcers which will destroy the sight of the eye.

CONJUNCTIVITIS

The most common form of infection of the eye is conjunctivitis, which means an inflammation of the conjunctiva, the covering which lines the eyelids and runs onto the eyeball. This may become infected by any one of several different germs. Generally there are burning and smarting of the eyelids, formation of pus, intense reddened appearance of the lids which may spread to the eyeball, and, usually associated with this, sensitivity to light, and the pouring out of tears.

New ointments and drops for use in the eye containing sulfa drugs or antibiotics with other useful remedies now make conjunctivitis quickly controllable.

PINK EYE

The treatment given by the physician varies according to the character of the germ that produces the infection and according to the extent of the infection. One germ produces the condition called "pink eye." Shortly after this germ gets into the eyes they become reddened, the lids will be found glued together in the morning, and there will also be swelling and puffiness. Sometimes this disease is transmitted by the use of a common towel, and in other cases by soiled hands. In treating such infections the doctor usually advises hot fomentations which are put on the eyes for five minutes at a time; sometimes recommending that boric acid or witch hazel be added to the hot water. It is not well, however, to take such infections lightly. It is safer to be certain of the exact nature of the condition. Again the new antibiotic drugs bring quick elimination of such infections.

TRACHOMA

Trachoma is a serious infection also affecting the eyelids, and there are infections by the gonococcus. These infections may spread to the cornea, causing large ulcers, with partial or complete loss of eyesight. It may be necessary to use treatment that is practically constant day and night, to save the eyesight. Indeed, most physicians recommend that the patient be put in the hospital. Sulfadiazine and other drugs and streptomycin have also been found useful in controlling trachoma.

STYES

There are numerous small glands in the eyelids which secrete oily material so that the eyeball is lubricated when the eyelid passes over it. When one of these glands becomes infected it is filled with pus. This is the common condition called stye, also known scientifically as hordeolum. In a few days the stye, like any ordinary pimple, comes to a head and breaks; then the pus

escapes. If the stye is not properly treated and the source of the infection eliminated, one stye will follow another, and they persist for a long time. If the stye
does not open itself, and if it is not opened, it will tend to be cleared up from
within, in which case a hard lump may be left which is filled with scar tissue.
This tends to enlarge, and it is best under such circumstances to have the lump,
called chalazion, removed by a physician. Repeated formation of styes indicates that the body has little resistance against infection. Under such circumstances, it is well to guard the general health by suitable diet and cleanliness.

TEAR DUCTS

A chemist said to his wife, "Your tears have no effect on me; they are simply
salt and water." Tears keep the eyes moist so that the delicate tissues, of
which they are made, are preserved. If the eyes are not constantly kept moist,
the tissues dry and are much more easily attacked by bacteria.

In a little bony notch on the inner side of the eye there is a gland called the
tear gland or lacrimal gland. From this, six or more little tubes carry the tears
to the eyes. There is another tube, which is known as the nasal duct, which
carries fluid from the eyes to the nose. Hence, whenever a person cries or his
eyes water, his nose runs simultaneously. When the amount of moisture is so
great as to overflow, the excess comes down through the nasal duct until there
is so much that it falls on the cheeks. Most of the time there is just enough
moisture to keep the eye in the proper state of softness and luster.

Occasionally a tear duct becomes blocked because of the presence in it of a
cinder or a hair. Under such circumstances, it is necessary to open it up. This
requires special instruments and the care of a physician who knows how to do
the unblocking correctly.

In other instances the gland and the duct become infected. Then there is a
reddened swelling in the inner corner of the eye and the discharge of a small
amount of pus. Pressure over the swelling will force out most of the pus. It is
sometimes possible to get relief by treatment, but in other instances it may be
necessary to cut into the gland, and there are instances in which it has to be removed surgically.

Tears have always had a romantic interest. In 1581 a Latin writer described
a girl sixteen years old whose tears resembled blood. Other cases have been
described in many countries. Apparently in such cases there has been a leaking
of red blood cells out of the blood vessels into the tear gland. In some instances
in which bloody tears appeared, the women concerned had not experienced the
normal changes that occur to girls. In other cases there were tumors of the
eyelids.

ULCER ON EYE

The most dangerous infection of the eye is the ulcer on the eyeball. This may
be due to any kind of infection, but the worst forms are those due to the germ
that causes pneumonia, the pneumococcus, and the one that causes gonorrhea,

the gonococcus. In both of these types there is rapid destruction of the tissue of the eyeball. If there is penetration or perforation due to such destruction, the interior of the eyeball is also infected, and then there is complete loss of vision.

There is another type of infection of the cornea or covering of the eyeball which occurs most frequently in young children who are undernourished and have frequent colds, and particularly in those who have tuberculosis. In such cases there is an excessive flow of tears and a great aversion to light. This symptom is called photophobia. Because of the aversion to light, which produces blinking and pain, the person is likely to keep the eyelid shut on the inflamed eye. If the eye is studied, it will be found full of little flecks of material deposited by the inflammation.

Another type of inflammation of the cornea is due to the second great venereal disease, syphilis. This is a most serious condition when it affects the eye, as well as when it affects any other part of the body. For this reason, the physician who treats the disease treats not only the eye but also the infection as it concerns the rest of the body.

It must be remembered that there are various ways in which germs can attack the eye. They may come in from the outside or from the inside. The same germs that cause inflammation in the joints or in the nervous system, coming from infection in the tonsils, or the teeth, or the throat, may also be carried by the blood to the eyes and bring about serious infection there. Under the circumstances, the mere healing of the condition in the eye is not sufficient. It is necessary to find the systemic cause responsible and to take care of that as well.

People with tuberculosis, infections of the teeth, the tonsils or the sinuses, with high blood pressure, kidney disease, or diabetes may have symptoms affecting their eyes directly related to the other diseases that have been mentioned, and the diseases of the eye will not be improved until the other conditions are brought under control.

INFLAMMATION OF THE IRIS

The iris is the colored circle surrounding the pupil. Any condition which affects the surface of the eye may also attack this tissue. The condition is likely to come on insidiously. Then there are persistent redness of the eye, pain, dimness of vision, and aversion to light. Such an infection is dangerous because there is a tendency for adhesions to form between the edge of the iris and the lens. This will produce a deformity of the pupil and interfere with vision. It is, of course, necessary for a physician to find out as soon as possible the cause of the infection and to control it.

CATARACT

The lens does not have blood vessels or nerves but receives its nourishment from the fluid material in the eye. The lens is entirely surrounded by a capsule which acts as a filter, keeping out undesirable material. Should this capsule be broken, the lens is infiltrated with material from the fluid of the eye; then it becomes cloudy, and the person has what is called traumatic cataract. As people get very old, the capsule gradually becomes less efficient, and the nutrition of the lens is interfered with. As the lens becomes clouded, it gradually becomes cloudy from the outside toward the center. When finally the center becomes clouded, it is exceedingly difficult for the person to see. This condition is called senile cataract.

It must be remembered that the human eye is like a camera. It has a lens; it has a shutter, which is the iris. The pupil is the hole in the shutter through which the light enters. At the back of the eye is the retina or sensitized plate on which the image is cast.

Most cases of cloudiness or cataract of the lens, such as have been described, occur in people between fifty and seventy years of age. The only treatment for senile cataract is surgical. There are no drugs, no drops of any kind, no exercise or treatments which are successful in stopping the slow development of a cataract. Nevertheless, such methods of treatment have been used by vast numbers of quacks to get money from people who fear approaching blindness because of cataract.

There are numerous operations now developed which are relatively simple and which are quite safe in the majority of instances. Moreover, good vision follows in 97 per cent of the operations for cataract. After the cataract is removed, the person wears what are known as cataract glasses. These are made so that they help in focusing the image properly on the retina.

The person who has been unable to see for some time because of the development of clouding, who has been unable to play golf or get about, and who then recovers his sight by a simple operation that any competent specialist in diseases of the eye can perform, is one of the most appreciative of all the people benefited by modern medical and surgical science. When the cataract is removed, the result is like defrosting a window or raising the window shade: the light comes in without obstruction, and the individual is able to see.

INFLAMMATION OF RETINA

The tissues of the eye behind the lens are also subject to infections and inflammations. There are the delicate membranes of blood vessels and pigments, the rigid outer coating, and the retina or membrane of light perception. The large cavity is filled with vitreous, the fluid of the eye. Normally, rays of light pass through the vitreous without any hindrance, but occasionally there are small pieces of tissue in the vitreous which cast a shadow on the retina, such shadows being seen constantly as specks. Inflammations which affect the retina and the delicate membrane associated with it may be associated with the changes that take place in the blood vessels or tissues in old age, with infections elsewhere in the body, and with specific damage to the tissue itself.

The physician uses an instrument called the ophthalmoscope to look into the eye and to observe any changes that have occurred in these tissues. When the vision of the eye becomes diminished, and without any pain, without any redness or inflammation, the physician looks for the cause. Sometimes he sees changes in the retina which indicate a systemic disorder, such as diabetes, tuberculosis, and high blood pressure. Obviously that condition must be taken care of before any attempts are made in relationship to the eye itself.

DETACHMENT OF RETINA

Sometimes the retina itself is loosened, so that the condition called detachment of the retina occurs. As soon as any part of the retina becomes detached from its bed, the vision controlled by that part is disturbed, and unless it is reattached in a short time the vision is lost permanently. The person who has had detachment of the retina should go to bed immediately. Sometimes competent control of fluid intake helps the situation. In other instances operations have been developed which appear to be useful in aiding reattachment of the retina. Several competent authorities say that reattachment with recovery of vision occurs in about 15 per cent of the cases.

GLAUCOMA

One of the most dangerous of all of the diseases of the eye is glaucoma, a condition responsible for a large proportion of blindness that exists today. The cause of this disease is unknown. Its principal manifestation is an increase of pressure inside the eye. Glaucoma causes about 15 per cent of all the blindness that occurs, and about one half of all the blindness that occurs in adults. The blood that comes into the eye to nourish it must pass out, or the fluid accumulates, in which case there is a sense of pressure with pain, the eye gets hard and red and, from the front, appears gray and cloudy.

In other cases, the fluid goes out partially but not completely, so that the increased pressure and the loss of sight take place gradually. A competent physician can actually measure the pressure in the eye by means of a special instrument called the tonometer. He can also look into the eye with the ophthalmoscope to see whether there has been sufficient pressure to cause a depression in the optic nerve tissues as they come into the eye.

As the glaucoma develops, the person can see in front of him but not so well on the sides. Gradually his field of vision becomes narrow, with final loss of sight. The expert can determine the narrowing of the field of vision by the use of the apparatus called a perimeter. If untreated, glaucoma leads certainly to blindness. It is difficult to control. Excessive pressure on sensitive tissue, such as of nerves, produces degeneration.

Here are some warning signals that indicate the need of an examination of your eyes:

Inability to adjust your vision to changes of illumination.

Inability to see well even after frequent changes of glasses.

Loss of vision toward either or both sides.

Blurred or foggy vision with rainbow colored rings around lights.

Physicians treat glaucoma by use of drugs which lower pressure in the eye and contract the pupil. Such a condition cannot be treated by the use of glasses. If medical methods fail, it is customary to use surgery to establish proper drainage and to keep the pressure in the eye permanently low.

A substance called Diamox is now prescribed for eliminating excess fluid from the body. It lowers tension within the eye and helps the symptoms and preparation for operation.

TRANSPLANTING THE CORNEA

One of the most sensational medical procedures has been transplantation of the transparent membrane which covers the surface of the eye and which is known as the cornea. Sometimes a scar appears in this tissue as a result of an infection or an injury or a burn, and as a result the vision is prevented as if a curtain were drawn over the pupil of the eye.

Not every case of scarring is suitable to such an operation. Failure of the operation may lead to severe emotional disturbances. Hence the surgeon and the specialist must choose the cases according to a wide variety of considerations which vary with every case. There are many diseases of the eye in which the scarring over the pupil is simply incidental. If there are severe scars, such as result from powder burns or burns by lime, involving all of the layers of the cornea, the transplant is seldom successful. Certain eyes are exceedingly sensitive to surgical procedures, and secondary inflammation may result in complete loss of sight.

Eye banks have been established from which the ophthalmic surgeon obtains the necessary material for use in the transplant. Frequently the material to be transplanted is obtained from the eyes of stillborn infants. Of special importance is the great amount of care necessary to be given to such eyes following an operation, because obviously secondary infection might not only damage the results of the operation but leave the patient with an eye worse off than the eye he had before the operation. The eye bank in New York City now supplies about twenty-five eyes each year, but its facilities have been increased so that tissue for transplantation is now available for as many as two hundred eyes each year. The operation of an eye bank is an exceedingly costly and difficult matter, requiring technical services that are not generally available.

EYE EXERCISES

For a good many years now attempts have been made to get people to train their eyes by exercises to improve the strength of the eyes in various ways, and thus to permit these people to avoid glasses. The original slogan was: "Throw away your glasses and have perfect sight."

The majority of experience of eye specialists during the past twenty years has inclined definitely to limit the extent of usefulness of eye exercises as a means of improving vision. The modern ophthalmologist or specialist in conditions affecting the eyes knows the limitations and insists that such methods cannot be applied indiscriminately to all sorts of defects of the eyes. Certain disturbances are not affected in any way whatever by exercises, including cataracts, destruction of the optic nerve, opaque scars of the cornea, and serious changes in the retina. A cataract is a cloudiness of the lens of the eye. The nerve must be alive and normal to permit vision. An opaque scar of the cornea is like drawing a window blind over a window so that such scars render vision impossible. The retina is the tissue in back of the eye which is responsible for vision, and obviously permanent change to the retina means permanent damage to vision. Exercises can do nothing to help such vision.

The psychologic treatment associated with education of the eyes helps to reconcile people to difficulties with vision even though it does not cure them.

In certain instances skillfully chosen exercises can improve the ability to see. Studies made with patients who are color blind show that it is possible by education to improve the ability to discriminate between colors, but it is impossible to cure color blindness since the condition is due to permanent changes in the tissues concerned.

People who are extremely nearsighted can be taught how to make better use of their vision, but it is not possible to reduce the nearsightness by any kind of exercise.

The One-eyed Worker

Occasionally people lose the sight of one eye without realizing it for some time, simply because it is quite possible to get along with only one eye and to carry on most of the general activities of life.

In Great Britain a specialist studied the psychologic reactions of 102 soldiers who had lost the sight in one eye. More than three fourths of these men had abnormal psychologic reactions. They were affected both by social prejudices and by emotional difficulties. In fear of making mistakes, they began to shun social contacts. Furthermore, the man with only one eye is likely to develop a fear of blindness, because he knows that any injury to the good eye may result in total blindness. Because of this, people with one eye frequently complain of pain in the eyes, eye strain, difficulty in standing the light, and similar symptoms. Among the 100 soldiers who were studied, 26 had such anxiety, 11 had exaggerated self-pity, and 10 had great anxiety about the future.

The specialist in conditions affecting the eye will want to make a special study of the good eye as well as of the one that has lost its sight. Even though the eye is blind, there is resistance to removing it. Nowadays, however, artificial eyes are available which are almost indistinguishable from the remaining good eye.

Another study of people with one eye was made to find out how many industrial firms would employ a one-eyed worker. Most small firms do not require employees to pass eyesight tests and will employ a one-eyed worker who can show his competence. Many firms do employ such workers, even knowing of the lack of sight. All of the firms which employed one-eyed workers expressed satisfaction with their work and with their accident records.

People who lose the sight of one eye in early childhood learn to accommodate quite well for the loss of vision. When, however, the sight of one eye is lost late in life, the accommodation may be much more difficult. Recovery is slower. In almost three quarters of all people the right eye is the dominant or master eye. For that reason, studies must be made of workers with only one eye to find out whether the eye that has lost sight is the master eye.

CHAPTER XXVII

The Ear, Tongue, Nose, and Throat
MORRIS FISHBEIN, M.D.

DISORDERS OF THE EAR

THE OUTER ear differs but little from other external portions of the body in the things which may disturb it. It may be the subject of small tumors which, of course, must be removed if they show the slightest tendency to growth or irritation. Sometimes cysts form which are nonmalignant tumors but which continue to swell or grow as long as the opening is blocked. These should be opened and the wall of the cyst removed, if there is not to be a recurrence.

ERYSIPELAS OF EAR

In erysipelas the ear will swell to tremendous size. Obviously it must be protected to prevent breaking down of the tissue due to the swelling and irritation. In frost bite of the ear it should be gradually warmed until the circulation returns. Then the skin must be protected to prevent infections with ulcers.

TIN EAR

One of the most common forms of injury to the ear is what is commonly called "tin ear" of the pugilist. Repeated blows on the ear result in the pouring out of blood between the cartilage of the tissue and its surrounding membranes. At first such swellings are bluish-red; they feel like dough, and they are opaque, so that light will not pass through. In some instances, it may be advisable for the surgeon to open the tissue and to remove the clot of blood, and, in that way, to prevent permanent thickening and swelling. It is sometimes necessary to plan the use of bandages which mold the ear and hold its shape while such surgical treatment is being undertaken.

Modern ideas of beauty demand that the ear lie fairly close to the head and that it be relatively small. Hence the plastic surgeons, particularly the bogus plastic surgeons, are likely to induce people to try all sorts of operations to hold the ears back or to lessen their size. Such operations are in many instances of doubtful value and may result in permanent changes which are harmful.

They should never be undertaken unless the person's occupation is such as to make slightly protruding or large ears a menace to earning a livelihood.

In addition to the diseases that may disturb the outer ear, there are disturbances which affect the canal up to the point of the eardrum. Almost any infection may involve the outer canal of the ear. Under such circumstances it is necessary to remove the infection and to prevent its recurrence by the use of proper antiseptics which a physician can supply and which should be used only after he has given proper instructions.

There is a good rule in medicine: namely, never put anything in the external ear any smaller than the elbow. The tissues are most delicate and may be seriously harmed by the use of wires, toothpicks, earspoons, or similar irregular or unsterilized devices. A scratch of the lining of the canal may result in the formation of a boil, which is exceedingly painful and which is difficult to handle in such an inaccessible part of the body.

The cerumen or wax of the ear is easiest removed, when it becomes hardened, by the use of a syringe with slightly warm water. This need not be done often, and harm can be done by needless or too frequent syringing. The syringe should always be sterilized by boiling before using, and the water should be previously boiled and then used warm. Before a person attempts to syringe an ear for himself or for a child, he should learn the technic.

The person whose ear is to be syringed usually sits in good light. It is customary to put a towel or cape around the neck and tuck it in over the collar to prevent soiling of the clothing. A kidney-shaped pan is held at the edge of the ear so that the fluid returning will run in the basin and not down the neck. In an adult the ear is pulled up and backward in order to straighten out the passage. Then the nozzle of the syringe, which has been filled and had all the air expelled, is placed just inside the outer opening. The water is then projected along the back wall slowly and without too great pressure, so as to permit return of the flow as the water goes in.

After the ear has been washed, the head may be turned on one side and the extra fluid allowed to run out. A person who understands the technic may then wipe out the canal with a small wisp of cotton. If a permanent antiseptic, softening material, or lotion is to be used, the physician can prescribe the proper one, and this is held in place with a little wisp of cotton, never inserted under pressure.

A foreign body in the external ear will seldom cause much discomfort unless it is a living insect. Cases are on record in which living insects have entered the ear and remained for many years, gradually being surrounded by hardened wax or cerumen, to the point at which a person lost his hearing entirely. The damage from foreign bodies in the external ear lies in rough attempts to remove them. If a living insect gets into the outer ear, a physician can destroy it by the use of a little chloroform vapor, under which circumstance the insect will either come out of its own accord or be killed and removed by a syringe.

It is not well for anyone to attempt to remove a foreign body from the outer ear if it cannot be syringed out, unless he has had special training in this type of work. Several interesting technics have been developed for removing foreign objects, one being the use of a device with an adhesive material at the end which sticks to the body that is to be removed. It is then gradually withdrawn.

A foreign body that is infected may produce irritation and serious infection with the formation of boils or abscesses which, in the external ear, are a menace frequently to life itself. A boil in the external ear demands the immediate and competent attention of an expert, who can arrange to open it in such a manner as to permit the infectious material to escape, to withdraw the pus, to relieve pain by a prescription of proper remedies, and to prevent the spreading and recurrence through the use of suitable antiseptic preparations.

EARACHE

When there is an infection of the nose or throat the bacteria sometimes get into the ear behind the eardrum through the Eustachian tubes, the passages leading from the mouth and nose cavities into the ear. Therefore, many infections of the ear may be prevented by properly cleansing infected noses and throats with mildly antiseptic and alkaline sprays and washes.

Emphasis must be placed on the word "properly" because such washes, as generally applied, force fluid, pus, and bacteria into the ear. These nasal douches should never be taken with any but the most gentle pressure, perhaps slightly snuffling the warm, alkaline fluid into the nose.

The early diagnosis of infection of the ear is important, if inflammation of the mastoid bone, behind the ear and contiguous to the brain, is to be prevented. The ears should always be examined if a child is ill and has fever. The presence of fever, bulging drum, and the symptoms mentioned are sufficient reasons for the physician to incise the eardrum to save the hearing of the child and to prevent burrowing of the infected pus into the mastoid region. When the diagnosis and the proper treatment of an infected ear are delayed, the results are likely to be extremely serious.

The first symptom of an infection in the ear is usually pain in the ear, and in some cases this is the only symptom. It must be remembered, however, that pains in the ear also are found in connection with presence of boils in the ear canal. Sometimes a pain in the ear may be associated with an unerupted wisdom tooth and inflammation of the joints of the jaw and severe tonsillitis or an infection of the sinuses around the nose.

OTITIS MEDIA

The doctor makes up his mind as to the presence of an acute infection of the ear by taking the temperature, which in these cases usually is high. However, special examinations in such cases of acute infections of the ear are made by direct inspection of the eardrum, using a magnifying device and a light. This device is called an otoscope, meaning a device for seeing the ear.

In most instances, a physician called to such a case and making a diagnosis of severe infection within the ear will arrange to open the eardrum promptly. This not only relieves the pain, but also makes it less likely that the infection will spread to the mastoid.

Application of heat often brings relief. For persistent infections the antibiotics in powder form have been helpful. Infections of the middle ear are being tremendously reduced by treatment of infectious diseases with antibiotic drugs. Moreover, early detection permits immediate injection of such drugs and prevention of ear infections sufficient to require opening of the ear drum.

MASTOIDS

If the condition spreads into the mastoid, mastoiditis develops and constitutes a much more serious condition than infection of the internal ear alone. When the infection spreads to the mastoid, great tenderness will be found in that region, and also pain on pressure. The physician watches carefully this development. From the very first, the mastoid bone may be tender on pressure because of the swelling on the inside. Whenever pain is severe and there is fever, the physician knows that the infection is serious, and he is likely to recommend immediate incision of the eardrum. The operation is not difficult and, if performed soon enough, is likely to prevent more serious complications.

People have strange notions about perforation of the eardrum, believing that this will interfere with hearing and cause other damage, whereas actually the eardrum heals promptly after the infection disappears, and hearing is likely to be just as good as it was previously. It is far less dangerous to hearing to incise the eardrum than to postpone the incision too long.

THE TONGUE AND ITS DISORDERS

The tongue is an organ which has always aroused the interest of the medical profession. Doctors of an earlier day used to pay a great deal of attention to the appearance of the tongue because of the relationship of such appearances to disturbances of the rest of the digestive tract.

Occasionally the tongue is abnormal in its construction at birth so that the condition of tongue-tie is produced, and there are other cases in which that portion of the tissue holding the tongue is abnormally long, permitting actual swallowing of the tongue with occasional asphyxiation. In some conditions the tongue becomes too large for the mouth and protrudes beyond the lips. This is particularly the case in the large tongue of the child that has deficient thyroid secretion with the development of cretinism.

GEOGRAPHIC TONGUE

Sometimes the surface of the tongue is marked by long, deep furrows instead of being smooth. There is a common condition called "geographic tongue" because the surface of the tongue looks like a relief map. In this condition there are grayish thickened patches on the surface. Apparently it is a mild inflammatory disorder which tends gradually to improve, the treatment usually including merely the washing of the mouth at fairly frequent intervals with mild antiseptic and alkaline mouth washes.

INFLAMMATION OF TONGUE

The tongue may be suddenly inflamed from a number of different causes, such as injuries, burns, insect bites, and occasionally association with such serious infectious diseases as scarlet fever, typhoid fever, or smallpox. Whenever the tongue is infected, the lymph glands in the region also become infected and swollen. In very serious cases death may result from such inflammation of the tongue, but in the vast majority of cases mild treatment tends to lead to recovery.

There are many nervous disorders or conditions affecting the nervous system in which there is pain in the tongue or burning of the tongue without any visible evidence in the neighborhood of the tongue itself. This condition sometimes occurs in locomotor ataxia, in hysteria, and in all sorts of nervous upsets of one type or another. Under such circumstances a physician may make sure that the condition is functional and not due to any destruction or inflammation of the tissues concerned. If he discovers actual disease of the nervous system, the case is treated by the well-established methods. If such disease is not discovered it may be necessary to use psychologic methods in controlling the symptoms, not only as they affect the tongue, but probably as they affect other parts of the body as well.

The tongue is primarily responsible for the sense of taste which is, at the same time, a composite of the sense of smell and the feel of food on the tongue. Loss of the sense of taste may result from inflammation or swelling of the tongue; it may be associated with hysteria. In the same way there may be exceeding sensitivity to tastes so that a person is constantly tasting sweet, sour, salt or bitter; and in other instances foods taste different from what they should.

In every such case it is necessary to make a most careful study of the entire patient, his surroundings and environment, and particularly his emotional condition.

THE NOSE

The nose is, in general, the least ornamental of the features of man. It is the mark for more insults and injuries than any other adornment of the human countenance. It is unnecessary to locate it geographically, since it presents itself. Remarkably, however, modern living conditions have made the nose, in more ways than one, a center of interest.

Actually, there is not much to the organ itself. It is composed of some small bones and cartilages and certain soft tissues which go to surround the two cavities. Of equal importance with the nose and inevitably to be considered with it are the nasal sinuses. These sinuses are cavities in the bones in the head which connect with the inside of the nose by means of small openings. There are, of course, nerves which take care of the motor and sensory functions of the tissues and which may be involved in any condition affecting the nose.

The most important of the structures in the nose from the point of view of disease is the mucous membrane or tissue which lines the cavities. It is one of the most sensitive tissues in the body, and when bruised or hurt in any way may respond with considerable trouble for the possessor. Not infrequently, minor infections occur, particularly in the hair follicles or in the roots of the hairs which are in the nose. These hairs have the purpose of filtering out dust or infectious material which comes into the nose with the air.

It is now generally well known that common pus-forming germs, such as staphylococcus and streptococcus, are widespread and easily get into the human body whenever they come in contact with a tissue that has been damaged in any manner. They may set up an infection which eventually may spread throughout the body. The pernicious habit of picking the nose, pulling out the hairs, or trying to squeeze out pimples or other infections may result in most serious inflammations or other disorders.

HYGIENE OF NOSE

The right way to take care of the nose is to remove carefully, by proper use of a handkerchief, such materials as can be reached easily. Those which cannot be reached may be washed out by the use of a mild spray, without pressure. There are now generally available all sorts of mild sprays of inert oils and small amounts of camphor, eucalyptus, or menthol, which serve this purpose conveniently. Under no circumstances should such materials be put in the nose under high pressure. If a spray is not convenient, the simplest method is to drop one or two drops into the nose.

An infection in the lining of the nose manifests itself by redness, swelling, discomfort, and pain, which increase steadily. The tip of the nose becomes swollen, and sometimes the swelling may even extend up to the eyelids. In the presence of any serious swelling involving the nose, it is well to have an inspection by a physician, who will determine the presence or absence of a localized spot of infection such as a boil or pimple, who can arrange to cause the infectious material to be released, and who will provide suitable dressings of warm antiseptic or saline solutions tending toward recovery.

When for any reason the nose is lost entirely, the facial expression naturally suffers. When the bridge of the nose disappears, as sometimes occurs in certain forms of disease, a saddle nose is caused which is anything but beautiful. The frequency of automobile accidents has resulted in damage to many a proboscis. Falls, industrial accidents, railroad wrecks, and gunshot wounds also produce damages that require medical attention, and the results of pugilism are a constant source of income to specialists in nasal reconstruction.

Mother Nature brings many a break into prominence by bestowing upon it a hump, a knob at the tip, or a deviation to one side or the other. In street fights anything can happen to a wayfaring nose, and medical literature records several instances in which the tip of one has been bitten off by an agitated opponent—male or female.

Forms of the nose have been described as long and short, upturned and downturned, humped and flat, wide and narrow, pointed and saddle-shaped. It is just as well that people do not worry too much about their particular type of nasal appearance. As soon as they get their minds fixed on this, they look into the looking glass until it gets tired of reflecting their appearance. The experts find that almost any amount of repairs and reconstruction is never satisfactory to the person who once embarks on the paths of nasal improvement.

PLASTIC SURGERY OF NOSE

If the loss of tissue or destruction of tissue causes damage to the health of the person concerned, the case certainly demands surgical attention. There are many ways of building up a broken-down or absent bridge. Some surgeons transplant bone and cartilage, some use celluloid, and others use ivory. Humps are removed by dissection and scraping or cutting. The best way to take care of a deformity from an accident, however, is to give it the best possible attention immediately after the accident. It is much easier to secure a good result if such care is given at that time than to attempt a complete rebuilding operation when tissues have healed in the wrong manner.

FOREIGN BODIES IN NOSE

Children not infrequently push all sorts of things into the nasal cavity. The character of things pushed into the nose is limited only by the size and the possibilities. Insane people also occasionally indulge in a similar performance. Among some of the common substances that have been found by physicians are chalk, buttons, seeds, and pieces of wood.

Occasionally the nasal cavity becomes infected with worms. Among others are maggots and screw worms, and indeed almost any of the worms which can live in the human body. Worms are seldom found in a normal nose. However, in the presence of any disease with an associated odor, flies are attracted which may lay eggs or in other ways convey the larvæ of the worms to the nasal cavity. Among the first signs of infestation of the nose by worms are irritation, sneezing, and an increased amount of discharge usually streaked with blood. The removal of worms from the nose is not a serious matter. The nose may be washed repeatedly with solutions containing proper antiseptic substances.

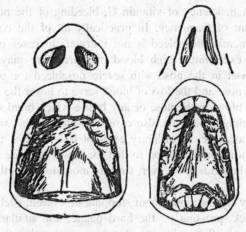

Fig. 51. *Left*: Normal jaw and nasal cavity. *Right*: Effect long-standing nasal obstruction.

The removal of inanimate foreign bodies not infrequently requires the greatest skill of a competent specialist. It may be necessary to use an anesthetic, to apply various solutions which will constrict the tissue of the nose, to employ the X-ray to localize the foreign body exactly. Once this is done, the doctor merely grasps the foreign body with a forceps and withdraws it, endeavoring to cause as little damage to the soft tissue as possible.

POLYPS IN NOSE

Sometimes growths in the nose, like polyps, are difficult to distinguish from foreign bodies. Usually the discharge coming from the nose as a result of the presence of a foreign body comes only from one side. Sometimes the removal of polyps or similar tumors is followed by the disappearance of chronic infection in the nose and sometimes also by the removal of asthmatic symptoms. It is not possible for the average person to diagnose the presence of nasal polyps for himself. The condition can, however, be diagnosed by a physician following an examination of the nose, in which he looks directly into the nasal cavity.

NOSEBLEED

There are many causes of bleeding from the nose, because the blood supply to the tissues is generally rich and the tissues themselves quite delicate. In many diseases in which the tendency to bleed is great, such as hemophilia and purpura, two conditions in which the elements of the blood are so altered that bleeding occurs frequently and coagulation of the blood takes place with difficulty, bleeding from the nose is a common symptom.

In the presence of severe infection and in the condition called scurvy, which is due to a deficiency of vitamin C, bleeding of the nose also occurs with a fair amount of frequency. In practically all of the conditions which produce severe anemia, nosebleed is not unusual. In cases of hardening of the arteries with exceedingly high blood pressure there may be rupture of a small blood vessel in the nose with severe nosebleed for some time. The bleeding from the nose and the loss of blood serve to lower the blood pressure.

Of course, any blow on the nose or any bruise which breaks a blood vessel will result in bleeding. There are also cases in which tumors within the blood vessels cause hemorrhage. In ordinary cases of nosebleed, if the person is at once placed in a horizontal position so that the blood pressure is lowered, and if he is kept cool, he tends to recover, since in most instances the bleeding will stop promptly.

There are many superstitions about stopping nosebleed, such as dropping a key down the back, pressing on the hard palate, and similar performances. However, there is no efficacy in such measures, except that they serve to distract the attention of the person whose nose is bleeding and keep him from being too much frightened during the short interval that usually elapses before the bleeding stops.

In more serious cases, however, physicians use measures which have a greater degree of certainty, such measures including packing of the nose with sterilized gauze, direct inspection with pinching of the bleeding vessel, cauterization with some substance like silver nitrate or chromic acid, and the use of various solutions which temporarily constrict the blood vessels, giving the blood opportunity to clot. In general, physicians avoid leaving packing in the nose for long periods of time because of possible dangers to the ears through blocking of the tubes that pass from the nasal cavity to the ears, and because of possible effects from blocking the nasal sinuses.

It should be borne in mind that the bleeding from the nose is not in itself a disease, but rather a symptom of disease; that it may be the warning sign for the onset of a serious disorder, such as a change in the blood, or even a tumor of the adrenal glands. On the other hand, it may merely be due to increased mental or physical excitement or any other condition that suddenly raises the blood pressure. In most cases the amount of blood lost is small, but if the person has repeated hemorrhages the amount lost may be sufficient to cause anemia and to demand special treatment for restoring the blood.

Sometimes hemorrhage from the nose in children is overlooked, because the blood goes back in the throat and is swallowed. In most cases of bleeding from the nose, even severe cases, the hemorrhage stops of itself in approximately ten minutes. If the hemorrhage continues longer, or if it is repeated, the condition is most serious and demands efficient attention. It is especially important to remember not to blow the nose after the bleeding has stopped, because that will dislodge clots and start the bleeding over again.

New blood coagulating remedies have been discovered which the doctor can apply in plenty of time to prevent loss of serious quantities of blood.

SINUS DISEASE

The sinuses are air spaces surrounding the nose. Because of their direct contact with the exterior, they frequently become infected with the common pus-forming germs. Because they do not drain easily, the infections tend to become chronic. Associated with such infections are feelings of tiredness, loss of appetite, pains in the joints and limbs.

The mucous membrane of the nose becomes deranged from a variety of causes, either by a bad diet which is deficient in vitamins, by sensitivity to various protein substances, or by some disorders of the glands of internal secretion.

The changes that take place in the mucous membranes make it possible for germs to invade them easily, and then infection begins. In cases when there is sensitivity to various food substances, the mucous membranes swell and are much more likely to be invaded by germs. In the same way, disorders of the glands of internal secretion are reflected by changes in the mucous membranes.

If the underlying cause is removed, the infection may be brought under control, but in the vast majority of cases correct treatment involves not only control of the underlying cause but also treatment of the infection. If the vitamins are insufficient, they may be supplied through giving a well-balanced diet. For the sensitivity, it is necessary to make diagnostic tests, which will indicate the special substance to which the person may be sensitive.

Disorders of the glands of internal secretion must be carefully investigated. There are some cases, for instance those in which the thyroid is deficient, in which it is possible to supply the deficiency through proper preparations.

Persons who work indoors in crowded rooms where the air is bad and the temperature too low or too high are more likely to develop infection of the sinuses than those who spend a good deal of time outdoors.

A constant discharge from the nose, particularly a discharge of pus, is one of the most certain indications of infection in the sinuses. Sometimes when discharge from the sinus becomes blocked there is swelling of the forehead, dizziness, and even ringing in the ears. There are several sinuses, each of which must be studied individually by the physician in order to determine the extent and nature of the infection. Such a study involves a thorough examination through the nose of the openings of the sinuses into the nose, washing of the sinuses to obtain the discharge, transillumination in a dark room which indicates whether or not the sinuses are clear, and the use of the X-ray, which indicates whether or not there is thickening of the walls of the sinuses or any amount of material present in the cavity.

People with chronic sinusitis never recover without treatment. Many of them have low-grade infections in which surgical treatment is not advisable, and these patients can be helped by drainage, frequent washing, and the application of various antiseptic substances.

Recently infected sinuses are being treated with forced inhalations of mists of penicillin and streptomycin and forced evacuation of the sinuses simultaneously by a negative pressure device. This method of treatment, developed by Alvin Barach, is perhaps the most promising of any yet discovered. Many patients with sinus disease improve by changing from moist, cold climates to warm, dry climates. Use of aerosols of antibiotics has increased rapidly but all these methods must be prescribed for the individual by the doctor.

In other cases, however, the infection of the sinus persists to such an extent that it involves danger to surrounding tissues. Cases are known in which the sight of an eye has been lost because of infection in a neighboring sinus. There are other instances in which the infection extends from the Eustachian tubes to the ear and thus involves the mastoid process. The constant inhalation of pus may set up bronchitis or pneumonia. The continuous slight fever results in a loss of vigor and in disturbances of digestion.

There are even cases in which loss of memory or neurosis has occurred because of the constant infection and irritation. It has been well established that an infection in the nose may be carried by the blood to other parts of the body, resulting in serious inflammations of joints, infection of the heart and the kidneys, and even meningitis.

In children, chronic infection of the sinuses may be associated with enlarged adenoids and tonsils. The removal of the adenoids and tonsils may eliminate the source of the infection and end the trouble. At the same time, it should be emphasized again that correction of the diet to include a proper amount of vitamins A, B, C, and D is of importance.

There are, of course, cases in which the same child may have an enlargement of the tonsils and adenoids, and associated with this a sensitivity to various protein substances. Obviously attention to both conditions is necessary if complete recovery is to be secured.

In older people, when the antrum is involved, the large sinus on each side of the nose, it may be necessary to remove all infected teeth in relation to the antrum and to clean out the infected bone at the roots of the teeth. An opening into the antrum from the mouth permits drainage and the healing of the diseased membrane. If such measures fail, it is possible to employ a surgical procedure, which involves a wide opening of the sinuses or even complete obliteration; such methods are, however, so delicate that they should be undertaken only by those especially competent, and then after the most careful consideration.

THE SENSE OF SMELL

Everyone knows that there are some odors that are pleasant and others disagreeable. In many instances the sense of pleasure or of discomfort is associated with some previous experience of the person concerned. For instance, the perfume called attar of roses is generally much more pleasant than that of asafetida. There are persons, however, to whom the smell is not altogether pleasant. Some odors seem exceedingly pleasant at the first whiff and then tend to become more unpleasant the longer they are present. This is because of their intensity.

In the University of Edinburgh, Dr. J. H. Kenneth has undertaken a series of researches, including twenty-nine men and thirty-four women who were examined as to their response to odors of many different substances and combinations of substances. The state of health of the person concerned seems to have something to do with the enjoyment of odors or with disagreement.

Psychological study was also made of associations with various smells. One man who was given camphor to smell immediately felt distressed and visualized the odor of a wardrobe and then a feeling of suffocation or being in the dark. It appears that the odor reminded him of an incident in 1892 when he was placed in a closet because of some youthful misdemeanor. In the closet were clothes which had been supplied with camphor as a moth preventive.

A girl who smelled xylol visualized herself on board a vessel in a harbor in Ceylon. The odor of xylol resembles that of benzol which comes from harbor launches. The odor of cedar-wood oil was associated with a summer evening on the Norwegian coast, with a cigar box in which money had been placed, with a road in the country. Later investigation indicated that the person had been in the habit as a child of walking along this road chewing the end of a cedar-wood pencil.

To one woman the odor of cedar-wood oil brought up the idea of spring cleaning and the cleaning of floors with a cedar-wood mop. Another girl told of the playing of the music of Chopin when she smelled vanilla; another thought of Ireland's song, "Sea Fever," when smelling pine oil.

The usual thought associated with asafetida was garlic or onions. One person thought of a street car in Edinburgh, and it was discovered that these cars were formerly lighted by acetylene gas which gives off a similar odor. The odor of orris root brought to one girl the idea of smelling an elephant at a distance. These investigations are of the greatest importance as an aid in the psychologic studies of the human reaction. They seem to offer further opportunity for more of the interesting home psychological games in which so many people now indulge.

The nose, like many other organs of the body, is lined with tissue called mucous membrane that secretes mucus. Sometimes these cells over-grow, and when they do, little tumors are formed which hang down into the nose and interfere with breathing; also by the obstruction they cause they may aid in setting up infection. Hence, it is desirable that they be removed. Sometimes even after they are removed they return, and since the exact cause of such tumors is not known, there is nothing to do but keep on removing them.

In general, the causes of tumors are not definitely known, although certain contributory factors are recognized. Several observers believe that polyps never occur except in the presence of infection, although others are convinced that the infection follows the polyps.

It is generally well established that the use of radium following the removal of tumor cells may prevent the formation of additional tumors. Hence, it has been suggested that the removal of nasal polyps be followed by mild treatment with radium element in order to prevent their return. The radium is usually applied in the form of a screen container several days after the polyps have been removed, when the inflammation due to the surgical procedure has subsided. Sometimes the polyps form in the sinuses rather than in the nasal cavity itself. Under such circumstances, a physician can detect their presence by injecting into the sinus a substance which is opaque to the X-ray, such as lipoidal. Then an X-ray picture is taken, and this reveals the presence of the tumor or growth inside the sinuses, preventing their filling completely.

THE THROAT

There are general inflammations of the throat associated with redness, swelling, and excessive discharge of mucus due to many different causes. Most common, of course, is exposure to cold, an extension of inflammation from the tonsils, the adenoids, or the nose. Excessive use of tobacco; excessive exposure to dust, smoke, irritating fumes, and sudden changes in temperature; excessive dryness, and similar atmospheric conditions may cause irritation of the throat. People who are sensitive to certain food substances sometimes react with blisters on the tissues of the throat, which become secondarily infected and produce irritations and inflammation.

There may be severe pain asosciated with swelling and inflammation of the throat, including pain in the ears because of blocking of the tubes which lead from the nose to the ears; there may also be a sense of fullness or obstruction, with much hawking and spitting.

The first thing to know about any inflammation of the throat is its cause. If the condition happens to be due to diphtheria, prompt action is necessary, including the giving of diphtheria antitoxin. If, however, it is due to some other type of germ, other methods of treatment are employed.

SORE THROAT

The pain of an inflamed throat is best relieved by use of an ice bag filled with cracked ice. Most doctors are now convinced that gargles seldom go deep enough in the throat in sufficient quantity or strength to permit them to have much effect in killing germs or in curing disease. They have the value of washing out everything they reach. They serve to relieve some of the dryness of the mouth and throat that is usually present with inflammation. They sometimes substitute a good taste in the mouth for a bad one, although some of the gargles themselves taste so bad that they make a bad taste worse. To have a definite effect from any antiseptic in the throat, it is necessary to apply

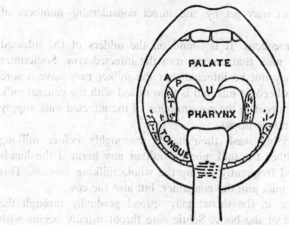

Fig. 52. Diagram showing palate, uvula, tonsils,
pharynx, and tongue.

it directly to the infected or inflamed part. This is best done by spreading material with a cotton swab or by using an atomizer properly. In order to get the antiseptic into the back of the throat, it may be necessary to hold the tongue or to use a tongue depressor.

MOUTH WASHES AND GARGLES

The primary purpose of a mouth wash or throat wash is to clean and soothe. A good cleaning mouth wash is merely salt solution made by adding a fourth of a teaspoon of salt to a half glass of warm water. If there is much mucus, the addition of a quarter of a teaspoon of bicarbonate of soda or ordinary baking soda may be beneficial. Most mouth washes and gargles sold in drug stores contain water, salt, baking soda or boric acid, with flavoring material and dye substances of various kinds. Many of them contain alcohol. Alcohol is astringent, cleansing, and somewhat antiseptic. Ordinarily, mouth washes may contain one part of alcohol to four or five parts of water.

There are innumerable lozenges now available which can be dissolved on the tongue. These have a soothing effect or slightly anesthetic effect. They also serve to moisten the mouth, but their antiseptic value is little, if any. Modern lozenges containing antibiotics like penicillin and streptomycin actually destroy the common germs that infect the throat.

The dryness that occurs in the mouth during any inflammation of the throat may be alleviated by drinking some effervescent water, such as ginger ale or vichy, or by chewing gum, or by the use of lozenges.

The most serious form of sore throat, next to diphtheria, is called epidemic septic sore throat. This is spread frequently by infected milk. When the milk supply is properly pasteurized, virulent organisms are destroyed. If, however, there is any carelessness whatever in the process of pasteurization, the germs causing septic sore throat may get by and infect considerable numbers of people.

This germ is a streptococcus. It is found on the udders of the infected cows and infects all the milk that comes from the infected cow. Sometimes the udder of the cow may not be infected, but the milker may have a sore throat. The milk that has become infected is then mixed with the general milk supply, and anyone taking part in the consumption of the infected milk supply is likely to develop septic sore throat.

Milkers should invariably wash their hands thoroughly before milking cows, and it will do neither the milk nor the milker any harm if the hands of the milker are washed frequently during the whole milking process. This will protect not only the milk and the consumer, but also the cow.

Infections of this type in the throat may spread gradually through the throat, involving the rest of the body. Septic sore throat usually begins with fever, chills, and a rapid pulse. These, however, are equally the symptoms of numerous other disorders of an infectious character. The fact that there are numerous other cases in the community at the same time helps to indicate the epidemic character of the disease. In most instances, investigation by the health department will serve to indicate that practically all the cases occur on the route of one distributor of milk. The study is then made to find which of the employees concerned is himself infected. An examination is also made of the herds of cows to determine whether or not any of the animals have infected udders. Not infrequently epidemic sore throat is mistaken for influenza. One epidemic has been described in which the condition was traced to infected ice cream rather than infected milk. Such epidemics are becoming infrequent. The antibiotics quickly control the streptococcus of epidemic sore throat.

TONSILLITIS

No one has ever determined exactly why we have tonsils. Apparently they serve some purpose in taking care of the infectious organisms that come into the throat. However, their response to infection is prompt swelling and inflammation with pain, soreness, difficulty in swallowing, swelling of the glands in the throat, high fever, a rapid pulse, a general weakness, and serious illness generally. Not infrequently the germs which develop in the tonsils are carried by the blood to other parts of the body and there set up inflammations, the regions particularly affected being the joints, the heart, and the kidneys.

The germ that is most frequently responsible for tonsillitis is the streptococcus, which is also responsible for various forms of heart disease, for erysipelas, and for similar conditions. When the tonsils have once been seriously affected, they apparently are likely to become infected again and again.

In children particularly it is exceedingly important to make sure that the condition is tonsillitis and not diphtheria. Tonsillitis produces a throat that is purplish-red and swollen, whereas diphtheria produces a grayish-white mem-

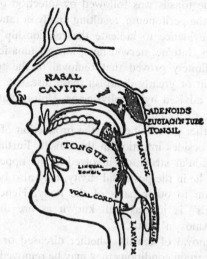

NASAL
CAVITY

ADENOIDS
EUSTACH'N TUBE
TONSIL

TONGUE

LINGUAL
TONSIL

VOCAL CORD

PHARYNX

OESOPHAGUS

LARYNX

Fig. 53. Lateral diagram of head showing relation of adenoids, tonsils, nose, ear, and larynx. Observe how close to the ear the adenoids are. Again observe that the floor of the nose and the adenoids are in the same horizontal plane. Also, discharge dropping down from the adenoids could easily fall on the vocal cords causing such disturbances as laryngitis and croup.

brane. The special importance of the distinction lies in the fact that the control in diphtheria depends on early diagnosis and the proper administration of a sufficient amount of suitable antitoxin.

The patient with tonsillitis should go to bed promptly. A physician will usually apply directly to the place of infection suitable antiseptics to destroy the germs that are on the surface. He will also control the fever and provide medication which may be helpful. The application of an ice bag or hot packs will give relief from the pain and soreness. A gargle with a small amount of baking soda helps to clear out the adherent mucus.

Chronic tonsillitis is especially dangerous because of the secondary effects. For this reason, physicians advise surgical removal of the tonsils in all such cases. Tonsillitis itself is seldom fatal, but the possibility afterward of an infected ear, or infected joints, or heart disease is so serious that a sore throat should never be neglected. Many years have passed since the medical profession first recognized the importance of removal of infected tonsils because of their relationship to disease. Tonsils are sometimes removed simply because they are so greatly enlarged as to interfere with swallowing and breathing. Between this simple enlargement and the severe states of infection in which the tonsils are filled with pus there is a wide variety of possibilities.

Much investigation has been done to prove that the infection in the tonsils may be carried by the blood to other parts of the body and there set up secondary infections which threaten life. There are well-established cases in which infection of the tonsils was followed by infection of the heart, of the kidneys, and even of the peritoneum, resulting finally in fatal peritonitis. There is also considerable evidence to indicate the relationship of infected tonsils to colds, infected ears, fatigue, nervousness, and rheumatic symptoms.

If it could be definitely proved that removal of the tonsils early in life would entirely prevent or greatly diminish these diseases, routine removal of the tonsils would be advised by all physicians. Unfortunately absolute proof of this fact cannot be provided.

There are many other possibilities for the production of colds, of nervousness, and of fatigue besides infection in the tonsils. Furthermore, the tonsils are not the only glandular structures involved in the upper respiratory tract. The adenoids, which lie in the postnasal cavity, may also be seriously infected and transmit infection to other parts of the body. Hence the combination "tonsils and adenoids" is just as well known as are the combinations of ham and eggs and Amos 'n' Andy.

The wholesale removal of tonsils, whether diseased or related to disease, is not warranted. In certain conditions they may be removed for definite effects, which experience has shown may certainly be secured. At present, the vast majority of physicians are convinced that the correct method for removal of the tonsils is complete surgical removal rather than the use of slow destruction by electricity or any other recently introduced method.

CHAPTER XXVIII

The Venereal Diseases
MORRIS FISHBEIN, M.D.

THE VENEREAL DISEASES are among the most common that afflict mankind. They spread from person to person in response to satisfaction of the biologic demand of the glands of man, but also occasionally through perfectly innocent sources, such as contaminated utensils, towels, and other appurtenances intimately used by human beings.

One fact must, however, be constantly kept in mind: both major venereal diseases, syphilis and gonorrhea, are caused by germs. The germs must be transmitted in order to transmit the disease. Every case of either one of these diseases comes from another case. Until a patient with one of these diseases is satisfactorily treated and his infection brought under control, he is a menace to everyone around him, including his wife—if he is married—his children, his friends, or associates.

The diseases are not new with man. They have probably existed since the earliest times, certainly since the Middle Ages. Everyone should have knowledge of the nature of these diseases and means of transmission, means of prevention, and correct method of treatment. Proper dissemination of such knowledge seems to be the only hope for their ultimate control.

SYPHILIS

Whether or not syphilis existed previous to 1493 is not established with certainty. About that time it appeared in Barcelona among Spanish sailors who had returned from Haiti. It reached Italy with the army of Charles VIII, and from Italy spread throughout Europe. At first it was called "Neapolitan disease" or the "French pox." The name spyhilis was given to it in 1530 by a writer named Fracastorius. Since that time, physicians have studied the disease constantly. Even before the modern era doctors had learned to treat syphilis with a fair degree of success with mercury. However, it was the discovery of the organism of the disease, and later the discovery of specific methods of treatment, that offered the first promise of complete control. The organism of spyhilis, known as "spirochaeta" or "treponema," was definitely established as the cause of the disease by the investigator Schaudinn in 1905. The organism is seen only with the microscope, and is found in the sore which is typically the first sign of infection with this disease.

TRANSMISSION OF SYPHILIS

In the vast majority of cases syphilis is transmitted from one human being to another during sexual relations. There are, however, records of accidental infection, such as those which occur on the hands of surgeons and midwives who have not properly protected their hands during their work; such as occur on the lips from infection through kissing, and such as occur occasionally on the breasts of wet nurses. Occasionally also the child may be infected before birth from its mother, in instances even when the mother herself is not actively diseased.

These facts should not frighten anyone into a phobia or constant fear of syphilis, since the disease is not transmitted as easily as the description may seem to suggest. Hotel beds, public lavatories, bathtubs, door knobs, books, utensils used in public eating places are not easily infected. Moreover, the germs do not live easily in the presence of dryness. Finally, it is necessary for the organism to get into a sore or an easily infected spot in order to invade the body. In most instances, thorough washing with soap and water does much to remove danger of infection. When it seems likely that one has been directly exposed to the development of the infection with syphilis, the rubbing of mercury ointment into the exposed area has been proved to be a protective measure of great value. It is well, however, to emphasize again that syphilis is rarely acquired by those who observe the elementary laws of personal hygiene and who have sexual relations only with those who are free from the disease.

FIRST SIGNS OF SYPHILIS

The first sign of syphilis is usually the appearance of a sore on the genital area or on the finger or wherever the germs gain entrance into the tissues. These sores develop slowly. At the same time the lymph glands in the region near by become swollen. A physician who sees such a sore makes his diagnosis certain by taking some of the fluid from the sore and studying it under what is called the dark field microscope. By reflected light he is thus able to see the spirochaetes wriggling in the fluid. He may also spread some of the secretion on a glass slide and stain it with suitable stains which make the organisms visible with the ordinary microscope.

The healing of the primary sore or its removal will not, however, prevent syphilis from invading the body. Usually, by the time the organisms are found freely in the sore, the body has already been quite fully invaded and it is necessary to give general treatment to control the condition. If immediate treatment is given before the appearance of the secondary symptoms, these are not likely to appear. Hence, the physician urges emphatically that every case of syphilis be treated at the earliest possible moment; in fact, that every case diagnosed from the symptoms be treated even before getting the results of the Wassermann test, so as to be certain that the control will be brought about at the earliest possible moment.

The test known as the Wassermann test, and a similar test, known as the Kahn test, are means of examining the blood so as to determine whether or not it contains a substance opposing syphilis, which is present only if syphilis has invaded the body. These tests are positive in more than 95 per cent of cases in an early stage. By their nature they enable the physician to determine whether or not improvement is taking place, and later whether or not the patient has been cured.

Venereal diseases can be cured, provided treatment is given sufficiently early and with sufficient intensity and for a long enough period of time. Modern treatment is based on use of adequate amounts of penicillin or other antibiotic drugs.

The secondary symptoms of syphilis appear about the time when the first sore is disappearing. These symptoms represent invasion of the body as a whole. Now the person is usually sick, he may be jaundiced, and eruptions may appear about the body. Frequently the hair falls out in spots, and occasionally serious sores develop on the skin. There may even be inflammation of the eyes, of the mouth, of the joints, or of the nervous system in this stage of syphilis. Because these symptoms may come and go, some patients are inclined to neglect treatment in the second stage of syphilis. This, however, should never be done. It is easier to treat the condition in this stage than in the third stage, in which the brain and nervous system become involved.

In the secondary stage there has seldom been destruction of the tissues of the body, so that treatment in this stage is more likely to be effective. Under no circumstances should the patient believe that the gradual disappearance of the symptoms represents cure of the disease. He should have a definite statement by a competent physician after that physician has made sufficient laboratory tests to venture an opinion with reasonable certainty.

In the third stage of syphilis, there occur not only destruction of tissues, but growths within various organs of the body, inflammations of the blood vessels, hardening of some of the organs, and other serious changes. In fact, the lesions of this disease are so varied that Sir William Osler once said that one who knew all of syphilis really knew all of medicine. The third stage grows constantly worse unless sufficiently treated. Fortunately, the third stage of syphilis is not likely to be as dangerous to other people as are the first and second, because in this stage the lesions are buried deeper within the body, so that the organisms are not so easily transmitted outside the body.

In the later stage of syphilis, it affects the nervous system. As a result come those two exceedingly serious diseases which are responsible for much disability and death: locomotor ataxia or tabes dorsalis, and paresis, also called general paralysis of the insane and dementia paralytica. In these conditions, other methods of treatment are required besides those commonly used for syphilis in the early stages. It may be necessary to apply treatment directly to the spine or to the brain. It may be necessary to infect the patient with malaria, which has been found to have special virtue in the attack on general paralysis, or to use the heat treatment, which has come to be well established as a useful method.

FACTS ABOUT SYPHILIS

Among certain facts which should be known to everyone relative to syphilis are the following:

This disease does not cause pimples.

It does not cause itching conditions of the skin.

It may cause ulcers of the legs, but more frequently these are due to varicose veins.

It may be responsible for failure to produce children, but there are also other conditions which may produce such failures.

It is not a form of blood poisoning, but testing of the blood will show whether or not the patient has syphilis.

It is not responsible for the vast majority of cases of baldness, but some cases of loss of hair not only of the head but of the entire body may be due to syphilis.

It has not been established in any way that syphilis is the cause of cancer or that these two conditions are in any way related.

INSTRUCTIONS FOR THOSE WITH SYPHILIS

If you have any sore on your genitals, no matter how small, or if you think you have syphilis, consult your physician. Do not under any conditions rely on the "blood medicines" that promise to eradicate syphilis, and do not be caught by advertising doctors—quacks—who try to get your money by promising to cure you quickly. Do not let druggists prescribe for you; they are not qualified to treat syphilis.

Do not hesitate to tell your doctor or dentist of your disease. Later in life if you get sick at any time, you should tell your doctor that you have had syphilis, since this fact may furnish a clue to treatment on which your cure depends.

Live temperately and sensibly. Do not go to extreme in any direction in your habits of life.

Try to get a reasonable amount of sleep—eight hours is the amount needed by the average person. And as a safeguard to others, sleep alone. Avoid possible contamination of others by contact with your secretions or excretions.

Absolutely do not use alcoholic liquors. All experience shows that drinking —even moderate drinking—is bad for syphilis.

Take good care of your teeth. Brush them two or three times a day. If they are not in good condition, have them attended to by a dentist. But when you go to him, tell him that you have syphilis.

Do not have sexual intercourse until you are told by your physician that you are no longer contagious. It will interfere with the cure of the disease, and it is criminal, for it is likely to give the disease to your wife.

You must not marry until you have the doctor's consent, which cannot be properly given until at least two years have passed after cure seems complete. If you do, you run the risk of infecting your wife and your children with syphilis.

Early in the course of syphilis, while it is contagious, the greatest danger of infecting other people is by the mouth. Because of this danger, do not kiss anybody. Particularly, do not endanger children by kissing them.

Do not allow anything that has come in contact with your lips or that has been in your mouth to be left around so that anybody can use it before it has been cleaned. This applies to cups, glasses, knives, forks, spoons, pipes, cigars, toothpicks, and all such things. It is better to use your own towels, brushes, comb, razor, soap, etc., though these are much less likely to be contaminated than objects that go in your mouth.

If you have any open sores—you will not have any after the first week or two, if you are treated—everything that comes in contact with them should be destroyed or disinfected.

To live up to these instructions will only require a little care until you get used to them; after that, it will be easy. If you do live up to them, there is a good prospect that syphilis will not do your health permanent harm or cause injury to others; and you will have the satisfaction of knowing that, after your misfortune, you have acted the part of an honest man in your efforts to overcome it.

Remember, the antibiotic drugs, particularly penicillin, are now known to be efficient in controlling syphilis. Often the condition is fully controlled in a few weeks. The number of cases has dropped to one-tenth what it used to be. To insure future safety, treatment must be continued until every evidence of the disease has disappeared. For your own good, you must see to it that you do not neglect your treatment after the first few months.

Penicillin, terramycin, and aureomycin are most important in the treatment of syphilis. By intensive treatment, patients may be free from the danger of infecting others in a few days. In early cases, the disease is apparently brought under full control within a week or ten days. Treatment demands, however, complete control by the physician during the period of treatment. Penicillin taken by mouth or in other ways is not safe or efficient. Patients must return frequently for repeated examinations and tests to be sure the condition is completely controlled.

WHEN PEOPLE WITH SYPHILIS MAY MARRY

One of the questions most frequently asked by a patient with syphilis is whether or not he may marry. Most physicians are convinced that a patient should be free from all syphilitic symptoms for at least one year before marriage should be contemplated. In some American states the bridegroom is compelled to furnish a medical certificate to show that he has been examined and found free from venereal disease. This has been, for instance, the law in Alabama, Louisiana, North Carolina, North Dakota, Oregon, Wisconsin, and Wyoming. However, none of these states requires a certificate from the prospective bride. The marriage of a person who has a contagious venereal disease is forbidden in Delaware, Indiana, Maine, Michigan, Nebraska, New Jersey, Oklahoma, Pennsylvania, Utah, Vermont, Virginia, and Washington. However, there does not seem to be any good evidence that any of these states secures adequate evidence from those applying for a license to marry.

The treatment of this condition is one of the most intricate problems that can confront a physician. He must use his remedies in relationship to the reaction of the patient and the response of the patient to them. No one with the disease should ever discontinue treatment until he is pronounced by a competent physician free from danger of transmitting the disease and cured to the extent that the condition is brought absolutely to a halt in his body. Persistence in the use of the new remedies that are available under proper control will yield a successful result in the vast majority of cases.

GONORRHEA

Gonorrhea has existed certainly since Biblical times. Although it is a widespread and serious disease, it is not a killing disease. As a cause of ill health, it ranks among the leaders, but as a cause of death it is not especially prominent. Many people believe that gonorrhea concerns only the sex organs, whereas the germ which causes it, described by the investigator Niesser in 1879, may invade any part of the human body. Like syphilis, it is spread mostly by sexual contacts. However, there are infections of the eyes sustained during childbirth or in other ways which attack mostly infants at birth. There are infections of the tissues in women associated with the use of bathtubs and toilet devices not properly cleansed, which are accidental infections with this disease. Little girls are occasionally infected by soiled hands of mothers or nurses.

Gonorrhea is responsible for a considerable percentage of all cases of blindness. It is one of the common causes of infection in the female abdomen, resulting in necessary surgical operations and occasionally removal of the female organs. It is responsible for a considerable amount of sterility in men due to infections of the various parts of the sex tracts. It is found not only among the poor but in all classes of society.

FIRST SIGNS OF GONORRHEA

From three to five days after a sex contact with a person who is infected the first signs of the disease may appear. These usually are a feeling of burning or stinging at the time of urination, associated with redness and soreness, and associated also with the formation of pus or matter which drips from the sex organ. This material is highly infectious and should not be allowed to come in contact with the eyes or sex organs of any other person.

If a physician is consulted immediately, he may be able to stop the disease in these early stages, when it is confined to the lower portion of the sex organs. If, however, it is not stopped at this time, the germs get farther back into the glands of the male and into the organs and tissues of the female. To the extent to which these organs and tissues are involved, gonorrhea is a serious disorder. The physician may make his diagnosis by an examination of the matter under the microscope, in which case he can actually find the germs, and also by tests of the blood. Occasionally the condition affects the joints, and it is also largely responsible for painful heels, causing outgrowths on the large bone of the heel.

TREATMENT OF GONORRHEA

In treatment, the physician uses many types of remedies, including antibiotics such as penicillin and terramycin given by injection into the muscles or blood stream. Gonorrhea is now controlled in 48 hours. Military authorities prevent gonorrhea by giving penicillin to men going on leave.

ADVICE TO THOSE WITH GONORRHEA

Persist in treatment until your doctor tells you you are cured.

Do not try to treat yourself.

Do not use a patent medicine or some "sure shot" that may stop the discharges but will not cure you.

Do not let an advertising doctor—a quack—get your money, and do not let a drug clerk treat you.

If you have had gonorrhea and you suspect that it is not cured, report to your medical officer.

During the acute stages keep quiet and take little exercise. As long as you have any discharge avoid violent exercise, especially dancing.

In order to avoid chordee, while the disease is acute, sleep on your side, urinate just before going to bed, and drink no water after supper.

Never "break" a chordee. To get rid of it wrap the penis in cold wet cloths or pour cold water on it.

Except at night, drink plenty of water—eight or ten glasses a day.

Do not drink any alcoholic liquors; they always make the disease worse and delay its cure. Also avoid spicy drinks such as ginger ale.

Do not eat irritating, highly seasoned, spicy foods, such as pepper, horse-radish, mustard, pickles, salt and smoked meats, or fish.

Always wash your hands after handling the penis, particularly in order to protect your eyes. Gonorrhea of the eyes is very dangerous; it will produce blindness if not at once treated, and the infection is easily carried to the eyes on the fingers.

Keep your penis clean. Do not plug up the opening with cotton or wear a dressing that prevents the escape of the pus from it. Wash the penis several times daily.

Burn old dressings, or drop them into a disinfecting solution.

Never use anybody else's syringe or let others use yours. While you are using a syringe keep it clean by washing it in very hot water, and, when you have finished with its use, destroy it.

Avoid sexual excitement. Stay away from women. Do not have intercourse. It will bring your disease back to its acute stage, and it is almost sure to infect a woman. Sexual intercourse while you have gonorrhea is a criminal act.

You are likely to obey instructions while your gonorrhea is acute, because it causes so much pain. Persist in them after pain is gone; by so doing you will prevent relapses, make your cure much easier and more certain, and expose no one else to the disease.

MODERN TREATMENT OF GONORRHEA

Penicillin is effective not only in venereal gonorrhea but also in gonorrhea affecting the eyes, the joints or the heart. Whereas this disease was formerly considered well nigh incurable, with penicillin cures seem to be almost 100 per cent.

MARRIAGE AFTER GONORRHEA

As regards marriage after an attack of gonorrhea, the patient should be examined at weekly intervals to determine whether or not any infection is present following treatment. The results should be negative three consecutive times before he can be considered definitely cured. It should be remembered that self-treatment with drug-store remedies is just as dangerous as complete neglect of treatment.

Prevention in gonorrhea is far better than cure. The chief factor in prevention consists in the avoidance of sex contacts when infection is present, and infection is likely to be present in any promiscuous woman, either commercial or private. There are various methods of protection against the possibility of infection, such as the use of rubber devices and injections of various antiseptics immediately after sex contact, these antiseptics being held in the organs until the antiseptics have sufficient amount of time to act.

CHAPTER XXIX

The Care of the Teeth
MORRIS FISHBEIN, M.D.

THE CARE OF BABY'S TEETH

FEW MOTHERS realize that the first attention to the teeth of the child must begin before it is born. The mother should visit the dentist early, keep her teeth clean and well cared for, and eat the proper food so that the child's teeth will be properly developed. The proper foods include plenty of milk, fresh vegetables, eggs, fresh and cooked fruits, the coarser cereals, and a sufficient amount of calories to provide energy. Foods to be avoided are the sweets in excess, meat in excess, pastries, and highly seasoned foods.

During the early months it is not necessary for the expectant mother to eat more than her usual amount of food, but during the last four months the amount of food must be increased slightly in order to provide a sufficient amount of material for building the tissues of the child.

There used to be a notion that it was not safe for a prospective mother to visit her dentist, but it is now realized that the dentist can do the necessary dental work without serious harm or shock, and that it is better to take care of the teeth immediately than to permit bad conditions to go on for months.

Of special importance for building sound teeth are vitamins C, D, and A. Vitamin C is found plentifully in orange and tomato juice and in the fresh vegetables; vitamins A and D particularly in cod-liver oil and egg yolks. The physician should see the prospective mother just as soon as she knows that she is going to have a child and advise her regarding the taking of cod-liver oil or of excess vitamins in the form of concentrates.

The baby that is nursed by its mother gets the best food a baby can get. If it is not nursed by the mother, it will have to have a diet arranged so as to include the necessary substances. The basis of all baby diets is milk, but milk is deficient in certain necessary substances, and these the doctor can provide for through modifications of the diet. He will tell the mother when the baby is to have orange and tomato juice and cod-liver oil and the amount of each it should have. The vegetables are the first foods to be added to the baby's diet, and they should be started slowly in very small quantities. By the time the child is one year of age it can eat most vegetables; it can also be having fresh milk, fruit, and Zwieback or toast.

Many physicians and dentists believe that coarse foods strengthen the jaws and help in hardening the gums. When a new tooth is about to come in, the coarse foods serve as a resistance against which the gums may work in order to permit the tooth to cut its way through. If the child is excessively irritant when the teeth are coming in, it is wise to have the advice of the dentist or family physician.

The first teeth come in at the front of the mouth between the fifth and eighth months, as a rule. If they happen to be a little early or late, there is no cause for worry. The next teeth come in between the eighth and tenth months, and the others about the time of the first birthday. Until the first teeth appear, the mouth of the child does well if let alone. After the first teeth appear, the gums and teeth may be wiped daily with a soft clean cloth dipped in water to which a little salt has been added. It is well to be exceedingly gentle.

About the eighteenth month a soft toothbrush may be substituted for the soft cloth, and as soon as the child is old enough it should learn to brush its teeth for itself. If the child likes the taste of toothpaste, it may have toothpaste. If it prefers the water with added salt, it may have that. Most physicians and dentists are convinced that a toothpaste is of service only in cleaning and polishing the teeth and has little, if any, special value for preventing infection or counteracting acid.

The chief reason for preserving the baby teeth is to keep the mouth in the right shape for the second teeth. All of the twenty teeth that are called temporary teeth are usually in the mouth by the time the child is three. Behind the first set is the second set. In order to have the second set properly developed, the food must be right and the mouth free from infection. The only certain way to control infection is to have dental care when it appears.

The most important permanent tooth comes in between the fifth and sixth year of life and is known as the six-year molar. It comes in six teeth back from the one in the front of the mouth in center.

There are four six-year molars, one on each side of the upper and lower jaws. They should have the most careful attention. Once gone, they are not replaced except with artificial teeth. If they decay and are removed without proper dental attention, the entire expression of the face and of the mouth may change. In the absence of the proper molars, food is not sufficiently ground before entering the stomach.

Every child should see a dentist following the appearance of the six-year molars. Only a generation has passed since dentists first began to give special attention to the teeth of the child. Now the subject is so important that there are many dentists who specialize exclusively in children's teeth. They are concerned with seeing that all of the teeth are straight, that they fit properly against the opposites in the other jaw, that they do not grind off surfaces that are meant to stand, and that they remain firmly and are not pushed into the wrong positions.

With the help of the X-ray, the dentist is able to see that the teeth are sound at their roots. By personal inspection he finds tiny spots which indicate the beginning of decay. These can be filled and polished and their decay stopped. The additional cost of the X-ray pictures means future saving. Preventive dentistry done early is cheap. Curative dentistry, done after decay has proceeded far, after the teeth have gotten into wrong positions, after some teeth have been lost, may be expensive and can be prevented.

Many communities are now adding fluorides to the community water supply as a means of preventing dental caries. There seems to be no doubt that this helps prevention though other causes persist and cases appear even when all children get fluorides.

ORTHODONTIA

Within recent years a new specialty has arisen in dentistry and in medicine called orthodontia. The word means "straight teeth." It means literally to arrange crooked teeth in a more harmonious and symmetrical curve so that they will function better and improve the facial appearance. It is, of course, necessary to realize that back of all health are proper nutrition and growth. Unless the child has a diet which contains a sufficient amount of calcium, phosphorus, vitamins A, C, and D particularly, it is not likely to have good teeth.

Unless the baby teeth have been suitably controlled and well taken care of, the teeth that come in thereafter will not be properly developed and distributed. Dentists are convinced that there are a considerable number of bad habits that are associated with development of malocclusion, which means improper closing of the teeth and jaws. Breathing through the mouth, sucking the thumb, and similar bad habits may be associated with bad formation of the teeth, the bones of the jaw and the muscles which control them.

The twenty baby teeth of infancy begin to disappear around the age of six, at which time also the four big six-year molars appear. Unless there is a full number of healthy teeth in the mouth at each age, they will not be properly arranged nor will they close properly. Each tooth depends on the one next to it for support. If any groups of teeth are pushed out of position, the whole set becomes irregular.

The orthodontist is a specialist in producing regularity of the teeth. Through gradual changes exercised at certain points the teeth are brought into proper position. This is done by the use of wire and of gold, and must be done slowly and carefully so as not to destroy the teeth in the process. It is a specialty within dentistry which concerns the ordinary care of the teeth. It is no longer necessary for any girl to appear in public after she has grown to mature age with teeth crossing over one another or with the protruding snaggle teeth that gave so many women a comical appearance in the past. Science in this way does much for human happiness.

THE CARE OF ADULTS' TEETH

The care of the teeth in the adult involves not only a suitable diet, but also a certain amount of simple dental hygiene. The popular slogan that a clean tooth never decays is probably correct if associated with the right definition of a "clean tooth." It is equally true that millions of unclean teeth never decay. Of course, unclean teeth are not desirable, because they permit the growth of bacteria that are usually associated with foul breath, they are unesthetic in appearance, and they are associated with irritations of the gums, cheeks, and tongue that may be serious.

About 1890 it was shown that certain acids formed by the action of mouth bacteria on a substance containing sugar when held in contact with enamel of the teeth for a certain number of hours would cause the enamel to fall apart and open the way to destruction of the softer dentine substance beneath. Since the acid must exist in concentrated form in order to do such work, the process usually goes on only in the tiny pits, fissures, or other defects in the enamel, or in the spaces between the teeth. The exposed surfaces of the teeth seldom decay because the natural movements of the lips, cheeks and tongue help to keep them clean.

Associated with the cause of tooth decay are errors in the diet. It is useless to take in large amounts of calcium unless the calcium is assimilated. Apparently phosphorus, the products of certain glands, ultraviolet rays, and the vitamins are involved in the use of calcium by the body and must be taken in the diet in order to permit the process to go on satisfactorily.

Once decay begins, once the enamel of the tooth is broken down, bacteria, constantly present in the mouth, aid the destruction. Chemical changes occur that are disastrous. The most that anyone can do is to keep teeth clean by the best methods possible, to overcome acids by the use of proper alkaline washes or pastes, and to see that the diet is of the proper nature to keep the teeth in a state of satisfactory nutrition.

TOOTH DECAY

The University of Chicago summoned four experts who have been devoting themselves to research on teeth to discuss the problem of constant decay of the teeth which is a disease of our modern civilization. Apparently people who live in remote areas of the globe under native or natural conditions are more free from tooth decay and have fewer cavities than do civilized men. When these people come into contact with the civilization of the white man and adopt his manner of living and his diets, their teeth begin to decay immediately and apparently tooth decay progresses rapidly.

The United States now has a national institute of dental research which is under the direction of the United States Public Health Service. Dr. H. T. Dean who is director of this institute of dental research says that the acids of the mouth have a great deal to do with the amount of decay. However, modern medicine and dentistry have apparently failed to find any specific method of changing the reaction of the material around the surfaces of the teeth or of making the surfaces of the teeth more resistant to the actions of the acids. Several methods have been suggested, including various technics for getting rid of the bacteria in the mouth, but apparently none of these is yet well established. Dr. F. J. Orland who is assistant professor of dental surgery in the University of Chicago has made a special study of the bacteria of the mouth and he is convinced that the acids created by these bacteria can harm the enamel of the teeth.

Dr. Conrad A. Elvehjem of the University of Wisconsin, who is widely known as an authority in the field of diet, pointed out that the bacteria in the mouth break down sugars into acids and he believes it is the acid that causes the trouble. He says that a good diet will prevent dental decay.

Dr. J. R. Blayney, professor of dental surgery of the University of Chicago, said that the chief problem is the development of a technic that will check the decay of teeth, and that the three conditions necessary for decay include a susceptible tooth, foods in the mouth that are constantly present, and bacteria. The discussion proceeded along the lines of these three factors. No one knows now just why the teeth of some people seem to be much more susceptible to decay than are the teeth of others.

TOOTHBRUSH

In cleansing the mouth a good toothbrush is necessary. Most of the toothbrushes sold today are too large for efficient brushing. There are all sorts of shapes available with many strange distributions of bristles, but so far as is known it is impossible to make a toothbrush that will conform exactly to the shape of the dental arch inside and outside. Some toothbrushes are made with bristles higher in the center and low at the ends, some with the bristles high at one end and low at the other end, some with bristles lower in the middle and high at both ends.

This seems to make little difference, the only necessity being that the brush be small and that the handle be such that it can be manipulated so that the bristles will reach the front, back and sides of every tooth. The toothbrush demands proper care to give it long life and to prevent its acting as a carrier of infections rather than as a preventive.

When a toothbrush is split, when bristles begin to break off and come out, the toothbrush should be thrown away. A new toothbrush should be put in a strong salt cold-water solution for two hours before using. Cold water should be used to moisten the brush before using and to rinse it thoroughly after the teeth are brushed. The brush should then be hung in the open air in such position that the bristles will not come in contact with anything else for twenty-four hours before the brush is used again.

Obviously, therefore, persons should have two brushes, one for morning and one for evening use. If a toothbrush is kept moist for too long a period of time or kept in an airtight container, the bristles are quickly destroyed. Most important, however, is the fact that bacteria grow on warm, moist toothbrushes, and that the use of the brush before it has dried thoroughly will merely add new bacteria to those taken from the mouth in the previous washing.

TOOTHPASTES, MOUTH WASHES, AND TOOTH POWDERS

One of the most debatable questions in medicine and dentistry today concerns the exact value of toothpastes, mouth washes, tooth powders, and similar mixtures for the health of the mouth and the teeth. Many physicians and dentists are convinced that the most any toothpaste can do is to keep the teeth clean and polished, and that therefore any good soapy preparation that tastes well serves the purpose. However, the preparations that are available are complex in their formulas and extraordinary in their claims.

Some toothpastes are widely advertised because of their alkaline content, since it is urged that alkalis tend to counteract the tendency of the mouth to become acid. It has not, however, been proved that there is any serious tendency in this direction, nor that an opposite tendency is especially valuable.

Another preparation is sold with the argument that it duplicates normal saliva and that the presence of normal saliva prevents tooth decay. It has been argued that sugar helps to cause decay of the teeth and that food particles between the teeth increase dental caries. The disadvantage associated with food particles and sugar is that these provide mediums on which bacteria grow and that bacterial products are injurious to the teeth.

Some toothpastes are sold with the special claim that they kill the germs in the mouth on contact, but most physicians realize that the first mouthful of food or the first breath of air will bring new germs into the mouth. Some toothpastes contain abrasive substances which scratch the enamel, and this is bad, since anything that makes a scratch or an abrasion may produce a spot in which germs may enter more easily.

Another toothpaste is sold with the claim that it contains a substance which digests away food particles and mucus, and another is sold with the claim that it contains enough of certain antiseptic to sterilize the gums and keep them sterile. The important thing for the average person to remember is the fact that most of these preparations are kept in the mouth not longer than a few seconds and that any effects which they may accomplish are quite temporary.

Most recent additions to toothpastes are ammonia preparation for preventing decay and chlorophyll for preventing odors. The evidence in support of these additions is not generally convincing to most scientists.

PYORRHEA

Pyorrhea means a flow of matter. However, the flow of matter or, to speak of it scientifically—pus—is not the most significant thing about this disturbance of the mouth and teeth. The important fact is that the condition becomes chronic and that as a result of this the tissue of the gums separates from the roots of the teeth. When they have once separated they are not likely to become attached again. Moreover, a constant presence of infectious matter leads to secondary disturbances in the body which may be exceedingly serious.

The blood picks up the germs from the pus pockets around the teeth and carries them to other parts of the body, where they set up new infections. Because the teeth are loose and the mouth is foul, the person with pyorrhea is likely to lose his appetite. He is unable to chew food satisfactorily, his digestion is interfered with, and he becomes in general much sicker than he would be with a clean mouth cavity.

Because the mouth is easy to get at, because the gums are tough, and because the saliva keeps the mouth constantly lubricated, the tissues stand a great deal of punishment before the condition becomes so severe that it is impossible to delay attention. For this reason, pyorrhea is usually a chronic rather than an acute disease.

For this reason also it is necessary to remind people again and again that the mouth should be looked at by a competent dentist at least once in every six months in order that such conditions may be detected early and given adequate care before they become so serious that the only hope lies in removal of all of the teeth, surgical attention to the gums, and the provision of artificial plates.

Among the causes of infections of the gums are continuous irritation from the edge of rough crowns or of fillings. A good dentist will see to it that a crown or a filling is absolutely smooth and continuous with the surface of the tooth to which it is applied.

Food particles may accumulate between the teeth and set up spots of local irritation and decay. The regular use of the toothbrush and of dental floss is necessary to prevent such an occurrence. Toothpicks, and especially pins, knives, forks, or other objects used in lieu of toothpicks, do severe damage to the delicate tissues when manipulated by a careless hand.

Tartar deposits are just as irritant as rough fillings. Moreover, they are easily susceptible to the accumulation of bacteria. Pyorrhea is one of the most menacing diseases known to man, and its prevention depends on constant vigilance.

Fortunately, antibiotic drugs, applied locally to infected mouths and also taken internally, help to eliminate pyorrhea.

HALITOSIS OR BAD BREATH

Bad breath, now politely referred to as halitosis, is offensive. There is little excuse for anyone to permit himself to become obnoxious for this reason to

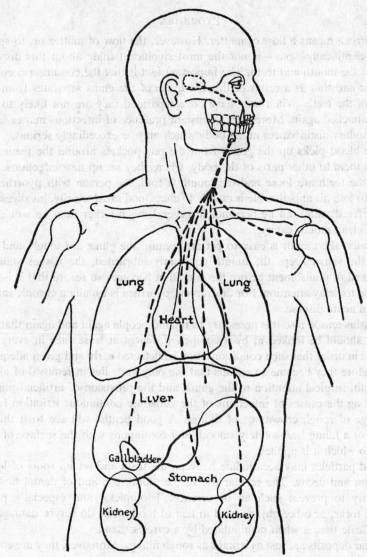

Fig. 54. Effects of abscessed teeth.

everyone around him, since it is possible to prevent the presence of such odors. The most frequent cause is related to the teeth, which may be subject to cavities or which may simply be surrounded with accumulations of decaying food products. Cavities should be filled and tartar deposits should be removed at least once every six months. The teeth may be kept clean by the use of dental floss and by the regular use morning and evening of a toothbrush with proper powder or paste. A high fat diet may be related to halitosis.

There are innumerable mouth washes containing antiseptics, alkalis, or acids, that may be used after the teeth have been brushed. Weak hydrogen peroxide solutions are sometimes of value. It is best to use strong solutions only on the advice of a competent physician or dentist.

After the teeth as the cause of bad breath have been eliminated, the tonsils must be examined as to the presence of infection. Another frequent cause of bad breath is infection in the nose or in the space behind the nose. The formation of crusts and of accumulations of infected material is bound to produce foul odor of the breath. Halitosis may also result from chronic disturbances of the stomach and of the intestines. If the tongue is constantly coated, if there is eructation of sour material from the stomach, the person concerned should consult a physician. Claims are now made that chlorophyll preparations control all sorts of body odors but the claims still need to be verified. Most recent evidence fails to support the claims for chlorophyll.

FALSE TEETH

The person who is compelled to wear any form of removable appliance in the mouth to replace natural teeth has special problems to which dentists have been giving concern. False teeth, artificial teeth, removable bridges, and plates are included in this category.

The person who is going to lose his natural teeth by extraction because of infections or due to any other cause should have a thorough study by the use of the X-ray before any natural teeth are removed. The dentist who is going to make the artificial denture can then advise intelligently which teeth may be saved and which should be extracted. This is particularly important because he wants to restore the patient's natural appearance, and he wants to retain everything possible to permit the making of the most suitable denture.

To do this, he takes impressions of the mouth, makes a record of the patient's profile and facial contour, studies the natural color of the teeth and similar factors. It is sometimes possible in making an artificial denture to correct deformities or abnormalities of the lower portion of the face. When a person is fitted with an artificial denture his experience is similar to being fitted with a suit or a dress. It may not be exactly right the first time, and some adjustments may be necessary.

When the work is completed the patient should not assume that it is permanent. The human body is a growing and changing organism which differs from year to year. This means that dentures should be studied from time to time if they become uncomfortable so that old ones may be refitted or new ones substituted. If this is not done there actually may be changes in the appearance of the face, deep lines and wrinkles being associated in some instances with the constant wearing of unsuitable dentures.

Artificial plates and teeth must be given even more care than natural teeth.

They should be brushed carefully and thoroughly after each meal and on going to bed at night. In this cleaning, cold or lukewarm water should be used—never hot water. It is just as important to be careful about handling dentures as handling expensive eyeglasses. The dentists suggest that when removing the dentures from the mouth the wearer should lean over a washbowl filled two-thirds full of water and hold the plates close to the water when brushing them. Then the water will break the fall if he happens to drop the artificial plate.

It is not advisable to try to crack nuts with artificial teeth. Biting threads, eating hard candy, and chewing on bones are sometimes responsible for ruining expensive dentures.

Just as soon as the teeth are secured, the person will do well to go into a private place and practice reading aloud in order to get used to the feel of the teeth and to their weaknesses. When the false teeth are first inserted, the facial expression may seem to be changed, but this is due to the effort of the muscles to take care of the plates. Just as soon as the false teeth become properly adjusted, the effort will disappear, and the expression will become natural again.

Naturally, the hardest thing to do with the false teeth is to eat. The person who has the teeth thinks that he has to manipulate both the teeth and the food. He will, therefore, do well to begin with food that requires little chewing and to avoid steaks and chops for the first few days. Small bits of food chewed slowly will easily be taken care of. Big masses of food may cause trouble. Until one learns to manipulate the teeth, and until the gums and the ridges have become hardened, one need not expect to eat everything and anything that is offered. If there are spots in the gums and the ridges have become excessively sore, the dentist should be consulted immediately to make the necessary changes and to prescribe the necessary treatment.

Artificial teeth, when out of the mouth, should be kept moist. The best arrangement is to put them in a salt solution, boric acid, or some favorite mouth wash.

CHAPTER XXX

Advice on the Diet

SOLOMON STROUSE, M.D. and CARL D. STROUSE, M.D.

INTRODUCTION

AN OLD-FASHIONED *proverb says, "Tell me what you eat and I will tell you what you are." Modern medicine has learned both the truth and the fallacy of this proverb. Our modern knowledge of nutrition has eliminated a great many of the fads in diet of an earlier day. It has, at the same time, brought to light the importance of diet for the control of disease as well as for the maintenance of the body in health. The questions of deficiencies of the human diet in their relationship to specific diseases are fully discussed in the chapter on deficiency diseases.*

The following chapter by Dr. Solomon Strouse and Dr. Carl D. Strouse calls attention to the important constituents of an average diet; the relationships between proteins, carbohydrates, fats, mineral salts, and vitamins; the importance of the relationship of acids to alkalis, and similar topics. It traces the progress of food through the digestive tract and then discusses specifically the value of such substances as meats, fish, sugars, milk, cereals, fats, fruits, vegetables, and other substances.

The chapter is supplemented by some tabular data, indicating the protein yield of various foods, the caloric yield of various foods, and the distribution of protein, fat, and carbohydrates for food used in normal diets. These diets are still further supplemented by other tabular data, describing the essentials of a normal diet as well as diets for special purposes.

M. F.

THE DEVELOPMENT OF THE NORMAL DIET

When Adam and Eve first walked in the Garden of Eden, some unconscious power led them to pick and choose the proper herbs and vegetables. When the children of Israel wandered through the desert, they too found what they needed. It seems rather a remarkable coincidence that the selective power has been such as to permit man to survive.

There is a sound basis for most of the Mosaic laws of food (now about three thousand years old). The first law, which prohibited the use of animals that did not chew the cud and had cloven hoofs, excluded all but herbivorous animals. The reason was that the carnivora ate flesh which might not be good, and therefore the flesh of the carnivora itself would become polluted. The second law restricted the eating of sea food to that with fins and scales. This, of course, excluded the mollusks, which were soft meat and which easily went into decay. The third law, restricting birds, especially enumerated all regarded as carrion eaters, the reason being obviously the same as for the law of animals. The fourth law, regarding blood, was based on the belief that blood potentially was the carrier of any pollution of the animal. The kosher method of killing simply removes blood from the animal as completely as possible. Others of the Mosaic laws which were developed during the later years of the history of the Jews cannot be explained either on the basis of modern knowledge of nutrition or on what was known of the Jews at the time. Probably many of these were mere superstition and taboo. Certainly they cannot be explained on the basis of our present knowledge of foods. Yet on the whole the remarkable historical continuity of the Jews indicates that their laws of living were based on sound concepts. This history is perhaps the most outstanding tribute to the trial-and-error method of which there is knowledge.

No formulation of a normal diet can be considered fairly without the realization of this and similar historical facts. Traditional, racial, and hereditary factors are of importance. Despite all that science has taught in recent years regarding the value of balanced diets, such knowledge alone is insufficient for the formulation of a normal dietary. The experiences of the human race might have been quite different, the result might have been much better, if modern dietary knowledge had been correct procedure five thousand years ago. Not as many infants would have died; people would have lived to a riper age; and the whole history of the world might have been different. Yet the fact remains that the world has survived.

The basis of the survival has been the old adage that the appetite is the guide to nutrition. This adage is, of course, only partially true. Given an abundant food supply, it is probable that appetite will guide the individual to a normal diet. However, the appetite easily becomes perverted. Whereas the infant who has not tasted sugar may pick out the best foods for his or her development, later in life, when the appetite has already been changed by poorly selected foods, it no longer is a guide.

Just at this point the truly marvelous contributions made by experimental nutritionists and physiologists come to help. The lessons of history cannot be excluded in constructing a diet, nor is it possible to achieve the optimum result without knowledge of the nutritional studies. The dietary aim naturally is an ideal, an ideal of perfect health for everybody, an ideal which aims to save the lives of infants and prolong the lives of adults, to prevent illness, improve general health, and to increase the store of human happiness. This ideal, of course, cannot be realized; practical considerations stand in the way. Just as the physician cannot send the stevedore with heart disease to California for the winter, so he cannot always prescribe an ideal diet on a limited budget. However, the task of prescribing an ideal diet is not nearly as difficult as it might seem to the uninitiated. In this chapter an attempt is made to simplify and clarify the situation and to show how a few fundamental facts and procedures make it possible for any person of average intelligence to eat fairly normal food.

FOOD FADS AND FANCIES

One of the great troubles with the tremendous interest in food has been a willful ignorance or malicious effort on the part of faddists and propagandists to obscure the issue. It might be just as well to start this discussion of food with comment on some of the present-day fads and fancies which seem to have an all too powerful hold on the imagination of many individuals. The propagandist spirit of the American advertiser, coupled with the gullibility of the reading public, made it possible to flood the world with all kinds of foolish dietary advice, most often not based on scientific evidence, usually completely erroneous, at times dangerous, and inevitably useless. The public has certain ideas on food; individuals or groups follow dietary regimens as they would worship idols.

Fortunately, the development of high standards by the Pure Food and Drug Laws and by the Council on Foods of the American Medical Association has prevented extravagant claims for many foods. Nevertheless, some of the so-called dietary principles which have gained vogue seem to have the backing of "medical authority (?)." Consider the roughage habit. According to the adherents of the roughage school, it is necessary to load the intestines with all kinds of indigestible and unassimilable substances like bran, which form an irritating bulk in the large intestines, and which may, although not always, lead to irritation of the intestines. Whereas a certain amount of indigestible residue is necessary to normal action of the bowels and evacuation, this is a long step removed from the rather violent loading of a weak bowel with a mass of unnecessary work.

Before 1880 wheat was milled almost entirely in local communities, and the milling process left the food value almost intact, but more refined milling processes have removed important parts of the vitamin B group from flour and thus from bread, rolls, and all flour products. White bread, which is the most attractive bread for most Americans, is actually the one bread from which most vitamins have been removed.

The Food and Drug Administration in 1941 established official standards for enriching flour with the B vitamins to replace those natural vitamins which had been removed. During World War II such vitamin addition became compulsory. With these additions, white flour is nutritionally adequate, and there is no evidence of anything harmful to humans in the present method of processing white flour. "Enriched bread" which contains added vitamins and minerals is nutritionally adequate, as can be seen from this table.

	Minimum	Maximum
Thiamin		
Riboflavin	1.66 mg.	2.5 mg.
Niacin	1.2 mg.	1.8 mg.
Iron	6.0 mg.	24.0 mg.
Vitamin D	250 units	1,000 units, optional
Calcium	500 mg.	2,000 mg., optional

Certainly, in America in the last decade, there has been a tendency toward the lessening of the meat intake, with a resulting theoretic possibility at least of considerable danger to the organism. The fear of meat is difficult to explain; perhaps it is the result of a rather widespread restriction of animal protein in the diet of people with high blood pressure. "Blood pressure" is a common complaint, made much of by physicians, insurance examiners, and the public in general; for years meat was taboo to such an illness. The aping mannerism of following one's neighbor perhaps caused Jones to follow Smith, and Brown to follow Jones, in lowering the meat intake. As a matter of fact, there has been some scientific work to prove that this tendency actually results in protein deprivation and a resulting condition that does not make for the best health.

When scientific pioneers, about twenty-five years ago, tried to show that meat in moderate doses was rarely harmful, even to a person with high blood pressure, they were not listened to. Today we no longer are fearful of meat, but are more fearful of the dangers of protein restriction. Two dangers of protein restriction are: protein edema and poorly balanced diet. It is a common observation of physicians that a person who is not permitted sufficient protein in his diet makes it up in either fat or carbohydrate. This may result in an unbalanced diet, of which more will be said later, or in an increase of weight which might not be advisable for that particular person. In people with high blood pressure, it is known that increase of weight is an undesirable burden, yet this extra trouble may immediately follow protein restriction. The intake of protein, from whatever source, may vary within wide limits, and healthy life can continue on an intake varying roughly from two ounces up to as high as five ounces of pure protein daily. The meat habits of a group are determined by the original habits of their ancestors, the environment in which they live, the quantity of meat in comparison to other foods, and other extraneous factors. The dangers of either over- or under-indulgence are grossly exaggerated.

Perhaps another important basic reason for the development of food fads and fancies lies in the well-established fact that certain people have idiosyncrasies or may be sensitive to certain foods. One of the best known physicians in the United States told this story of one of his early patients, a charming young lady who had been sick for many weeks and who had already had several medical advisers. As he walked into her room he was greeted with the question, "Doctor, would you mind if I asked you a question before you started on me?" He replied, "Of course not." Whereupon the young lady said, "Tell me confidentially what foods you dislike." When the doctor informed this patient that he had no particular dislikes for food, he naturally inquired the reason for her question. He was then told that each one of the previous doctors had restricted the particular article of diet which, as far as the young lady was concerned, disagreed with the particular doctor.

Physicians no longer prescribe diet on this basis, but the rocking-chair brigade of the hotel summer resorts and the ubiquitous lay medical adviser are only too apt to give free instruction to anyone who will listen. There is such a thing as food idiosyncrasy. There are individuals to whom bananas or strawberries or cabbage or any other perfectly normal food may act as a poison. This is not due to the food but is due to a state of "sensitization" of that particular individual to that particular food, and has nothing whatever to do with the construction of a normal diet for normal persons. It is not always known why a person becomes "sensitized"; the fact that he is compels him to avoid certain foods.

FOOD POISONING

At this point food poisoning can be discussed. There have been serious epidemics of food poisoning, usually due to some error in the transportation or handling of the food. This may occur in canning, in improper refrigerating, or in numerous ways, but when food poisoning occurs it affects everyone who eats this lot of food. Individual cases of poisoning by food are so extremely rare as to be negligible. In many communities mild epidemics of food poisoning occur, usually due to some carelessness in the handling of the product. Most of these epidemics are due to bacterial contamination of the food, and only rarely are the chemicals used for spraying trees responsible. The old diagnosis of "ptomaine poisoning" is no longer made, and from the standpoint of diagnosis the last thing to think of in the presence of a "bellyache" is the food. Most abdominal pains are caused by something wrong in the insides of the person. Rare instances of green-apple bellyache or similar insults to the stomach do occur, but it is fairly safe to assume that some organ of the body rather than the food is at fault.

EXTRANEOUS FACTORS IN DIET

To return to the fundamental considerations which must be borne in mind in the development of the normal diet, certain extraneous factors which lie beyond the field of actual digestion, assimilation, or scientific food values must be recognized. The three most important "outside" influences are the source of the food supply, heredity, and tradition. A study of dietary habits of a people living in the midst of plenty shows that such persons are apt to eat more of their local supply. For instance, in the tropics, where fresh fruits and vegetables are abundant and cheap, those foods form the major part of the dietary of the tropical races. On the other hand, in Alaska, where fat is the most available food, fresh fruit and vegetables are rarely, if ever, seen in the dietary, whereas, in the more temperate zones between the two extremes, where the source of food supply depends only on the rapidity of transportation, a more generalized diet will be found in common use. It is not difficult to bring California and Florida fruit and vegetables to the New York market in midwinter, but it would be difficult to carry them to Alaska. During the seasons when local truck farms and orchards are producing, local districts will be found to consume the products of the local markets. The use of foods frozen where grown is becoming increasingly popular, and the experience with them has been generally satisfactory. This method of handling food products retains the original appearance and flavor.

The ability to buy food is also important in establishing a normal diet. Even in the midst of plenty, availability of food has little interest for the man who cannot buy it. During periods of economic depression and general unemployment, insufficient funds interfere with the purchase of proper foods, and this naturally has a bad effect on nutrition.

Heredity and tradition cannot be discounted in the consideration of normal diet. The tradition of certain of the Italian localities to take their carbohydrate in the form of spaghetti and ravioli forms a contrast to the Slavic tradition of coarse rye bread. Yet both spaghetti and rye bread furnish an excellent source of cereal carbohydrate. The same is true, for instance, of certain of the Orientals in whose diet raw fish is a staple, whereas to the average Occidental such food is so distasteful as to be practically impossible of assimilation. Inconsistently, however, raw oysters and clams are well tolerated. In a population with as mixed an origin as the American people, it would be quite natural to anticipate such wide ranges in dietary construction. It would be obviously ridiculous to demand that the American citizen of German, Scandinavian, or Italian descent be compelled to consider a piece of white bread as the standard form of starch.

THE NEED FOR FOOD

The body needs food for two purposes: as fuel to supply energy, and to repair the waste of body tissues which goes on in the daily wear and tear of life. Considering the fuel aspect of food first, one starts with a discussion of the significance of the word "calorie." This word seems to be shrouded in mystery, yet there is no mystery attached to it. Calorie is simply the name given to the fuel value of anything that is burned up. Large establishments using a great deal of fuel do not buy coal by the ton but by the number of heat units or calories furnished per dollar. Food plays the same rôle in the human machinery as does coal in the furnace or gas in the motorcar. The first purpose of food is to furnish fuel; if this fuel in the form of food were not available to the body, the body would naturally immediately start to consume itself. Starvation is the result of the fires of human life burning human life itself. Therefore, in con-

FOOD VALUES
CALORIES

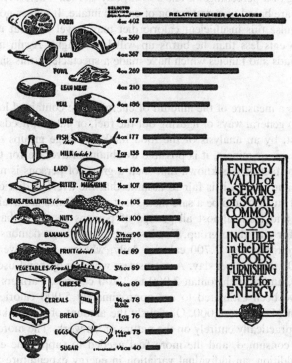

RELATIVE NUMBER of CALORIES

	SELECTED SERVING	
PORK	4 oz	402
BEEF	4 oz	369
LAMB	4 oz	367
FOWL	4 oz	269
LEAN MEAT	4 oz	210
VEAL	4 oz	186
LIVER	4 oz	177
FISH (fat)	4 oz	177
MILK (whole)	1 oz	138
LARD	½ oz	126
BUTTER, MARGARINE	½ oz	107
BEANS, PEAS, LENTILS (dried)	1 oz	103
NUTS	½ oz	100
BANANAS	3½ oz	96
FRUIT (dried)	1 oz	89
VEGETABLES (fresh)	3½ oz	89
CHEESE	½ oz	89
CEREALS	¼ oz	78
BREAD	1 oz	76
EGGS	1½ oz	73
SUGAR	½ oz	40

ENERGY VALUE of a SERVING of SOME COMMON FOODS INCLUDE in the DIET FOODS FURNISHING FUEL for ENERGY

Fig. 55. Calory chart.
(Courtesy of National Live Stock and Meat Board)

tructing a diet it is always essential that sufficient calories be given to maintain ody weight and to supply fuel for the energy consumed by the body.

Frequently the human body is compared to a machine. This analogy must ever be allowed to go too far, because the machine, built of noninflammable naterial, simply goes out of commission when the necessary fuel is withheld. he fundamental concept, however, of the use of food for fuel in the human ody is exactly the opposite. As soon as insufficient fuel is furnished in the orm of insufficient calories, the machine continues to work, using its own naterial as fuel, and if the procedure is allowed to continue too long, death evitably results. The main difference, then, between the human body and a nachine of metal is that the machine of metal is a thing apart from the sub-tance fed to it as fuel, whereas the human body is of the same substance as ie fuel, and therefore its life depends entirely on sufficient outside fuel being rnished to prevent its consuming itself.

The practical importance of this idea extends not only into the life of normal human beings, but is of particular importance in the life of overweight or obese persons. Loss of weight means loss of body tissue, and this in turn is equivalent to the burning of a percentage of one's own body as fuel. Therefore, all reduction methods are based on a restriction of caloric intake. It makes no difference under what guise this insufficient caloric diet may travel or what it contains, anybody who eats less than he burns up will lose weight. Again attention is called to the fads and fancies which have made a spectacle of this simple law.

CALORIES

A calorie is a measure of the amount of energy value contained in any food. There are two general ways of figuring out the fuel, or caloric, needs of any individual. First, by an analysis of the food intake of large groups of soldiers, schoolmistresses, or miners, it is possible to obtain an average for that group. As a matter of fact, if it is known that such a group of persons is maintaining life, activity, and health, it is fair to assume that the average diet obtained in this statistical study would be a safe diet. Plenty of statistics are available from all countries and from almost all groups of persons to give a basis for the average diet for any given group. For instance, it has been demonstrated that tailors use approximately 2,700 calories daily, whereas woodsawers may use 5,000 to 6,000 calories per day. A seamstress working by hand uses approximately 2,000, and a washwoman 2,900 to 3,700 calories. Farmers in various countries have been estimated to use approximately 5,000 calories, whereas lumbermen in Maine use 8,000. Obviously the amount of food taken by anyone depends practically entirely on the nature of his work. The more work, the more energy consumed, and the more fuel needed to supply the energy. But there is, in addition, an individual variation in energy expenditure which permits one person to do a certain amount of work while eating less food than his neighbor doing similar work. This is explained by individual differences in the function of the human body, and it explains in part why certain persons have difficulty controlling their weight. Second, the amount of fuel needed by the body can also be determined by a study of the individual needs. A person of certain general type of body, height, weight, age, and occupation is in general similar to another person with the same qualifications. Mere existence, which includes the act of breathing, the beating of the heart, the involuntary movements of the body—activities which continue even during sleep—consume energy. All interchanges of energy are grouped under the general name of metabolism. And the energy of mere existence is called basal metabolism.

Today basal metabolism can be estimated for any person by means of a simple breathing machine. In this machine the patient is allowed to breathe oxygen for a certain length of time. The amount utilized is carefully measured, and on the basis of some comparatively simple calculations the rate of energy consumed by this individual can be estimated. This is all that is meant by basal metabolism, and it is comparatively easy to find out just how much any person of a given age, height, and weight will need to sustain mere existence. Many

Height (inches)	5	6	7	8	9	10	11	12	13	14	15	16	17	18	19
							Years								
38	34	34													
39	35	35													
40	36	36													
41	38	38	38												
42	39	39	39	39											
43	41	41	41	41											
44	44	44	44	44											
45	46	46	46	46	46										
46	47	48	48	48	48										
47	49	50	50	50	50	50									
48	----	52	53	53	53	53									
49	----	55	55	55	55	55	55								
50	----	57	58	58	58	58	58	58							
51	----	----	61	61	61	61	61	61							
52	----	----	63	64	64	64	64	64	64						
53	----	----	66	67	67	67	67	68	68						
54	----	----	----	70	70	70	70	71	71	72					
55	----	----	----	72	72	73	73	74	74	74					
56	----	----	----	75	76	77	77	77	78	78	80				
57	----	----	----	----	79	80	81	81	82	83	83				
58	----	----	----	----	83	84	84	85	85	86	87				
59	----	----	----	----	----	87	88	89	89	90	90	90			
60	----	----	----	----	----	91	92	92	93	94	95	96			
61	----	----	----	----	----	----	95	96	97	99	100	103	106		
62	----	----	----	----	----	----	100	101	102	103	104	107	111	116	
63	----	----	----	----	----	----	105	106	107	108	110	113	118	123	127
64	----	----	----	----	----	----	----	109	111	113	115	117	121	126	130
65	----	----	----	----	----	----	----	114	117	118	120	122	127	131	134
66	----	----	----	----	----	----	----	----	119	122	125	128	132	136	139
67	----	----	----	----	----	----	----	----	124	128	130	134	136	139	142
68	----	----	----	----	----	----	----	----	----	134	134	137	141	143	147
69	----	----	----	----	----	----	----	----	----	137	139	143	146	149	152
70	----	----	----	----	----	----	----	----	----	143	144	145	148	151	155
71	----	----	----	----	----	----	----	----	----	148	150	151	152	154	159
72	----	----	----	----	----	----	----	----	----	----	153	155	156	158	163
73	----	----	----	----	----	----	----	----	----	----	157	160	162	164	167
74	----	----	----	----	----	----	----	----	----	----	160	164	168	170	171

Fig. 56. Height and weight at various ages.

thousands of control experiments of the nature of the one just outlined have given standards of comparison. The results are expressed in terms of either plus or minus variations from the standard. In other words, if the report reads "basal metabolism, plus 15 per cent," it means simply that that individual is consuming 15 per cent more energy than the normal.

It is further known that every activity of the body, whether it is walking, talking, eating, playing golf, or mining coal, increases the amount of energy consumed by the body. Therefore, having found the basal requirements of an individual, the doctor can, by the addition of the demands of the individual's other activities, compute what his total needs for the day will be.

CLASSIFICATION OF FOODS

However, in addition to the fuel value of food there are certain other demands that food must fill. The need to repair body waste is one of the most important; there must be a sufficient supply of mineral salts and vitamins and water. Protein supplies the material to replace tissue waste and, to a certain extent, energy. The main source of energy, however, is in the fats and carbohydrates of the diet, since fats provide double the calories of proteins.

The main food elements are grouped under several big headings: protein, fat, carbohydrate, water, mineral salts, and the so-called accessory food factors, vitamins. Usually food as it is eaten is composed of a mixture of these main food elements, frequently with one predominating. A study of food analyses will show, for instance, that beef or the meat of any animal, including fish and poultry, consists mainly of protein with a varying amount of fat. Protein is the one element of food that contains nitrogen, and for that reason is the only food that can replace tissue lost in the body. Many foods contain small amounts of protein, but not in the proportions available in animal matter. Proteins are chemically complex substances made up of a number of so-called amino acids. The nature of a specific protein depends on the kinds and amount of amino acids and the manner in which they are combined. For this reason not all proteins have the same nutritional value. Some of the basic components (amino acids) are necessary for metabolism and are not supplied by all of the proteins. The most common and important proteins and their sources are: albumin from egg, the protein of wheat and corn, the protein of milk, of meat, and the glandular organs. Some cereals, vegetables, and nuts also contain available and utilizable protein.

The carbohydrates are the starch or sugar parts of food; they are indispensable for rapid use as fuel. They are found in fruits, vegetables, cereals, and milk. Ordinary sugar is the most concentrated type of carbohydrate available. Sugar is found in pure form in fruits and to a lesser extent in some of the vegetables. Starch is a higher combination of sugars and furnishes the main ingredient of the various cereals. Bread contains a large amount of starch. From the standpoint of actual utilization of sugar, it makes no difference whether the carbohydrate is obtained in the form of starch or of the simpler sugars. The simpler sugars are absorbed as such or after slight chemical change, whereas starch needs a longer process of digestion to make it available. This is of importance particularly in the treatment of diabetes mellitus. Vendors of certain artificial food products advertise them as being free from sugar, which is partially true;

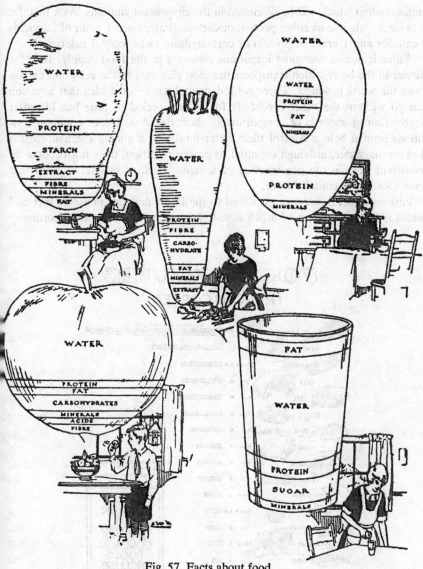

Fig. 57. Facts about food.

ut when such articles of food contain liberal amounts of starch, they must be
lassed in the same category as straight sugars.

Fats, of course, are known as such: meat fats, oils, and butter fat being the
ost obvious members of this family. They are found both in animal and plant
fe, and whatever their derivation are potentially equal energy producers. The
ame amount of fuel value is attached to an ounce of butter, olive oil, cotton-
ed oil, or oil derived from maize. There is, however, a difference in their vi-

tamin content which will be discussed in the chapter on vitamins. As a fuel, fat is twice as valuable as either protein or carbohydrate, since 1 gram of fat yields 9 calories and 1 gram of protein or carbohydrate yields only 4 calories.

Water is one of the most important elements in the food supply. It is the carrier in the body which transports the food elements to the cells and carries away the waste products. There is fundamental truth in the idea that a person can go without the other foodstuffs for a long period of time but life after deprivation of water is of comparatively short duration. Under common conditions human beings control their water intake by a simple mechanism; for that reason water, although essential to proper nutrition, does not become an important item in the construction of a menu. It is, of course, recalled that most solid foods contain water.

Various mineral salts are also vital to the body, and this phase of diet and health is still the subject of much investigation. The common use of ordinary

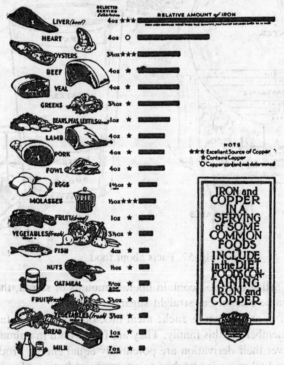

Fig. 58. Iron and copper chart.
(Courtesy of National Live Stock and Meat Board)

table salt is a direct result of the need of man for this material. Other elements, however, are just as vital, and among the most important are iron, calcium, iodine, and phosphorus. A carefully balanced dietary regime concerns itself with the salt content of foods which, as might be anticipated, varies greatly.

In certain districts of this country, notably the areas around the Great Lakes, a definite deficiency of iodine in the diet and water supply has been demonstrated. In these districts a rather large number of children develop enlargement of the thyroid gland (goiter). This deficiency has been met by the addition of iodine to table salt.

ELECTROLYTES AND THE ACID-BASE RATIO

"Electrolytes" is the name given to a group of inorganic chemical substances which keep the body from becoming too strongly acid or alkaline. A normal diet contains electrolytes such as sodium chloride (table salt), potassium, phosphate, bicarbonate, and others. The body also manufactures some electrolytes by chemical breakdown of foods. In the past emphasis was placed on the total effect of all electrolytes on the body, and the diet was calculated in terms of acid or alkaline residue. As our knowledge of the rôle played by each of these substances has unfolded, we no longer think in terms of the total effect, but rather in terms of the need of each individual electrolyte.

Salt (sodium chloride) is the most widespread and most important of all electrolytes. A normal person can eat much or little salt without harm. Heat prostration results from excess loss of salt through perspiration, so that persons working in extreme heat need extra salt. In certain diseases of the heart and kidney, especially, salt is frequently retained in the body with water so that a condition generally known as "dropsy" results. In another disease—failure of the adrenal glands—extra dietary salt is a necessary part of treatment. Potassium, like sodium, may be harmful in excess in certain conditions, or may be needed in extra amounts in certain other diseases such as in diabetic coma or diarrhea in infants. In certain kidney conditions such as stones or infections, the acidity of the urine may be changed by diet or medicine, but this change has little effect upon the body as a whole.

Ulcers of the stomach usually are associated with an increased amount of stomach acid, and treatment is approached from the viewpoint of neutralizing this acid by foods or medicines. Foods will themselves absorb some of the stomach acid while at the same time they increase the formation of acid. Certain alkaline drugs are effective by combining and neutralizing the stomach acid. Some of these chemicals are themselves electrolytes.

Body alkalinity is quite different from stomach acidity. The layman frequently confuses these two states. The fruit juices, which when they enter the stomach are acid, are usually poor food for a person who has already too much acid in his stomach, but such stomach acidity may have nothing whatever to do with the general body reaction. The fruit juices, acid in the stomach, become valuable alkali when they reach the blood stream and the tissues.

In health, true acidosis does not occur. But the body mechanisms maintaining chemical balance are so accurate that the frequently expressed fear of acidity is practically never justified. A normal well-balanced diet will take care of this problem without any special attention.

VITAMINS

From a nutritional point of view, the first fifty years of this century may well be labeled, "The Age of the Vitamin." The name was coined in 1913, but before then it was known that certain so-called accessory food factors were nec-

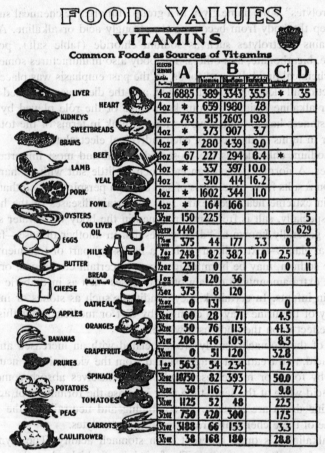

FOOD VALUES
VITAMINS
Common Foods as Sources of Vitamins

	SELECTED SERVINGS (Edible Portion)	A	B			C†	D
LIVER	4oz	6885	389	3343	35.5	*	35
HEART	4oz	*	659	1980	7.8		
KIDNEYS	4oz	743	515	2603	19.8		
SWEETBREADS	4oz	*	373	907	3.7		
BRAINS	4oz	*	280	439	9.0		
BEEF	4oz	67	227	294	8.4	*	
LAMB	4oz	*	337	397	10.0		
VEAL	4oz	*	310	414	16.2		
PORK	4oz	*	1602	344	11.0		
FOWL	4oz	*	164	166			
OYSTERS	3½oz	150	225				5
COD LIVER OIL	½oz	4440				0	629
EGGS	1¾oz	375	44	177	3.3	0	8
MILK	7oz	248	82	382	1.0	2.5	4
BUTTER	½oz	231	0			0	11
BREAD (Whole Wheat)	1oz	*	120	36			
CHEESE	7/8oz	375	8	120			
OATMEAL	½oz	0	131			0	
APPLES	3½oz	60	28	71		4.5	
ORANGES	3½oz	50	76	113		41.3	
BANANAS	3½oz	206	46	105		8.5	
GRAPEFRUIT	3½oz	0	51	120		32.8	
PRUNES	1oz	563	54	234		1.2	
SPINACH	3½oz	18750	82	393		50.0	
POTATOES	3½oz	30	116	72		9.8	
TOMATOES	3½oz	1125	52	48		22.5	
PEAS	3½oz	750	420	300		17.5	
CARROTS	3½oz	3188	66	153		3.3	
CAULIFLOWER	3½oz	38	168	180		28.8	

* Not determined but present in small amounts.　† A portion of the vitamin C is destroyed in cooking.
§ Evaporated milk diluted with an equal amount of water has the same value as pasteurized milk.
(1) Thiamin: 1 microgram — ⅓ International Unit
(2) Riboflavin: 1 microgram — ⅓ Sherman-Bourquin Unit
(3) Ascorbic Acid: 1 milligram — 20 International Units

Fig. 59. Vitamin chart.
(Courtesy of National Live Stock and Meat Board)

essary for proper growth and development. In the eighteenth century, a dietary experiment was performed by one William Stark, a friend of Benjamin Franklin, who killed himself in an effort to prove the value of a so-called "simple" diet of bread, water, and olive oil. In the sixteenth century, the value of lemon juice as a curative for scurvy among seamen was discovered by the Dutch, and at the end of the eighteenth century the introduction of citrus fruits and vegetables in the British Navy's food rations led to the disappearance of this disease among British sailors.

The original experiments on the need of these accessory food factors were done on animals, experiments similar to the one William Stark performed on himself. After animal experiments proved the necessity of these substances for the animal diet, the research was extended to human beings, and physicians proved that certain human diseases resulted from a deficit of certain vitamins. Probably today the best known and most thoroughly understood vitamins are vitamin A and carotene, vitamin D, vitamin K, vitamin C, the various ingredients of the B complex and vitamin B_{12}.

The recognition of clear-cut cases of vitamin deficiency is a comparatively easy procedure. The real trouble lies in minor instances of such deficiency. Vitamins are used much too frequently on self-prescription or advice of the druggist, a procedure certainly not entirely harmless. In the first place, a false sense of well-being may arise and obscure serious, masked illness, and, second, excessive use of some vitamins may be harmful. The extent of this abuse of a good thing may be illustrated by the fact that in 1950 over $200,000,000 worth of vitamins were sold at retail over counters. This figure does not include vitamins and vitamin concentrates sold to manufacturers for products eventually marketed to the consumer as enriched foods or feeds.

There is a definite field for the use of vitamins when a deficiency is proved. There is absolutely no physiological difference between natural vitamins in foods and those sold over the counter. If a normal diet is taken, such as outlined by the Food and Nutrition Board, National Research Council, 1950, extra vitamins rarely will be necessary.

Milk	1 pint
Eggs	1
Meat, fish, poultry, or cheese	1 or more servings
Fruits	2 servings, one citrus or tomato
Vegetables	2 servings, green or yellow
Potato	1 serving
Cereal and bread (whole grain or enriched)	4 servings
Cream	2 ounces
Butter	1 ounce
Dessert	1 serving

The size of the servings is somewhat arbitrary, and other foods may be added if needed to complete the meals. It is our belief that if you have no other disease and if you eat according to this table, you probably will not need those extra tailor-made vitamins.

DIGESTION, ASSIMILATION, ABSORPTION

In order to understand how the body uses food for its own purpose, one must have a basic knowledge of the processes of digestion, assimilation, and absorption of the material eaten. Before such a complex substance as a piece of meat or such a comparatively simple one as a glass of milk can be utilized by the body, profound chemical changes are initiated. These changes start as soon as food passes the lips. The mouth actually "waters" when food is brought near, and this watering process is due to the secretion of juices by the digestive glands surrounding the throat. These juices perform two functions; first, to moisten the food, and, second, to take part in the breaking down of some of the starches.

The teeth are a definite part of the digestive system. Proper chewing of the food, which is constantly being moistened by the salivary juices, means a better preparation of such food for the work of the stomach and intestines. These two initial procedures in the use of food are frequently considerably underemphasized. Food then passes into the stomach, where digestion and mixing continue further. The stomach digestion is not extensive, being limited in the main to a partial attack on protein by the pepsin of the stomach and to the coagulation of milk. Yet stomach digestion is an important second step, in some respects the most important. It is the stomach which responds most to stimulations from outside the body. Appetites may be made or broken by the smell of food that is distasteful. Hunger pains can be stimulated in the stomach by the sight or smell as well as taste of the food.

From the stomach, food is passed on into the intestines, where more ferments, especially those from the pancreas, continue digestion. The intestines also have the function of continuing the forward movement of the food. During the passage of foodstuffs through the intestines chemical processes have changed them into a condition in which they are now suitable to be absorbed into the body. Absorption of these simplified end products of digestion into the lymph and blood streams is followed by a rebuilding process in the body. This rebuilding process involves the construction of new units which can be assimilated as part of the body or can be burned as fuel by the body. What is left of the food passes along the intestinal canal, and the unusable remnant, in addition to a certain amount of secretions of the large intestine, forms the feces, or material that is excreted.

PREPARATION

Frequently the food question is approached too scientifically. The same group of protein, fat, carbohydrate, mineral salts, vitamins, and calorie units may be assembled into a meal which when presented to a normal or particularly a sick person becomes almost useless. If the meat is burned, the eggs are stale, the vegetables are tasteless, or the tray dirty, few people care to eat. It is not only the appeal to the taste and sense of nicety that concerns us in the preparation of food; there is also a sound physiologic principle involved. The digestion and assimilation of food substances depend to a large extent on the so-called psychologic effect.

THE DINNER TABLE

Not only are the preparation and serving of food important factors in consideration of proper diet, but the whole atmosphere of the dinner table may make the difference between a well absorbed, well utilized meal, and one which causes distress and perhaps even illness. Many patients with "upset stomachs" do not recognize that the source of their trouble is actually some irritation while they are eating, such as a fretful child, the college student son returned from vacation with a bad report of his year, or even less significant episodes like a constant hacking cough. The meal should be a place for friendly greeting, pleasant conversation and complete relaxation.

We have been in the habit of eating three meals a day, assuming that this is the best procedure. It is probably true, however, that a more even distribution of food throughout the working day would result in increased efficiency and a greater sense of well-being. In fact, some work has been done to prove this. It is well known, for instance, that golf players can maintain a better average playing ability if they take a certain amount of sugar or candy during the game, and it is also known that soldiers on the march usually carry some concentrated food. It certainly is advisable not to undertake physical activity for too long a period on an empty stomach.

BUILDING THE DIET

In considering the need of the body for food, the most important factor involved is the one already mentioned: namely, the need of fuel to supply energy. Without a sufficient supply of fuel the body will burn itself up; therefore, the amount of food consumed by the body must at least furnish enough energy to equalize the amount spent by the body. In addition, however, there is always a certain amount of wear and tear on the body tissues which must be replaced by food. This wear and tear can only be made up by protein, and therefore every normal diet must contain sufficient protein to equalize the amount lost in the daily body activity. When sufficient calories are furnished in the diet, no matter by what kind of food, wear and tear is considerably diminished, but when the total amount of calories furnished is insufficient, there is increased destruction of body tissue.

The adult human body is pretty well stabilized, but the growing body of childhood or adolescence represents a constantly increasing demand to keep pace with growth. In feeding children, therefore, the amount of protection that is required to prevent loss of body tissue is greater than it is in adult life. It is an accepted principle of infant and child feeding to use comparatively large amounts of protein in the normal diet. In adult life, however, provided sufficient total food is given, there is apparently a wide variation possible in the protein intake. Work done in America on the explorers Stefansson and Anderson indicates that high protein-fat mixtures, to which these explorers were accustomed in their sojourn in the Arctic regions, when continued under experimental conditions in America did no demonstrable damage to the organism.

During and following both World Wars a clinical disease picture became evident which probably resulted from insufficient protein—the so-called protein edema or watery swelling of the tissues. Whenever insufficient protein was available to meet basic needs, otherwise normal human beings developed an anemia and edema or dropsy which disappeared subsequently when an adequate diet became available. This was the first striking mass illustration of the dangers of too little protein and called attention to the probability that too little protein might be more dangerous than too much. In general, if a mathematical protein requirement has to be fixed, it is perfectly safe to say that a minimum of from 0.6 gram to 1.5 grams of protein per kilogram or two pounds of body weight should be sufficient protection against either under- or overindulgence in this necessary article of diet.

VARIETIES OF MEAT IN THE DIET

A cursory study of any food tables will indicate that a large supply of protein is found in animal products, dairy products, and vegetables. The protein from all meats, including fish and fowl, is essentially the same. There is certainly no difference between the red meat of steer and the red meat of lamb. Experimental evidence suggests that in certain kidney diseases animal protein in excess is not handled by the body as well as non-animal protein. But poorly informed people go beyond this. Individuals who think they are eating too much meat stop at beef and take lamb, fish, chicken, or even eggs. There can be no more absurd contradiction in fundamental ideas than this all too common practice. There is one slight difference between red meats and white meats, and that is in the so-called extractives found in the uncooked red meat.

An effort to explain the widespread belief in the essential difference in meats leads nowhere to a scientific basis. This idea represents one of the erroneous unfounded traditions current in much thinking on diets.

Another source of protein is the organs of animals. These differ from muscle protein in their chemical structure, but in the normal diet they can replace other perhaps more expensive portions of the animal. In certain diseases the doctor will advise against the use of these organs because of the difference in their chemical structure. Since the use of liver in the treatment of anemia and of pancreatic extract or insulin for diabetes, the price of these two organs has risen so as to make them no longer economical articles of food. There remain, however, heart, spleen, brain, and kidneys as easily available portions of the animal.

In neighborhoods where fresh fish is abundant and cheap it frequently replaces other forms of animal protein in the normal diet. It has exactly the same value qualitatively and practically the same quantitively, and therefore can well replace meats which have to be brought from other districts. The same thing, of course, is true of farm lands where poultry is easily accessible. In such neighborhoods poultry will form a cheaper protein than would be obtained from other kinds of animal life. Like fish, it has the same value as has beef protein.

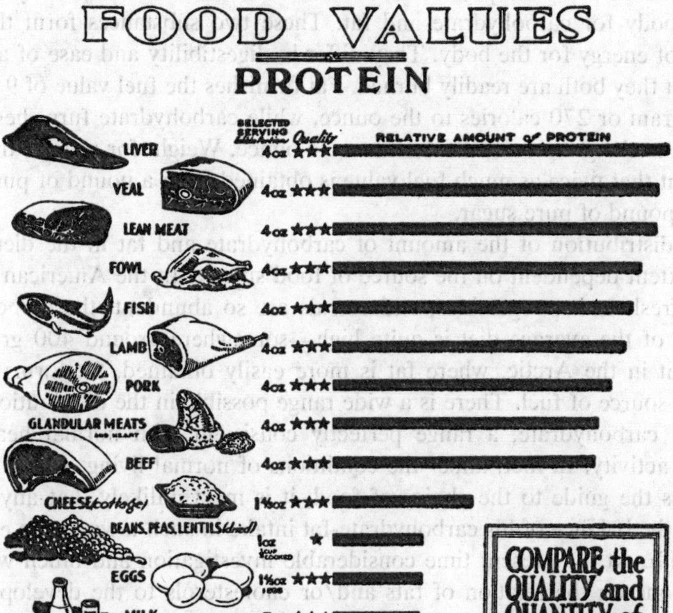

Fig. 60. Protein chart.
(Courtesy of National Live Stock and Meat Board)

Eggs, consisting as they do of protein and fat, can likewise replace meat in the dietary. The white of the egg is almost pure protein, and the yolk is almost pure fat. Two eggs will contain approximately the same amount of protein and fat as will a piece of round steak 3 inches by 3¼ by ¾ inch, and can be substituted in that way. The high fat content of egg yolk makes it not an exact substitute for meat products in the normal diet and in certain diseases.

CARBOHYDRATE AND FAT

There are other sources of protein available for the body, particularly in some of the dairy products, cereals, and vegetables. Therefore, before continuing on the protein aspect of these foods, it is wise to review briefly the need of the body for carbohydrate and fat. These two substances form the great source of energy for the body. They differ in digestibility and ease of assimilation, but they both are readily burned. Fat furnishes the fuel value of 9 calories to the gram or 270 calories to the ounce, while carbohydrate furnishes only 4 calories to the gram or 120 calories to the ounce. Weight for weight, then, it is apparent that twice as much fuel value is obtained from a pound of pure fat as from a pound of pure sugar.

The distribution of the amount of carbohydrate and fat in the diet is to a great extent dependent on the source of food supply. In the American dietary, where fresh fruits, vegetables, and cereals are so abundant, the carbohydrate content of the average diet is quite high—somewhere around 400 grams per day. But in the Arctic, where fat is more easily obtained, fat forms the important source of fuel. There is a wide range possible in the distribution of the fat and carbohydrate, a range perfectly consistent with normal health and normal activity. In fact, under the conditions of normal living, where appetite becomes the guide to the choice of food, it is most unlikely that anyone will change the balance of his carbohydrate-fat intake in such a way as to endanger his health. At the present time considerable investigation and much writing is being done on the relation of fats and/or cholesterols to the development of diseases of the arteries. Right now the subject is too confused to permit any dogmatic statement.

In analyzing the average food supply, one notes that the source of fat in the American dietary is to a great extent from butter, cream, eggs, meat, olive oil, vegetable oil, and nuts. Carbohydrates are derived to a large extent from sweets of all kinds. Far-reaching changes have occurred in the American dietary as a result of our varying consumption of sugar. About 100 years ago our annual consumption of sugar was not more than 10 pounds per person. Since the Civil War, and especially from 1910 until wartime sugar rationing, this increased progressively so that our prewar consumption of sugar was over 100 pounds per person each year. During World War II it diminished to 78 pounds. Now that sugar rationing has been discontinued, the expected increase in sugar consumption has resulted.

MILK

Milk, which is such a stable article of diet for the growing child, is not used as extensively in the dietary of the American adult as it should be. Milk is a natural food, and it occupies the unique position of being almost a complete food. It contains protein, fat, carbohydrate, salts, some vitamins (depending upon whether the milk is whole, pasteurized, or skimmed), and serves in the ordinary dietary, both of the child and the adult, as the most constant source of calcium. In children calcium is necessary for the healthy development of normal bones and teeth, and in adult life for the preservation of the teeth and in the regulation of the nervous system. The milk proteins supply all the amino acids necessary, and milk may replace meat in the diet. Carbohydrate is present in the form of lactose or milk sugar, which is easily assimilable. *Cream* differs from milk only in that it contains a markedly increased amount of fat and a

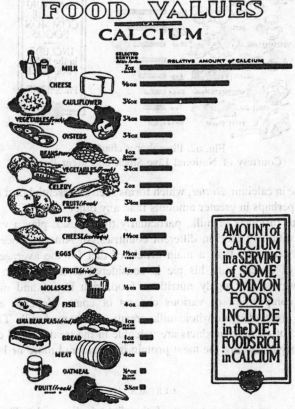

Fig. 61. Calcium chart.
(Courtesy of National Live Stock and Meat Board)

FOOD VALUES
PHOSPHORUS

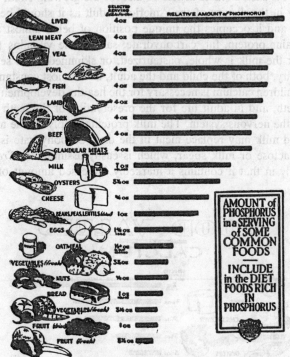

Fig. 62. Phosphorus chart.
(Courtesy of National Live Stock and Meat Board)

slight increase in calcium. *Butter,* which forms such an essential part of the diet, is consumed perhaps in greater amounts than any other fat.

The various products of milk, particularly the *cheeses,* play a varying rôle in the composition of food in different countries. In America cheese is more apt to be an accessory than a main article of diet for the average citizen; a small block of cheese with his pie is considered to add zest to the meal. Cheeses, however, are highly nutritious food, rich in fat and mineral elements. The composition of various cheeses of course depends entirely on whether they are made from whole milk, cream, or skimmed milk. The proteins of cheese and of all milk products are valuable in the treatment of certain diseases, such as gout, where the meat protein is considered more or less toxic to the system.

CEREALS

Cereals form an important part of the diet of all people. The old time-honored use of the word "bread" as a synonym for all food is eloquent testimony to the extremely important rôle that bread plays in life. As a matter of fact, the bulk of the world's supply of food is furnished by the cereal grains. As a class, they are rich in carbohydrate and protein. They are comparatively easily grown and transported, and in comparison with other foods are economical. Before the milling process, most of the cereal grains contained both mineral salts and vitamins. This makes no difference whether the grain is wheat, rye, barley, oats, or rice. There are minor differences in the composition of these various grains, but from the broad standpoint of their use as sources of food they are practically equal. They contain a very high carbohydrate, varying usually around 75 per cent and protein varying from 7 to 15 per cent. The fat content is relatively small. However, when one stops to consider that bread is almost always eaten with butter, when butter is available, and the cereals as such are supplemented by milk or cream, the deficiency in fat is soon made up.

The protein of cereals is not considered as complete a protein as is that of milk or meat, because it does not contain all of the necessary amino acids. There is considerable variation in the quality of proteins found in the various grains. Usually each cereal grain contains some but not all of the necessary amino acids. Of the vitamins, B is contained in abundance in the whole grain, but it is almost entirely removed in the process of milling. A is present only in small amounts. The mineral salts are not present in the cereal grains to a great enough extent to be of real value in the diet. There is present, however, cellulose, which, while without food value, has a rôle in digestion in that it produces peristalsis and assists in the evacuation of the bowels.

Of recent years various processes have been developed for the commercial production of oils from grains. These oils are having a wide use because they are cheaper than butter and olive oil, which formerly were used almost exclusively. Oils are also being made from vegetables. Except for the difference in vitamins, there is no essential difference between the newly developed vegetable and cereal oils and butter. They are practically identical in fuel value and may be used interchangeably if supplemented by vitamin-containing foods, such as fresh fruits, vegetables, and milk.

From what has already been said regarding their essential similarity, it must be evident that there is no necessity for standardizing the kind of cereal grains that form the basis of diet. As a matter of fact, history and current international practice clearly demonstrate the equal efficiency of American white bread, German rye bread, Russian black bread, Italian spaghetti, and Oriental rice.

SUGARS

The common table sugar is cane sugar or sucrose. This may be derived from most fruits, from the sugar cane, the sugar beet, or from various other sources. By the time sugar is refined, there should be no practical difference in its composition or its value as food. Milk sugar is somewhat different, but from the standpoint of the body use, is practically identical. The simpler sugar known as grape sugar or glucose is usually commercially derived from corn syrup. It has practically the same value as has cane sugar, since cane sugar is split by the body into glucose before it is absorbed.

Other forms of sugar are molasses, which contains cane sugar, maple syrup, and honey. From a standpoint of body chemistry, these are equally valuable.

Sugar is the most easily burned form of fuel. It is burned up more quickly than fat, and for that reason it is sometimes known as a stimulant. Tired athletes or weary soldiers frequently go out of their way to obtain candy. This is physiologically sound because exercise results in the quick burning up of the sugar available in the body, and the need for replacement is made evident by fatigue.

The carbohydrate of the cereal grains, which has already been discussed, is, however, in a more complicated chemical structure, which requires considerable treatment by the body before it can be utilized. Such digestion by the body requires a longer time to make starches and higher carbohydrates ready for absorption. This is the only essential difference between such higher carbohydrates and plain sugar. Potentially a cereal contains 75 per cent carbohydrate, exactly equivalent to an equal amount of 75 per cent sugar solution. This fact is of particular importance in dealing with the disease diabetes. In this disease the gullible patient reads that a certain patent food product contains no sugar—and gets into all kinds of trouble because of the high content of starch.

FRUITS

Among the common sources of carbohydrate are fruits and vegetables. The fruits are practically a mixture of water, sugar, certain of the vitamins, minerals, and indigestible residue. From a practical point of view, they are fat free and protein free. Their main use in the dietary is in the supply of vitamins A, B, and C. As late as 1885 the disease scurvy was a common threat of long sea voyages, when the diet was lacking in all fruits. There is no more striking episode in the history of food than the discovery by Takaki that the addition of orange and lemon juice to the diet prevented the appearance of this disease. Fruits are also mild laxatives. Nowadays the stabilization of the fruit industry is such that fresh fruits are available almost throughout the year, and the process of canning and freezing has reached such perfection that there is no excuse for any diet at any time to be without fruit of some sort.

VEGETABLES

The vegetables have the same value as the fruits in their supply of vitamins and cellulose. In addition, most of them have an important mineral content, and many are much higher in food value than the fruits. The leafy vegetables, such as spinach, lettuce, cabbage, are not important as sources of energy or of protein; but some of the seed vegetables, such as beans and peas, are valuable for their protein and carbohydrate. Some of them contain a small amount of fat. Potatoes are in a class by themselves, containing mainly water and about 20 per cent carbohydrate, as well as a negligible amount of protein and a valuable ash. Potato peel contains a large amount of cellulose, which is helpful to peristalsis. The main value of potato, particularly the white potato, is that it furnishes an abundance of carbohydrate and mineral salts at a low cost. Most of the other vegetables fall somewhere between the descriptions of the leafy vegetables and the seed vegetables, and their actual composition can be seen in any food table.

NUTS

Nuts vary a great deal in their food content and as a rule are rich in protein and fat and poor in carbohydrate. In the American dietary they are used mainly as additional portions of the diet.

FATS

In the discussions of the various foodstuffs mention has been made of their fat content. The rôle that fat plays in the body is that of fuel and a carrier of many important vitamins. As fuel, it is the most concentrated food we have, its caloric value being twice that of an equal portion of carbohydrate or protein. Probably the most important fats are butter, butter substitutes, cream, meat fats, and the oil of some of the vegetables and cereal grains. In addition to supplying available fuel, the concentrated nature of this food makes it one of the best articles of diet for building up undernourished individuals and for preventing loss of weight. It must be emphasized that, although the fuel value of all fats is practically identical, their complete availability as food depends to a great extent on their vitamin content, which varies greatly in the different fats.

CONDIMENTS AND SEASONING

Some other less important elements go to make up the normal diet. Seasoning is a necessity if food is to be palatable. Table salt, which is the commonest article used for seasoning, is necessary for complete living, yet can be harmful when taken to excess in the presence of certain forms of heart disease. Some of the other condiments, such as vinegar and spices, have no particular value except as stimulants to the appetite. The various caffeine and theobromine drinks such as coffee, tea, cocoa, and chocolate are stimulants, which in the case of tea and coffee are without food value. Cocoa has slight food value, but since it is usually made up as a milk drink, it forms a very nourishing and substantial article of diet. None of these beverages is necessary. In many instances they add to the zest and joy of living, and for the average healthy individual are certainly without danger when taken in moderate amounts. Taken to excess, it is possible that the amount of stimulant may have a deleterious effect.

ALCOHOL

As a food, alcohol has a caloric value of 7 to the gram, is easily oxidized, and therefore is a valuable food. It is not easy to evaluate all the studies on alcohol into material permitting dogmatic statements. However, it can be said that alcohol in moderate amounts ordinarily does no harm. The word moderate, however, is a relative term, and moderation for one person may mean excess for another. Certainly, excess of alcohol, like excess in any article of food, should be avoided. There is a difference between the danger from excess of alcohol and that from other food products in the fact that alcohol, in addition to being a food, has a definite poisoning influence when taken in too large amounts. Another disadvantage of excess of alcohol lies in the fact that the person who overdrinks will avoid other more nutritious and necessary foods.

THE NORMAL DIET

The normal diet described on p. 781 will form a basis of good living and will take care of the body needs. The necessary basic considerations of normal diet are few and simple. First, there must be enough fuel to supply the energy expended by the body. This fuel is furnished by the three major elements, protein, fat, and carbohydrate, but more efficiently by the fat and carbohydrate. Second, sufficient protein must be supplied to replace tissue waste. Third, water, mineral salts, and vitamins come in as of major importance qualitatively, but of minor importance quantitatively. The proportions of the different foods may vary within comparatively wide limits, yet an excess of a single food factor may produce deficiency of some other food which it replaces. In other words, balancing of all the elements in a diet is important. The amount of protein needed is an inconstant factor. The carbohydrate and fat may be distributed according to the source of supply and their availability. The necessary vitamins and usually the mineral salts are furnished by milk, fresh vegetables, fresh fruits, butter, and cereals.

A steadily rising wave of advertising propaganda in books, magazines, and over the radio and television has resulted in a one-sided attention to the vitamins. Also it is a fact that almost all dietary advances in the past ten years have been associated with the isolation and study of these most important accessory food factors. However, they are not the only essentials of a good diet, and any general discussion of human nutrition must include the consideration of other equally important dietary factors. The aim of all scientific food research is to determine the diet for the individual that will create and maintain the highest degree of health. It is true that the majority of the people of the past survived in spite of their ignorance of all the facts of modern dietary science; but it must be added that their survival was dependent upon the selection by the trial-and-error method of those foods which today modern scientific investigation has definitely established as the constituents of the normal diet. This so-called normal diet is a very simple one, consisting of a palatable mixture of common foodstuffs. On p. 781 will be found the Normal Diet outlined by the Food and Nutrition Board, National Research Council, in 1950.

There are many combinations of food which meet these new requirements. America is fortunate today that it has a large number of trained nutritionists who can translate these allowances into terms of foods available and practical in many parts of the country.

The table below shows that a moderately active man should have 3,000 calories of food per day; a very active man, 4,500 calories per day, and a man who leads a sedentary life should have 2,500 calories a day. A woman, because of her lesser weight, takes 2,500 calories a day, if she is moderately active; 3,000 calories if she is very active, and 2,100 calories if she leads a sedentary life. The woman who is nursing a baby needs as many calories a day as the woman who is very active—3,000 calories a day.

RECOMMENDED DAILY ALLOWANCES FOR SPECIFIC NUTRIENTS
(Committee on Food and Nutrition, National Research Council)

	Calories	Protein, Gm.	Calcium, Gm.	Iron, Mg.	A.* International Units	Thiamine (B¹),† Mg.	Ascorbic Acid (C),† Mg.	Riboflavin, Mg.	Nicotinic Acid, Mg.	D. International Units
Man (70 Kg.)										
Moderately active	3,000	70	0.8	12	5,000	1.8	75	2.7	18	
Very active	4,500	..	...	..	....	2.3	..	3.3	23	•
Sedentary	2,500	..	...	..	....	1.5	..	2.5	15	
Woman (56 Kg.)										
Moderately active	2,500	60	0.8	12	5,000	1.5	70	2.2	15	
Very active	3,000	..	...	..	....	1.8	..	2.7	18	•
Sedentary	2,100	..	...	..	....	1.3	..	1.8	13	
Pregnancy (latter half)..	2,500	85	1.5	15	6,000	1.8	100	2.3	18	400-800
Lactation	3,000	100	2.0	..	8,000	2.3	150	3.0	23	400-800
Children up to 12 years										
Under 1 year ‡	100 per Kg.	3-4 per Kg.	1.0	6	1,500	0.4	30	0.6	4	400-800
1- 3 years	1,200	40	1.0	7	2,000	0.6	35	0.9	6	
4- 6 years	1,600	50	1.0	8	2,500	0.8	50	1.2	9	
7- 9 years	2,000	60	1.0	10	3,500	1.0	60	1.5	10	•
10-12 years	2,500	70	1.2	12	4,500	1.2	75	1.8	12	
Children over 12 years										
Girls—13-15 years	2,800	80	1.2	15	5,000	1.4	80	2.0	14	
16-20 years	2,400	75	1.0	15	5,000	1.2	80	1.8	13	•
Boys—13-15 years	3,200	85	1.4	15	5,000	1.6	90	2.4	16	
16-20 years	3,800	100	1.4	15	6,000	2.0	100	3.0	20	•

These are tentative allowances toward which to aim in planning practical dietaries. These allowances can be met by a good diet of natural foods; this will also provide other minerals and vitamins, the requirements for which are less well known.
* Requirements may be less than these amounts if provided as vitamin A, greater if chiefly as the provitamin carotene.
* One mg. of thiamine equals 333 international units; 1 mg. of ascorbic acid equals 20 international units (1 international unit equals 1 U. S. P. unit).
† Vitamin D is undoubtedly necessary for older children and adults. When not available from sunshine, it should be provided probably up to the minimal amounts recommended for infants.
‡ Needs of infants increase from month to month. The amounts given are for approximately 6 to 18 months. The amounts of protein and calcium needed are less if from breast milk.
¶ Allowances are based on the middle age for each group (as 3-3, 6 and so on) and for moderate activity.

ESSENTIALS OF A NORMAL DIET

1. Calories—
   a. Bed rest .... 1000 – 1200   c. Light work .... 1800 – 2500
   b. Invalidism .... 1500 – 2000   d. Moderate work .... 2300 – 3000
   e. Heavy work .... 3000 – 4000
2. Water—6 to 8 glasses
3. Carbohydrate .... 250 – 325 Gms.
4. Protein .... 60 – 75 Gms.
5. Fat .... 125 Gms.
6. Roughage—6 to 10 servings of bulky food
7. Vitamins—adequate amounts of A, B, C, D, E, and P. P. factor
8. Salts or minerals

	Adults	*Children*
Calcium	.68 to 1 gm.	1 gm.
Phosphorus	1.32 gms.	1 gm.
Iron	.015 gm.	.015 gm.
Sodium chloride	2 gms.	

PROTEIN YIELD OF VARIOUS FOODS

Food	Amount*	Protein, Gm.
SOUPS (canned—diluted as directed)		
Asparagus	6 oz.	2
Bean	6 oz.	11
Beef	6 oz.	10
Bouillon	6 oz.	5
Celery	6 oz.	3
Chicken	6 oz.	3
Chicken gumbo	6 oz.	7
Clam chowder	6 oz.	7
Consommé	6 oz.	6
Julienne	6 oz.	5
Mock turtle	6 oz.	11
Mulligatawny	6 oz.	5
Mutton	6 oz.	9
Oxtail	6 oz.	7
Pepperpot	6 oz.	8
Printanier	6 oz.	8
Pea	6 oz.	9
Tomato	6 oz.	3
Vegetable	6 oz.	6
Home-made cream	6 oz.	6 to 10
Split pea	6 oz.	19
FISH		
Codfish	2 by 2 by ¾ in.	5
Haddock	2 by 2 by ¾ in.	5
Halibut	2 by 2 by ¾ in.	6
Salmon	2 T.	7
Sardines	4 small	7
Tuna	2 T.	7
Clams	6	9
Crab meat	¼ cup	7
Lobster meat	¼ cup	8
Oysters	7 medium	6
Shrimp	12	15
MEAT		
Roast beef	Av. serving	12
Tenderloin steak	Av. serving	17
Bacon	3 strips 5 in. long	5
Corned beef		9
Dried beef		6
Lamb chop	1 chop	14
Mutton chop	¾ in. thick	19
Pork chop (lean)		31
Veal chop		24
Fowl	3 by 3 by ¼ in.	6
Frankfurter		8
Ham (boiled)	4 by 3 by ¼ in.	10
Beef liver	4 by 3¼ by ⅜ in.	16
Calves' liver	4 by 3¼ by ⅜ in.	16
Chicken liver	Average size	12
Pork roast	2½ by 2 by ¾ in.	13
Pork tenderloin	4 by 3½ by ¼ in.	19
Round steak	2 by 1 by 1 in.	13

*In the tables, t. indicates teaspoonful; T. indicates tablespoonful.

Food	Amount*	Protein, Gm.
BEVERAGES		
Whole milk	6 oz.	6
Skimmed milk	6 oz.	6
Buttermilk	6 oz.	5
Evaporated milk	6 oz.	12
DESSERTS		
Gelatin cream desserts	Av. serving	7 to 10
Cornstarch puddings with egg	Av. serving	7 to 10
Rice tapioca with egg	Av. serving	8 to 11
Fruit gelatins	Av. serving	4
Ice cream	Av. serving	4 to 7
FRUITS		1 to 2
VEGETABLES (fresh)		1 to 4
CHEESE		
American	1 cubic inch	6
Cottage, dry	2 T.	6
Cream, Philadelphia	⅓ cake	2
Limburger	1 cubic inch	5
Roquefort	1 cubic inch	5
Swiss	1 cubic inch	6
Pimento	2 T.	4 to 7
MISCELLANEOUS		
Breads	Av. slice	3
Egg	1	6
Cereals	Av. serving	1 to 4

DISTRIBUTION OF PROTEIN, FAT, AND CARBOHYDRATE

Meal	Amount*	Gm. or Cc.	Protein, Gm.	Fat, Gm.	Carbohydrate, Gm.	Calories
BREAKFAST						
Stewed prunes	6 t.		2	..	34	144
Cream of wheat	½ cupful (20 Gm. dry)		2	..	14	64
Sugar	2 t.	10	..	..	10	40
Cream	¼ cupful	60	2	12	2	124
Soft eggs	2	100	13.4	10.5	..	150
Toast	1 slice	30	3	..	16	78
Butter	½ t.	2½	..	2	..	18
Coffee						
Cream	1 T.		0.5	3	5	31
Sugar	2 T.	10	..	..	10	40
Milk	6 oz.	180	6	7.5	9	128
LUNCHEON						
Cream of corn soup	Av. serving		5	9.5	18	178
Crackers	2	14	2	2	10	66
Crisp bacon	3 strips 5 in. long	23	4.5	7.5	..	86
Fruit salad without dressing	Av. serving		..	..	16	64
Entire wheat bread	1 slice	30	2	..	14	64
Butter	1½ T.	2½	..	2	..	18
Milk	6 oz.	180	6	7.5	9	128
Prune custard	1		8	7	56	316

*In the tables, t. indicates teaspoonful; T. indicates tablespoonful.

Meal	Amount*	Gm. or Cc.	Protein, Gm.	Fat, Gm.	Carbohydrate, Gm.	Calories
DINNER						
Chilled tomato juice	3 oz.	90	..	..	3	12
Roast chicken		120	24	20	..	268
Stuffed baked potato	1		5	2	28	150
Squash (½ teaspoonful butter)	Av. serving		2	2	10	66
String beans (½ teaspoonful butter)	Av. serving		1	2	3	34
Hard roll		30	3	..	16	76
Butter	½ t.	2½	..	2	..	18
Cucumber and radish salad	Av. serving		1	..	4	20
Orange ice	Av. serving		..	..	66	264
Black coffee						
Crackers	2	14	2	2	10	66
American cheese	1 cubic in.	20	6	7		87
			100.4	107.5	358.5	2,798

CALORIC YIELD OF VARIOUS FOODS

Meal	Amount*	Protein, Gm.	Fat, Gm.	Carbohydrate, Gm.	Calories
BREAKFAST					
Stewed prunes	6	2	..	34	144
Sugar	2 t.	..	..	10	40
Farina	½ cupful	2	..	14	64
Sugar	2 t.	..	..	10	40
Whole milk	¼ cupful	2	2.5	3	43
Soft egg	1	6	6	..	75
Butter	1 t.	..	4	..	36
Toast	1 slice	3	..	16	78
Butter	1 t.	..	4	..	36
Coffee					
Cream	1½ T.	7	4.5	0.7	46
Sugar	2 t.	..	..	10	40
Milk	6 oz.	6	7.5	9	128
LUNCHEON					
Vegetable soup	Av. serving	1	11	9	139
Crackers	2	2	2	10	66
Crisp bacon	3 strips 5 in. long	5	11	..	119
Fruit salad	Av. serving	..	15	16	199
Entire wheat bread	1 slice	..	..	14	64
Butter	1 t.	..	4	..	36
Milk	6 oz.	6	7.5	9	128
Caramel pudding	Av. serving	3	3	52	247
Sugar	1 t.	..	..	5	20
Milk	¼ cup	..	2.5	3	43

*In the tables, t. indicates teaspoonful; T. indicates tablespoonful.

Meal	Amount*	Protein, Gm.	Fat, Gm.	Carbohy-drate, Gm.	Calories
DINNER					
Chilled tomato juice	3 oz.	..	..	3	12
Broiled steak	3½ by 3 by ¾ in.	17	25	..	293
Stuffed baked potato	Av. size	5	2	28	150
Squash	Av. serving	2	4	10	84
String beans	Av. serving	1	4	3	52
Hard roll	1	3	..	16	76
Butter	1 t.	..	4	..	36
Cucumber and radish salad ..	Av. serving	1	..	4	20
Orange ice	Av. serving	..	..	66	264
Black coffee					
		71.7	123.5	354.7	2,818

CONSTIPATION

Constipation is most frequently the result of taking a diet of foods which have little or no undigested residue in the intestines. The three types of constipation are:

1. Atonic.   2. Spastic.   3. Obstructive.

1—Atonic Constipation is the usual type and one in which there is lack of muscle tone, resulting from lack of exercise and incorrect diet.
To correct.
1. Regular daily bowel movements should be established.
2. Six to eight glasses of water a day.
3. Enemas and cathartics should be avoided.
4. A diet with 800 grams bulk of fruit and vegetables may be taken daily which is equivalent to:
   ½ cup of 9 per cent vegetables.
   3 cups of 3 to 6 per cent vegetables.
   ⅔ pound of fruit.
5. Vitamins B and C are of great importance in any disease of the gastro-intestinal tract, so it is advised that an abundance of food containing these vitamins be included in the diet.

Sample Diet

BREAKFAST

Fruit—2 large servings.
Whole grain cereal if cereal is used.
Egg, bacon, ham, or similar food.

Whole grain bread—butter.
Hot beverages.

LUNCHEON

Cream soup, cottage cheese, or other protein food.
Vegetables—2 or 3 servings.

Fruit—1 large serving.
Whole grain bread—butter.
Milk.

DINNER

Fruit cup, grapefruit or melon.
Meat, fish, or fowl.
Potato.
Other vegetables—2 or 3 servings.

Salad.
Fruit or any dessert made with fruit.
Whole grain bread—butter.
Any beverage.

*In the tables, t. indicates teaspoonful; T. indicates tablespoonful.

Additional Suggestions:

1. Fruit or fruit juice may be taken between meals and before retiring.

In giving a diet with considerable bulk care should be taken to supply sufficient protein.

2—Spastic Constipation is characterized by irregular spasms accompanied by severe pain. It may result from continued use of condiments, excessive use of tea, coffee, or tobacco.

The diet should

1. Avoid irritation which would increase spasm.
2. Assist in evacuation.
3. Improve general nutritive condition of patient.

Sample Menu

BREAKFAST	LUNCH	DINNER
Strained orange juice.	Vegetable broth.	Cream potato soup.
Cream of wheat.	Soft boiled egg.	Cottage cheese with cream.
Dry toast.	Dry toast.	Dry toast.
Cocoa or milk.	Plain jello.	Baked custard.
	Milk.	Milk.

If milk is not thoroughly digested, it may be peptonized or boiled.

Puréed vegetables and soft cooked fruits may be added when condition is relieved.

3—Obstructive Constipation—Obstruction may be caused by cancer, tumor, or adhesions.

1. The diet should omit all foods with an indigestible residue.
2. Avoid gas-forming foods.
3. Omit meats which putrefy easily.
4. Avoid serious underfeeding if patient is to be operated upon.

(Compiled from various sources.)

Bland Diet

DIETETIC PRINCIPLES

1. Weak peristaltic stimulants.
2. Sub-acid foods.
3. Moderately low and smooth residue foods.
4. Regular and simple meals.
5. Avoidance of:
   a. Coarse, raw foods.
   b. Stimulating condiments and spices.
   c. Gas-forming foods and mixtures.
   d. Extreme temperatures in foods.

FOODS ALLOWED

Soups—strained.

Meat—fish or fowl with short fiber.

Milk and milk products—in all forms including cream cheese.

Eggs—soft cooked, eggnogs.

Vegetables—mild, sieved, and potatoes.

Fruit juices—pear, blueberry, peach—sub-acid.

Cereals—without bran; and Italian pastes.

Breads—without bran.

Dessert—custards, simple puddings, jello, blanc mange.

Beverages—weak tea, coffee.

FOODS NOT ALLOWED

Meat sauces, pickles, highly seasoned foods, excessive use of condiments, salads, coarse raw vegetables, fried foods, acid fruits and fruit juices, hot breads, strong tea, coffee and cocoa.

DIET	MENU
BREAKFAST	**BREAKFAST**
Bland fruit juice.	Pear juice.
Cooked cereal (without bran).	Strained oatmeal.
Soft cooked egg.	Poached egg.
White bread (toast)—butter.	White toast—butter.
Weak coffee, tea or cocoa.	Weak coffee.
Small amount sugar.	Small amount sugar.
	(10:00 A.M., eggnog.)
LUNCH	**LUNCH**
Cream soup strained.	Cream asparagus soup.
Cottage cheese or other cheese or	Cottage cheese.
entrée—starchy food.	Sieved carrots.
Sieved vegetable.	Custard.
Simple dessert.	White bread toast—butter.
White bread toast—butter.	Milk.
Milk.	(3:00 P.M., milk.)
DINNER	**DINNER**
Cream soup or clear soup.	Chicken broth.
Meat.	Lamb chop.
Potato or starchy food.	Baked potato.
Sieved vegetable.	Puréed peas.
Simple dessert.	Tapioca cream.
White bread toast—butter.	White melba toast—butter.
Milk or weak tea.	Milk.
	(8:00 P.M., weak cocoa.)

NOTE: Milk may be given at 10:00 A.M., 3:00 P.M., and 8:00 P.M.

DIET FOR HYPERACIDITY

DIETETIC PRINCIPLES

1. Sub-acid fruits and fruit juices.
2. Weak secretory and peristaltic stimulants.
3. Moderately bland and nonirritating foods.
4. Adequate nonstimulating proteins.
5. Foods which bind acids.
6. Low salt and moderately high fat.
7. Regular meals.
8. Frequent feedings in some cases.
9. Avoidance of:
   Stimulants, condiments and highly seasoned foods, meat extracts, uncooked foods except tender lettuce, very hot and very cold foods.

FOODS TO USE

Soups—cream.
Meats—tender.
Milk and milk products—all milk modifications and cheeses.

Eggs—soft cooked.
Vegetables—all cooked and easily digested.
Fruits—sub-acid fruits and fruit juice, such as pears, apple sauce, etc.
Salads—cooked with bland dressing.
Cereals—in small amounts.
Breads—white and whole wheat.
Dessert—simple puddings and ice creams.
Beverages—weak tea, coffee, and cocoa, and alkaline mineral waters.

FOODS TO AVOID

Strong meat stocks; rare meat; coarse raw and cooked strong vegetables; acid fruits and fruit juices, coarse fruits; sour or lactic acid milk; hot breads; concentrated sweets, condiments, spices, stimulants; fried foods; and strong tea and coffee.

DIET

BREAKFAST

Sub-acid fruit.
Cooked cereal, cream.
Soft cooked egg, or bacon.
Toast, butter.
Milk or weak cocoa.

LUNCHEON

Cream soup.
Cottage cheese or meat.
Vegetable.
Salad—cooked fruit or vegetable.
Simple pudding or cooked fruit.
Bread, butter, and milk.

DINNER

Meat, tender, well cooked.
Potato, butter.
Vegetable, two or cooked fruit or
   vegetable salad.
Simple dessert.
Toast, butter.
Rich milk.

MENU

BREAKFAST

Apple sauce and pear juice.
Cereal, cream.
Soft-boiled egg.
Toast, butter.
Milk or weak cocoa.

LUNCHEON

Cream of mushroom soup.
Lamb chop.
Carrots and peas.
Pear and cheese salad.
Rice custard, whipped cream.
Bread, butter, and milk.

DINNER

Steak or fish.
Baked potato, butter.
Squash.
Asparagus, hot or as salad.
Custard.
Melba toast.
Rich milk.

FEEDINGS BETWEEN MEALS

10:00 A.M., 3:00 P.M., 8:00 P.M., milk and cream drinks.

DIET FOR HYPO-ACIDITY

DIETETIC PRINCIPLES

1. Natural acid foods.
2. Strong secretory stimulants.
3. Low residue, smooth foods.
4. Restrict liquid intake if motility is impaired.
5. Thorough mastication.
6. Regular and preferably small simple meals.
7. Rest after meals.
8. Avoidance of:
   a. Bacteria-carrying foods.
   b. Extremes in hot and cold foods.
   c. Foods containing sodium bicarbonate, carbonated waters.
   d. Fermentable sugars and sweets.
   e. Excessive use of fats and proteins.

FOODS TO USE

Soups—clear meat or vegetable broths.
Meats—broiled or roasted chicken, lamb, beef, fresh-water fish, raw oysters.
Milk and milk products—sweet and sour.
Eggs—soft cooked.
Vegetables—sieved beets, carrots, celery, peas, potatoes, sweet potatoes, tomatoes, asparagus tips, and squash.
Fruits—cooked and all fruit juices.
Cereals—cooked or dry cereal, rice.
Breads—plain bread or toast.
Dessert—simple puddings, jello, and cooked fruits.
Beverages—weak tea, coffee, cocoa, lemonade, and all sour fruit juices.

FOODS TO AVOID

All raw, coarse fruits, vegetables, fried and greasy foods; pork and all smoked and preserved meats and fish, all iced drinks, frozen desserts, and all very hot foods or drinks. All fermentable sugars and sweets, hot breads, candies, nuts, pies, and all cheese except cottage cheese.

DIET	MENU
BREAKFAST	**BREAKFAST**
Sour fruit juice.	Grapefruit juice.
Cooked fruit.	Apricots.
Cereals.	Puffed rice—cream.
Egg or bacon.	Poached egg.
Toast—butter.	White toast—butter.
Coffee or tea—cream and sugar.	Coffee or cocoa.
LUNCH	**LUNCH**
Meat broth.	Beef broth.
Cottage cheese or meat.	Cream sweetbreads.
Sieved vegetable.	Sieved beets.
Bread and butter.	Melba toast—butter.
Simple dessert or cooked fruit.	Lemon gelatin with whipped
Tea with lemon, lemonade, grape-	cream.
fruit juice, or fruit juice.	Tea with lemon or lemonade.
DINNER	**DINNER**
Soup or broth.	Roast beef.
Meat.	Mashed squash.
Vegetable.	Sieved spinach.
Salad.	Cooked grapefruit salad.
Bread and butter.	Boiled dressing.
Cooked fruit or simple dessert.	Peeled baked apple.
Tea, coffee, lemonade, or fruit	Tea, coffee, or lemonade.
juice.	

CHAPTER XXXI

Posture
MORRIS FISHBEIN, M.D.
Adapted from an article by R. TAIT McKENZIE, M.D.

GOOD POSTURE will cure some conditions and certainly prevent many others. In infancy its preventive value has the greatest influence on the ensuing life of the baby, though much can be done, by means of persistent exercise, to overcome faults of posture in later life.

The home and school can coöperate effectively in training children to observe the rules of correct posture. In the school, however, most can be done in providing desks and seats of correct height and size, as well as the instruments for gymnastic exercises.

The need for proper seating cannot be too greatly emphasized, because of its direct effect on the spine. Desks should be designed to fit the abnormally large or small, as well as the normal-sized child. The seated pupil should not use a seat so low that his shoulders perforce become rounded, his head droops, and his chest is flattened. The elbows should be able to rest on the desk without stooping or unduly elevating the shoulders, and the edge of the desk should overlap the edge of the seat. Many schools have a certain number of specially adjustable desks and seats for the express use of children who are above or below the average size.

Perfectly fitting seats are not everything. A child cannot sit still long. It is not in his nature to do so. He will become weary unless sufficient opportunity is allowed for exercising and changing the posture during school hours. If he sits too long, the upper part of the body leans forward on or against the desk, constricting the chest, crowding the abdominal organs, and impeding the circulation in the veins. The weight is supported by the arms, and the head, neck, and spine hang by the muscles of the shoulder blades in abnormal curves. To relieve this overstrain of the back and shoulder muscles the pupil slumps back until his weight rests on the shoulder blades and lower end of the spine, leaving the center of the back unsupported. The back sags down in a single long curve, the chest contracts, the breathing is made shallow, and the circulation slows up. This position stretches the muscles and ligaments of the spine, rounds the back and shoulders, and shoves forward the chin.

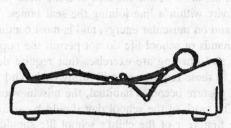 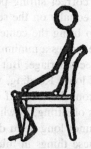

Fig. 63. Lying down requires the least energy.   Fig. 64. Sitting requires 4 per cent more energy than lying down.

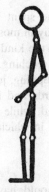 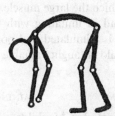

Fig. 65. Standing requires 12 per cent more energy than lying down.   Fig. 66. Bending requires 55 per cent more energy than lying down.

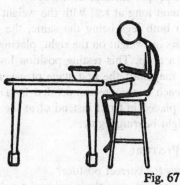 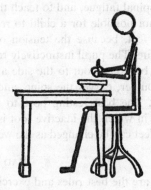

Fig. 67

Poor posture.   Good posture.

CORRECT SITTING POSTURE

The correct sitting posture is one in which the pupil sits erect, the pelvis resting equally on the seat, with the arms beside the hips and the head poised so as to bring the center of gravity within a line joining the seat bones. This posture makes a minimum demand on muscular energy, and is most conducive to correct carriage. But the demands of school life do not permit the pupil to keep it long. Reading, writing, and drawing are exercises that require deviations from the ideal. If we add to these requirements ill-fitting desks and long periods of sitting, in which bad posture becomes habitual, the mischievous result cannot long be in doubt. The work of the school day should be arranged with these things in mind. The first year of the child's school life should not have more than one third of the time in confinement at the desk.

KINDERGARTEN TRAINING

Short periods of sitting, followed by double that time spent in muscular activity out of the seat, should be the rule. This activity may in most cases consist of movements correlated with intellectual exercise. In the kindergarten exercise is admirably combined with mental culture by the teaching of imitative games in which the large muscle groups are exercised in hopping, jumping, and running, and in imitating with the arms the flight of birds and insects. The circulation is stimulated and postural faults are prevented, while at the same time the child is taught valuable lessons in natural history in which his interest never flags.

TRAINING IN HIGHER GRADES

The school day of children in the higher grades should have two five-minute periods of corrective exercise at least, in addition to the games of the recess, previously described. These exercises should be designed to promote quick, strong, muscular control; to expand and enlarge the chest by deep breathing; to bring the blood from the abdomen out into the extremities; to correct spinal fatigue, and to teach the proper carriage of the body.

It is not possible for a child to remain long at rest with the weight equally on both feet, because the tension on both legs being the same, the muscles rapidly tire. The pupil instinctively rests his weight on the right, placing his left leg with bent knee out to the side as a prop. This resting position lowers the right shoulder, curves the spine, and may start the first stage of a permanent scoliosis. The best resting pose to teach is that recommended by Dr. Eliza Mosher, in which the inactive foot is placed in front instead of at the side. In this the feet can be changed as the weight-bearing leg tires.

BAD POSTURE

What are the best rules and exercises for correct posture?

There is a test now widely used by which even the untrained teacher may

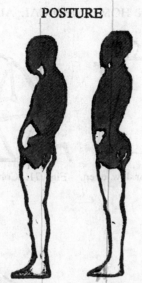

Fig. 68   Fig. 69.

Fig. 68 shows the relation of the head, thorax, and pelvis in the incorrect standing position. Fig. 69 shows the relation of the head, thorax, and pelvis in the
correct standing position.

form an accurate estimate of a child's posture. The first part of the test is
designed to find the pupil's ability to take the erect attitude. The long axis of
the trunk should continue the long axis of the head and neck. To assist the eye
of the observer, a vertical line may be dropped from the front of the ear to the
forward part of the foot. In poor posture the axes of the head, neck, and trunk
will form a zigzag instead of a straight line.

Another simple way to estimate the extent of the deformity is to stand the
child beside an upright pole or rod. The variations from correct posture are
three: the so-called fatigue, or gorilla type, in which the head is thrust forward,
the chest sunken, and the abdomen protruded; the round-back posture, in
which the hollow at the small of the back is obliterated, a posture cultivated by
faults of seating already described; and the bantam, or pouter-pigeon type, in
which the chest is pushed forward and upward, and the lower spine over-
extended, forming a marked exaggeration of the natural lumbar curve. This
posture is always the result of faulty teaching and is an exaggeration of the
correct standing posture caused by the mistaken efforts on the part of the
teacher to overcorrect the first two faults.

ENDURANCE TEST

A child who can assume a good posture may not be able to sustain it. Some
kind of endurance test is therefore an aid whereby faults of posture may be discovered and eliminated by having the children march. As the march proceeds,
old muscle habits reassert themselves, and many pupils who could hold the correct posture for a few minutes fall back into habitual faults. Heads will drop

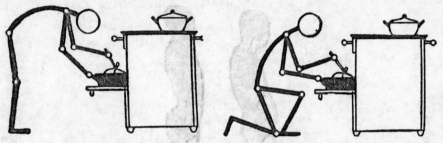

Fig. 70. Incorrect posture for low oven. Fig. 71. Correct posture for low oven.

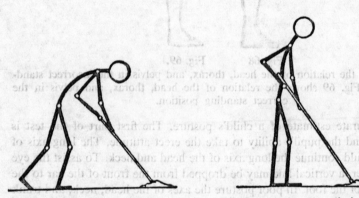

Fig. 72. Handle too short. Fig. 73. Longer handle eliminates stooping.

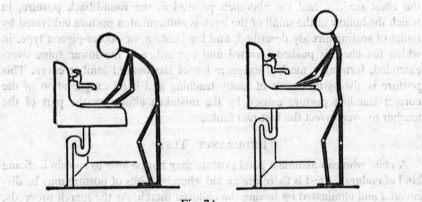

Fig. 74.

Sink too low. Sink correct height.

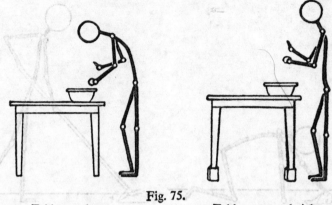

Fig. 75.

Table too low.   Table correct height.

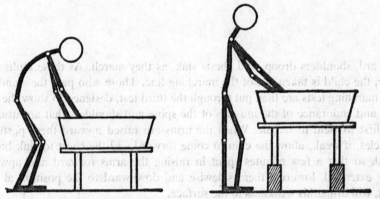

Fig. 76. Washtub too low. Correct height obtained through blocks.

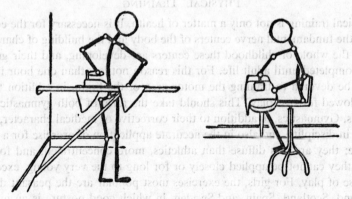

Fig. 77. Standing is fatiguing. Sitting is more comfortable.

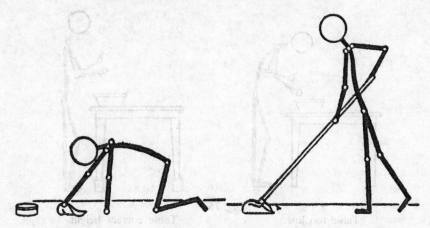

Fig. 78. Kneeling is fatiguing. Suitable equipment saves strength.

forward, shoulders droop, and chests sink, as they march. As these faults appear, the child is taken out of the marching line. Those who pass the standing and marching tests are then put through the third test, designed to show the action and endurance of the muscles of the spine and shoulders that are usually the first to yield to fatigue. When the arms are raised upward these postural muscles, if weak, allow the chin to come forward and the chest to sink backward, so that a few minutes spent in raising the arms forward and upward fully extended, lowering them sidewise and downward to the position at the start, will bring this weakness to the surface.

PHYSICAL TRAINING

Physical training is not only a matter of health. It is necessary for the education of the fundamental nerve centers of the body and the building of character. During the whole of childhood these centers are developing, and their growth is not completed until adult life. For this reason not less than one hour in five should be devoted to training the motor area of the brain, in addition to the time allowed for free play. This should take the form of both gymnastics and athletics. Gymnastics, in addition to their corrective or medical character, have a value in discipline and also in the accurate application of exercise for a given purpose; they are less diffuse than athletics, more concentrated, and for this reason they cannot be applied closely or for long to the very young, except in the guise of play. For girls, the exercises most popular are the peasant dances of Ireland, Scotland, Spain, and Sweden, in which good posture is an integral part of the dance, and agility and grace are developed.

POSTURE OF STUDENTS OF COLLEGE AGE

The necessity for good posture at college age is a logical sequence to the valuable habits learned in childhood. The college student's remediable defects must be corrected, and his physical powers trained to the highest point of efficiency. He must be taught that graceful carriage characteristic of the well-bred man. His powers of self-preservation and efficiency must be increased. If he has not learned it already, he must be given the opportunity for physical recreation through a knowledge of sports and games, for athletic activity should be the safety valve of a sedentary life, and should also teach, in addition to those social and moral qualities which can be cultivated so well in no other way, the lesson of gracefully carrying the body. That is why a university course in physical education should begin with a careful examination to find the exact bodily condition of the student and so to give an intelligent foundation on which to base advice and instruction. Nor is the examination of the student complete without a test of his ability to accomplish certain muscular feats that cover the main activities of the body, in exercises of maximum effort and of endurance.

PHYSICAL EDUCATION FOR WOMEN

Physical education for women too often follows slavishly the scheme planned for men, not because it is best for women, but because it is the same. This is a deplorable mistake, because bodily training of the two sexes must differ radically in order to fit each for its own future life and environment. It cannot, with impunity, ignore the psychologic and physiologic differences between the boy and the girl and between man and woman.

In these days of professional freedom for women, with its consequent demand on their efficiency and endurance, there is much reason for women to practise good posture. Many women suffer from the effect of faulty attitude with its direct relation to pain, like backache and headache.

The first twelve years of a girl's life need differ little from that of a boy's in physical activity. She may lead the same outdoor life, climbing, swimming, running, playing ball, and nothing will prepare her so well for the great physical and mental change which takes place with the attainment of puberty. Outdoor games and exercises establish nervous stability and poise and give the best possible foundation on which to build her future womanhood.

GAMES FOR WOMEN

Women cannot stand prolonged physical or mental strain as well as men, but with frequent rests they can in the end accomplish almost as much. Certain games, such as football, boxing, pole vaulting, and heavy gymnastics, are obviously unsuited to them; but in dancing, swimming, calisthenics, archery, skating, and fencing they come much nearer to competing with men on equal terms. While they are less adapted to arduous muscular work, their vital endurance is better; so that the disadvantage they have in other activities is made up for by this greater tenacity to life. With a few exceptions, girls accustomed to athletics and gymnastics can continue exercise without detriment during menstruation, though they should refrain at that time from too exhausting contests or competitions.

Swimming is one of the best exercises for women, calling into action most of the muscles of the body, but sparing those of the back so generally overworked in standing and sitting postures.

Finally, it is quite as important to take occasional hours of absolute rest, in the recumbent position, at it is to exercise, especially when the nervous and muscular system is overwrought.

POSTURAL EFFECT OF CLOTHING

The importance of proper clothing for men, women, and children has a high place in the promotion of good posture that cannot be overemphasized, although in these days of greater freedom and simplicity in dress there is not so much need to belabor the point as there was a few generations ago. Any tendency to return to the constricting, overweighted, and too numerous garments of a few decades past should be greatly deplored.

Proper shoes have a definite effect on posture, in both children and adults. It has been found that the ground plan of the human foot varies so that it may be straight, inflared, or outflared; therefore, no one type of shoe will be suited to all types of feet. Deformities of the feet, either from the construction of the footwear or from the breaking down of the longitudinal and lateral arches of the feet, have a vital influence on posture. The balance of the foot, either flat or on a high heel, also affects the posture, although this is not so serious as was formerly supposed, if the shoe is so made that the weight rests on the heel instead of slipping forward and crowding the toes into the forward part of the shoe.

The advantage of the upright position is somewhat offset by the frequency of deformities due to a yielding of the structures concerned with support. The body may yield at the spine, at the knee joints, or at the arch of the foot, which becomes broken down and flattened, causing the deformity known as flat-foot. A typical case of flat-foot shows a turning out of the line of the heel, a convexity of the inner contour of the foot, and a concavity of its outer margin. A tracing of the foot would show no instep. The great majority of such cases are what might be termed static and are found in nurses, clerks, waiters, barbers, motormen, and all others whose long hours of continued standing keep the muscles and ligaments of the foot constantly on the strain. The pernicious habit of standing with the toes turned out always makes it worse. Flat-foot is also found in the very fat, whose weight is too much for their ligaments. Bernard Roth, in his series of 1,000 cases of twisted spine, found flat-foot in 76 per cent of them. In an examination of 1,000 supposedly normal students I have found it in 217 cases. Lovett has found many cases among hospital nurses, who are peculiarly susceptible to it. The symptoms are varied. A considerable degree of flat-foot may be present without causing much irritation, and again great pain may be caused by a comparatively slight degree of this deformity. In any case, the close association between footwear and posture must always be kept in mind. The Posture League has designed shoes of the straight, inflared, and outflared types, providing for this natural variation in the normal foot, and at the same time correcting or preventing a position which would tend to drop the arches and produce pain or deformity.

CLOTHING AND ROUND SHOULDERS

Another frequent postural deformity caused or aggravated by improper clothing is round or uneven shoulders. Clothing which is supported by suspenders bearing on the points of the shoulders tends to pull them downward and forward. It is a common deformity among school children, and occurs in almost 20 per cent of university students uncomplicated with other postural defects. It is frequently discovered in girls about the age of puberty, when especial attention is apt to be paid to their figure and carriage. Round shoulders are not likely to be outgrown, and patients usually become permanently and structurally set in the faulty posture, with flattened chest walls and distorted figure.

The clothing should be examined, and when found to be supported from the tip of the shoulders the garments should be altered to bring the pressure in toward the root of the neck, instead of out on the shoulders. It has been pointed out that the cut of most ready-made clothing causes pressure on the back of the neck and tip of the shoulders, constantly tending to produce this deformity. Such clothing, especially men's and boys' suit coats, and men's, women's, and children's top coats, should be bought with particular care that the shape of the shoulders and backs of these garments do not have a tendency to encourage poor posture.

EXERCISES FOR FAULTY POSTURE

The following six exercises are recommended for the correction of the ordinary case of faulty posture:

1. With the patient standing in his habitual faulty position, place the hand about one inch in front of the sternum and tell him to raise the chest and shove it forward to touch the hand without swaying the body. He will at first try to draw the shoulders back, but this fault must be overcome at the very beginning, and the shoulder muscles must be kept relaxed. Gradually increase the distance to which he can bring the chest forward, repeating it again and again until he

can take the position without difficulty and without contracting the muscles of the back. While in this position make him breathe deeply five times and then relax. This should be done before a mirror, so that he will recognize the feeling of the correct posture and associate it with the proper attitude as seen in the glass. He should then try to take it without looking at the mirror. This posture should be drilled into him until it becomes habitual and until he can maintain it without discomfort. R. J. Roberts, of Boston, used to tell his young men to press the backs of their necks against the collar button, considering this as the keynote of the position. In whatever way it is accomplished, the object is to get the proper relation between the thorax and the pelvis.

After repeating Exercise 1 twenty times, take:

2. Arms forward raise, upward stretch, rise on tiptoes, inhale. Sideward lower, slowly press the arms back, and exhale. This exercise, when done correctly, expands the chest, bringing in all the extensors of the back and levators of the shoulders.

3. The patient stands, arms downward and backward, fingers interlocked and palms outward. Extend the neck, roll the shoulders backward and forearms into supination, the palms being first in, then down, and then out. Reverse to starting position and relax. This exercise is valuable for projecting the chest forward, stretching the shortened ligaments, and drawing in the abdomen. Care should be taken to have the chin pressed backward when the arms are brought downward and turned outward. In resistant cases, where this exercise cannot be done with the fingers interlocked, a handkerchief tied in a loop may be substituted and held in the fingers.

4. Patient stands with the arms at the sides. Arms sideward raise, upward stretch, inhale, forward bend, and rise. Arms sideward, lower, exhale. In this exercise the lungs are filled when the chest is in the most favorable position for expansion. The breath is retained when the trunk is flexed, forcing the air into the cells of the lungs under pressure. The bending and rising bring into powerful action the extensors of the back and neck and the retractors of the shoulders.

5. Patient lies prone on a couch with the feet strapped, or upon the floor with the feet caught on the edge of a bureau or other article of furniture. Hands clasped behind the head. Raise the head and extend the spine, pressing the elbows backward. This exercise is a severe one on the back and shoulders. Follow with a deep breathing exercise.

6. Patient lies in similar position as in Exercise 5, arms at the sides. Raise head, bring arms forward and imitate the breast stroke.

In this exercise the spine is kept in static contraction, while the retractors of the shoulders are alternately contracted and relaxed.

ADDITIONAL EXERCISES

Here are some simple exercises which help to strengthen the muscles of the back and abdomen and thus improve posture:

1. Lie on the back, hands back of the neck. Take a deep breath and raise chest high; keep chest up and exhale by pulling abdomen in. *2.* Same position; knees bent, feet pulled up. Pull abdomen in hard and then relax part way. *3.* Sit in a chair, trunk bending forward. Incline trunk forward from the hips, keeping spine straight. This exercise may be done standing. *4.* Standing; abdominal retraction. Stand with the heels four inches away from the wall but with the hips, shoulders, and head touching the wall; flatten the lower part of the back against the wall by pulling in the abdominal muscles. Holding this position, come away from the wall with the weight well forward on the balls of the feet. *5.* Standing; leg raising. Stand with hands on hips, back flat, and chin in; raise leg forward without bending the knee; lower it; repeat with other leg. This exercise teaches how to hold the back flat. *6.* Carrying the head forward; clasp hands behind the head. Force the head back against their pressure, keeping chin in. This strengthens the muscles of the back of the neck. *7.* Spinal curvatures. "Stand tall," holding the back straight. Rise on the toes with the arms extended forward and up, stretching the arms and the body. *8.* Distended abdomen. This condition may be prevented and largely overcome by doing exercises 2 and 4.

CHAPTER XXXII

The Foot

PHILIP LEWIN, M.D.

T HE FOOT makes one of the important contacts between man and the
world in which he lives. Because the human being's predecessors walked on
four feet, men, women, and children are often unstable on two. Man's feet
and ankles are constructed so that he has stability when standing, moves
easily, and there is comfort in standing, walking, and running. The tissues
themselves must be healthy. This requires adequate circulation of the blood
and normal nerve supply. It is surprising how small the degree of motion in
the ankle joint can be consistent with adequate walking. However, some degree of painless, free motion is essential, particularly if you desire grace and
spring to the step. Compare the beautiful stride and grace of movements about
the stage of leading actresses with the awkward motion of limbs and feet of
less accomplished performers, and you will realize how important a graceful
gait is to present the general impression of beauty.

The disorders and defects which affect the feet include those which are
present at birth, deformities which are acquired due to accidents, diseases of
the bones, joints, muscles, and nerves, and disturbances of the circulation of
blood to and from the feet.

Many children are born without a full quota of toes, with webs between
the toes like a duck, with extra toes, with overgrowth of the leg and foot,
and sometimes with one toe lapping over another. Some of these disturbances
are of slight importance, but they make it difficult to walk satisfactorily, even
in special shoes. Surgical attention is necessary in some cases.

Deformities of the feet may result from tuberculosis, syphilis, infantile
paralysis, other infections, breaking down of the arches, and inward or outward deviation of the foot. Each of these conditions demands special consideration. If you fall landing heavily or off balance on a foot, or if the foot
is given a hard blow, one or more bones may fracture. If the foot is suddenly
twisted, a dislocation or a sprain may occur, and sometimes portions of the

bones pull apart. Then, too, the surface of the foot may be subjected to the occurrence of warts, small tumors, or the development of corns due to either irritation or other disturbances.

The foot is so definitely associated with the posture of the body generally and with the jarring of the tissues within the abdomen and skull, that any interference with its normal function may affect the whole body. Many disturbances in the leg, the knee, the hip, and the back may be associated with disturbed physiologic action of the feet. When the ancestors of human beings walked on four feet, they dwelt in fields and meadows. With the development of the city have come hard floors, cement sidewalks, and asphalt streets; with the growth of civilization have come shoes and stockings; with changes in transportation, automobiles and streetcars. All these affect the use of the feet and may be partially responsible for some of the difficulties which are commonly seen by orthopedic surgeons and other specialists in diseases affecting locomotion.

FUNCTIONS OF THE FEET (PHYSIOLOGY)

There are two chief functions of the feet: (1) To bear the weight of the body; (2) to permit easy walking. The weight-bearing line is determined by dropping a plumb line from the center of the hip joint through the middle of the kneecap; this falls through the middle of the mortise bone of the ankle and through a point between the first and second toes. The two large bones of the foot are this mortise bone, between the leg and the foot, and the heel bone. The heel bone or os calcis serves as the attachment for the largest tendon in the body, known as the Achilles tendon. It will be remembered that in the Greek mythology the weak point of Achilles was in his heel. The heel bone furnishes the initial bearing surface of the foot as it strikes the ground in walking.

The feet are among the most abused portions of the human body and are probably responsible for about as much agony as human beings can sustain. Fashion takes no account of foot comfort or foot health. Modern shoes, particularly for women, bring about extraordinary malformations. Hiking crazes cause large numbers of people to undertake long walks with poor equipment. Motorcars keep many people from walking enough to give the feet adequate exercise.

SHOES

Millions of words have been written about shoes, and everyone who manufactures them seems to have his own ideas. There are shoes with flexible shanks and shoes with rigid shanks, as well as shoes with semi-flexible and semi-rigid shanks. People without any foot troubles may do well in flexible shank shoes. Those who have foot trouble, however, and who require both exercise and support, will usually feel much better with shoes with a rigid shank. It is believed that the best type of shoes have round toes, medium-width shanks, and are made over a last with a straight inner border. Extremes in the height of heels are undesirable, and a good heel is neither too low nor too high.

Few people understand how to take care of their shoes properly. Shoes will last much longer and give much better service from the point of view of protecting the feet if they are changed daily. The pair that is not in use should be kept on a suitable shoe tree. The rubber heel has proved its value in minimizing shock to the feet and thereby to the other organs of the body.

The circulation to the feet must be adequate if the toes are to be healthy. Such circulation is not maintained when the leg is constricted by tight garters or by rolling the stockings in a hard ridge or knot. Such constriction causes interference with the normal flow of blood and tends to break down the valves in the veins, resulting in bulges (varicosities).

HYGIENE OF THE FOOT

Feet must be kept clean if they are to maintain a good state of health. They should be bathed once daily, using a non-irritating soap. After being dried, the foot may be dusted with a simple powder. In exceptional conditions it may be desirable to have other types of powders, but these should be selected by a physician. These powders frequently contain salicylic and boric acids. Long applications of medicaments of this kind to the feet may result in maceration, or softening and burning of the skin.

A simple measure for aiding the circulation of the legs and feet in health is the use of the contrast bath. Two large buckets big enough to hold both feet and perhaps to reach up halfway to the knees are needed for the purpose. One bucket is filled two-thirds full of warm water. The other bucket is filled two-thirds full of cool water. The person who is taking the contrast bath sits between the two buckets. He first places both feet in the warm water for one minute, then removes the feet and places them in the cool water for one minute. This procedure is alternated for ten minutes. The alternating dilatation and contraction of the blood vessels is helpful and aids the circulation in the tissues. The same effect may be secured by spraying alternately with hot and cold water for one minute each.

There is nothing so restful as massage of the feet, particularly after a tiresome day. The feet may be kneaded with rotary movement of the fingers. Cold cream, olive oil, cocoa butter, or similar ointments, may be used to lessen irritation. In many instances, when the foot is tired and irritated because of excessive walking or standing, hot applications in the form of moist dressings of a saturated solution of epsom salts are helpful.

Most feet get enough exercise simply by walking. For the abnormal foot with weakness of the arches, many special exercises have been developed which are exceedingly useful in strengthening the tissues. These are adapted particularly to the treatment of flat-feet.

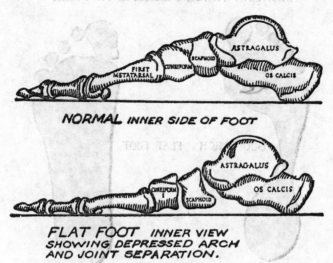

FLAT FOOT INNER VIEW
SHOWING DEPRESSED ARCH
AND JOINT SEPARATION.

Fig. 79. Showing what happens in case of a fallen arch.

FLAT-FEET

The exact cause of flat-feet is not known, but it is believed that there is a hereditary tendency, since they tend to run in families. Moreover, some races tend to be more flat-footed than others. The feet of the baby should be examined soon after birth, perhaps not later than at six months, and then again each year to make certain that they are developing properly, and that corrective measures in the form of suitable shoes, supports, or braces are not needed. When the feet grow rapidly, especially in young adolescent girls, and when improper shoes are worn at the same time, flat-feet are likely to develop.

Flatness of the feet appears most commonly in fat people; first, because the feet carry excessive weight and there is a disproportion between the weight carried and the size and strength of the feet; second, because there may be associated disturbances of the glands that control metabolism in children who are overfat. Such disturbances are likely to be associated with deformities in the growth of the bones and ligaments.

In many instances flat-feet may be the result of accidents, such as falling suddenly from a height. The child with flat-feet may be found to be under par, so far as its general muscular condition is concerned. These children frequently have knock-knees, the back is rounded, and the mother says that the child is awkward. The shoes are "run over" unnaturally. The foot is usually not painful in the child, because it is still flexible, but the child manifests a disinclination to run and to play.

A competent study of the feet by one who knows how to evaluate the arch and to determine its functional condition will usually reveal the character of the disturbance. A mere print of the foot, the type of examination frequently given in those shoe stores which promote "health" shoes on a pseudo-

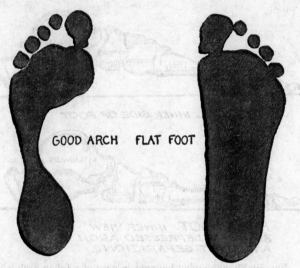

Fig. 80. Footprints indicating quality of the arch.

scientific basis, is not sufficient examination to indicate the real nature of flat-foot. The specialist in care of the feet first determines the extent of the disorder and then applies his treatment specifically to the causes and conditions found. His purpose is to teach proper walking, to increase the power of the supporting structures, to stimulate the circulation of the blood, and to

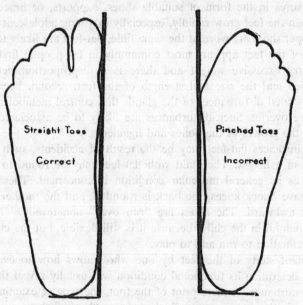

Fig. 81. Straight toes and pinched toes.

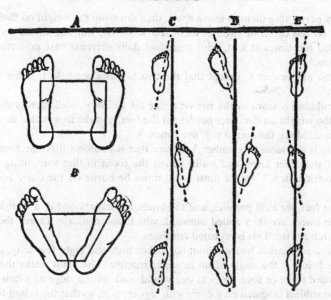

Fig. 82. Right and wrong foot postures. A. Correct standing position. B. Military standing position—incorrect. C. Correct walking position. D. Military walking position—incorrect. E. Indian position, walking.

:orrect conditions associated with flat-feet, such as knock-knees and bowlegs.

Children who have flat-feet must be taught to walk with the feet parallel or toeing in slightly. In walking, the weight comes down on the heels and is tilted toward the outer borders of the feet, coming up on the toes with a pring. In few instances of flat-feet is it necessary to have shoes made to order. A competent physician can arrange the heels in such a manner with pads and supports as to compel a child to walk over the outer border of the foot. This also forces the ankle into a correct position with relation to the leg. In some instances it is necessary to insist on high shoes and perhaps even to re-enforce he uppers, to aid weak ankles.

The usual gymnasium shoes should be worn for gymnastics only. Ballet lippers should be worn only for dancing, and sometimes it is desirable to insert supportive pads in these shoes. Children with flat-feet should not go bare-oot, except in the sand, nor should they wear bedroom slippers around the louse. The shoe is a corrective measure and should be worn at all times vhen the feet are in use.

Most authorities recommend a series of exercises which are helpful in orrecting flat-feet. It is difficult frequently to get children to use these exer-ises, but if they are taught as a game, the child is likely to participate with njoyment. The list of exercises includes:

1. Stand barefooted with the feet parallel and about two inches apart, strad-dling a seam or a line in a rug. On the count of one, "force" the feet apart with-

out really permitting them to move apart, thus throwing the weight on their outer borders; on the count of two, let them roll in slowly, but not all the way. This is repeated ten times at first, with a gradual daily increase that may run up to twenty-five.

2. Same as number 1, except that the two big toes are held together and on the floor.

3. Straddling a seam in the rug or a line on the floor, walk across the room with all the weight on the outer borders of the feet, and the toes curled downward and inward. Make the round trip five times.

4. This is the same as number 3, except that the subject lifts one foot to the height of the other knee, and walks across the room in that way, using the so-called "ostrich step." Weight must at all times be borne on the outer border of the foot.

5. The feet are held parallel, and the knees are maintained in a straight position. The knees are then rolled outward, which automatically causes the longitudinal arch to rise. This is repeated ten times.

6. Use a supination board, about six inches high and eight feet long, its sloping sides being at the angle of an isosceles triangle. The child walks the length of the board three or four times as one would walk on the ridge of a house roof.

7. The subject is seated on a chair with legs crossed, so that the raised foot can relax. He then holds the foot at right angles with the leg and not turned in or out. The exercise is done in four counts. On the count of one, the foot is allowed to relax into the position of toe-drop. On the count of two, it is swung in; on the count of three, it is forcibly pulled upward; and on the count of four, it is brought back to the starting position, describing a half circle. This is performed ten times.

8. This is a resistive exercise. The subject sits on a table, and a second person sits on a chair. The subject forcibly swings his foot inward and upward, and holds it in this position with all his power. The second person attempts to swing the foot outward and downward. This effort on the part of the second person is resisted by the subject. The exercise is carried out ten times. At no time should the second person use as much power as the first.

9. Older children and adults can perform this exercise as follows: The right foot is turned inward and upward and held in that position firmly. The left foot is placed against the right, and attempts to force the right outward, which effort the right foot resists. Then the feet are reversed. After each of these exercises the subject relaxes his foot.

Occasionally operations are necessary to lengthen heel tendons in muscle-bound feet, but in the majority of cases of flat-feet a surgical operation is seldom indicated.

A few special exercises have been developed for stretching the Achilles tendon of the heel:

1. Simply walking on the heels across the room five times.

2. From the standing position with the feet parallel, the patient squats down to the position of sitting on the heels, maintaining the heels and toes on the ground. This is done in two counts.

3. The patient stands facing the wall with the toes twenty-eight inches from it. The toes are placed together and the heels as far apart as possible. With the hands placed against the wall and the heels maintained on the floor, the entire rigid body is allowed to fall forward as far as possible by bending the elbows, and to remain in this position a few seconds before returning to the starting position. This is done in two counts, about ten times.

4. The apparatus for this exercise consists of two handles fastened to the wall and a heavy wooden block three and one-half inches high, twelve inches wide, and seven inches in depth, fastened to the floor. The patient faces the wall, standing with the forward parts of both feet on the block, and holding onto the handles. On the count of one, the heels are allowed to touch the floor, the body being kept parallel with the wall. On the count of two, the return is made to the starting position. The exercise is carried out from ten to twenty times, this number being attained gradually.

5. The patient stands with the forward half of each foot on a stair, facing upward and holding the balustrade, and allows the heels to drop. He then returns to the starting position.

"Fallen" Arches

Feet may become painful because of stress and strain. This is particularly the case in the condition commonly called fallen arch, which occurs in both sexes. People who stand long hours on their feet, such as policemen, motormen, tailors, or saleswomen, are especially likely to be disturbed by painful feet due to extraordinary stress on the arches. There are pain and rigidity of the tissues and at times even spasms of the muscles in the effort to overcome the strain. Any general affection may be reflected in the feet.

In case the arch has fallen, relief frequently occurs when the person is able to stay off the feet. Hot applications and massage of the feet are helpful. The padding of the shoes in such cases is comforting. The shoes must be fitted so as to aid in supporting the arch with a rigid shank of medium width. A competent authority will insert felt pads to support the depressed structures.

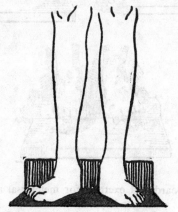

Fig. 83. Example of rigid flat-feet.

METATARSAL ARCH DISORDERS

A series of exercises has been developed for the purpose of building up the tissues that support the metatarsal arch. The following exercises have been found of special value:

1. *Doorstop Exercise.* Two old-fashioned doorstops, obtainable at the hardware section of one of the 5-and-10-cent stores, are prepared for use by removal of the rubber tips with a pair of nippers. Then they are screwed into a board about fourteen inches long, eight inches wide, and two inches thick. The centers of the doorstops should be six inches apart. A heel rest two and three-eighth inches high is attached.

The board is placed on the floor, and the subject sits on a chair in front of it. Each foot is placed on a doorstop with slight pressure just behind the metatarsal bones. On the count of one, the toes relax slowly. This is continued until one has counted two hundred. (This number should be attained gradually.)

2. *Towel Exercise.* The subject sits in a chair. A large hand towel is spread on the carpet, with the narrow edge facing the patient. Both feet are placed on the towel so that half of each foot is on the towel. The towel is grasped with the toes of one foot, then with the toes of the other. As the toes of one foot grasp, those of the other foot relax. This is continued until the entire towel has been dislodged.

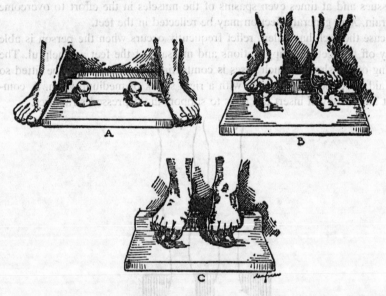

Fig. 84. Doorstop board and exercise for metatarsal arch. No ankle valgus is permissible.
(Lewin, Courtesy of *American Journal of Surgery*)

3. *Golf-ball Exercise*. A golf ball is placed on the rug and rolled under the metatarsal arch for one minute. Then it is picked up with the toes of one foot and placed under the toes of the other foot, and the exercise is repeated for another minute. The subject alternates in this manner six times.

4. *Marble Exercise*. Marbles of various sizes are placed on a rug. The subject sits on a chair and picks up the marbles with the toes and throws them forward.

5. *Pencil Exercise*. A round pencil is placed on a hard floor, and by means of the toes curled downward the subject pushes and pulls the pencil around the floor with short, quick movements.

Feet that are improperly fitted with shoes are frequently subject to other conditions such as corns, calluses, bunions, or hammer toes. Excessive perspiration and infection with ringworm or "athlete's foot" are other problems.

SPRAINED ANKLE

A sprained ankle is one of the most common injuries affecting human beings, again chiefly because they were not intended to walk originally on two feet. A slight failure of complete support throws the weight of the body unnecessarily on a group of ligaments never planned to bear that much weight, and a sprain frequently follows. A sprain represents stretching or tearing of the tissues of the joints. It must not be confused with fracture, which is a breaking of bone. In many instances fracture is overlooked and the condition diagnosed simply as sprain, with the result that healing may be delayed.

It is, therefore, exceedingly important to have X-ray pictures taken in every doubtful case. Sometimes several pictures are necessary to determine the presence of very small fractures of the bones. Some authorities treat sprains by putting on a plaster cast for a few days, elevating the foot and leg, and then applying suitable adhesive straps to give the foot complete rest.

After a period of from seven to fourteen days, when irritation and pain have subsided and healing has begun, an elastic anklet may be worn. These anklets may be removed each morning and evening for contrast baths—that is, alternating baths of one minute each in hot and cold water, for ten minutes. Passing an electric current through the tissues by means of diathermy tends to hasten subsidence of inflammation and helps to promote recovery.

A simple outline for the treatment of sprained ankle follows:

1. Put the person at rest in bed immediately.
2. Elevate the leg and ankle.
3. Apply ice bags.
4. Apply a snug resilient bandage.
5. Call a physician.

When the physician arrives, he will probably arrange to have X-ray pictures made, if necessary. He will arrange for strapping the ankle with adhesive, or, if the sprain is severe, he will put on a plaster-of-Paris cast. In less severe cases he is likely to apply a snug bandage. Under no circumstances should the feet be allowed to hang for long periods, since this will tend to permit the accumulation of fluid and produce more pain and swelling.

PAINFUL HEELS

A painful heel may be due to many causes; sometimes there is inflammation of the heel tendon. Under such circumstances, it is desirable to prevent at once all bearing of weight on the heel bone and to apply a suitable bandage or cast so as to make certain that there is a relaxation of the pull of the tendon on the muscles of the calf and on the heel bone. In addition, there must be suitable baths and massage to stimulate the tissues and aid recovery. If the condition is very slight, elevation of the heel by the use of pads of felt or sponge rubber reduces the degree of strain.

In certain infections within the body, such as infection of the teeth, tonsils, or other portions, there may be associated secondary trouble in the feet. Associated with this there may be injury to the tissues due to falling on the feet or the wearing of improper shoes. As a result of the continued irritation there may be a growth of bone on the lower, inner surface of the large bone of the foot, the heel bone, and the production of what are called "spurs." Occasionally the development of these spurs is associated with infection, but this is by no means constant.

It is, of course, exceedingly important first to determine the presence of any infection and to control that. Associated with the growth of the spur and infection there are pain, tenderness, swelling, and a tendency to limp. These come on gradually, and the pain and tenderness usually seem to be felt first along the inner border of the heel. Since painful heel may be due to a wart, to inflammation of the covering of the bone, or to an injury, it is well first to inspect very carefully the outside of the foot, and then, if the cause cannot be found, to have an X-ray picture which will promptly reveal the presence of a spur.

If the foot is then placed at rest and suitably treated with heat, the pain and sensitiveness will disappear. The use of felt pads tends to relieve pain in the weight-bearing portions of the foot. In some cases operative removal of spurs may be necessary.

CLUB-FOOT

About 75 per cent of all club-feet, which are present at time of birth, are of the type in which the toes point downward and inward. This occurs once in a thousand births; 65 per cent are in males, and in 57 per cent of cases the deformity is present only on one side. The exact cause of club-foot is not known, but it is said to be due sometimes to a wrong position of the child previous to birth. In previous decades, such children were permitted to go crippled through life. Nowadays this is not tolerated, because it is realized that early and effective treatment by a competent physician will bring about cure. The chance of cure depends on the age of the child when first seen, the type and degree of the deformity, the persistence of the treatment, and other factors. Active treatment may be necessary for months, and care and supervision for years.

The first treatment for club-foot is usually applied at birth or during infancy. The object is to correct the deformity as soon as possible and to maintain the correction until proper use of the foot has made the correction permanent. In correcting club-foot, a competent orthopedic surgeon is likely to manipulate it so as to get it in proper position and to hold it in place by suitable bandages, adhesive straps, splints, plaster-of-Paris casts, or braces.

After the correction has been established, massage, exercise, and modification of the shoes tend to hold the feet in proper position. In some instances it is impossible to control club-foot by manipulative measures and the use of casts and braces alone. In these cases it may be necessary to perform surgical operations for readjustment of the tissues or even complete reconstruction.

Ingrown Toenails

When a foot which has been neglected from the point of view of hygiene develops a complication like ingrowing toenails, the owner of that foot is in for an exceedingly painful time. The large toenail is the one usually concerned in the ingrowing procedure. Almost everyone thinks himself competent to advise on the handling of ingrown toenails. Therefore, the patient usually has tried all sort of poultices, antiseptics, and ointments on his toe before coming to the physician. When he finally does come, the nail and the toe will be found red and swollen. Pus may be exuding from under the nail. Not infrequently the infection is brought about by the practice of clipping the toenails with sharp scissors that are seldom sterilized before use.

Some simple suggestions for treatment include:

1. Stop all attempts at the use of poultices, liniments, and soaking of the foot in baths.

2. Apply an antiseptic solution to the infected portions of the nail where it comes in contact with the skin.

3. Do not attempt to manicure the nail with the intricate technic used for fingernails.

4. Use a pair of surgical scissors with rounded ends, which will not lacerate the skin or do much damage if the scissors slip. Cut a shallow "v" or "u" in the middle of the nail.

5. A *tiny* rolled-up wisp of cotton should be carefully tucked under the edges of the nail and saturated with castor oil.

As dressing for an ingrown nail, it is merely necessary to use a piece of surgically clean gauze, to wear stockings thick enough to afford protection, and shoes loose enough to prevent pressure but not so loose as to cause rubbing. If this procedure is followed repeatedly, the ingrown toenail gradually returns to normal, and proper hygiene thereafter will keep it in that condition.

WARTS

Among the most common growths on the human skin are warts of various types. Almost everybody has a "cure" for warts and some have rather fantastic ideas of how they originate. Warts sometimes disappear spontaneously, but the disappearance is usually credited to the fact that someone has murmured a potent charm at midnight in a cemetery or buried a string containing as many knots as there are warts. A wart causes little trouble, but it can grow very large in the eyes and mind of the person who owns it. The only time warts cause trouble is when they are situated in places where pressure makes them painful.

There seems to be some evidence that the wart is an infectious condition caused by a filtrable virus, or an organism so small that it cannot be seen under the microscope. However, it cannot be highly infectious, since there are many people who are in contact with warts but never get them.

The ordinary wart can be removed by many methods; sometimes merely through softening by the application of corrosive chemicals; sometimes by cutting or sandpapering, and sometimes by the application of an electric current which kills the blood supply and causes the wart to fall off. This last process is painful, but the pain may be eliminated through the use of local anesthetics. The X-ray will cause the disappearance of a wart. Various strong acids are also used. There is always the danger, however, that the burning will extend deeper than the wart, and as a result an unsightly scar will remain.

One of the most painful types of warts is that which occurs on the sole of the foot, "plantar wart." There seems to be plenty of evidence for believing that these are infections, since they occur particularly in young people in schools and gymnasium classes who go barefoot around the gymnasium or the swimming pool or wear each other's stockings. Such warts may become so painful as to interfere with walking. Their treatment demands careful consideration of a competent physician. The hard skin on the bottom of the foot must be softened, the wart removed, and the damaged tissue protected by proper antiseptics and dressings during the process of healing. Sometimes the electrical needle is used to destroy these warts, but this also demands the help of an expert. Operation may be necessary.

BUNIONS

During the period from 1917–24 about 300 operations were done in a New York hospital for the relief of bunions. In this work some 25 surgeons cooperated, and one of them has recently reviewed the results of 200 operations performed on 108 patients. Ninety per cent of the patients were women. Pain was the chief reason for operation in more than half the cases, but one fourth of them had the operation because the foot was badly deformed by the bunions. Indeed, one of the patients had had bunions for thirty-five years, and five of them had had them for more than twenty years.

Most of these patients had tried wearing broad shoes, arch supports, and other devices, before they finally decided to have the bunion removed by an operation.

While the operation is simple, it is necessary for the patient to stay in the hospital in bed for from twelve to eighteen days in order to permit good recovery before an attempt is made to walk on the foot. In most instances the operation consists in the removal of part of the overgrown bone that is responsible for the pain and the deformity. After the operation patients are able to move the great toe freely and are free from pain.

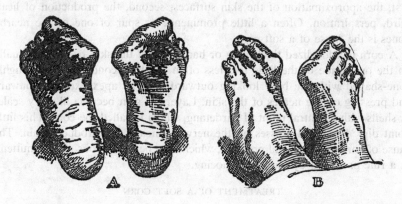

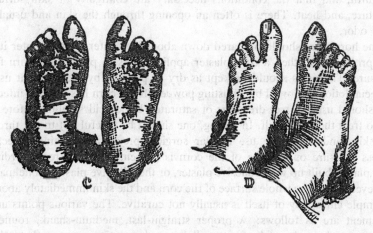

Fig. 85. Severe bunions and hallux valgus treated by Porter operation.
(Porter, Courtesy of *Surgery, Gynecology, and Obstetrics*)

In many instances the bunion may be associated with a chronic inflammation of the joints that has localized to a certain extent in the great toe. When this is the case, operative removal of the bone does not always insure complete elimination of the condition. A physician who is thoroughly informed as to the general condition of the patient is therefore able to decide whether or not the operation should be recommended in any case. The proper selection of the operative procedure in each individual case is of the greatest importance.

CORNS

Corns are of two varieties: hard corns which occur on the exposed irritated surfaces, and soft corns which occur between the toes, usually between the fourth and fifth. The conditions necessary to produce a soft corn are, first, the approximation of the skin surfaces; second, the production of heat; third, perspiration. Often a little prominence or spur of one of the nearby bones is the cause of a soft corn.

A corn is a localized thickening or hardening of the skin occurring usually on the outer side of the little toe, less often on the second toe. It is roughly cone-shaped with the base looking outward and the apex extending inward and pressing on the nerves of the skin. Layers of skin become like dry scales or shells with a central point of hardening, which is called the core. This little point dips down and presses on the nerves beneath and produces pain. The cause of corns is abnormal pressure, which may be continuous or intermittent, as a rule produced by improper shoeing.

TREATMENT OF A SOFT CORN

In order to understand the treatment for soft corns, it is important to remember that they occur only between the toes, usually between the fourth and fifth, and that the conditions necessary are contiguity of skin surfaces, moisture, and heat. There is often an opening through the skin and usually a fetid odor.

The horny rim should be pared down about the center, or the center itself, if it projects, and then a corn plaster applied so as to protect the corn from pressure. The parts should be kept as dry as possible by the frequent use of a special lotion, followed by a dusting powder. If the corn has become infected, one should use hot wet dressings of saturated boric acid solution before trying to treat the corn itself. In paring, one should be careful not to cut through the skin, and of course use regular surgical precautions against infection. Unless pressure on the site of the corn is prevented, it will recur; ordinary corn plaster built up with adhesive plaster, or the adhesive plaster alone may be laid evenly over the whole surface of the corn and the skin immediately about it.

Simple chiropody of itself is usually not curative. The various points under treatment are as follows: A proper straight-last, medium-shank, round-toe shoe; second, in these shoes a small felt pad, exerting pressure behind the heads of the metatarsal bones; third, special exercises to strengthen the supporting structures of the metatarsal arch; fourth, a simple dusting powder between the toes three or four times a day; fifth, the preparation of a stocking, making a stall for the fifth toe, as a thumb in a mitten; sixth, X-ray treatment; seventh, radium treatment; eighth, electrical treatment; and ninth, operation, consisting of removal of the soft corn and the opening in the skin, if present, and the removal of a bony spur.

Soft corns should be kept clean and dry. They should be washed frequently with alcohol, dried and powdered. The application of strong acids must be left to the physician.

The treatment of an ordinary hard corn is in most cases unsatisfactory, as after removal it recurs when pressure is again applied. A time-honored remedy is salicylic acid in collodion or ointment. The most important prophylactic measures are correctly fitted proper shoes and hosiery. Palliative treatment consists of immersion in hot water and soap, after which the lesion is pared and covered with adhesive strips or a protective ring-shaped pad.

PERSPIRING FEET

Hyperhidrosis or excessive perspiration of the feet is a common and troublesome condition. It is most commonly found in overweight individuals—both children and adults—in whom there seems to be a glandular disturbance of some kind. The treatment consists in local applications of aluminum chloride solution painted on the surface of the foot three nights in succession. The patient should discontinue the treatment for about a week, when he should resume the application for three nights in succession again. Washing the feet two or three times daily is helpful. Chromic acid may be used as a foot wash, this to be followed by dusting powder on the foot and in the hose. X-ray treatment is usually successful. Some cases are so resistant to treatment that surgery is required.

FOOTNOTES AND FOOTSTEPS

"The future of the race moves forward on the feet of little children."—
Phillips Brooks—Parents Magazine.

One pair of feet must last a lifetime.

Feet are among the first structures to show age, wear and tear and stress and strain.

A man may be as old as his arteries but he acts as old as his feet.

When your ankles roll in, your foot troubles begin.

Put your pride in your pocket and your feet in good shoes.

Fit the foot, not the eye.

Put your better foot forward; then make the other one just as good.

Bad feet are good barometers of failing health.

He who is no longer "upon his toes" will soon be "down on his uppers."

Take the arch out of your back and put it in your feet.

Foot care is foot insurance.

It isn't the load that breaks us down, it's the way we carry it.

The height of the longitudinal arch does not determine the strength or the usefulness of a foot.

A flat-foot may give a good performance, whereas a high-arched foot may be incompetent.

Flat-feet are not necessarily painful feet.

Flat-feet plus "rheumatic" feet are painful and stiff.

Overeating is usually reflected in the form of painful feet as well as pain in the abdomen.

Obesity throws additional strain on the feet.

Overeating may cause "foot dyspepsia."

It never hurt a person with painful feet to be put on an anti-obesity, anti-gout diet for a short period.

There is no shoe too small for a vain foot.

It should not be necessary to "break in" shoes.

The size of the foot changes during walking, but the shoe does not.

Every foot has two sizes: one while sitting, another while standing.

Your feet may be larger after tramping around all day, but your shoes are not.

If we had more correct shoes, we wouldn't need so many "corrective" shoes.

Cramping your feet will cramp your natural style.

In each of the forty-eight states every blacksmith must have a state license to shoe a horse. In no state does a shoe fitter have to have anything but a yardstick, a shoehorn, and a glib tongue. It doesn't sound like horse sense, does it?

A flexible shoe is sufficient for those who need only exercise, but for those who need both exercise and support, it is insufficient. It may be used "part time" to alternate with a rigid-shank shoe.

Shoe trees are indispensable.

The child walks on the same hard surfaces that adults do, namely, hard floors, cement sidewalks, and asphalt streets—therefore, he should have the same protection.

Many children outgrow but never outwear their shoes.

One of the worst sitting positions is that in which the child sits with his legs folded so that the heels nearly touch the buttocks and the feet are in flat-foot position.

Flat-feet and a weak back are often found in the same child.

Teach your child to place his or her feet "squarely" on the ground or squarely on the floor, whether they are sitting, standing or walking.

A slight degree of "pigeon-toes" may be desirable.

The purposes of exercises are to strengthen the supporting structures of the arches and to stimulate the circulation.

CHAPTER XXXIII

Nervous and Mental Disorders

GEORGE K. PRATT, M.D.
Revised by MORRIS FISHBEIN, M.D.

INTRODUCTION

ABOUT 9,000,000 people in the United States are suffering from mental illness and other personality disturbances—about 6% of the present population, or about 1 in every 16 people. Of this number, about 1,500,000 are suffering from mental illness. About 7,500,000, it is estimated, have other personality disturbances. In addition, there are about 1,500,000 mentally deficient people—conservatively about 1% of the population.

There are about 650,000 patients in mental hospitals. In addition, there are about 120,000 mentally deficient and about 20,000 epileptic patients in institutions for the mentally deficient and epileptic.

Each year about 250,000 new patients are admitted to mental hospitals. In addition, about 100,000 more are admitted who have been in mental hospitals before. Thus new admissions and re-admissions total about 350,000 a year.

About 30% of all the patients who go to general hospitals, and about 50% of all the patients who go to general practitioners suffer from mental illness and other personality disturbances or physical illnesses associated with mental illness and other personality disturbances.

Mental illness or other personality disturbances are usually significant factors in criminal behavior, delinquency, suicide, alcoholism, narcotic addiction, and often in cases of divorce.

At What Age Do Mental Illness and Other Personality Disturbances Occur?

Mental illness and other personality disturbances occur at all ages. Few cases of psychosis occur before the age of 15. The various psychoses have "preferred" age ranges for their initial development. They do not all affect the same age brackets to the same extent. Schizophrenia (dementia praecox) is the "psychosis of youth and early adult life." This disorder begins as a rule between the ages of 15 and 30. Few people develop it after 50. The most common psychoses of the middle age group—between 35 and 60—are manic-

depressive psychosis, general paresis, alcoholic psychosis, paranoia and involutional melancholia. The first three develop most frequently between the ages of 40 and 50. The last two are most common in their initial incidence between the ages of 50 and 55. The "psychoses of old age" are senile psychosis and cerebral arteriosclerosis. The great majority of cases develop after 60.

Emotional Health

Most people have minor emotional disturbances that are not recognized but have medical significance because of their effects on the general health. Many people in industry, in labor and in public life get along although they suffer at all time with difficulties of adjustment to their environment. From 30 to 60 per cent of all the people who come to the doctor as patients come primarily because of complaints due to emotional disorders, which are reflected as physical disorders. Frustrations, anxiety and fear may appear as headaches, ulcers of the stomach, asthma or similar conditions. Treatment is not fully satisfactory unless it takes care of the mental as well as the physical factors.

Our population has become an aging population. People live much longer than was common 50 years ago. As people get older they tend to develop more emotional experiences, and this has greatly multiplied the need of psychiatric help. One out of every twenty people will need advice or guidance from an expert for severe emotional illness at some time during his lifetime. This is proved by the fact that more than one-half of all the veterans in veterans' hospitals are psychiatric patients. Thirty-seven per cent of the men released from the army for medical reasons were for psychiatric disorders. A total of 51 per cent of all medical separations from the military service were due to personality disturbances. In addition people who are mentally disturbed constitute about one-half of all the patients in hospitals in the United States.

Often human beings become mentally and emotionally disturbed because of self-condemnation related to problems which they do not understand. The social and cultural considerations which regulate human sex behavior are far more rigid than the biological considerations. These considerations define what is moral much more definitely than do biologic and medical science.

In various portions of the United States the attitudes of people vary a great deal as to the ordinary relationships between the sexes. In some portions of the country it would be considered a gross violation of domestic relations for a married man to have lunch with a married woman other than his wife. In other branches of American society, and this refers of course particularly to our larger cities, such ordinary meetings are within the pattern of every day social existence.

When a young man moves in the United States from one community to another he may require several months to find out the restrictions on conduct which are considered suitable to the new community. Up to 1915 people paid very little attention to inhibitions and did not fret much about these matters. Since that time public education on psychological subjects has created fear among many people of being considered inhibited.

*People who are infantile in their emotional attitudes are likely to be de-
pendent on their parents or substitutes for the parents as for instance a govern-
ess or nurse and to expect infinite amounts of services and tolerance from
the parents. Sometimes men and women of advanced years retain this infantile
attitude until the death of the parent or some forced separation which may be
quite tragic in their lives. Thus a woman 38 years old who was subject to repeated moody spells had that kind of dependence and had to have someone
strong on whom to lean in all her difficult situations. The child who has been
"teacher's pet" as he grows up will have to be the "boss's favorite" when
he gets a job.*

*The child develops some sense of personal responsibility but can always
get rid of it by an excuse. The child still has to have complete trust in some
other person. People who grow up and maintain their childish level are people who always find excuses for the failures, alibis for their weakness and
who "pass the buck" whenever confronted with difficult situations. The child
who passes the period of puberty with its development of secondary sexual
characteristics really goes through two periods which may be called early
adolescence and late adolescence. The child in early adolescence begins to
have a drive for self assertion and begins to resent parental domination. Just
as the male animal shows his best characteristics for the attraction of the
female, so also the boys in early adolescence begin to show off and to indulge
in contests in which they can demonstrate their superiority. The boy's room
begins to be filled with trophies won at the track or in the swimming pool
or at other sports. The girl's room begins to be decorated with programs of
dances, souvenirs of parties and knickknacks accumulated on dates.*

*As late adolescence develops "dating" becomes the most important aspect
of life. If this passes on to what boys and girls call "going steady," difficult
mental situations may develop. Parents frequently try to dominate the situation because of economic, religious or purely emotional reactions. These situations may lead to emotional disturbances in the young that may mark the
life of the growing youth for many years thereafter.*

*Finally, adults are supposed to have a balanced perspective and to adjust
themselves to various social roles but adults still need affection, security and
well established relationships toward other people. If the adult has failed to
mature and depends heavily on the affection of others, if he requires definite
signs of favoritism, he is unlikely to be able to develop a satisfactory marriage
and may react emotionally to situations which he himself cannot solve.*

*Suitable adjustment of workers to their surroundings is important in estab-
lishing a smooth-running condition in any business or industry. Ask the
average businessman if he needs a psychiatrist in his business, and he will
think you are mentally disturbed. Psychiatrists, most people believe, spend
practically all of their time finding people who need to be confined in institutions because they are wholly irresponsible.*

Most large industries have employment interviewers who have knowledge of the positions to be filled, of the persons in the department and, therefore, of the kind of employee who will fit best and serve most satisfactorily under the circumstances. Most employment interviewers can recognize easily a prospective employee who is so far "off the beaten path" from a mental point of view as to be unsatisfactory for any job. No one suggests that employment interviewers should be replaced by psychiatrists or psychologists. What a businessman wants is a worker who can respond to the particular problems and procedures of the job for which he is employed. The boss seldom wants to be troubled about the general personality of an employee or the question of how he gets along with his wife. Nevertheless, that very situation may be important in relation to the quality or amount of work. Problems may arise which are due to a neurosis or psychosis in some employee whose mental condition has not been recognized.

Mental hygienists are convinced that training ought to be made available to employment managers or to the workers in the personnel divisions of industries. Workers are frequently transferred into personnel departments because they appear to be able to get along well with other people, but sometimes because they are hard and skeptical. Generally they work out their own technics, whether for the handling of personal problems or for the selection of new employees.

Already there are plenty of reports of instances in which employees who failed to respond acceptably to their executives were given scientific study and thus saved for the organization. We have learned how to modify the attitudes of parents and to improve their relationships with their children. Similar tactics are needed for executive businessmen to improve their relationships with their employees.

M. F.

Abnormal mental conditions were not always regarded as sickness. Departures from average mentality in bygone centuries were usually considered to be religious or legal problems. Not until well into the seventeenth century did medicine acknowledge responsibility for "insanity" as a variety of sickness. Not very much was known about its symptoms (except a few of the more violent, spectacular ones) and still less was known about what caused it or how to cure it. For a long time the best doctors could do for mental patients was to see that they were given humane care in suitable institutions and were no longer maltreated or subjected to the abuse that formerly was the lot of the insane in practically every country of the world. For this reason these institutions were called "asylums."

Gradually, physicians came to be interested in the mentally sick people and to engage in scientific research. First it was discovered that mental disease was not just one sickness, but was, instead, a term that applied to a large number of sicknesses; second, these various kinds of mental disease often had quite different symptoms; and third, some cases always seemed mild while others were severe. As a result it became possible to classify the different kinds of mental disease and to pin labels on them. For a long time physicians devoted most of their attention to describing, classifying, and diagnosing the many divisions and subdivisions and sub-subdivisions that were coming to be recognized.

Unhappily for the patients, this describing and classifying failed to do much in a practical way toward getting them well. At last the doctors called to their assistance certain other sciences, particularly psychology and philosophy. Between them they commenced to study the problem of *why* people acted as they did and what it was that made them say the things they said.

Some physicians attacked the problem from the conventional angle of physical medicine. They searched in the physical make-up of the patient's body for the motives that underlay human behavior. In many mentally disturbed people they were able to find physical diseases—or at least disorders of physical functions—that seemed to account for the symptoms. Thus, in that type of mental disease known as general paresis they saw with the microscope and often with the naked eye certain areas in the patient's brain where the consistency of the tissue was altered and partially liquefied. They also discovered (much later) that the cause of all the trouble in these cases was the tiny microorganism of syphilis which had invaded the brain and central nervous system. But when all was said and done, there yet remained a majority of all the known abnormal mental conditions for which the most scientific study failed to find any adequate physical cause.

Other doctors attacked the problem from the functional rather than the organic point of view. If unusual displays of behavior do not seem to have a physical cause, then let us begin with some of the cases in institutions that seem free from any organic disease and see what we can learn by studying, not just the structure and physiology of their organs, including their brains, but also their psychology. In other words, let's study man as a *whole*. This was a novel medical idea in those days, for up to that time most physicians had devoted their efforts to studying anatomical fragments of the patient such as heart or liver or lungs, and what these fragments did and how they acted. Now it was proposed to study, not so much what these special organs did, but what *the whole patient did* who owned these organs. This method finally became known as the study of "total reactions" and is the method that is being given increasing attention today. Essentially this is psychosomatic medicine.

The symptoms exhibited by men and women with various types of mental disorder have a close (if slightly disguised) resemblance to the basic personalities and traits of character that had marked these persons for many years before they became mentally sick. The mental disease symptoms, when properly interpreted, are seen to be but exaggerations of similar symptoms in evidence, perhaps, from childhood, but milder, of course, at that earlier age, and unrecognized then as anything more significant than "queer" or annoying or fussy habits of personality. There usually is a close connection between adult mental disorder and the development of unhealthy "patterns" (or habits) of personality during the plastic years of childhood, when personality is in the process of being molded. Often it is possible today to predict whether a child will grow up to become an adult who develops some form of mental disease, or whether he will go through life with his mental health unimpaired. Thus, a child whose "patterns" of personality are so sound and sturdy that they enable him to meet in a healthy manner disappointment in life, failure, or frustration is the child who will probably become an adult free from mental disorder. But another child may develop patterns that prove feeble reeds on which to lean when disappointment or failure confront him. As a consequence, he is unable to adjust himself in a wholesome manner to these trying experiences and is forced instead to flee into some form of mental disease as a sort of compromise adjustment.

CAUSES OF MENTAL DISORDERS

Why do people behave as they do? One patient was supposed to have become mentally sick because he lost his job and all his money. Another's mental disorder was attributed to a disappointment in love. As knowledge of psychiatry (which is that branch of medicine dealing with nervous and mental diseases) began to grow, it finally became evident that many of these alleged causes were not the real basic causes at all but merely *precipitating* causes. That is, the loss of money or the disappointment in love were only the last straws to break the camel's back—the final strains on an adjustive capacity that had never been strong in the first place. Otherwise, everyone who lost his money or was disappointed in love might be expected to develop mental disease as a result. The great majority of men and women faced with similar difficulties managed to adjust to them. So far as most functional mental disorders are concerned (those in which it is not possible to find a physical cause) the true and basic cause is a failure on the part of the patient to adjust himself to certain of the mental conflicts that beset him.

When a child is born into the world he brings with him a variety of psychological baggage. Part of this consists of his intellectual endowment, but at the moment we are more concerned with another part which might be called certain emotional tendencies inherited from his immediate ancestors—parents and grandparents. Still a third part—one that is beginning to receive a great deal of serious attention nowadays—consists of an assortment of primitive, savage instincts and "drives," which he also inherits as his share of the heritage of all mankind. These might be thought of as racial tendencies which the whole human race inherits from its ancestors of millions of years ago. These primitive instincts or "drives" include the instinct of self-preservation as well as that of race-preservation and many others. In those days, countless ages ago when man was first beginning his long painful struggle toward his present stage of development, there were few niceties. People did about as they pleased. If one cave man was hungry and his neighbor had a fresh piece of bear meat, the first man killed him—if he could—and took what he needed to keep himself alive. If a second cave man took a fancy to the woman of a third, he seized her—if he could—and henceforth she was his, at least until a still stronger cave man took her away from him in turn. Life probably was a pretty simple, crude (according to present standards), direct sort of affair. Men and women did what they wanted to whenever they felt like it with little to hinder them except the one restraint of superior physical strength, and there was scant place in the tribal code of that day for those more civilized feelings of altruism and unselfishness.

But slowly man came to be civilized. Slowly he came to realize that the first stirrings of finer needs within him could not always be satisfied by brute force alone, and that it was to the broader interests of that new, finer part of him, as well as to the interests of his group as a whole, to make a place in his scheme of things for regulations, prohibitions, and self-imposed restraints. This was not accomplished, however, without protests from the other part of him that longed for the "good old days" when there were no restraints and man did as he pleased unless someone stronger prevented. Here, then, developed mental conflict—a conflict between desire versus duty; between the savage, primitive instincts that formerly were expressed in crude, direct form with no pretense at disguising them, and the dawning realization that the demands of individual and social progress called for the repression or the transformation of some of these primitive instincts into more socially acceptable ones.

In the tens of thousands of years that have elapsed since this conflict first began, advancing cultural development has succeeded in annihilating these raw, primitive "drives" whose direct display had become, by this time, quite taboo. But here is where another discovery of modern psychiatry throws an interesting light on human behavior. Doctors know that the human body today harbors several vestigial remains or remnants of organs that have no known function in a 1950 model body, but which are believed to have served a vitally necessary purpose in the human body of millions of years ago. Thus, the human appendix has no known useful function in this day and age, unless, as some wag once remarked, it is to enable surgeons to ride in limousines. But in the psychological field something of the same thing is believed also to have occurred, and psychiatrists insist that modern man carries with him in the unconscious part of his mind certain vestigial remains of ancient instincts and impulses that once served a useful purpose when given frank, direct expression, but which thousands of centuries of civilization now demand be modified.

This is what is meant when we say that a child is born into the world with psychological baggage that includes—'way down deep in his unconscious— the carry-over of some of these primitive "drives." And this is why every modern nursery school teacher will tell you that the very young child is completely selfish (selfish, that is, when viewed from our adult standards) and completely antisocial as well. For the first two or three years of his life the child wants to do what he wants when he wants, without any interference. His tiny mental life for this period is much nearer that of his primitive cave-man ancestors than it is of his immediate generation, and at first he tries to act accordingly. He demands immediate gratification of all his desires. If he is hungry for food, he demands to be fed—instantly. If he is hungry for attention, he insists on being cuddled. If he is uncomfortable from a full bladder, he wets himself at once and in any place. He has no consideration for the feelings of others, and his chief aim in life is to get pleasure and avoid pain.

But as he grows older his mother begins to train him in food and toilet habits. She tries to teach him to control his wants, to wait for more appropriate times for their expression. She also, lovingly but firmly, gets it across to him that he can't always have his own way; that self-gratification is only possible through some consideration of others, or is dependent on the will of someone who is stronger. And so gradually he is required to submit to that process known as the "civilization of instinct," and he becomes a more socialized creature. But do not make the mistake of thinking that because he gradually checks some of his primitive desires and shows a willingness to give in to others, he has lost these desires or that he has become altruistic all of a sudden. To be sure, he has learned it is to his advantage to make concessions to this mother-person who has the power to bestow or withhold pleasure; who can approve or punish. And he likewise comes to the conclusion that gratification of his pleasure needs often must come in a roundabout manner, after first placating mother, who stands in the rôle of authority. That is how genuine unselfishness and altruism have their beginnings. The child learns that full gratification requires the coöperation of others, and he becomes altruistic only as he comes to realize that it pays to be altruistic because one gets the most pleasure out of life that way. Nevertheless, while he may submit gracefully to the "civilization of instinct" with a minimum of protest, the savage instincts are always there under the surface of consciousness, and the individual, no matter how old he grows to be, is forever trying to shape his mental life in accordance with what the followers of the school of dynamic psychology call the "pleasure principle." But opposed to this pleasure principle is another called the "reality principle." Both are pulling, in the unconscious mind of the person, in different directions. Swayed by the pleasure principle, he seeks to act in a way that will insure immediate gratification of primitive desires but avoids as much unpleasantness in the process as possible. In the opposite direction he experiences a pull from the reality principle which tends to shape his mental life according to the demands of necessity as personified at first by the stronger power of the parents and later by the customs of society. Dr. Abraham Myerson, a distinguished psychiatrist in Boston, writing about these conflicts, has this to say about them:

Every human being is a pot boiling with desires, passions, lusts, wishes, purposes, ideas and emotions, some of which he clearly recognizes and clearly admits, and some of which he does not clearly recognize and which he would deny. These desires, passions, etc., are not in harmony with one another; they are often irreconcilable, and one has to be smothered for the sake of the other. Thus, a sex feeling that is not legitimate, an illicit forbidden love has to be conquered for the purpose of being religious or good, or the desire to be respected. So one may struggle against hatred for a person whom one should love—a husband, a wife, an invalid parent, or child whose care is a burden—and one refuses to recognize that there is such a struggle. So also one may seek to suppress jealousy, envy of the nearest and dearest; soul-stirring, forbidden passions; secret revolt against morality and law which may (and often does) rage in the most puritanical breast.

In the theory of the subconscious these undesired thoughts, feelings, passions and wishes are suppressed and pushed into the innermost recesses of the being, out of the light of conscious personality, but nevertheless, acting on that personality, distorting it, wearying it.

For these reasons we say the real task of childhood is to bring about a balance between primitive, biologic desires on the one hand, and the demands of society as symbolized by mother and father, on the other. If a child can bring about such a balance, we say he is well adjusted and has good mental health. But if he cannot, then the degree of resulting maladjustment depends on the strength of the primitive impulse that grips him, as well as on the severity of the social demands made on him.

ADJUSTMENT OF BEHAVIOR

This ability to adjust one's self to experiences that thwart one's desires or primitive "drives" is an ability partially acquired during childhood. This may sound strange to those brought up to believe that mental disorders or emotional disabilities were a sort of curse visited on the patient through the processes of inheritance by an indiscreet ancestor. There *is* such a thing as heredity figuring in the causation of certain types of mental disorder, of course, and it would be incorrect to assume that the modern psychiatrist wholly disbelieves in heredity. Nevertheless, it has been too great a temptation in the past to attribute practically every display of human behavior we don't happen to like to this factor. Scientists have been forced in recent years to admit that much of the knowledge that exists about the laws of heredity in laboratory white mice and guinea pigs is not necessarily applicable to human beings. Indeed, there are few *facts* about human heredity known to science, and a vastly greater amount of research will be necessary before we will be in a position to say definitely what traits man inherits and what ones he forms after birth as imitations of or reactions to similar traits displayed by his parents.

Modern opinion, therefore, is veering around to the belief that the type of training a young child receives from its parents during the flexible years when its personality is in the process of being shaped determines pretty much how successful he is going to be in harmonizing the conflicts we have just mentioned, and how well he adjusts. For this reason increasing attention is being paid today to problems of mental hygiene and child guidance among normal boys and girls. Mothers, fathers, school teachers, and others may help the child form habits or "patterns" of personality so staunch and sound that these will aid him in meeting and adjusting to the inevitable frustrations in life that come sooner or later to each of us.

The formation of sturdy patterns of personality in these early years helps to explain why one person is able to adjust in a reasonable, healthy way to some distressing experience such as the loss of a loved one, loss of job, or the inability to attain some cherished ambition, while another, faced with a similar experience, cannot adjust to it and expresses his resulting maladjustment in terms of symptoms of some kind of mental disorder. A boy of six is taught by his parents to develop the healthy pattern of making his own tiny decisions and of finding his childhood security in the products of his own accomplishments rather than in having to depend for success on the personal favoritism of others. As this boy grows older and passes into adolescence these patterns remain with him, and he is able to cope with the mixture of adolescent emotions (made up of the desire to grow up and be independent, versus the wish to remain in the sheltered, protected state of childhood) with a minimum of difficulty. This ease of adjustment will likely be true also of his adult years when he will find himself able to meet adult responsibilities, disappointments, and rebuffs without having to run away from them by developing neurotic symptoms.

On the other hand, another boy of six may have a mother whose own emotional satisfaction in life can be gratified only by realizing that someone needs and depends on her. As a result she may develop what has come to be called an overprotective, oversolicitous attitude toward her child which keeps him emotionally tied to her and fails to allow him to become normally independent. As the physical and intellectual growth of such a child continues apace, his emotional growth tends to remain stunted. He reaches the physical age of adolescence, but because his principal patterns of personality are still the dependent childish ones of an earlier age period he is unable to adjust to adolescent demands and produces a variety of symptoms to express his maladjustment. Symptoms of this sort sometimes take the form of quarrelsomeness, defiance, or rebellion; or they may express themselves in the quieter but more ominous form of causing the youth to withdraw into a seclusive, shut-in, and solitary existence in which he forsakes the discomfort of trying to adjust to the world of reality in favor of retreat into a daydream world of fancy and imagination.

MENTAL TRAINING IN CHILDHOOD

Proper mental hygiene training in childhood, therefore, becomes extremely important if good mental health is to be maintained and mental disorder avoided. One of the most vital things of all in the process of helping a child form healthy patterns of personality is to assist him in creating a feeling of security for himself. By this is meant, not so much a feeling of physical or economic security as of *emotional* security. To feel emotionally secure a person must develop at least two firm convictions: first, that he is recognized as a person valued by others, and that he really belongs to and is accepted and needed by the group of which he is an intimate part. This means, first of all, by his family, then by schoolmates, next by the neighborhood in which he lives, and lastly, by society in general. The second conviction is that he can be confident of success in doing at least one thing really well. It matters little what this thing is providing the person is able to do it by means of his own efforts and is not dependent for success on the favoritism of someone else. To be able to do this gives a legitimate feeling of accomplishment and provides that poise and self-confidence that are the external signs of security.

DEGREE OF MENTAL DISORDERS

At the left-hand end of the line shown below exists a condition of normal or average mental health such as most of us enjoy. As we travel toward the right side of the line some interesting changes begin to appear. For example, somewhere in the vicinity of the point on the line marked (1) we may find that average mental health begins to show a flaw or two in its soundness. This may be manifested by nothing more unusual than the habit of temper tantrums or perhaps of chronic timidity in a child, or possibly by habitual irritability or a feeling of "touchiness" in an adult.

| MENTAL | (1) | (2) | (3) | MENTAL |
| HEALTH | | | | DISEASE |

But as we journey farther along the line toward the right, departures from average mental health become more obvious. At the point labeled (2), for instance, an individual may come to be thought of by his neighbors as "queer" in some way. Perhaps he shows a fanatical streak about religion or politics or some of the healing cults. If it happens to be a woman, maybe she is "queer" about keeping such an immaculate house that everyone in it is uncomfortable; or else she may go around with a perpetual chip-on-the-shoulder attitude, complaining that everyone else is trying to get the better of her. While still retaining more or less of the good mental health they started out with, such persons nevertheless show by their "queerness" that they already have traveled some distance from the left-hand end of our line.

At the point marked (3) mental health becomes unmistakably impaired, and the efficiency of the individual becomes correspondingly lessened. Now the symptoms are much exaggerated. If, previously, these people may have complained that the world has not given them a square deal, now they may develop definite delusions of persecution and arm themselves against their "enemies." Or it may be that other curious notions have crept in. They can't go into closed places or mix with crowds, or else they grow panicky when required to ride on the subway, or are obsessed with distressing ideas that they are going to faint or die.

At last the right-hand end of the line is reached. Here mental health vanishes completely and mental disease reigns supreme. Now the person is "insane," his patterns of adjustment broken down entirely.

There is no sharp or clear-cut line that divides mental health from mental disease. Mental health may be thought of as excellent, good, fair, or poor, grading imperceptibly to the right of this line toward the point where mental disease may be said to enter the picture. This point is extremely difficult to locate on the line because standards differ in different groups, and what might pass for merely a poor or even fair degree of mental health among one group of people or in one section of the world might well be labeled a mild degree of mental disorder in another. Moreover, it is only when mental disease has progressed from mild to extreme that we are justified in calling a person "insane."

INSANITY

"Insanity" is purely a legal term. It has no medical standing. It simply means that a given person's symptoms of mental disorder have grown so serious and his sense of judgment has become so faulty that the law steps in and makes it possible for others to decide for the patient what measures are necessary for his proper treatment and the safeguarding of his property. Although in this country alone there are more than three hundred thousand such "insane" persons in mental hospitals, there are doubtless twenty to thirty times as many others who display some signs of maladjustment or mental disorder of such lesser types as probably will never bring them to a mental hospital. While not in good mental health and often "queer" and hard to get along with, the great majority of these persons are never thought of by their fellow citizens as mentally sick. And yet, according to modern psychiatric conceptions of what constitutes mental disorder, the fears, worries, spells, and what not of these men and women are made of precisely the same stuff, although of course in lesser degree, as that from which definite mental disease is made.

This modern psychiatric conception of what constitutes mental disorder is explained admirably by Dr. C. Macfie Campbell, professor of psychiatry at Harvard Medical School, in the following:

A disorder is a mental disorder if its roots are mental. A headache indicates a mental disorder if it comes because one is dodging something disagreeable. A pain in the back is a mental disorder if its persistence is due to discouragement and a feeling of uncertainty and a desire to have a sick benefit instead of putting one's back into one's work. Sleeplessness may be a mental disorder if its basis lies in personal worries and emotional tangles. In fact, many mental reactions are indications of poor mental health, although they have not usually been classed as mental disorders.

Thus, discontent with one's environment may be a mental disorder if its causes lie, not in some external situation, but in personal failure to deal adequately with one's emotional problems. Suspicion, distrust, misinterpretation are mental disorders when they are the disguised expression of repressed longings into which the patient has no clear insight. Stealing sometimes indicates a mental disorder, the odd expression of underlying conflicts in the patient's nature. The feeling of fatigue sometimes represents, not overwork, but discouragement, inability to meet situations, lack of interest in the opportunities available. Unsociability, marital incompatibility, alcoholism, an aggressive and embittered social attitude; all these may indicate a disorder of the mental balance which may be open to modification.

How different is this conception from the older one that held there were only two varieties of people; the sane and the insane!

MENTAL DEFECT

Before going any further it is important that we digress for a few pages to explain about another kind of abnormal mental condition. This is not a condition of mental *disease,* but instead, of mental *defect.*

After talking with someone who is seriously mentally sick or "insane" many people are astonished to discover that the patient remembers things, knows what they are talking about, and that in general his intellectual faculties are usually not affected by his illness. This is due to the fact that most kinds of mental sickness are disorders of the patient's feeling or emotions and not of his intellect. To be quite accurate, there are a few kinds of mental disease (especially those associated with physical changes in the brain) in which the more advanced stages are accompanied by a lessening of intelligence, but for the most part patients ill from mental disease tend to retain much of whatever original intellectual ability they once possessed.

FEEBLE-MINDEDNESS

With mental defect, however, this is not true. A person who is mentally defective ("feeble-minded" is another term meaning the same thing) is one whose intelligence has never developed properly. Mental defect and mental disease, therefore, are two quite different things and should not be confused with each other. The illustration of two balky automobiles might be used to explain this difference. One auto balks and falters because the driver does not know how to manage its complicated machinery. This might be compared to mental disease where in most instances the auto itself (the human machine) is sound enough, but where the driver has not learned how to coördinate the use of brake, clutch, and gas throttle. On the other hand, a second auto may balk and falter despite excellent driving because there is a defect or flaw somewhere in the original machinery. This is comparable to a person with a condition of mental defect whose intellectual processes have been deficient since birth because of faulty heredity, birth injury, or the onset of infectious disease (measles, scarlet fever, "sleeping sickness," etc.) early in childhood.

In a very simple little pamphlet the late Dr. Walter Fernald, one of the great pioneers in this country in the study of mental deficiency, describes the symptoms of feeble-mindedness as follows:

The symptoms of mental defect vary according to the degree of defect. In extreme cases the defect is observable in early infancy. The baby does not "take notice" or follow sounds or bright lights, or smile, or grasp objects with his fingers, or have vigorous muscular movements, or nurse properly, and so forth. As he grows older his teeth may not appear at the usual age, or he may learn to walk late and with an awkward, shambling gait, or he may be late in using his hands, or his untidy habits may persist for a long time. He is very apt not to talk until he is three or more years old. In general he remains a baby for a long time.

In less severe cases the above symptoms may be less marked or absent and the defect may not be recognized until the child is found to be unable to learn in school at the usual school age, and cannot be promoted from year to year like other children.

He usually shows his defect in other ways. He may not be able to get along with other children in games and sports. He is often teased and picked on by playmates of his own age, but since they do not regard him as an equal he usually associates with children younger than himself. He is usually easily influenced and shows poor judgment and reasoning power. In general he is not able to meet new situations.

As he grows older he is apt to be led into mischief, since he finds it hard to resist temptation. If neglected or allowed to associate with evil companions they are rather more likely than normal persons to acquire immoral or vicious habits, although this tendency has probably been overstated. Some mental defectives seem innately vicious and troublesome from early childhood, but the majority seem about as amenable to proper associations and proper bringing up as do normal children.

In mental deficiency, whether the cause be inherited or acquired, medical science knows of nothing to do to repair the damage to brain tissue that is responsible for the condition. Consequently, it can never be cured. In this respect, also, mental defect is not like mental disease, where cure is often accomplished. But if mental defect cannot be cured, at least there is much that can be done to help the feeble-minded person make a reasonably satisfactory adjustment to life with whatever limited intelligence he possesses. In the higher grades (there are three recognized degrees of feeble-mindedness: the *moron* who is next to the normal in intelligence; the *imbecile,* who is next lowest on the scale, and lastly the *idiot*); in the higher grades early recognition of the defect will enable parents and teachers to avoid making too many demands that the child keep up to the standards of normal children. This will help him to maintain his morale and prevent him from developing feelings of inferiority as a result of encountering nothing but failure in life. Likewise, he can be trained in good habit formation that will stand him in good stead when his impulsive judgment threatens to fail him. Later, training in simple trades and occupations within their capacity of accomplishment is possible for children of the moron and upper imbecile groups. But like all people with unaverage mental conditions, the mental defective needs *individual* treatment. What works with one fails with another, and each case must be dealt with as a special problem requiring individual methods.

PREVENTION OF MENTAL DISORDER

What can be done about mental disorders? Modern psychiatrists are far more interested in learning why the patient had to take recourse in mental disease, and what his symptoms mean, instead of merely what they are. Instead of talking about the differences in symptoms of dementia praecox, or hysteria, or epilepsy, or some of the many other mental disorders, suppose we review briefly some of the important points already brought out and then proceed to a final discussion of what can be done to prevent or cure mental disorders.

The following outline of important viewpoints already mentioned may help to clarify the situation:

1. Mental health and mental disease blend into one another like the colors in the rainbow, with no sharp line of separation.

2. Since mind affects body, and vice versa, the *whole* patient must be studied, not just one detachable part of him.

3. Mental disorders never come suddenly. Except for those caused by an organic physical disease they have been in the process of making for many years before finally appearing.

4. Symptoms of mental disorders usually are but exaggerations of attitudes or traits of personality present in the patient for many years previously.

5. While there are thousands of different precipitating causes for mental disorders, most of them have one basic cause in common in an inability to adjust to certain inner conflicts or to the demands for conformity of the outside world.

6. This basic cause is practically always in the unconscious part of the patient's mind, and he is, therefore, unaware of what it is about.

7. Mental *defect* should not be confused with mental *disease*. The first has to do with impaired intelligence. The second with mismanaged emotions.

TREATMENT OF MENTAL DISORDER

Now for something about prevention and treatment. To do this it will be necessary to make a rough division in our material between children and adults, but with some inevitable overlapping. In childhood the job has two aspects. One is to help the child's parents help him to build up sound and sturdy mental health. The other consists in helping parents to nip in the bud before they get well established certain traits and attitudes which experience has taught will grow into some kind of mental maladjustment in later years. Please note the difference in the nature of these jobs. The first has to do with insuring mental *health*, while the second is concerned with preventing mental *disease*. One is like building a fireproof house from the ground up. The other is comparable to calling the fire department early before the fire gets completely out of control. The mental hygiene movement in this country has performed a valuable service to parents and teachers in the past with the second aspect of this job, but until very recently no one in the mental hygiene movement has attempted the more difficult task of building health in contrast to preventing disease.

By the time adult years are reached, there is relatively little that can be done by way of preventing mental disorders, except, perhaps, to keep milder ones from growing more serious. The treatment task also grows more difficult as the mental disorder becomes more deeply entrenched.

But to return for a moment to the maladjustments of children. These are expressed in a variety of ways. Temper tantrums, fussy, dawdling food habits, timidity, shyness, overconscientiousness, bed-wetting (in older children), bullying and aggressiveness, stealing, lying, truancy; all these should be regarded as danger signals pointing to some underlying conflict which must be sought out and discovered before anything practical can be done by way of permanently remedying the condition. But unlike the methods of treatment in other branches of medicine, the treatment of behavior disorders and undesirable personality traits in children can seldom be successfully undertaken by directing treatment to the child alone. His annoying behavior is a symptom of maladjustment somewhere within his emotional apparatus and is invariably bound up in some manner with the attitudes and emotional reactions displayed toward him by his parents. The treatment of the behavior problem, therefore, will require that these parental attitudes be taken into account. Indeed, so thoroughly is this believed by mental hygienists that they have created an axiom to the effect that "you cannot change the child's behavior until you first change the parental attitude that caused the behavior." Treatment primarily, then, *is directed toward the parents*, and this treatment consists largely in endeavoring to get them to modify the undesirable attitude that unwittingly and with the best of intentions they have adopted.

But what about the adult? And what kind of treatment is indicated for his mental disorder? Obviously, the answer must depend on the nature of his problem. In general, however, adult treatment can be thought of as comprising two main varieties: treatment of the basic emotional difficulty whenever this proves possible, and treatment of symptoms. One should never be satisfied with restricting treatment of mental disorders to symptoms alone unless there is nothing else to be done. Unhappily, in numerous cases of serious mental disease or "insanity," the case has progressed so far before psychiatric assistance is called that there remains little to do except to treat the symptoms. But with less severe cases—the psychoneuroses, for example, with their many fears, compulsions, anxieties, etc.—it is often quite possible to get at the roots of the trouble and effect a cure by means of a special type of treatment known as "psychotherapy." This method does not make use of medicines or physical kinds of treatment like massage, baths, etc., but relies for its effectiveness instead on a special emotional relationship between patient and psychiatrist. There are several different kinds of psychotherapy. One in particular is called "psychoanalysis" about which a great deal of misunderstanding exists. Only a comparatively few kinds of mental difficulty are suitable, at this stage of our knowledge, for psychoanalytic treatment. Moreover, as yet there are not many psychiatrists in this country who have had the indispensable special training that is necessary before one is competent to use psychoanalysis. But for the particular cases it is suited for, and in the hands of a well-trained psychiatrist, psychoanalysis enables us to explore the unconscious mind of the patient and, after locating the source of the conflict, is a most helpful procedure in the process of emotional reëducation which, if successful, restores the patient to an improved degree of adjustment.

PSYCHOTHERAPY

Other forms of psychotherapy are used for cases that do not require so deep an exploration into the unconscious. Thus, various kinds of suggestion are sometimes made use of, and occasionally even hypnosis, although most psychiatrists have come to the belief that hypnosis at best is of value only in the temporary relief of symptoms and is powerless to bring about a lasting cure. For this reason it is very little used by capable physicians.

The treatment of more serious conditions of mental disorder, like "insanity," where institutional care is required, is very complicated. Suppose we trace the treatment of an imaginary case of "insanity" and see what happens in an up-to-date hospital for mental disease. First of all, the patient has been, in all probability, behaving queerly for some months before the family has gotten courage to seek medical advice. He may have been depressed, or he may have been excited. Perhaps he has had delusions that others are following him, or that something has been placed in his food, or that "voices" speak to him, or what not. It makes little difference. The point is that the family at last recognize he is "not right." The family physician is consulted. He makes a careful examination, both physically and mentally, and either recommends that the patient be treated in a suitable public or private hospital for mental diseases, or, if the case is an unusually puzzling or obscure one, he may ask that the family authorize him to call into consultation a capable psychiatrist.

Some cases of this kind can be cared for at home, but in an overwhelming number of instances it is far better for patient and family alike if the former is removed to a hospital. This is a hard decision for relatives to make, for there still exists a great deal of cruel and unwarranted stigma about people who require mental hospital care. But it is almost certain that much of the patient's underlying conflict—the reasons for his becoming mentally sick—are tangled up in family relationships, and if he can get away from the well-meaning but unwholesome family atmosphere for a time his chances of early cure are improved.

So we will assume that the family agrees to hospital treatment. Next is the matter of commitment. This is merely a legal device to safeguard the interests of the patient. It consists in making application to a court for an order to have the patient admitted to a hospital in order that he can receive the special treatment available at such a hospital. In most states commitment can be made without undue publicity, the judge (unless he be vindictive or a stickler for the letter of the law) waiving the right to have the sick man haled before the court, and accepting the legally sworn-to certificate of the committing physicians who give their professional opinion that the patient is mentally sick and needs mental hospital care.

The patient arrives at the hospital. In modern, well-equipped state hospitals for the mentally sick he is first taken to the receiving ward, where he remains for ten days to several months, depending on the nature of his condition. While in the receiving ward he is examined very carefully by a number of physicians, and treatment for his immediate needs is prescribed. This may be rest in bed, plenty of nourishing food, and an occasional sedative, if sleepless or restless. But sometimes the patient is wildly excited on admission. Then it is likely that a special kind of treatment known as the "continuous bath" will be ordered by the doctor. This consists in greasing the patient's body with vaseline and then placing him in a specially constructed tub through which flows a gentle stream of water heated to whatever temperature is indicated. Usually it is just above body heat. A canvas sheet is placed over the tub to prevent the patient from getting out and an attendant or nurse is stationed near by to see that the sick man or woman does not hurt himself or slip under the sheet.

After a time the patient relaxes under the influence of the warm water. His excitement begins to subside, and he may even go to sleep. The continuous bath is a far more humane method of controlling excitement and violence than any other kind of restraint known, including hypnotic drugs and the strait-jacket. All up-to-date hospitals have them, and in better hospitals of this kind straitjackets, camisoles, and similar devices for confining the arms and legs of patients have been abandoned. Indeed, in many modern hospitals the only place a straitjacket can be found is in the hospital museum.

But perhaps the patient is depressed instead of excited. Possibly he has no appetite and refuses to eat, or maybe he has delusions that he has committed all sorts of fantastic crimes. He may accuse himself of having brought ruin on the family, or of being responsible for all the misery in the world, or of having committed the "unpardonable sin," whatever that may be. At any rate, he is deeply depressed, and the doctors understand that the chances are in favor of his contemplating suicide, if, indeed, he has not already expressed the intention of taking his own life. It is necessary, therefore, to safeguard him from self-injury. Such patients are usually very clever in managing to evade the nurse or others who are on the watch for attempts at suicide, and this is another reason why home care is dangerous, especially for depressed patients. Even under the most constant attention a patient may elude his nurse and dash through a window, or cut himself, or in some other way do away with himself. Eternal vigilance is the price of safety in such cases.

Sometimes the patient won't eat, and then another method of treatment is necessary. If he gets to the point where his refusal to take food threatens to retard his recovery, or if, as not infrequently happens, it comes down to a question of actual starvation, the doctor inserts a soft rubber tube through the patient's nostrils into his stomach and slowly pours down it a mixture of milk and eggs at necessary intervals.

But gradually the patient improves. Now he is transferred from the receiving ward to another. Here he will find other patients whose behavior is like his own and in various stages of recovery. Seeing other patients whose condition has improved is an incentive for our patient to make further progress. Presently he is encouraged to take walks on the ground outside and in company with a nurse or a group of others. He is given an opportunity to visit the occupational therapy department at frequent intervals, where, under skilled supervision, he can get his mind off his troubles and reëstablish habits of concentration and industry.

At last he is well enough to go home. And modern science has another victory to its credit. Unhappily, the hospital course of some patients is not as successful as the one we have described. Some mentally sick men and women are not allowed by their relatives to come to the hospital until their illness has reached such an advanced stage that little but kindly custodial care can be given them. Moreover, some kinds of mental illness seem to be of such a stubborn nature from the beginning that the case is almost a chronic one from the start. Nevertheless, it is astonishing to observe how the rate of recovery is steadily increasing. At the present time about 25 per cent of all first admissions to mental hospitals are completely cured, while an additional 15 per cent are able to return home, after a time, well enough to live in the outside community even though they are not completely recovered.

This recovery rate, however, depends to some extent on the kind of hospital the patient is treated in. Modern, up-to-date hospitals have no difficulty in maintaining this rate, but less progressive ones are usually able to do little more than provide custodial care for their patients. This is why there has come about a technical distinction between *treatment* hospitals and *custodial* ones. In the former every modern form of medical and psychiatric treatment is used to cure the patient. The staffs of doctors are recruited from alert, progressive men and women; the scientific equipment is the last word in efficiency, and the laboratories allow no promising method of treatment to go untried.

COMMUNITY HOSPITALS FOR MENTAL DISORDER

It must be confessed, however, that not all our state hospitals for the mentally sick are of this variety. There still exist backward hospitals where the superintendent is a political appointee whose professional skill has not advanced since his early medical training. In these institutions scientific apparatus is meager, and little or no advantage is taken of recent psychiatric discoveries.

In the last analysis the responsibility for backward mental hospitals rests on the community. It is an axiom as true in this field as in any other that a community gets just about what it is willing to pay for, in the way of public service. If citizens of a community are too negligent to insist on a high quality of psychiatric service, then they must be willing to take what is possible. A well-equipped and modern mental hospital costs money to run, but it also restores a much higher percentage of its patients to health. Any community can have this high quality of service if it wants to.

And now, just a word in closing about state hospitals in contrast to private hospitals or sanatoriums. Any generalizations are sure to do an injustice to certain institutions, but so far as generalizations are permitted, it may be fair to say that a modern *treatment* state hospital is likely to be a more effective place for a mentally sick patient than a *custodial* private one. There are a few private sanatoria not run primarily for commercial profit where some of the best scientific work in the country is being done. These hospitals are at least partially endowed by private funds, so that they are not wholly dependent on patients' fees for support. But if we except these (as well as a handful of commercial ones), then most of the others cannot afford the elaborate and expensive equipment or the legitimately higher salaries commanded by physicians of superior skill.

The modern state hospital, on the other hand, deals with several thousand patients instead of fifty or a hundred or so. It receives its funds from the state government and is thereby enabled to equip itself in the most effective manner. Furthermore, while the salaries of its staff are often lower than those of some private sanatoria, the progressive scientific spirit permeating the whole atmosphere and the opportunity to use adequate equipment tend to attract to it the better medical men and women in the psychiatric field. On the whole, therefore, if expense is a serious matter for the family to consider, it will be well for them to consider the state hospital (but *only* if it is a modern, progressive one) in favor of a small, inexpensive but custodial private one.

This story of mental disorders comes now to a close. Mankind has traveled far since those days, centuries ago, when sufferers from "insanity" were regarded as being afflicted with demons and evil spirits and chained in dungeons.

The mystery of mental disease has been stripped away, and now we are able to recognize it as a kind of sickness, often amenable in some measure to psychiatric treatment and curable in an increasingly large number of cases.

Modern psychiatry has new technics like the insulin shock and metrazol shock treatments, which are applied in cases of dementia praecox or schizophrenia and depressive forms of insanity. Similarly, electric shock to the brain has been tried. One of the latest technics is the removal of a portion of the frontal lobe of the brain for depressive forms of insanity. All of these methods are still highly experimental and should be used only by experts working in institutions.

A new apparatus called the encephalograph enables the doctor to determine if the activities of various areas of the brain are proceeding as the normal brain does. Most important is to detect the symptoms of mental disorder early. The earlier treatment is begun the better the chance for recovery.

CHAPTER XXXIV

Old Age

MORRIS FISHBEIN, M.D.

A LTHOUGH ONE HUNDRED YEARS of life is possible to human beings, only 30 people in 3,000,000 reach that age. And more than two thirds of the persons who do reach that age are women. The reason for this latter fact is that women are usually less exposed to accident and infection and, what is more important, are more apt to lead temperate lives.

Census figures from Great Britain show that the average number of persons more than 100 in the British Isles is about 110, and that 80 of this number are women.

These figures are not absolutely accurate, since most old people are proud of their age and tend to exaggerate. For example, in nearly every census, more people who give their ages as over 91 are found than people who give their ages as between 85 and 90. British health authorities assume that many jump from 85 to 91 in a year or two.

THE SPAN OF LIFE

However, the span of life is gradually increasing. And in time we may expect to have more and more people above 90. The chief reason for this remains the rapid decline in death rates for infants. Thus, a man born in 1854 had a life expectancy of 40 years. Now he may reasonably expect to live to be 68. Having reached the age of 60, a man's expectancy of life is now 14½ years, and a woman's 16 years.

Since heredity seems to play a large part in longevity, it is conceivable that encouragement of intermarriage between families that tend to live long would produce stock that tended to live long. However, such experiments among humans are almost impossible, and this theory must remain largely a matter of conjecture.

One of the real problems we have to face is to make the lives of the aged happier and healthier. They must realize their own shortcomings in regard to

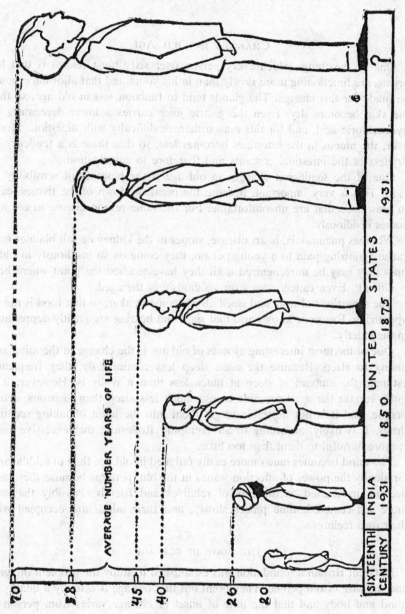

Fig. 86. Life expectancy.

strength and ability to throw off disease, while those around them should always take into consideration the changes which come with advanced age. If older persons observe the simple rules of health, there is no reason why their declining years should not be happy.

Changes in Old Age

One of the things which every person over sixty must realize is that his organs are functioning more slowly than in his youth and that allowances must be made for this change. The glands tend to function less in old age, so that the skin becomes dry. Even the gastric juice carries a lower percentage of hydrochloric acid, and for this reason there is difficulty with digestion. Moreover, the mucus in the intestines becomes less, so that there is a tendency to dryness of the intestinal contents and therefore to constipation.

One of the significant changes in old age is the blunting of sensibility to pain. This is very important, because the breaking down of the tissues leads to sensations that are uncomfortable. For the same reason disease in old age comes insidiously.

Whereas pneumonia, heart disease, stones in the kidney or gall bladder may cause agonizing pain to a young person, they come on so insidiously in older ones they may be unrecognized until they have reached the point where help is difficult. Even cancer comes on insidiously in the aged.

The sensations of taste and smell also become weaker, so that food is not so appetizing. Everyone knows also that sight and hearing are greatly depreciated in the elderly.

One of the most interesting aspects of old age is the change in the mind and ability to sleep. Because the aged sleep less continuously, they frequently estimate the amount of sleep at much less than it really is. However, it is quite certain the aged are able to use much less sleep than vigorous, active people, and it is not desirable to get them into the habit of taking sedative drugs. It is likely, according to Sir Humphry Rolleston, that excessive sleep is more harmful to them than too little.

The mind becomes much more easily fatigued in old age than in middle age. Gradually the power of affection wanes in the old, perhaps because they have become habituated to the loss of relatives and friends. Possibly they are more self-centered; time passes slowly, and their minds are occupied with their own feelings.

THE BODY IN OLD AGE

In Great Britain a foundation was established to study the problem of aging and the care of old people. They point out that old age is actually a quality of mind and body and that the time of onset of old age varies from person to person. For a number of reasons old age has been taken to begin at 60 for women and 65 for men, and these figures are taken as standard in pension acts.

People in advanced years require more medical attention than do those of younger ages. Nevertheless, one fourth of all the old people studied had gone for three years or more without seeking medical aid and in many instances had virtually never required any. More than 12 per cent of the people had gone so long since seeing a doctor that they could not remember when the last time was, and more than 7 per cent were certain that they had 20 years or more of good health.

They found relatively little undernourishment among the old people; in fact, only 3 per cent were classed as undernourished. The chief nutritional disturbance was a lack of iron, which affected about 5 per cent of the women.

It was found also that men tend to remain normal in body build as they grow old, whereas women show much growth variation in the direction of either leanness or stoutness. Twenty-five per cent of women over 85 years of age were undeniably obese.

As people grow old, they find more or less difficulty in getting around as well as they used to. Only 2½ per cent of the people over 60 years of age were confined to bed, and it was thought that the figure was low because old people who live at home have in most instances to help in looking after themselves. For that reason, if the aged find it necessary to be continuously in bed, they are transferred to institutions.

Almost one-fourth of the old people were capable of only limited getting about in their immediate districts. After 70 years of age the specific symptoms of old age are likely to become emphasized. These include weakness, dizziness, difficulty with traffic, inflammation of the back and lack of confidence.

Caring for old people at home puts a severe burden on the younger generation, many of whom carry this strain for years and years without relief.

Stairs are a particular problem when old people are concerned and when they are in poor health. At least one-third of old people have trouble getting up and down stairs or both ways. Stairs are especially a hazard when they are steep and when they lack a rail. Whenever old people are compelled to use stairs, there should be a rail to help them. Over 6 per cent of old people were unable to use stairs at all. The trouble with stairs was especially hard on old women because of their desire to participate in housework. Old people themselves recognize the special problem that is presented by stairs, and a large majority think that bungalows are the ideal type of home.

Among the medical conditions that affect old people most are rheumatism or arthritis, the effects of falls or accidents, and bronchitis.

Almost half of all old people are troubled with coughs, and men more than women. Rheumatic conditions of one kind or another affect more than half, and they vary from just twinges of pain to crippling incapacity from involvement of the joints. Women are more frequently affected than men, and this is particularly hard on them because of the nature of their work in the household.

Men have a liability to gout nearly ten times that of the women. Pain in the feet affects nearly 40 per cent of the old people and women twice as often as men. Another symptom that causes much distress is frequency and urgency of emptying the bladder. This affects one-third of all the old people. It is commoner in women than in men, and it makes shopping difficult.

Difficulties in hearing affect men more than women. Some dizziness is experienced by at least 75 per cent of the women over 85 years of age, and difficulty in getting about in the dark is a symptom for more than 90 per cent of women over 85. However, in general, old people are extremely unsteady in walking, some of it due to dizziness, some to failure to lift the feet properly.

DISEASES OF OLD AGE

Even premature senility may occur in youth. Heart disease, atrophy of the brain, and hardening of the arteries may also occur in comparatively young people. However, most of the diseases that occur in the aged are the result of gradual breaking down of the tissues. These include hardening of the arteries, heart failure, hardening of the liver, enlargement of the prostate, cancer, obesity, and indigestion. However, old age does modify any disease, so that it is different from the same condition in youth.

Measles, scarlet fever, typhoid, and diphtheria occur very rarely in old people, probably because they have been infected in youth and thereby developed immunity from these diseases. The form of sick headache called migraine usually becomes less troublesome as age advances and may disappear with increasing years. A recent conception of this disease indicates that it may be the result of sensitivity to some protein food substance, and perhaps the repeated attacks eventually bring about desensitization.

Even when an aged person is in good health, he must keep a close watch for the diseases to which his age makes him particularly susceptible. Happiness for all elderly persons is principally a matter of health, and so health must be guarded more and more closely as time goes on.

The changes that occur in the skin of the aged are due to gradual loss of activity on the part of the glands and of the tissues responsible for immunity. Because the aged are likely to be a little less scrupulous in the care of the skin, slight infections occur repeatedly. There are also bed sores. Itching is a stimulus to severe scratching and secondary infections take place in the scratches.

The blood vessels may lose their contractile power, and there are occasionally tiny hemorrhages under the skin. One of the most severe conditions that affects the aged is the reaction called herpes zoster. It is a form of shingles which develops along the course of a nerve and which in the aged may be exceedingly painful. Moreover, once the attack has passed, the pains may continue and return at intervals without the eruption. These conditions must be watched closely and treated immediately.

Of course, the aged suffer frequently with dizziness due to many possible causes. Sometimes it is due to accumulated hard wax in the ear, sometimes to changes that have taken place in the internal ear; frequently it is associated with high blood pressure, hardening of the arteries, and changes in the circulation of the blood in the brain. Sometimes the result is a difficulty of coördination between the eye, the ear, and the sense of balance, so that the aged may stagger or fall when the eyes are raised suddenly or under some similar stimulus.

One of the diseases more likely to occur in the aged than in the young is paralysis agitans, or the shaking palsy. Although this disease may occur in youth, the vast majority of cases occur in people between fifty and seventy years of age. The disease occurs twice as often in men as in women. It is marked by tremor of the hands, with a pill-rolling movement, and it tends to progress, running a complete course in from ten to fifteen years.

The aged should be especially careful to consult a good physician when any of the symptoms described in this article occur. While they may be simple results of old age, without more serious implication, they should be checked at frequent intervals by the family doctor.

EXERCISE AND HYGIENE

Old people have particular difficulty in walking, for many reasons. First, there may be weakening in the circulation; sometimes pain in the muscles results from imperfect circulation. Often older persons walk with short steps, because in this way they are better able to control their sense of balance.

While the aged may have high blood pressure, it is not so serious as in youth.

Of course, old people suffer with disturbances of digestion because of the changes that have taken place in their secretions, and also because they have difficulty in keeping infection away from their teeth and because they do not chew the food properly. The constipation of old age is now largely controlled by the taking of mineral oil which serves the purpose of softening the intestinal mass and making elimination easy. This remedy is practically harmless and adds years of health to many older persons. Hemorrhoids are frequent in the aged and are, of course, associated with constipation.

There was a time when the teeth of the human being gradually fell out as he grew older so that he found himself, by the time he reached old age, able to take only liquid food or food that was soft. Modern dentistry has made it possible for the aged to chew steaks or vegetables of considerable fibrous content. It is for this reason that the aged must frequently resort to laxatives or to mineral oil in order to aid the weakened intestinal muscles in handling the waste material.

The aged are likely to suffer particularly with accumulations of mucous material in the lungs; with diminished power of the lungs to repair themselves, small areas of degenerated tissue break down, and the material accumulates and has to be coughed out of the lung. The continued inhalation and coughing results in disturbances such as bronchopneumonia or similar complaints.

The elderly are particularly prone to varicose veins, to inflammations of the joints, and to fixed joints which follow inflammation.

CANCER IN OLD AGE

Cancer has always been recognized by the medical profession as a disease of old age. More recently it has seemed to occur fairly frequently among younger people, and there are many explanations advanced for this fact. It is recognized that heredity plays a large part in cancer, and that inbreeding may bear some responsibility. The British statistician, Karl Pearson, found that the maximum incidence of cancer occurs at the age of forty-six in women, and of fifty-six in men. The chief cancer period is from forty-six to sixty-four years.

It is well established that cancer is associated with long continued irritation of susceptible spots in the tissue. Obviously aged people are more subject to long continued irritation than are the young. Men suffer, of course, much more frequently than do women with cancer of the lips and tongue, perhaps because of their smoking habits. Even though women have begun to smoke cigarettes regularly, it is unlikely that they will suffer as much with cancer of the lips and tongue as do men, because women are much more careful about the state of their mouths and teeth. Men suffer with cancer of the prostate; women with cancer of the organs particularly concerned with childbearing.

There have been many attempts to explain cancer in old age, but all of them are theoretical. In old age the degenerative process in the cells leads to the formation of new tissue, and the repeated demands made on the cells in this way may result in the sudden rapid growth that is called cancer. Warthin, eminent pathologist, considered cancer to be merely a sudden rapid aging of a group of cells.

Whatever the cause may be, older persons should be especially careful to treat all slight infections and to visit a physician if these irritations do not respond readily to treatment.

The chapter on cancer in this book gives the most recent and reliable information available.

THE CRITICAL AGE FOR MEN

Pediatricians say that the first year of life is the most critical. Others insist that the first 10 years are the hardest. Some call adolescence with the transition from childhood to adult life the most critical period.

The great control that is now asserted over infant mortality and the elimination of many of the diseases that used to affect youth make the majority of doctors today think that the most serious age is the period of transition from maturity to old age. Men enter the most critical period of their lives at 50. This is the time when they begin to need glasses to read the print in the telephone book. Now they begin to get tired a little earlier in the afternoon.

Occasionally, the onset of these conditions induces resentment. Many a physical culture expert or the proprietor of a health institute or a gymnasium has earned an excellent livelihood from the fact that these men take up exercise and try to prove to themselves that they are better than they really are. The wise man will realize that aging is a natural process and that the conditions that come with advancing years must be treated with respect. If the thyroid gland, the sex glands and the pituitary are less efficient, the deficiency will be reflected in the body generally. A doctor can prescribe glandular substances to overcome such deficiencies in part.

Hardening of the arteries and high blood pressure are two of the most important symptoms. Many years ago a wise physician said that a man is as old as his arteries. Incidentally, men are more frequently affected with hardening of the arteries than are women.

Arthritis is another condition that occurs many times to people after the age of 40 and which cripples and disables a good many older people.

Medicine can do a great deal for these disturbances if they are brought soon enough to medical attention. But man is not immortal and the wise man will recognize the aging process and conduct himself accordingly.

THE OLD MAN AND THE JOB

Women in the home keep on at their job of running the household and taking care of the family as long as they are able. Many of them find work ready to handle even up to seventy-five or eighty years of age. By contrast the man retired at anywhere from sixty to seventy years of age may find himself full of the desire to work and produce and to contribute to the public good and yet be shut out of his opportunity to do the work that he can do best.

The professional man who can serve as a doctor, a lawyer, a clergyman, an artist or a writer can keep on without too much difficulty. The worker in industry finds the situation much more difficult, regardless of his physical or mental age. As a man gets older he loses speed and those who operate machines find that they cannot keep up. Furthermore, the conditions of industry do not provide for continued work at a lesser wage but insist that the full wage be paid regardless of advancing years. Insufficient study has been given to the kinds of work that are especially suited to the older worker, aside from employment as a timekeeper or foreman or administrator. If the old men are kept on too long the younger men complain that there is no opportunity to rise in the establishment. Power and increased income are likely to go with promotion and few old men wish to go back to positions of less influence or income.

Many men anticipate with the greatest of pleasure the day when they are to retire from work. These are the men who dislike the job to begin with, and who have an avocation which gives pleasure and to which they can devote themselves after retirement.

Physicians are convinced that a busy rather than an aimless life is the ideal prescription for old age. For too many instances are known of fairly young men who retired only to die within a few years from what seemed simply to be the ultimate effects of boredom and self-neglect.

A survey in Britain showed that the care of the aged for the most part rests on the family, and then the neighbors where there is real community life and spirit. In one community 57% of the burden rested on one daughter and there was little indication that multiple daughters shared the responsibility. Usually it was the youngest daughter that carried the burden, and the older ones reserved the right of criticism.

EMOTIONAL PROBLEMS OF OLDER PEOPLE

An editorial in the American Journal of Public Health calls attention to recent scientific studies of the special emotional hazards that are characteristic of advancing years.

As people grow older they develop limitations on vision and hearing and a reduction of physical activity and of endurance. They also begin to have difficulties in remembering and in coördination. Fortunately the specialists in sight and hearing are now able to give great aid toward supplementing weaknesses in sight and hearing. We are also learning much about rehabilitation and measures for helping people who are failing physically.

Older people often begin to find incomes steadily reducing with expenses steadily increasing. True social security aims to help in meeting the situation but other trends incline toward putting older workers completely on the shelf.

Many older people having given up their steady occupations have failed to develop any hobbies or outside interests to which they can turn their attention. Their lives assume continuous boredom and ultimate depression.

As a husband or wife is lost the friends of the family incline to fall away from the remaining member and social contacts diminish leading to loneliness and introversion.

In ancient societies the aged were viewed with respect and came to be the Nestors, advisers and counsellors. Our modern civilization drifts to an opposite extreme where all the emphasis is placed on youth.

The American Journal of Public Health says "we would do well to recognize the assets as well as the liabilities of senescence; to train ourselves in middle age for ripe and fruitful later years; to provide the medical and psychiatric and rehabilitative aids needed for healthy aging; and to regard the elderly not as outcasts but as essential and potentially valuable elements in the life of the family, the neighborhood and the nation."

CHAPTER XXXV

Drugs and Their Uses
MORRIS FISHBEIN, M.D.

Modern man is protected against disease, is relieved of pain, and occasionally cured by discoveries that have been made in the professions of pharmacology, pharmaceutical manufacture, and pharmacy.

HOUSEHOLD REMEDIES

Elsewhere in this book is a discussion of the family medicine chest with a list of the household remedies that are easily available and which may be used by any person according to his own judgment. For example, the laxatives like mineral oil, phenolphthalein, cascara, and substances like agar and psyllium seed which add bulk to the excretions. Included also are such mild antiseptic substances as iodine, mercurochrome, and similar preparations. For pain relievers there are combinations of aspirin, phenacetin, and caffeine, sold under a wide variety of names, as well as simple preparations which include aspirin alone or aspirin buffered or other products related to aspirin.

Most of the potent and possibly toxic preparations prescribed by doctors are not sold over the counter without a physician's prescription. The Federal Food, Drug and Cosmetic Act regulates the labeling of drugs. It prohibits certain statements from appearing on the labels and demands warning labels for other substances which may be habit-forming or which are especially toxic. A new drug cannot be introduced into sale between the states unless an application has been made for it. This application must show by adequate scientific evidence that the drug is safe for use under ordinary conditions.

PRESCRIPTION DRUGS

The American Medical Association's Council on Drugs publishes annually a volume known as "New and Nonofficial Drugs" in which drugs are classified as to their general character. If the product is manufactured properly and the claims made for it are justified it is described in this book.

ANESTHETICS

Anesthetics are not of course easily available except by prescription and are generally used only in the hospitals and in the doctor's office. Local anesthetics are substances which may be put on the skin or injected under the skin and thus produce freedom from pain in the areas concerned. One type of anesthetic is injected into the spine to block the nerves of the spine, thus preventing pain during childbirth. When the drug is permitted to flow in gradually during the childbirth, the method is described as continuous caudal analgesia.

The general anesthetics include a wide variety of substances, such as ether, nitrous oxide, oxygen gas, ethylene, cyclopropane, and several other substances which the anesthetist gives to the patient for inhalation. Another type of anesthesia is basal anesthesia in which drugs capable of blocking sensation are injected into the veins. These are usually derivatives of barbituric acid.

ANTIHISTAMINES

During allergic reactions a substance known as histamine is released into the tissues. The antihistamines are used in such conditions as hay fever, asthma, and rhinitis because they block histamine. When these substances are used in mild hay fever, particularly in the first part of the season, they are usually effective in relieving symptoms.

The antihistamine drugs are useful also in the prevention and treatment of general reactions such as the allergic coughs, the allergic inflammation of the nose, the eruptions of hives, and the itching which accompanies other allergic diseases.

Any of the antihistaminic drugs can occasionally produce undesirable reactions in some people. The physician must be aware of this possibility. Sometimes the antihistamines produce a tendency to deep sleep. In other instances they may produce inability to concentrate, dizziness, and disturbed coordination. The worst symptoms that may result are tremors, nervousness and even convulsions. These are some of the reasons why the antihistamines in large doses should be used only when prescribed by a doctor. Several antihistamines are available in drug stores and can be purchased without a prescription. These are usually used to stop excessive secretion from the nose during the beginning of a cold and sometimes are applied in ointments for ivy poisoning or other skin reactions.

MOTION SICKNESS DRUGS

Most of the effective motion sickness drugs are now dependent on an antihistamine action. Among the most common of these are Dramamine, Bonine, Marezine, and various other preparations of antihistaminic drugs.

For years derivatives of scopolamine and hyoscine have been used effectively in preventing motion sickness.

Since all of these drugs possess the possibility of harm, they should not be taken continuously unless prescribed by the doctor. On most ships and on airplanes the attendants usually have available some of these anti-motion sickness remedies and they will give one or two doses with the understanding that the dosage is not continued and is only for immediate relief over a short period.

ANTI-INFECTIVES

Certain substances have the power to stop the action of bacteria, to impede their growth, and sometimes to destroy them. For instance certain drugs are known to be effective in controlling the germ of tuberculosis. These include streptomycin, one called PAS or para-amino-salicylic acid and also isonicotinic acid derivatives of which the one most frequently mentioned is isoniazid. There are several forms of these drugs known by various names which the physician prescribes according to his choice.

A substance known as oxyquinoline is available in various forms and is used frequently against germs or fungi.

Another drug called mandelamine has the special property of being eliminated in the urine and acting as a urinary antiseptic.

Another chemical group is known as the nitrofurans. These substances and their derivatives are effective against a variety of diarrheal disorders, infections in the urinary tract, and infections throughout the body, particularly by the pus-forming germs.

Among the earliest and most important of the anti-infective substances were the sulfonamides, discovered by Domagk, for which he received the Nobel Prize. The sulfonamides are available in a variety of forms. The ones to be used in the control of a known infection are chosen according to their established ability to stop the growth of the germs that are concerned. Among the best known sulfonamides are sulfadiazine and sulfamerazine. Another is sulfamethazine. A newer form is sulfacetamide which is available in various forms, depending on the area of the body where it is to have its effect.

The modifications of the sulfa drugs are numerous. Still another is known as Kynex or Midicel. There are varieties of gantrisin which are designed to affect specific portions of the body and to be used either in tablets, capsules, or given by injection.

ANTIBIOTICS

The antibiotics are substances derived from various living organisms which can stop the growth of germs or destroy germs. The first to receive extensive use was penicillin. Then came many others of which about twenty are in common use. Their names are streptomycin, Chloromycetin or

Chloramphenicol, Bacitracin, Tyrothricin, magnamycin, Seromycin or cyclo-serine, Erythromycin or Ilotycin, Neomycin, Albamycin, Nystatin or Myco-statin which is used especially against monilia.

Another group includes oleandomycin which is especially active against germs like the staphylococcus, the streptococcus, and the pneumonococcus. It may also have effects in stopping the growth of the gonococcus and the meningococcus. Of this variety is Cyclamycin.

Penicillin is used in a variety of ways, either by tablets taken by mouth, or capsules, or by injections under the skin, according to what the physician thinks is best for the individual patient.

Among the variety of forms of penicillin is crysticillin (which is a com-bination of penicillin with a local anesthetic). Some forms of penicillin have been prepared so that they may be injected into the muscles and remain active over long periods of time.

Another new antibiotic is polymyxin, also ristocetin, and the various tetracyclines which include Aureomycin, Terramycin, Achromycin, and Panmycin. Most recent are Vancomycin and Viomycin.

Especially important is the fact that there are some two thousand possible antibiotics. One of the latest to be developed is an antibiotic which apparently can affect the growth of cancer cells. This is known as actinomycin D.

ANTIFUNGAL AGENTS

Various fungi may attack the human body, infecting the skin or the lungs or, indeed, other portions of the body. One substance which attacks them particularly is griseofulvin but there are other substances derived from chemicals such as Iso-par, Asterol, Sterisil, and Sodium Caprylate. Another is Triacetin, and one of the most frequently used is Undecylinic Acid which is commonly called Desitin.

ANTIMALARIAL AGENTS

Malaria is caused by an organism known as the plasmodium which occurs in various forms in the body. Quinine and various derivatives of quinine which have been developed act particularly against the malarial organisms. Among the important derivatives are Camoquin, Aralen, Primaquine, Dara-prim, and Atabrine, which was much used during World War II. Because these drugs are so powerful they are used only when prescribed by a physician and in the manner prescribed. The drugs may be used to cure malaria or even taken to prevent malaria.

ANTIPEDICULAR AGENTS

Pediculosis is caused by three varieties of lice, which are commonly called the head louse, the body louse, and the crab louse. A number of drugs have been developed which are especially active against lice and these are called pediculocides. These drugs are applied externally and great care is taken to see that they do not get into the eyes or on the mucous membranes.

DISINFECTANTS AND ANTISEPTICS

Among the most important of all disinfectants is chlorine. An ideal disinfectant has never been discovered because such a substance would have to have the power to destroy all forms of all infectious agents and still not be injurious in any way to human tissue cells or be capable of causing sensitization in human beings. Every antiseptic must, therefore, be used in relationship to its effects not only on the organisms that are to be destroyed but also on the human body. Various antiseptics and disinfectants depend principally on chlorine, mercury, silver, peroxides, carbolic acid, soaps, and similar substances.

VERMIFUGAL AGENTS

The human being is susceptible to infestation with a great number of worms, such as the pinworm, the whipworm, the tapeworm, and hookworm, the filaria, and even such strange worms as the loa loa. Drugs have now been developed which can rid the body of these worms but as with the disinfectants and antiseptics, they must be used with great care because of the danger of toxic reactions.

ANTICANCER DRUGS

Already there are available and in use under controlled conditions in hospitals a number of drugs which can destroy the cells of cancer. These are known as cytotoxic agents. Many of them are highly poisonous and, therefore, they must be used only under completely controlled conditions. Among older drugs which have been used in this way are derivatives of arsenic and urethan, also nitrogen mustards and substances derived from folic acid which stop metabolism. X-ray is used to destroy cancer cells and radioactive isotopes may be used directly in contact with cancer cells. There are also hormones like estrogens and testosterone which act against the spread of cancer cells.

AUTONOMIC DRUGS

Certain drugs act particularly against pain in the nerves, against the effects of stimuli coming along the nerves, and in the tissues of the brain. One class of these drugs is known as the autonomic drugs since they are concerned with the effects of nerve impulses coming through the autonomic nervous system. This is also known as the sympathetic nervous system.

Some drugs induce responses by the body which mimic the responses which come when stimuli pass along the nerves of the sympathetic nervous system.

One of the autonomic drugs is amphetamine or benzedrine. This acts to overcome depression. Its effects are opposed to those of the sedative drugs like the barbiturates. This drug has been found useful in depressing the appetite and it alleviates sleepiness and fatigue; however, it is not desirable to eliminate fatigue by destroying the sensation. The real answer to fatigue is rest. The dangers lie in the elimination of the warning signal of fatigue in people who are overdoing. There is also the possibility of habit-formation from continued use. And finally there are possible dangerous effects on the circulation of the blood.

Other drugs of similar type are Dexedrine, Paredrine, Octin, and Isoprel. The number of possibilities is considerable and perhaps a score of drugs acting in a similar way will eventually become available.

Some drugs are used to constrict the membranes of the nose—as adrenalin and Privine. An appetite destroyer is Preludin.

ADRENERGIC BLOCKING AGENTS

Drugs have been found which can block the stimuli coming through the sympathetic nervous system. These drugs act to oppose the action of adrenalin. They lower blood pressure by causing dilation of the blood vessels and they stimulate the action of the intestines. Usually they increase the heart rate.

Among the most well known of these drugs are ergotoxine, ergotamine, piperoxan, and dipenamine.

CHOLINERGIC AGENTS

These drugs act to produce effects such as occur when the parasympathetic nerves are stimulated. They can slow the action of the heart, dilate blood vessels, and increase gastrointestinal motion and secretion. Most of these drugs are derived from a substance called choline.

DRUGS USED FOR THE HEART

Cardiovascular drugs are those whose action on the heart and other portions of the blood vessel system affect either the total output of the heart or distribution of blood to various branches of the circulation. Some of these drugs affect the rhythm and output of the heart; others dilate blood vessels, and still others may act to affect hardening of the arteries.

Most important of all drugs for the heart is digitalis and associated with it a variety of preparations and derivatives.

Many substances have been discovered which have a specific effect on high blood pressure. All of these are potentially toxic and can be used only when prescribed properly by the physician. One of the best known is hexamethonium, also Apresoline, mannitolhexanitrate, Inversine, Ansolysen, and Metamine.

CENTRAL NERVOUS SYSTEM

Many drugs have their principal actions in depressing the central nervous system. These include anesthetic drugs, hypnotics, and sedatives. Here also come the anticonvulsants, the drugs used against cough, and the tranquilizing drugs.

The analgesics are used to relieve pain. For this purpose morphine is best known, but similar effects are had from milder salicylates like aspirin and phenacetin. These mild analgesics do not produce addiction and are usually considered safe for sale without a prescription.

The more powerful drugs which have been developed must be sold only with a prescription.

Many modifications have been made of opium and its derivatives, including morphine. All of these substances must be prescribed only with the use of a license to prescribe under the Anti-Narcotic Act.

Many persons have become accustomed to taking sedative drugs in order to encourage sleep. There are great numbers of barbituric acid derivatives which are used for this purpose. These are effective as sedatives and are used in insomnia, hysteria, nervousness, mental disturbances, and epilepsy. They act directly on the central nervous system.

Insomnia is of several varieties: One in which falling asleep is difficult; another in which sleep comes easily but is very quickly disturbed so that the person awakes frequently during the night or exceedingly early in the morning. Drugs should never be taken routinely for this purpose. Sleep may be promoted in a variety of ways. Perhaps it is best that sleep-producing drugs be used only when prescribed and only in the manner of use prescribed by the doctor. A very small dose of a sleep-producing drug may start the sleep and thereafter the person sleeps well throughout the night.

Many sleep-producing drugs are followed by hangover which seriously interferes with the usual activities.

ANTICONVULSANTS

Many drugs have been discovered which can stop the convulsions of epilepsy or other convulsive disorders. Among the best known are Dilantin, Peganone, Phenurone, Paradione, Tridione, Mysoline, Milontin.

These drugs are of the greatest importance because today thousands of persons with convulsive disorders are enabled to go months or even longer without a convulsion through proper use. Because of their potency, only a physician who has thoroughly studied the patient and who understands the nature of the convulsive disorder should prescribe the drug of his choice according to the needs of the individual patient.

Certain other drugs which act on the nervous system may prevent cough by their local effects on the nervous system and on the tissues involved in coughing. Codeine, a derivative of morphine, is a powerful drug in preventing coughs. There are, however, other drugs not derived from morphine which prevent cough through action on the nervous system.

The tranquilizing drugs include particularly Thorazine, Pacatal, Trilafon, Compazine, Sparine, Dartal, Vesprin, and Temeril. Under this group also come the derivatives of rauwolfia which includes Serpasil, Reserpine, and similar preparations. Most widely known of the tranquilizers is meprobamate which is also known as Equanil. This, however, is a relaxant drug rather than a depressant.

NERVOUS SYSTEM STIMULANTS

There are drugs which stimulate the nervous system and which are used to overcome depressions, to energize the body, and to oppose the actions of sedatives and tranquilizers. Many of these drugs are toxic in the sense that they may raise the blood pressure, stimulate the beating of the heart, and produce great breathlessness.

For years people have known that tea and coffee, which contain caffeine or theobromine or theophylline, have the power to stimulate. Students have taken caffeine or many cups of coffee to keep awake during study. Some derivatives of choline and of xanthine have effects of stimulating the central nervous system. New psychic energizers which control endogenous depression are Nardil Catron Tofranil and many more.

CONTRACEPTIVES

Contraceptives are used to inhibit the action of the sperm cells or to prevent the passage of the sperm into the uterus. They are of many varieties and are discussed under other sections of this work.

SKIN REMEDIES

The number of chemical substances used upon the human skin runs into hundreds. These are used to protect the skin, to control blemishes, to disinfect the skin, to stop itching, to take care of scaling and oiliness, to remove the skin, and for many other purposes. In the chapter on the skin many of these remedies are thoroughly discussed.

ALCOHOL DETERRENTS

Among the new remedies recently developed are drugs like Disulfiram or Antabuse which cause the person who takes them to develop unfavorable symptoms to drinking alcohol. Such a drug obviously must be used with the greatest of care because of the possible dangers from poisoning.

ENZYMES

Within the human body there are many substances produced which act to aid the functions of the body. For instance, one enzyme called hyaluronidase can limit the spread of fluids in the body and is used to prevent scar tissue.

Another enzyme can inactivate penicillin and is used when there are toxic reactions from the use of penicillin.

Some enzymes prevent clotting of the blood and are used to dissolve clots. One such enzyme, Chymotrypsin, is injected into the eye to loosen the tissues around a cataract.

STOMACH AND INTESTINAL DRUGS

Persons who suffer from excess acid can take drugs which stop the *flow* of acid. Other drugs protect the wall of the stomach against the *effects* of acids.

BLOOD DERIVATIVES

Many substances have been derived from blood and are used in medicine. These include the whole blood itself as is used for transfusion, the serum from the blood, the liquid portion of the blood (which is called plasma), the clotting material (which is called fibrin). Other substances such as heparin, dicumarol, and Tromexan prevent the clotting of blood and are used after coronary thrombosis to prevent further clotting. Some drugs have been developed which are used to prevent bleeding. These include Thrombin, which is derived from the blood itself.

Various drugs are used to stimulate the growth of red blood cells, including particularly iron, and various forms and modifications of iron. Also there are organic substances derived from liver and from the wall of the stomach which may stimulate the growth of red blood cells.

THE HORMONES

The glands of internal secretion include the pituitary gland, the thyroid, the adrenal glands, and the sex glands. From all of these, substances have been derived which have powerful effects. From the adrenal glands comes cortisone and hydrocortisone, also adrenalin, and aldosterone. From the pituitary gland comes pituitrin, ACTH, and various other hormones which stimulate the action of the breasts, the sex glands, the thyroid, or the adrenals. The sex glands which include the ovaries and the testes give rise to hormones which are of great importance in the functions of the body, including the function of growth.

The pituitary is believed to contain hormones which are important in affecting the color of the body and the growth of the body.

From the pancreas comes insulin, which controls the use of sugar by the body, and trypsin which is a digestive ferment. (See also Chapter XX, ENDOCRINOLOGY)

IMMUNOLOGIC AGENTS

By injection of various substances into the human body the blood produces substances which resist the proteins which have been injected. By such technics we derive various serums and antitoxins. Thus there are vaccines and serums against many diseases. These vaccines are now available against influenza, whooping cough, poliomyelitis, rabies, tuberculosis, and many other disorders.

Serums may be made against almost any type of germ but they are effective only according to the response of the animal to the toxic substance.

EDEMA-REDUCING AGENTS

Among the greatest of recent discoveries are drugs which can cause elimination of fluid from the body. Among these are particularly Diamox and Diuril. These have been found to be of the greatest importance in heart failure and in various other conditions in which fluid collects in the tissues. Before these new discoveries, various mercury derivatives were used and some are still used for the same purpose. On the other hand, a drug called Benemid derived from benzoic acid serves to block the renal tubules so that a drug like penicillin is held in the body until it can have its effect.

THE VITAMINS

Many vitamin preparations are now available to provide for the effects of these important substances when they are insufficient in the diet or when the body does not use them satisfactorily. They are fully discussed in Chapter XXX, ADVICE ON THE DIET.

CONCLUSION

Many of the drugs here discussed were first announced as miracles. Today the "miracle drugs" have become commonplace, but as a result of their use human beings have been freed from much pain and distress; lives have been saved from infections which were formerly invariably fatal.

The development of these drugs has given us a better world in which to live.

Index

191; scarlet fever, 205; tetanus, 225

Antixerophthalmic vitamin, 424

Antrum, 730

Anxiety (*see also* **Nervous tension; Stress**), hypertension caused by, 566

Aorta, 301, 561; function in circulation, 303; hypertension caused by coarctation, 565; hypertension cured by operation, 569; location (*fig.*), 320; origin of arteries, 319; renal artery connection, 368; rheumatic fever, 311; syphilis, 318–19

Aortic stenosis, 574

Aplasia of the marrow, 410

Aplastic anemia, 410

Appendix, diabetic should have removed if infected, 554; no known useful function, 825

Appendicitis, 352–53; bacillary dysentery mistaken for, 358; danger of using laxatives, 9; diabetic coma mistaken for, 554, 556; distinguishing from ulcers and gall-bladder disease, 353; dysentery distinguished by examination of blood, 232; mistaken for acute indigestion, 338

Appetite, drug to reduce, 854; guide to nutrition, 756; loss of, 188; pregnancy, 128

Apples, food elements in (*fig.*), 765

Apresoline, 572

Aralen, 236, 852

Arches, fallen, 809

Arc lights, 646

ARDERNE, 402

Arginine, 472

Argyrosis, 620

Ariboflavinosis, 428

ARISTOTLE, 373

Arizona, diabetes mortality, 509

Armpits, lymph nodes, 416

Arsenic, albuminuria may be caused by, 379; diarrhea caused by, 357; industrial poison, 610; insecticides, 621; liver injured, 351; lupus erythematosus, 681; nephrosis, 395; poisoning, 36, 601, 612, 615; scaling wax, 619; syphilis, 667; use against cancer, 853

Arsphenamine, 237

Arteries, 561; aorta, 301; circulation (*fig.*), 17; coronary, 301; hardening of. *See* **Arteriosclerosis;** heart, 300; pulmonary, 303

Arterioles, afferent, 394; emotional tension causes to tighten, 566; kidney, 368

Arteriosclerosis, cerebral, 569, 820; cholesterol may develop, 549; climate indicated, 264; diabetes, 548; diabetic gangrene, 551–52; hypertension, 564, 568; natural, 320; nosebleed, 728; old age, 844, 847; overeating may cause, 549; periodic health checkup important in detecting, 599; renal, 394; ulcers, 345

Arthritis, 287–96; amebic dysentery, 359; causes, 288–90; climate neither causes nor cures, 290; diet, 292; dysentery, 358–59; old age, 843, 847; physical therapy, 292–93; psoriasis associated with, 680; results of treatment, 296; rheumatism distinguished from, 287; symptoms, 290–91; treatment, 291–96

ARTHRITIS AND RHEUMATISM FOUNDATION OF NEW YORK CITY, 294

Artificial kidney, 390, 396

Artificial respirators, in infantile paralysis, 215

Artificial resuscitation, 23–25

Asbestos, 610; dust, 602

Asbestosis, 610

Ascites, meaning, 370; treatment, 392

Ascorbic acid (*see also* **Vitamin C**), 161; daily requirement, 781; deficiency produces scurvy, 428; foods as sources (*fig.*), 430

Asexual reproduction, 60

Asphalt, 610

Asphyxiation, first aid, 23–25

Aspirin, allergy to, 462; arthritis, 294; colds, 250–51; dosage, 14; gout, 294; hives caused by, 679; medicine chest, 13–14; menstruation, 46; pain reliever, 10, 849, 855; rheumatism, 294

Asthenia, neurocirculatory, 323–24

Asthma, 455–57; ACTH, 474, 502; adrenalin, 473–74; antihistamines, 473, 850; attacks precipitated by topics calling forth feelings of bitterness, regret, and failure, 281; children comparatively easy to treat, 466–67; chloride of lime may cause, 613; compounds E and F, 490; cortisone, 474; desensitization, 472; eczema also manifested, 459; emotional disorders

Birds, encephalitis, 241; psittacosis, 239; reproduction, 63

BIRKHAUG, KONRAD, 223

Birth (*see also* Caesarian section; Childbirth; Confinement; Pregnancy), delivery at home, 143–44; estimating date, 126–27; out of wedlock, 83–84

Birth control. *See* Contraception

Birthmarks, moles, 672–73; superstitions concerning, 148; vascular, 673–74

Bisexuality, 494

Bismuth, lupus erythematosus, 681; nephrosis, 395; syphilis, 667

Bisulphide of carbon, 611

Bites, first aid, 29–30; insect, 187, 670–71, 724; mosquito, 234–36; rat-bite fever, 236; tick, 237

BITTER ROOT VALLEY (MONTANA), 237

BLACK, DR., 217

BLACKALL, 376

Black-and-blue marks, 419

Black cancer, 580

Black damp, 621

Black eye, 709–10; first aid, 19

Blackheads, 659–60; acne vulgaris, 675; adolescent girls, 45; caused by heavy foundations and cake make-up, 642; female sex hormones decrease, 687; steaming, 646; treatment, 647; vitamin B₆ may help clear up, 631

Black urine, 400

Black widow spider, first aid, 30

Bladder, Aristotle believed to be chief site of urinary formation, 373; cancer, 120, 592; stones, 380, 425; ureters carry urine from kidneys to, 367

Bland diet, 786–87

Blanket, electric, 292

BLAYNEY, J. R., 749

Bleaching agents, hair, 694, 704

Bleeder. *See* Hemophilia

Bleeding (*see also* Hemorrhage), abnormal, 418–20; anemia caused by, 407; cancer danger signal, 119, 577; cancer of intestines, 585; control, 16–18; epinephrine, 489; first aid, 16; intestinal cancer, 585; leukemia, 595; lungs, 266; nipple, as evidence of breast cancer, 586; nose, 16, 46, 219, 727–28; shaving, how to stop, 12; time, determination of, 406; vitamin K, 440–41

Blindness, color, 718; gonorrhea causes, 742; prevention, 707–8; ultraviolet

rays may cause, 603; xerophthalmia causes, 425

Blisters, chicken pox, 210; fever, 667–68; hypersensitivity, 197; infectious diseases, 186; wet dressings, 645

BLOCH, 424

Blood, 403–20; anemia (*q.v.*), 406–11; banks, 412; brown-colored, 614, 617; cells. *See* Red blood cells and White blood cells; chocolate-colored, 614, 617; circulation, 303, (*figs.*) 302, 320; clots, 406, 857; composition, 303, 403–6; coughing, 254; count, 384, 404, 405, 407; daily flow through kidneys, 370; deficiencies as result of radiant energy, 603; effect of drugs on, 857; fibrin, 857; function, 403; germ identification, 184; groups, 412; hepatitis spread by transfusions, 349–50; injections to prevent disease, 190; plasma, 403, 857; platelets, 403, 405–6; poisoning, 187–88, 357, 396; pregnant women should know type, 120; pressure. *See* Blood pressure; response to germ invasion, 188; Rh (Rhesus) factor, 120–21, 412–13; serum, 191; storage, 412; sugar (*see also* Glucose; Dextrose), 533–34; supply (*fig.*), 320; tests, 403–6; types, 412; urine, 592; vessels, 300, 319

Blood derivatives, 857

Blood-lettings, polycythemia, 414

Blood pressure, 561–74; changes during stress, 283; high. *See* Hypertension; how recorded, 561–62; labile, 562; low. *See* Hypotension; lower diastolic, 561; machine, 562; mechanism, 561–62; normal, 562–64; regulation by drugs, 855; upper systolic, 561

Blowing the nose, 252

Blue color (blood not receiving enough oxygen), 254

Blue discoloration of skin, 609, 610

Blue moles, 673

Blushing, 626

B.O., 627, 658

Body, changes, interpretation of, 278; changes, related to feelings, 270; odor, 627, 658; response to germs, 188–89

Boils, 663; anthrax infection, 602; ear, 722; massage dangerous, 646; need not be cut, 664; occupational incidence,

603; scalp, 701; treatment, 664–65; wet dressings, 645

BOLLMAN, 388

Bombs. *See* **Atom bomb**

Bone marrow puncture, 404–5

Bones, brittle, 492–93; cancer, 594; cancer of bowels causes secondary growth in, 360; growth, 500; radiation may injure, 608; rickets, 182; skeleton (fig.), 17; tuberculosis, 188; tuberculosis germ in cattle, 262

BOOERHAAVE, 375

Borax solutions, poisoning, 37

BORDET, 208

Boric acid, antiseptic in first aid, 21; antiseptic in medicine chest, 11; cold cream, 643; dusting powders, 641; eye bath, 20, 201, 711; foot powders, 804; measles, 191; medicine chest, 11, 13; mouth wash, 733; pink eye, 712; poisoning, 37; rosacea, 677; scalp dermatitis, 696; skin antiseptic, 644; solution, how to make, 644; sunburn, 647, 656; wet dressings, 645

Boron, poisoning, 37

Borrelia vincentii, 228

BOSTOCK, 376, 443

BOSTON, diabetes mortality, 506; psittacosis, 239

BOSTON SAFE DEPOSIT AND TRUST COMPANY, 545

Bottles, in artificial feeding of infants, 170

BOUCHARDAT, 531, 546, 550, 559

Bowel movements (*see also* **Cathartics; Feces; Laxatives**), daily, 354–55; germ invasion, 188

Bowels, cancer, 360–61, 584–86; digestive hormones, 504; dysentery, 230–33; effect of insecurity and anger, 276; hemorrhages, 220; pregnancy care, 131

Bowlegs, 434, 807

Bowman's glomerular capsule, 367–68

Boys, adolescent, 82–89

"Boy-struck" period, 83

Bruces, arthritis and rheumatism, 293

Brain, arteriosclerosis, 569, 820; disease, 509; fever, 203; inflammation. *See* **Encephalitis, epidemic; meningitis,** 188

Brains, avoided in gout diet, 292

Brash, water, 342

Brass, ague, 612, 621; chills, 621; industrial poison, 611–12

Bread, enriched, 758; food values, 777; hepatic diet, 351; smooth diet for indigestion, 339

Breakfast, diabetic diet, 529; smooth diet, 339; standard test, 335

Breast feeding, 164–66; benefits, 145; calorie requirement, 781; cancer rate lower, 587; difficulties, 165–66; gallbladder disease may occur, 347; position, 146; rickets unlikely, 432; technic, 165; weaning, 147, 166

Breasts, caked, 164; cancer, 120, 578, 586–88; lump may indicate cancer, 577, 586; milk secretion, 496–97; monthly examination, 587, 599; nipples, fissuring of, 165; periodic examination for cancer, 587, 599; pituitary stimulates, 499; pregnancy care, 125, 137; soreness and swelling of, in adolescent girls, 45; swelling after birth, 145

Breath, bad. *See* **Halitosis;** water eliminated daily, 365

Bride (*see also* **Marriage**), 94–98; frigidity may be produced by groom's awkwardness, 114

BRIGHT, RICHARD, description of uremic state, 387; first reports of nephritis, 366; work, 375–76

Bright's disease (*see also* **Nephritis**), 394–95; defined, 366, 385; diarrhea caused by, 358; example of renal albuminuria, 378; term 125 years old, 371

Brittleness, in bones, 492–93

Bromides, boils, 663; folliculitis, 663; hypertension, 573

Bromine, allergy to, 462

Bronchial asthma, 444, 455–57

Bronchiectasis, asthma leads to, 457; phosgene may cause, 618

Bronchitis, albuminuria may follow, 379; asthma leads to, 457; cold may introduce, 252; cough may indicate lung cancer, 590; infants, 175; old people, 843; phosgene may cause, 618; sinus infection may cause, 730

Bronchopneumonia, old people, 845; vitamin A deficiency, 425

Bronze, industrial poison, 612

BROOKS, PHILLIPS, 817

destroyed by, 519; cancer treatment, 578

Cocaine, poisoning, 38

Cockatoos, psittacosis, 239

Coconut oil, shampoos, 693; soap, 640

Codeine, 856; colds, 251; shingles, 668

Cod-liver oil, infant's diet, 171; rickets, 183, 434; vitamin A, 424; vitamin D, 161

Coffee, as a stimulant, 856; hypertension may be aggravated by, 567–68; possibly undesirable for adolescent girls, 44

Coitus (*see also* **Intercourse, sexual**), incomplete, as contraceptive method, 122; trivial role in reproductive process of fish, 67–68

Colchicine, 294

Cold, allergy to, 462–63; occupational hazard, 600

Cold bath, 638; technic of conditioning against colds, 249

Cold cream, medicine chest, 13; senile freckles, 682; skin care, 642–43; soap substitute, 638; sunburn, 656; use more justified in middle life, 648

Colds, 244–57; albuminuria may follow, 379; allergic, 252; antiseptic solutions will not prevent, 11; beginning of infectious disease, 186; causes, 245–47; dampness as cause, 601; diet, 250–51; hayfever, 252; head, 247; infants, 173; nasal allergy confused with, 454; prevention, 247–50; respiratory disease, 253–57; rheumatic fever may recur after, 306; rose, 252; spring, 252; summer, 252; symptoms, 247; syphilis mistaken for, 666; treatment, 250–52; undulant fever mistaken for, 229; vaccines, 249–50; whooping cough resembles, 208

Cold sores. *See* **Herpes**

Cold wave lotions, 694

Colic, 165, 179

Colitis, 357–58; emotional tension may cause, 566; mucous, 465; polyps, 361; ulcerative, 276, 358

Collagen diseases, 312

College, medical, 1–2

College, education, amount required for studying medicine, 2

Colon (*see also* **Bowels; Intestines**), bacillus, 285; cancer, 360, 584–86; colitis,

357–58; digestive role, 330; disease, appendicitis confused with, 353; inflammation, 357–58; material in semisolid state, 354

Color blindness, 718

Colored glasses, 201

Colored people. *See* **Negroes**

Colostomy, 361

Columbian spirits, 616

Coma, diabetic, 505–6, 554–57

Combs, hair, 690

Combustion of food in body, 159

Comedones, 675

Common colds. *See* **Colds**

Communicable diseases. *See* **Infectious diseases**

Community mental hospitals, 838

Complexes, sexual, 115–16

Compound E. *See* **Cortisone**

Compound F. *See* **Dihydrocortisone; Hydrocortisone**

Concentration tests (kidneys), 383

Conception, fear of, as cause of frigidity, 114; prevention of. *See* **Contraception**

Condensed milk, 166–67, 168

Condiments, food values, 779; hepatic diet, 351

Confinement (*see also* **Caesarian section; Childbirth; Pregnancy**), 141–42

Congenitally defective hearts, 305

Congress, sexual. *See* **Intercourse, sexual**

Conjugal allergy, 449

Conjugal love (*see also* **Intercourse, sexual**), 101

Conjunctivitis, 712; acetylene torch work may cause, 609

Constipation, 354–57; cancer of bowels, 360, 585; colitis, 357; diet, 340, 356, 785; effect of dejection mistaken for, 276; functional significance, 277–78; gallstones, 348; hypertension may be aggravated by, 567–68; infants, 179–80; intestinal cancer, 360, 585; intestinal obstruction, 361; old people, 845; pellagra, 436; pregnancy, 131, 138; skin affected by, 633; typhoid fever, 219

Consumption. *See* **Tuberculosis**

Contactants (causes of allergy), 448

Contact dermatitis, 458–59; scalp, 695

Contagious diseases (*see also* **Infectious diseases**), 185

Devil's pinches, 420
DEVINE, MRS., 559
Dextran, 391
Dextrin, 167
Dextrose, absorbed and stored as glycogen, 477; artificial feeding of infants, 167; diabetics, 487
Diabetes insipidus, 400, 503, 511
Diabetes mellitus, 486, 505–60; ACTH or cortisone may cause, 502; age at onset, 516, 521, 548, 550; arteriosclerosis apt to occur, 568; arteriosclerosis of pancreas causes, 569; blamable, 511–14; blameless, 514–17; blood sugar, 523–24; blood test, 404; boils often accompany, 663; camps, 559; carbuncles may accompany, 664; cataracts, 548; caused in dogs by removal of pancreas, 485; coma, 554–57; coma distinguished from insulin reaction, 541; controllable, 520–21; coronary thrombosis, 548; death rate, 505–7, 510; defined, 510–11; destruction of pancreas results in, 476; detection, 521–24; diagnosis, 524; diet, 486, 524–31; dogs aid research, 520; employment of diabetics, 546–47; exercise, 531–32; eyes affected, 558–59, 714; folliculitis more common in diabetics, 662; foot care, 552–53; gangrene, 551–52; heredity, 508, 514–17, 549–50; Hospital Teaching Clinic, 559–60; hypodermic syringe not kept in medicine chest, 11; identification card, 556, (fig.) 542; improvement possible, 534; incidence, 508–10, 521; infections, 553–54; insulin and cortisone in rheumatoid arthritis, 295; insulin reaction distinguished from coma, 541; insulin treatment, 532–43; insurance for diabetics, 547–48; itching may be caused by, 661; life expectancy, 506–7, 511, 532–33; life expectancy before insulin, 517; lunches before retiring, 543; marriage considerations, 515–16, 550–51; medals for diabetics, 545, 548; menu (see also Diabetes mellitus diet), 529–30; nephrosis, 396; nervous troubles, 557–58; old age, 548–49; overweight often precedes, 512–14; pancreas is responsible, 517–18; pregnancy, 132, 550–51; prevention, 511–17; quack remedies, 392; reduces resistance to other diseases, 186–87; renal, 400; retina changes, 716; starch to be avoided as well as sugar, 778; thrombosis, coronary, 548; transmission of disease to offspring (see also Diabetes, heredity), 515; treatment, 524–43; ulcers relatively rare, 345; urine abnormal, 399–400; urine tests, 521–23, 531; usefulness, 543–46; vascular purpura, 420
Diacetic acid, testing urine for, 557
Dial, to produce sleep, 10
Diaparene chloride, 156
Diapers, washing, 156
Diaphragm, action, 30–31; contracted when anxious, 281
Diarrhea, 357–58; cancer of bowels, 360, 585; chronic, 358–59; death rate (fig.), 298; diabetic coma, 555; digestive causes, 331; drugs for, 851; dysentery, 231; functional significance, 277–78; gastro-intestinal allergy, 465; indigestion, 337; infants, 180–81; infants' malnutrition caused by, 182; intestinal obstruction, 361; kidney disease, 386; pellagra, 436, 630; radiation may cause, 608; reaction to stress, 276; typhoid fever, 219
Diasone, 266
Diastole, 301, 561
Diastolic pressure (see also Blood pressure), 561, 565
Diathermy, 811
Dichloro-difluoromethane, 614
DICK, GEORGE F. and GLADYS HENRY, 205
DICKENS, CHARLES, 148, 635
Dick test, 206
Dicoumarol, 406, 441, 857
Diet, 755–89; appetite as guide, 756; arthritis, 292; beverages, 339–40, 351; bland, 786–87; calorie requirements, 762–64; chicken pox, 211; classification of foods, 764–67; colds, 250–51; constipation, 340, 356, 785; diabetes, 486, 524–31; dropsy, 390; fads, 757–59; gout, 292; hair growth, 688–89; hepatitis, 350–51; hyperacidity, 787–88; hypo-acidity, 788–89; importance in control of dietary diseases, 327; indigestion, 339–40; infants, 158–71; infectious diseases, 191; kidney dis-

fancy should not be treated with, 173; flea bites, 30; herpes simplex, 668; nose hygiene, 725; psoriasis, 681; sunburn, 656

Menthol-camphor solutions, nose sprays for colds, 251

Menthyl salicylates, sunburn protection, 647

Menu (*see also* **Diet**), diabetic's, 529–30

Mercurial nephritis, 393

Mercurial nephrosis, 396

Mercurochrome, antiseptic in first aid, 21, 849; antiseptic in medicine chest, 11

Mercury, albuminuria may be caused by, 379; avoid use after iodine application, 644; dermatitis caused by, 653; bichloride of. *See* **Bichloride of mercury;** diarrhea caused by, 357; douches, 389; fulminate, 614; nephritis, 391–92; nephrosis, 395; poisoning, 616; syphilis, 737; vapor lamps, 433

MERING, VON, 517

Merthiolates, antiseptic in first aid, 21; antiseptic in medicine chest, 11

Mesothorium, 616

Metabolic disorders, arthritis or rheumatism may result, 289–90; gout, 288

Metabolism (*see also* **Basal metabolism**), hormones control, 567; tests, 484

Metallic salts, in powders, 642

Metamucil, 140; during pregnancy, 131

Metaphen, antiseptic in first aid, 21; antiseptic in medicine chest, 11

Metatarsal arch, (*fig.*), 805; disorders, 810–11

Methanol, industrial poison, 616

Methemoglobin, 609; nitrobenzene poisoning, 617

Methium, hypertension, 572

Methyl alcohol, 616

Methyl chloride, 616

Methylene blue, to test excretory ability of kidneys, 383; use for carbon-monoxide poisoning, 27

Methyl violet, 616

Metrazol shock treatment, 839

METROPOLITAN LIFE INSURANCE COMPANY, 507, 508, 510

Mexicans in Chicago, tuberculosis among, 258

Mica, industrial poison, 617

Mice, encephalitis virus, 242, 243; glanders, 238; psittacosis, 240

Microcentrifuge of proteins, 380

Microscope, 3; cancer research, 598; dark field, 738; germ identification, 184

Middle age, sex hygiene, 103–8

Midicel, 851

Migraine, allergic, 463–64; first aid, 32–34; old age, 844; reaction to stress, 283–84

Miliary tuberculosis, 266

Milium, 675

Milk, acidified, 169–70; allergy caused by, 447; artificial feeding of infants, 166–70; condensed, 166–67, 168; constipation diet, 356; digestibility by infant, 162; evaporated, 161, 166–67, 170; food elements in (*fig.*), 765; food values, 775–76; fortified with vitamin D, 161; goat's, undulant fever spread by, 229; infant's diet, 159; pasteurization, 221–22, 229; pregnancy diet, 128; rickets prevented by sufficient amount in infant's diet, 182; scarlet fever spread through, 204; septic sore throat spread by, 733; sugar, 180; tuberculosis diet, 267; tuberculosis prevented by pasteurization, 262; typhoid fever spread by, 219; undulant fever, 229

"Milk crust" on baby's scalp, 155–56

Milkers, should wash hands thoroughly, 734

Milk of magnesia, heartburn relieved by, 139; infants, 180; laxative, 9; laxative during pregnancy, 131

MILLER, JAMES ALEXANDER, 263

Milt, 62, 68

Mineral oil, burns 657; constipation, 356; dryness of skin, 661; laxative, 9, 13, 849; vitamin A depleted by, 633

Minerals, daily requirement, 781; infant's need, 159–60; nail brittleness caused by deficiency, 705; pregnancy diet, 128; rickets caused by deficiency, 182–83; skin requirements, 633

Mineral salts, function, 764, 766–67; infant's diet, 161–62; scarlet fever diet, 206; skin requirements, 633; whooping cough diet, 209

MINKOWSI, 517, 520

Para-aminosalicylic acid, tuberculosis, 266, 490, 851

Paracentesis, 392

Parakeets, psittacosis, 239

Paralysis, agitans, 845; benzine poisoning may stimulate, 611; encephalitis, 241; hardening of brain arteries, 569; infantile. See Infantile paralysis

Paranitraniline red, 619

Paranoia, 820

Paraphenylenediamine, dermatitis caused by, 653; hair dyes, 694–95; occupational diseases for furriers, 601

Parasites, intestinal, 362–63; skin, 668–71

Parathion, 618

Parathyroids, 491–93; location (fig.), 478; skin affected by, 634

Paratyphoid fever, infected water most common source, 357

Paratyphoid infections, in infants, 180–81

Paredrine, 474

Paregoric, in medicine chest, 11

Parents (see also Father; Mother), duties, 110

Paresis, age at onset, 820; syphilis microorganism causes, 823

Paris, psittacosis, 239

Paris green, poisoning, 40–41

Parkinson's disease (see also Palsy, shaking), encephalitis symptoms similar, 242

Paronychia, 705

Parotid glands, mumps, 212

Parotitis, epidemic. See Mumps

Parrot disease. See Psittacosis

Partridges, encephalitis virus, 242

PAS. See Para-aminosalicylic acid

Pasteur, Louis, 185, 193, 226, 227–28, 257

Pasteurella tularensis, 233

Pasteurization, 166; tuberculosis prevented by, 262; typhoid fever reduced by, 221–22; undulant fever controlled by, 229

Patch test, 451

Patches, red, infectious diseases, 186

Patent medicine, samples not to be kept in medicine chest, 12

Paul, Saint, 521

Paulus, Aegineta, 386

Peabody, Amelia, 545

Pearson, Karl, 846

Pechey, 391

Pediculoides ventricosus, 614

Pediculosis capitis, 702–3

Pediculus capitis, 669

Peeling of skin, scarlet fever, 204

Pellagra, 435–37; diarrhea caused by, 358; niacin, 427; pyridoxine, 428; result of shortage of niacin, 160; skin changes, 630–31; United States, 422, 423

Pelvic examination, 589

Pelvic organs, female (fig.), 48

Pelvis, girl's broader than boy's, 86; kidney, 367–68

Pemphigus, 681–82

Penicillin (see also Antibiotics), allergy to, 462; allergy treated by, 637; angina, Vincent's, 228–29; chicken pox, 211; diabetic gangrene, 552; diphtheria, 195, 198; enzymes prevent toxic reaction to, 857; erysipelas, 223; German measles, 204; gonorrhea, 743, 744; hemolytic streptococcic infection, 316; hives may be caused by, 678; impetigo, 662; infectious diseases, 192; kinds of, 851; pneumonia, 256; pus-producing skin infections, 664; rat-bite fever, 237; rheumatic fever, 316; scalp infections, 710; scarlet fever, 207; seborrheic dermatitis, 700; sinuses, 730; skin antiseptic, 644; skin eruptions caused by, 652; syphilis, 404, 667, 739, 741; tetanus, 226; throat lozenges, 733; Vincent's angina, 228–29; wens, 672

Penis (see also Circumcision), cleaning child's, 156; gonorrhea, 744; function, 69; how to get rid of a chordee, 743; washing, 117

Pennyroyal, poisoning, 40

Pepsin, 770; acts only in an acid medium, 329; digestive function, 335; gastric juice, 328

Peptic ulcers, gastritis resembles, 343; heartburn, 342; reaction during stress, 281; role of blood sugar in development, 345

Perborate, sodium, Vincent's angina, 229

Percomorph, 161

Perennial nasal allergy, 454–55

Perforation, ulcers, 346

INDEX

903

introduce, 238; secondary, 174; sinus infection may cause, 730; virus, frequently attacks patients with lung cancer, 591–92; whooping cough frequently precedes, 208

Pneumothorax, artificial, 259, 266

Podophyllin, 672

Poison gas, first aid, 26–27; pneumonia prepared by, 253

Poison ivy, 652–53; antihistamines, 850; dermatitis, 458; wet dressings, 645

Poison oak, 652–53

Poisoning, albuminuria may result, 379; antidotes, 35–42; arsenic, 601; blood, 187–88, 357, 396; first aid, 34–42; food, 34–42, 759; mercurial, 396; metallic, 34–42; nicotine, 601, 621; symptoms, 35–42

Poisons, body's response, 188–89; dangerous, defined, 7; diarrhea caused by, 357; germs develop, 187–88; industrial, 609–21; mistaken for acute indigestion, 338

Poliomyelitis, acute. *See* **Infantile paralysis**

Polish, nail, 705

Pollen, 61; hay fever, 452–54; injections, 453–54; spring or rose cold caused by, 252

Polley, Howard F., 287

Polycystic kidneys, 400–1

Polycythemia, 413–14

Polyposis, 361; cancer of intestines caused by, 586

Polyps, cancer of bowels, 360–61; nose, 727, 732

Ponds, country club, breeding places for mosquitoes, 235

Poplar, spring or rose cold caused by, 252

Pores, 624

Porter, Sidney, 327

Porter operation, 815

"Port-wine marks," 673–74

Postnatal care, 145–46

Postpartum care, 145–46

Postrenal albuminuria, 380; defined, 378

Postum, Instant, 339

Postural albuminuria, confused with true nephritis, 381

Postural orthostatic forms of albuminuria, 379

Posture, 790–801; adolescent girl, 44; athletics, 796; bad, 792–93; clothing affects, 798–99; college-age students, 797; dancing, 796; endurance test, 793, 794; exercises, 799–801; gymnastics, 796; physical training, 796; women, 797–98

Posture League, 799

Potassium (*see also* **Electrolytes**), in urine, 369

Potassium chloride, dropsy, 391

Potassium cyanide, poisoning, 38

Potassium hydrate, soap formed by, 640

Potassium hydroxide, poisoning, 35

Potassium iodide in table salt, 481

Potassium nitrate, dropsy, 391

Potassium permanganate solution, wet dressings, 645

Potassium tartrate, 363

Potatoes, food elements in (*fig.*), 765; hepatic diet, 351

Potato salad, germ carrier, 187

Pot-bellied minnow, mosquito larvae eaten by, 236

Poultice, mustard, colds, 251–52

Poultry, protein content, 773

Pouter-pigeon type of posture, 793

Powders, skin, 641–42; tooth, 750

Pox. *See* **Chicken pox; Smallpox**

P-P. *See* **Vitamin P-P**

Prairie itch, 614

Pratt, George K., 819

Pre-eclampsia, pregnancy, 397

Pregnancy (*see also* **Birth; Caesarian section; Childbirth; Confinement**), abortion during early months, 139; afterpains, 144–45; antepartum care, importance of, 124; appetite, perversion of, 128; asthma, 455; bathing, 135–36; belching, 139; beriberi, 427; bowels, care of, 131; breasts, care of, 137; cathartics, 131; clothing, 132–33; constipation, 131, 138; corsets, 132–33; cramps, leg, 140; delivery at home, 143–44; dental care, 745; diabetes, 132, 550–51; diet, 127–28, 129–30; disappearance of menstruation, 47; dizziness, 139–40; douches, 137; estimating date of birth, 126–27; exercise, 133–35; fainting, 139–40; fruits, 131; gall-bladder disease, 347; gastroposis, 343; genitals, care of, 137; German measles serious,

cia areata, 703; rheumatism, 288; skin disorders, 637; study of total reactions, 823

Psychotherapy, 835–38; allergic headache, 464; allergy, 469–70; nasal allergy, 455

Psyllium seed, constipation, 356; laxative, 9, 13, 849

Ptomaine poisoning, 759

Ptyalin, enzyme in saliva, 329

Puberty (*see also* **Adolescence**), acne vulgaris, 675–76; beginning of female's production of mature egg cells, 67; connection with menopause, 48; girls, 43; glandular change, 636; skin changes, 647

Pubic louse, 670

PUBLIC HEALTH SERVICE, 507, 508, 521, 549, 749

Puerperium, 144–45; rest necessary; 146

PUERTO RICO, rheumatic fever uncommon, 313

Pulmonary artery, function in circulation, 303

Pulmonary fibrosis, asthma leads to, 457

Pulmonic valve, affected in rheumatic fever, 311

Pulse, 561; irregularities, 325–26; rapid, in exophthalmic goiter, 319; test for danger of death from failure of respiration, 27

Puncture, bone marrow, 404–5; splenic, 418

Pupils (eye), 708; unequal size a symptom of brain injury, 28

"Puppy love," 88–89

Pure Food and Drug Laws, 757

Purgatives, constipation caused by habitual use, 356; digestive diseases, 363–64; flatulence caused, 339

Purine, avoided in gout diet, 292; gout results from body's inability to handle, 289–90

Purpura, due to absence of platelets, 419; nosebleed, 727

Purulent nephritis, 373

Pus, meant to protect the individual, 282; requires prompt medical attention, 21–22

Pus appendix, 352

Pus kidney, 373, 397

Pus-producing skin infections, 662–65

Putty, occupational hazard, 619

Pyelitis, 396; albuminuria may arise in, 380; infants, 176; pregnancy, 132, 397; prostate gland enlarged, 398

Pyelogram, 383; horseshoe kidney recognized by, 401

Pyelonephritis, 396–97; pregnancy, 397; prostate gland enlarged, 398; resulting from renal lithiasis, 397

Pyemia, endocarditis may occur, 317

Pylorus, 179, 354

Pyorrhea, 751

Pyramidon, agranulocytosis, 415; less safe than aspirin, 13

Pyrazidin, tuberculosis, 266

Pyrene, occupational hazard, 619

Pyrethrotoxic acid, in insecticides, 613

Pyrethrum, allergic diseases from, 613

Pyribenzamine, 473; psoriasis, 681

Pyridoxine (*see also* **Vitamin B₆**), 426, 428

PZI. *See* **Protamine zinc insulin**

Quacks, cancer treatment, 579; distinguishing from ethical physicians, 3; gonorrhea, 743; kidney disease, 392; syphilis, 740

Quail, tularemia, 234

Quarantine (*see also* **Isolation**), mumps, 212; whooping cough, 209

Quarter Century Victory Medal, 545

Quartz mercury vapor burner, 249

Quartz mercury vapor lamps, light baths, 646; ultraviolet rays in tuberculosis of larynx, 268

"Queerness," 829

Quinine, hives caused by, 679; malaria, 236, 852; occupational hazard, 619; poisoning, 41

Quinidine, poisoning, 41

Rabbit fever. *See* **Tularemia**

Rabbits, encephalitis virus, 243; glanders, 238; psittacosis, 240; tularemia, 233, 602; vaccine for rabies, 228

Rabies, 30, 226–28; control, 228; deaths, 228; incubation period, 226–27; meaning of words, 226; nervous system, 188; Pasteur treatment, 227–28; superstition concerning "dog days," 226; symptoms, 227; transmissible disease, 226–28; vaccine, 228, 468, 858

SHERMAN, 422, 423

Shingles, 668; chicken pox induces, 210; lesions may require ointments, 211; old age, 844

Shock, electric, first aid, 23–26; resulting from burns, treatment of, 22; treatment for mental patients, 839

Shoe-button spider, first aid, 30

Shoes, 803–4; ballet slippers, 807; bedroom slippers, 807; gymnasium, 807

"Shots," 250

Shoulders, round, 799

"Show" (discharge from vagina at beginning of labor), 143

Sickle cell anemia, 410–11

Sicknesses, infants', 171–83

Sigmoid, cancer, 360

Silica, 601; industrial poison, 619–20

Silicatosis, mica dust may cause, 617

Silicosis, 601–2; asbestosis resembles, 610; granite is common source, 614; occupational disease, 605; sandstone is a source, 619; siliceous materials cause, 619–20

Silver, occupational hazard, 620

Silver nitrate, erysipelas, 223; ringworm of the nails, 706

Silver salts, diarrhea caused by, 357

SIMMONDS, 422

Singeing the hair, 691

SINGER, KARL, 403

Single kidney, 400–1

Sinuses (*see also* **Nose**), 725; disease, 729–30; infections (*see also* **Colds**), 192; migraine, 32

Sinusitis, nasal allergy differentiated from, 454; pollen injections make hay fever patient less likely to develop, 454

Sister Kenny treatment for infantile paralysis, 215

Sitting posture, correct, 792

Sitz baths, during pregnancy, 136

"606," rat-bite fever, 237

Six-year molar, 746

Skeleton, human, showing arterial circulation (*fig.*), 17

Skin, 622–706; abnormal functioning, 658–62; adolescence, 647; adrenal glands, 634–35; aging, 624; allergy, 450, 457–61, 636–37; antiseptics, 643–44; bathing, 638–39; blue discoloration, 609, 610; body odor (*q.v.*), 658;

boils, 663; burning, how to relieve, 191–92; cancer, 579–80, 674; capillaries, 626; carbuncles, 663–64; care, 638–46; chafing, 654–55; change during stress, 270–71; chapped, 642, 654; childhood, 647; cold cream, 642; color, 625–26; constipation causes eruptions, 356; dermatitis from external irritants, 652–54; dressings, wet, 645; drug rashes, 652; dryness, 660–61; eczema, 648–52; emotional disorders, 637; endocrine glands, 633–36; eruptions caused by constipation, 356; eruptions caused by infectious diseases, 186; erysipelas inflammation, 222–23; excessive functioning, 658–62; feeding, 626, 628; folliculitis, 662; frostbite, 657–58; functions, 627–29; growths, 671–74; heat rash, 658–59; herpes simplex, 667–68; herpes zoster, 668; hydroquinone affects pigmentation, 615; hypersensitivity, 636–37; impetigo, 662; infancy, 646–47; infections, 662–71; inflammations, 648–58; inner layer, 622, 623–24; intestinal function, 633; itching, 661–62; itching, how to relieve, 191–92; lotions, 642; massage, 645–46; nervous tension, 637; nutrition, 626, 629–33; occupational disease, 601; oil glands, 625; oiliness, 659–60; outer, 622–23; ovaries, 636; parasites, 668–71; parathyroid, 634; peeling in scarlet fever, 204; perspiration (*q.v.*), 658; pigmentation, 615, 625–26, 682–84; pituitary gland, 635; pores, 624; powders, 641–42; pregnancy stretches, 624; prickly heat, 658–59; protection, 628; pus-producing infections, 662–65; rashes, 204, 652, 658–59; regenerative power, 629; ringworm, 668–69; scales, 205; scarlet fever, 204; scar tissue, 629; sebaceous glands, 625; seborrhea, 659–60; shingles, 668; soap, 639–41; spirochetes, 665–67; steaming, 646; structure, 622–26; sugar stored in, 511; sun baths, 646; sunburn, 655–57; sweat glands, 136, 624–25; sweating (*q.v.*), 658; syphilis, 665–67; testes, 635–36; tests do not harm children, 467; tests to determine allergy, 450, 637; tests to determine tuberculosis, 264–65; texture,

philiacs, 419; hepatitis spread by, 349–50; rheumatism, 294

Transmissible diseases (*see also main listing of each of the following diseases*), 218–43; amebiasis, 230–33; angina, Vincent's, 228–29; brucellosis, 229–30; dysentery, 230–33; encephalitis, epidemic, 240–43; erysipelas, 222–24; glanders, 238–39; hydrophobia, 226–28; lockjaw, 224–26; malaria, 234–36; parrot disease, 239–40; psittacosis, 239–40; rabies, 226–28; rat-bite fever, 236–37; Rocky Mountain spotted fever, 237–38; tetanus, 224–26; tularemia, 233–34; typhoid fever, 218–22; undulant fever, 229–30; Vincent's angina, 228–29

Transparent soaps, 641

Transplantation, gland, 104–5

Trauma, changes in heart caused by, 304

Traumatic cataract, 715

Traumatic injury to heart, 326

Travel, during pregnancy, 134

Traveling physician, not suitable as family doctor, 3

Tremors, encephalitis, 241

Trench foot, 657

Trench mouth. See Vincent's angina

Trench nephritis, 394

Treponema, 738; vincentii, 228

Trial diet test (for allergy), 451

Trichloracetic acid, warts, 672

Trichlorethylene, occupational hazard, 613, 621

Tricuspid locks (*fig.*), 302

Tricuspid valve, affected in rheumatic fever, 311; function in circulation, 303

Triethylenemelamine, Hodgkin's disease, 595; lymphosarcoma, 595

Trinitrophenol, 619

Trioxid, 621

Tromexan, 441, 857

TROUSSEAU, 400

Truth, importance in sex education, 79

Trypsin, in pancreatic juice, 329, 858

Tsetse flies, African sleeping sickness, 187

Tubercle bacillus, kidney disease, 385

Tuberculin tests, 259, 468; children, 264

Tuberculosis, 120, 257–69; ACTH contraindicated, 474; Addison's disease as one manifestation, 490; arthritis may result, 289; asthma mistakenly diagnosed, 450; beds available in United States, 259; beryllium poisoning produces similar changes in lungs, 611; bleeding lungs, first aid, 18; bones, 188; cattle, 261–62; cause determined, 184; climate in prevention and treatment, 262–64; cortisone contraindicated, 474; death rate, 261, 265, 510 (*fig.*), 257, 298; detected early in diabetics, 544; diabetes mortality lower, 509; diabetes seldom complicated by, 521; diet, 261; disordered action of the heart classified as, 324; drugs for, 851; endocarditis symptoms similar, 317; eye, 188; eye infection may accompany, 714; foot deformities may result, 802; health resorts, cost of, 262; heart disease less expensive in cost of human lives, 297; hypotension, 573; incidence, 191; joints, 188; kidneys, 388, 398; larynx, 268; lungs, 18, 188; measles lowers resistance, 202; menopause formerly believed to cause, 118; nervous system, 188; predisposition in children with congenitally defective hearts, 305; renal albuminuria, 379; resistance reduced by chronic disorders, 186–87; respiratory disease, 257–69; retina changes, 716; rheumatism may result, 289; scalp changes, 698; secondary invader in measles, 202–3; silicosis, 620; skin reaction, 628; symptoms produced by an allergy, 464; tobacco, 621; undulant fever resembles, 230; vaccine, 858; whooping cough frequently precedes, 208; young married couples, 100

Tuberculous meningitis, 266

Tuberculous nephritis, 393

Tubers, asexual reproduction, 60

Tubular insufficiency, 396

Tubular nephritis, 393

Tubules (kidney), 367–68, 370

TULARE COUNTY, CALIF., 233

Tularemia, occupational disease, 602; transmissible disease, 233–34; treatment, 234